third edition

Electrocardiography in Clinical Practice

TE-CHUAN CHOU, M.D., F.A.C.C.
Professor Emeritus of Medicine
Division of Cardiology
Department of Internal Medicine
University of Cincinnati College of Medicine
Attending Physician, University of Cincinnati Hospital
Consultant, Veterans Administration Hospital
Consultant, Children's Hospital Medical Center
Cincinnati, Ohio

1991
W.B. SAUNDERS COMPANY
Harcourt Brace Jovanovich, Inc.
Philadelphia London Toronto Montreal Sydney Tokyo

W. B. SAUNDERS COMPANY
Harcourt Brace Jovanovich, Inc.

The Curtis Center
Independence Square West
Philadelphia, PA 19106

Library of Congress Cataloging-in-Publication Data

Chou, Te-Chuan.
    Electrocardiography in clinical practice / Te-Chuan Chou. —
3rd ed.
        p.   cm.
    Includes bibliographies and index.
    ISBN 0-7216-3286-6
    1. Electrocardiography.   2. Heart—Diseases—Diagnosis.
I. Title.
    [DNLM: 1. Electrocardiography.   2. Heart Diseases—diagnosis.
WG 140 C552e]
RC683.5.E5C454   1991
616.1'207547—dc20
DNLM/DLC   91-8973

Editor: Richard Zorab
Designer: Ellen M. Bodner
Production Manager: Bill Preston
Manuscript Editor: W. B. Saunders Staff
Illustration Coordinator: Cecelia Kunkle
Indexer: Helene Taylor

Electrocardiography in Clinical Practice, 3rd edition   ISBN 0-7216-3286-6

Printed in the United States of America

Last digit is the print number: 9   8   7   6   5   4   3   2   1

To my wife Nora
for her continuing support

FOREWORD FROM THE FIRST EDITION

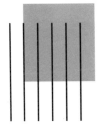

I am told that the purpose of a foreword is to say something good about a forthcoming book that the author would be too modest to say himself. In the case of Dr. Chou's new book this 'is easy to do. Dr. Chou, with Dr. Robert Helm, has already written a best seller in the field of vectorcardiography. I predict that this publication will be equally successful. One's first reaction upon hearing the title of a new book on electrocardiography is "What? Who needs another book on electrocardiography?", but this is not just another book on electrocardiography. It will be unique in the field. It is the kind of book that I would like to have written myself because I have long believed that there is a need for this kind of presentation.

Dr. Chou does not take the usual approach of a textbook on electrocardiography; namely, that of a discussion of electrophysiology, followed by the theory of the abnormalities in various major disease states, followed by a series of a small number of clinical examples. Rather, he has written a book of clinical correlations that is extensively illustrated.

Dr. Chou's book deals with clinical electrocardiographic correlations in every major field of medicine, ranging from the common ones of ventricular hypertrophy, myocardial infarction, and T-wave abnormalities to the more uncommon ones of hypothermia, and changes with cerebrovascular accidents.

I have read Dr. Chou's manuscript carefully, and would make the following comments: It is clear, well-written, inclusive, and extensively referenced. I think that everyone who is interested in clinical electrocardiography will find something of value in Dr. Chou's book, even the expert cardiologist. It is so well-referenced that it provides a source for intensive reading on any given clinical subject.

Dr. Chou has had a quarter of a century of experience in clinical-electrocardiographic correlations, correlations with autopsy findings, and correlations evaluated by clinical investigation in the Division of Cardiology of the University of Cincinnati. He has also had many years of interaction with Dr. Samuel Kaplan's group in pediatric cardiology at the Cincinnati Children's Hospital. His extensive knowledge, research, and wide reading are clearly evidenced in this book

NOBLE O. FOWLER, M.D.
Professor Emeritus of Medicine
University of Cincinnati College of Medicine

PREFACE TO THE THIRD EDITION

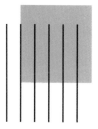

In keeping with the goals of previous editions, the third edition of *Electrocardiography in Clinical Practice* continues to emphasize the value and limitations of the electrocardiogram, the differential diagnosis of the electrocardiographic findings, and their correlation with the clinical and anatomical data. The chapter on myocardial infarction, injury, and ischemia has been extensively revised. The clinical and anatomical correlates of Q-wave and non–Q-wave infarction are discussed. Electrocardiographic changes after coronary reperfusion, prognostic value of the electrocardiogram in myocardial infarction, and the subject of silent myocardial ischemia have been added.

In the sections on cardiac arrhythmias, the discussion on the differential diagnosis of narrow and wide QRS complex tachycardia, especially the latter, has been expanded. The newer antiarrhythmic agents such as encainide, flecainide, propafenone, and adenosine, as well as the proarrhythmic effects of the antiarrhythmic drugs in general, are included.

A new chapter on traumatic heart disease and cardiac transplantation has been added to this edition. Some changes have been made in the discussion of artificial electronic pacemakers in keeping with the advances in pacemaker technology. A total of 54 new illustrations have been added.

It is hoped that this text will continue to serve as a reminder that the electrocardiogram, if used properly, is still one of the most important diagnostic tools in modern medicine.

I would like to thank Dr. Noble O. Fowler, Professor Emeritus of Medicine, Division of Cardiology, University of Cincinnati College of Medicine, for reviewing Chapter 26. As during the preparation of previous editions of this text, his comments and suggestions were most helpful. Drs. Winston Gaum and David Schwartz have kindly allowed me to use some of their patients' electrocardiograms from the Children's Hospital Medical Center, Cincinnati. Ms. Zenia Frantz has helped me in selecting instructive tracings from our Holter Laboratory. My other colleagues and fellows in the Division of Cardiology have continued to provide me with new case materials.

Mrs. Jean Johnson typed the manuscript and organized the references. Her many years of excellent secretarial support are appreciated.

TE-CHUAN CHOU, M.D.

CONTENTS

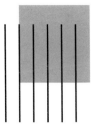

I NORMAL AND ABNORMAL ELECTROCARDIOGRAMS

Artery Disease: Sensitivity and Specificity ▪ Conditions Often Associated
With False-Positive or False-Negative Exercise Test for Coronary Artery
Disease ▪ Exercise Testing in Patients With Abnormal Resting
Electrocardiograms ▪ Prognostic Value of Exercise Testing ▪ Exercise
Testing for the Exposure of Ventricular Arrhythmias ▪ Safety of the
Exercise Test

II   THE CARDIAC ARRHYTHMIAS

of Antiarrhythmic Drugs ▪ Psychotropic Drugs (Phenothiazines, Tricyclic
Antidepressants, Lithium)

NORMAL AND ABNORMAL
ELECTROCARDIOGRAMS

I

Normal Electrocardiogram

1

P WAVE

Atrial activation begins in the sinoatrial (SA) node and spreads in a radial fashion to depolarize the right atrium, the interatrial septum, and then the left atrium[4,12] (Fig. 1–1A). The last region of the left atrium to be activated is the tip of the left atrial appendage, or in the posteroinferior left atrium beneath the left inferior pulmonary vein.[4] Three specialized pathways that contain Purkinje fibers have been identified to connect the SA node to the atrioventricular (AV) node. They are called the anterior, the middle, and the posterior internodal pathways. An interatrial pathway, the Bachmann bundle, connects the right and left atria. The role of these fibers in human atrial impulse conduction under normal circumstances is still unclear, however. For practical purposes, the early part of the P wave may be considered to represent the electrical potential generated by the right atrium, the late portion by the left atrium, and the midportion by both atria and the interatrial septum.

The results of recent studies of sinus node electrograms suggest that the sinus pacemaker may sometimes shift spontaneously within the SA node.[16] Atrial epicardial mapping during cardiac surgery also revealed that, in patients with "sinus" rhythm, the pacemaker impulse is sometimes initiated in the right atrium outside of the sinus node and may be multicentric in origin.[4] These findings may explain, at least in part, the changes in the morphology of the P waves often seen in healthy subjects during sinus rhythm.

In normal adults, the duration of the P wave, which represents the duration of the atrial activation, varies from 0.08 to 0.11 second.[6] In a study that involved a large population, a significant number of subjects had a duration of 0.12 to 0.13 second. Lepeschkin gives a mean duration of 0.085 second with a standard deviation of 0.015 second.[28] For practical purposes, a value above 0.11 second can usually be considered as abnormal.[19]

The P-wave axis in the frontal plane is directed inferiorly and leftward, which correlates well with the general direction of the spread of atrial excitation. The P axis determined from the limb leads varies from 0° to +75°,[24] with most falling between +45° and +60°. Therefore, the P wave is always upright in leads I and II and inverted in lead aVR. In lead III, it may be upright, diphasic, or inverted. When it is diphasic, the initial deflection is positive and the second component is negative. The P wave in lead aVL is also variable in polarity. A negative P wave is relatively common in this lead. When it is diphasic, it has a negative–positive deflection. In lead aVF, the P wave is usually upright, but a diphasic or flat P wave may occasionally be seen.

In the precordial leads, the P wave is often diphasic in leads V_1 and V_2. The early right atrial forces are directed anteriorly and the late left atrial forces posteriorly. Therefore, the diphasic P wave has a positive–negative configuration. An entirely positive or negative deflection may also be seen in lead V_1, but the P wave in lead V_2 is seldom entirely negative. In the rest of the precordial leads, the P wave is always upright because of the essentially right-to-left spread of the atrial activation impulse.

The normal P wave may show small notches or slurring. This is probably related to the transition from right atrial to left atrial depolarization. Some claim that, when the normal P wave is notched, the interval between the two peaks should not exceed 0.03 second.[52] In my experience, however, many healthy young individuals with notched P waves may have a peak-to-peak interval greater than this value, although it seldom reaches 0.05 second.

The amplitude of the P wave in the limb leads seldom exceeds 0.25 mV in normal individuals at rest. In the precordial leads, the positive component of the P wave is less than

0.15 mV. In lead V_1, the negative deflection is usually less than 0.1 mV. The total area of the negative component is a more accurate measure of the normality of the P wave in this lead, however. Morris suggested that the product of the maximum negative amplitude in millivolts and the duration of the negative deflection in seconds should not exceed 0.003.[34] During routine interpretation of the electrocardiogram (ECG), if the area of the negative component of the P wave in lead V_1 occupies one small square or more of the recording paper, the P wave is considered abnormal.

PR INTERVAL

The PR interval is measured from the beginning of the P wave to the beginning of the QRS complex. The term *PQ interval* is preferred by some electrocardiographers because it is the period actually measured unless the Q wave is absent. Electrophysiologically, the PR interval represents the interval between the onset of atrial depolarization and the onset of ventricular depolarization. In normal AV conduction, it involves the time required for the activation impulse to advance from the atria through the AV node, bundle of His, bundle branches, and the Purkinje fibers until the ventricular myocardium begins to depolarize (see Fig. 1–1B). It does not include the duration of conduction from the SA node proper to the right atrium.

In adults, the normal PR interval is 0.12 to 0.20 second.[28] The most common value is 0.16 second. It is generally shorter in children and longer in older persons. The interval also may become shorter as the sinus rate increases. Although lead II is usually used for this measurement, for the sake of accuracy, the interval should be taken from the lead with the largest and widest P wave and longest QRS duration. Such a selection avoids inaccuracies incurred by using the leads in which the early part of the P wave or QRS complex is isoelectric. Because most modern ECGs record several leads simultaneously, the points of onset of the P wave and the QRS complex can be verified by examining the other simultaneously recorded leads.

With His bundle recording, it has been

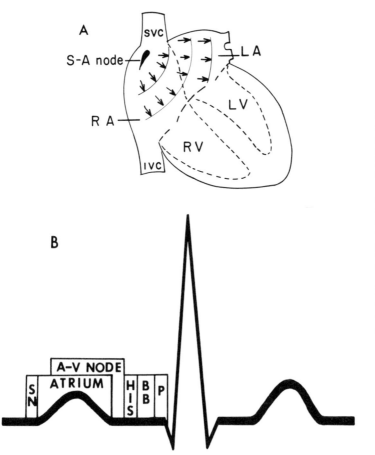

FIGURE 1–1. (A) Schematic diagram of the heart depicting the radial spread of atrial activation from the SA node. (Reproduced from Chou TC, Helm RA, Kaplan S: Clinical Vectorcardiography, 2nd ed, Chapter 3, p 31. New York, 1974, by permission of Grune & Stratton.) (B) Schematic diagram of a P-QRS-T complex illustrating the sequence of activation of the atria and specialized conduction fibers. SN = sinoatrial node; HIS = bundle of His; BB = bundle branches; P = Purkinje fibers. (Reproduced from Damato AN, Lau SH: Clinical value of the electrogram of the conduction system. Prog Cardiovasc Dis 13:119, 1970, by permission of the author and Grune & Stratton.)

shown that most of the AV conduction time is consumed by impulse conduction proximal to the His bundle. The AH time, the time between the intracavitary potential recorded from the lower part of the right atrium and the His bundle spikes, is between 50 and 130 msec.[8,11,36] The HV time, or the interval between the His spikes and the onset of ventricular deflections, is between 35 and 55 msec. Slower conduction through the AV node is mainly responsible for the longer AH time.

The PR segment is the horizontal line between the end of the P wave and the beginning of the QRS complex. Its duration depends on the duration of the P wave as well as the impulse conduction through the AV junction. Although the segment is usually isoelectric, it is often displaced in a direction opposite to the polarity of the P wave. It is, therefore, depressed in most of the conventional leads except lead aVR. The displacement is mainly due to atrial repolarization. In normal subjects, the amount of PR segment depression is usually less than 0.8 mm and the amount of elevation is less than 0.5 mm.[9] Taller P waves are more likely to be associated with a greater degree of PR-segment depression and smaller P waves with lesser PR-segment changes.

QRS COMPLEX

Ventricular Activation

The QRS complex represents the resultant electrical forces generated from ventricular depolarization. In the normal sequence of activation, the ventricular excitation begins at the middle third of the left interventricular septal surface. From there, the impulse spreads in a rightward direction. Using isolated human hearts, Durrer and associates[12] demonstrated early left ventricular activation also in the anterior and posterior paraseptal areas. The forces generated from these two areas are, however, in opposite directions and are mostly neutralized by each other. The right ventricle begins to depolarize shortly after the initiation of left ventricular activation. The excitation starts at the right septal surface near the base of the anterior papillary muscle, and the impulse spreads leftward. Because a much larger area of the left septum is depolarized in comparison with that of the right septum, the net effect of the septal activation is from the left toward the right.

Soon after the beginning of the septal activation, the impulse arrives at most of the sub-

endocardial layer of the myocardium of the apical and free wall of both ventricles through the Purkinje network. Within the inner layers of the ventricular wall, because of the deep penetration of the Purkinje fibers into the myocardium, the activation waves spread in all directions. Consequently, their effects cancel each other and little potential can be detected outside the area. The thickness of the layers to be activated in this manner has been estimated to be one third to two thirds of the entire wall. In the outer layers of the ventricles, the impulse spreads uniformly in the endocardial-to-epicardial direction. Because of the much larger muscle mass of the left ventricle, the result of its activity dominates that of the right ventricle.

The last areas of the ventricles to be depolarized are the basal portion of the septum and the posterobasal portion of the free wall of the left ventricle. The late arrival of the impulse can easily be explained by the rarity of the Purkinje fibers in these areas. The general direction of the spread of impulse in the ventricular wall is outward and backward. In the basal septum, the wave proceeds toward the base and moves from the left to the right.

In summary, because of its larger muscle mass the left ventricle contributes most of the QRS forces (Fig. 1–2). The initial left septal activation generates vectors directed rightward and anteriorly. The major ventricular forces from the free wall of the left ventricle are oriented leftward and inferiorly. The late activation of the posterobasal portion of the left ventricle is accompanied by terminal QRS

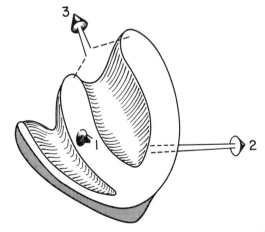

FIGURE 1–2. Representative resultant spatial vectors of ventricular activation. Vector 1 represents the resultant force of the initial septal and paraseptal activation; vector 2, the activation of the free wall of the ventricles; and vector 3, the basal portions of the ventricles.

forces directed posteriorly. Correspondingly, the polarity and amplitude of the various components of the QRS complex in the various leads are determined by the relation between these vectors and the lead axes.

QRS Duration

The duration of the QRS complex represents the duration of ventricular activation. It should be measured from the lead with the widest QRS complex, because in certain leads the initial or terminal vectors may be perpendicular to the lead axis and an isoelectric line is inscribed and the QRS may appear narrow. Although the interval traditionally is measured from the limb leads, the precordial leads, especially leads V_2 and V_3, may have the widest complex. Another difficulty in obtaining an accurate value arises from the fact that ventricular repolarization usually begins before the completion of depolarization. Therefore, there is an overlap and fusion of the terminal part of the QRS and the onset of the ST segment. The end point of the QRS is slurred. This problem is encountered more frequently in the precordial leads. If the leads are recorded simultaneously, the beginning and end of ventricular excitation can be identified more accurately. The interval so determined usually is slightly longer than that obtained from the single-channel trace. With the single-channel recording, it is my practice to choose the widest complex in any lead with the sharpest onset and termination regardless of whether it is a limb lead or a precordial lead.

In normal adults, the QRS duration varies between 0.06 and 0.10 second, and about half of adults have a value of 0.08 second.[24] A duration of 0.11 second sometimes may be observed in healthy subjects. Men tend to have slightly longer durations than women.

QRS Axis

By convention, the QRS axis represents the direction of the mean QRS vector in the frontal plane. It is determined by using the hexaxial reference system derived from the Einthoven equilateral triangle (Fig. 1–3). Two methods generally are used. One method is to find a lead with an isoelectric complex or a lead in which the algebraic sum of the deflections is zero. The QRS axis is perpendicular to this lead, and its positive terminus points toward the limb lead with the largest net positive deflection. The other method is to use the algebraic sum of the deflections in two leads, usu-ally leads I and III, to plot out the axis. The results obtained from these two methods are not necessarily the same. Furthermore, the direction of the axis may be different when a different pair of leads is used. A variance of up to $\pm 35°$ occasionally may be obtained in the same individual.[39] The main reason for the discrepancies is that the three standard limb leads do not form an equilateral triangle and the adjacent axes of the hexaxial reference system are not separated by a 30° angle. The electrical axes of the limb leads form a scalene triangle as described by Burger and van Milaan[5] (Fig. 1–4). A more accurate QRS axis (as well as P and T axes) can be obtained by using the hexaxial reference system derived from it. Langner further improved the reference system by modifying the scales of the leads to compensate for their unequal strength,[25] since the same unit potential applied to the various leads does not give the same magnitude of deflection. Although it is theoretically desirable to use the reference system based on Burger's triangle, most values given in the literature were determined from leads I and III by the traditional method.

The normal range of the QRS axis in the frontal plane is between $-30°$ and $+105°$.[19,43] Most people have values between $+30°$ and $+75°$. A significant difference is found among various age groups, with a leftward shift of the axis in older individuals. In an individual under the age of 30, the axis is seldom superior to 0°. After the age of 40, the axis is seldom to the right of $+90°$. Therefore, for clinical purposes, the normal limits for persons under the age of 40 are 0° to $+105°$, and for those over the age of 40, from $-30°$ to $+90°$. There also is an association between the QRS axis in the frontal plane and body weight. A thin person is likely to have a more vertical axis, and overweight individuals tend to have a more leftward axis. The trend of leftward shift of the axis with aging is particularly pronounced in overweight subjects. There is no significant sex difference in the axis even though older women generally have less leftward shift of the axis.

QRS Morphology and Amplitude

The morphology and amplitude of the QRS complex, as in the case of the QRS axis, are significantly affected by some of the constitutional variables. With advancing age, the amplitude of the QRS complex decreases, but the changes are less apparent after the age of 40.[17,40] Men generally have a larger QRS am-

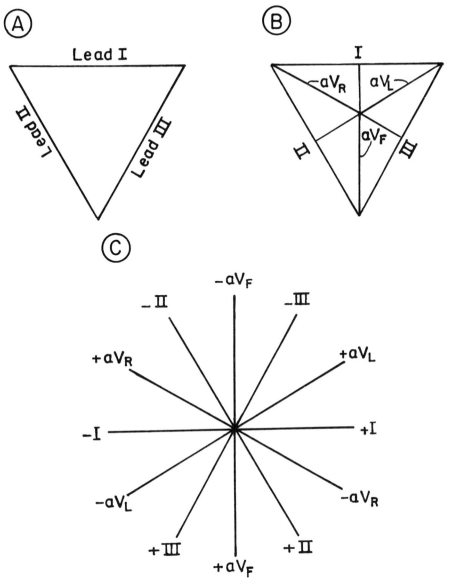

FIGURE 1–3. (A) Einthoven's equilateral triangle formed by leads I, II, and III. (B) The unipolar limb leads are added to the equilateral triangle. (C) The hexaxial reference system derived from B.

plitude than do women.[14] Blacks have higher voltage than do white subjects.[17,24,40] With increasing body weight, the QRS complex decreases in amplitude. The normal ranges of the amplitudes of the Q, R, S, and T waves in men and women of different age groups, as compiled by Lepeschkin,[28] are given in Table 1–1.* The morphologic changes other than those secondary to the change in QRS axis are less pronounced and are dealt with during the

discussion of the individual components of the complex.

LIMB LEADS

The morphology of the QRS complex in the limb leads depends on the orientation and amplitude of the instantaneous QRS vectors in the frontal plane. The polarity of its major deflection is related to the direction of the mean QRS vector or axis and is determined by the projection of the QRS vector on the lead axis in question. Because the normal range of the QRS axis is between −30° and +105°, lead I

---

*Minor differences exist between some of the values listed in the table and those discussed in the following paragraphs.

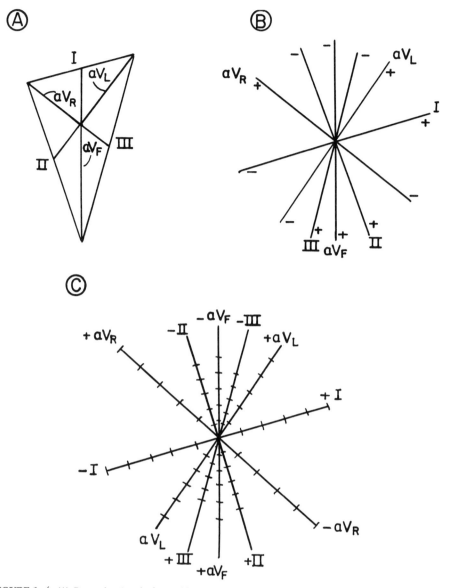

FIGURE 1–4. (A) Burger's triangle formed by the lead axes of leads I, II, and III, with the addition of those of the unipolar limb leads. (B) The hexaxial reference system based on Burger's triangle. (C) The hexaxial reference system with the addition of scales in proportion to the relative magnitude of deflection recorded with the same unit potential in the various leads.

usually records a dominant R wave, except in younger subjects with a rightward axis when an R/S ratio of less than 1 may be seen (Fig. 1–5). This is especially true in lead aVL, in which the entire QRS may be negative if the QRS axis is +90° or greater. Lead II invariably has a prominent R wave, since the projection of the mean vector is always on the positive side of the lead if the axis is normal. In contrast, the vector points toward the negative side of lead aVR, which, therefore, always records a negative deflection. An essentially upright complex is more common in lead aVF, especially in younger individuals.

Because of the orientation of the lead III axis, the morphology of the QRS complex in this lead is variable. The normal QRS vector may project on either the positive or negative side of the lead axis. Because the QRS axis is between +30° and +75° in most instances, the mean QRS vector is almost perpendicular to the lead. A slight shifting of the direction of the QRS vector may change its projection on the lead from the positive to the negative side or vice versa, with corresponding change in the polarity of the complex. The respiratory variation of the morphology also is most pronounced in this lead (Fig. 1–6). For the same

TABLE 1–1. Normal Amplitudes of Q, R, S, and T Waves: Means and Ranges (in Parentheses)*

Lead	Age (yr)	Q Wave	R Wave	S Wave	T Wave
I	12–16	1.0 (0–3.0)	5.9 (0–12.0)	1.3 (0–10.0)	2.4 (1.6–6.0)
	16–20	0.3 (0–1.3)	4.3 (1.8–9.5)	1.0 (0–3.5)	2.1 (0.2–3.7)
	20–30 ♂	0.3 (0–2.6)	5.7 (1.3–12.9)	1.3 (0–4.0)	2.1 (0.9–4.1)
	20–30 ♀	0.1 (0–1.0)	4.8 (1.3–9.5)	0.8 (0–3.2)	2.1 (0.5–4.0)
	30–40 ♂	0.2 (0–1.2)	5.4 (1.8–11.3)	1.2 (0–4.2)	2.0 (0.6–3.7)
	30–40 ♀	0.2 (0–1.1)	5.1 (1.4–15.0)	0.6 (0–2.9)	2.0 (0.9–3.8)
	40–60 ♂	0.2 (0–1.1)	6.0 (2.0–11.6)	0.7 (0–3.0)	1.9 (0.7–3.5)
	40–60 ♀	0.2 (0–1.2)	6.2 (2.0–12.5)	0.3 (0–2.1)	1.9 (0.7–3.2)
II	12–16	1.0 (0–2.5)	13.5 (3.5–24.5)	1.4 (0–7.0)	3.3 (−0.2 to +6.1)
	16–20	0.5 (0–2.8)	9.5 (2.9–15.8)	1.4 (0–6.3)	2.7 (0.2–5.7)
	20–30 ♂	0.5 (0–2.1)	11.7 (4.7–19.1)	1.4 (0–4.8)	2.9 (0.8–5.8)
	20–30 ♀	0.3 (0–2.2)	9.9 (3.9–15.9)	0.6 (0–2.9)	2.4 (0.7–4.4)
	30–40 ♂	0.3 (0–1.3)	9.3 (4.0–17.0)	1.3 (0–4.3)	2.7 (1.0–5.0)
	30–40 ♀	0.2 (0–1.3)	8.7 (2.1–15.5)	0.8 (0–3.2)	2.2 (0.6–4.9)
	40–60 ♂	0.3 (0–1.2)	7.5 (1.9–15.5)	0.8 (0–3.8)	2.3 (0.8–4.3)
	40–60 ♀	0.2 (0–1.5)	8.1 (2.6–15.3)	0.7 (0–3.1)	2.2 (0.8–4.1)
III	12–16	1.6 (0–5.0)	9.0 (1.0–26.0)	1.1 (0–9.0)	0.8 (−1.6 to +3.5)
	16–20	0.6 (0–4.6)	6.8 (1.2–15.0)	1.1 (0–4.9)	0.8 (−1.9 to +3.9)
	20–30 ♂	0.6 (0–2.6)	7.1 (0.8–15.8)	1.1 (0–6.0)	0.8 (−0.9 to +3.0)
	20–30 ♀	0.6 (0–2.2)	6.0 (0.5–14.2)	0.6 (0–4.3)	0.3 (−0.7 to +2.1)
	30–40 ♂	0.5 (0–2.0)	5.0 (0.3–12.4)	1.4 (0–8.5)	0.7 (−1.5 to +2.9)
	30–40 ♀	0.3 (0–1.0)	4.5 (0.1–12.7)	0.8 (0–4.5)	0.4 (−1.8 to +2.4)
	40–60 ♂	0.4 (0–2.4)	3.2 (0.1–11.9)	1.6 (0–7.5)	0.4 (−1.2 to +2.2)
	40–60 ♀	0.4 (0–2.0)	3.6 (0.1–11.8)	1.4 (0–6.0)	0.3 (−1.1 to +1.7)
aVR	12–16	7.9 (0–14.0)	1.2 (0–3.0)	2.5 (0–19.0)	−2.9 (−5.2 to −0.5)
	16–20	2.1 (0–9.0)	1.2 (0–4.7)	4.3 (0–11.1)	−2.0 (−4.8 to −0.1)
	20–30 ♂	2.5 (0–11.5)	0.6 (0–3.2)	9.0 (0–16.1)	−2.5 (−5.0 to −0.8)
	20–30 ♀	2.5 (0–11.5)	0.5 (0–1.8)	6.9 (0–11.6)	−2.2 (−5.0 to −0.7)
	30–40 ♂	2.1 (0–9.0)	0.6 (0–3.2)	7.6 (0–12.0)	−2.3 (−4.2 to −1.0)
	30–40 ♀	2.1 (0–9.0)	0.5 (0–2.2)	6.2 (0–14.6)	−2.1 (−3.5 to −0.9)
	40–60 ♂	2.0 (0–8.5)	0.5 (0–2.2)	6.8 (0–11.0)	−2.1 (−3.4 to −0.8)
	40–60 ♀	2.0 (0–8.5)	0.4 (0–1.6)	6.8 (0–12.5)	−2.0 (−3.6 to −0.7)
aVL	12–16	1.0 (0–6.0)	2.4 (0–12.0)	3.0 (0–20.0)	1.1 (−1.0 to +3.6)
	16–20	0.5 (0–2.5)	1.9 (0.2–6.0)	2.0 (0–8.0)	0.6 (−1.8 to +3.6)
	20–30 ♂	0.3 (0–3.5)	2.0 (0.1–8.3)	2.7 (0–8.7)	1.7 (−0.8 to + 2.1)
	20–30 ♀	0.3 (0–3.5)	1.9 (0.1–7.2)	2.0 (0–9.2)	1.0 (−0.4 to +2.2)
	30–40 ♂	0.3 (0–2.3)	2.4 (0.1–8.5)	1.8 (0–6.8)	1.8 (−1.0 to +2.1)
	30–40 ♀	0.1 (0–1.3)	2.3 (0.3–9.2)	1.0 (0–4.5)	1.0 (−0.4 to +3.0)
	40–60 ♂	0.2 (0–1.3)	3.4 (0.2–9.3)	1.1 (0–4.6)	1.1 (−0.5 to +2.2)
	40–60 ♀	0.2 (0–1.4)	3.3 (0.2–8.5)	0.7 (0–3.9)	0.7 (−0.1 to +2.6)
aVF	12–16	1.3 (0–3.0)	10.2 (0.1–21.8)	1.0 (0–4.0)	2.3 (−0.7 to +5.4)
	16–20	0.8 (0–3.8)	7.7 (1.8–14.0)	1.0 (0–4.9)	1.8 (−0.6 to +5.2)
	20–30 ♂	0.5 (0–2.2)	8.8 (1.0–16.9)	0.7 (0–4.9)	1.1 (−0.2 to +3.5)
	20–30 ♀	0.3 (0–1.6)	7.6 (1.8–15.6)	1.0 (0–2.1)	0.5 (−0.1 to +3.1)
	30–40 ♂	0.3 (0–1.3)	6.7 (1.0–14.8)	0.8 (0–4.4)	1.0 (0.4–3.8)
	30–40 ♀	0.3 (0–1.2)	6.2 (1.0–13.9)	1.2 (0–2.6)	0.5 (0.1–3.2)
	40–60 ♂	0.2 (0–1.2)	4.7 (0.3–12.6)	0.9 (0–4.1)	0.9 (0–3.1)
	40–60 ♀	0.2 (0–1.1)	5.3 (0.3–13.4)	1.0 (0–3.9)	0.8 (−0.2 to +2.6)
V_1	12–16	0	5.6 (0–16.0)	13.8 (5.0–26.0)	−1.5 (−4.0 to +7.0)
	16–20	0	4.6 (0.4–16.7)	11.7 (1.8–25.1)	0.9 (−3.5 to +6.0)
	20–30 ♂	0	3.3 (0.3–8.9)	11.4 (5.0–18.0)	0.9 (−2.2 to + 3.9)
	20–30 ♀	0	1.6 (0–5.3)	7.4 (1.6–14.2)	−0.7 (−2.1 to +2.0)
	30–40 ♂	0	2.2 (0.2–5.4)	9.1 (3.2–17.6)	0.7 (−1.4 to +3.3)
	30–40 ♀	0	1.6 (0–5.8)	7.6 (3.8–14.3)	−0.6 (−2.6 to +1.2)
	40–60 ♂	0	1.7 (0.1–4.9)	8.6 (2.9–16.7)	0.9 (−1.3 to +3.9)
	40–60 ♀	0	1.4 (0.1–4.0)	7.2 (2.3–15.1)	−0.2 (−1.9 to +1.5)

Table continued on following page

TABLE 1–1. Normal Amplitudes of Q, R, S, and T Waves: Means and Ranges (in Parentheses)*
Continued

Lead	Age (yr)	Q Wave	R Wave	S Wave	T Wave
V$_2$	12–16	0	9.1 (2.0–21.0)	20.1 (4.0–51.0)	4.5 (−4.3 to +13.5)
	16–20	0	7.3 (0.5–20.5)	16.2 (2.6–45.5)	3.9 (−3.8 to +14.1)
	20–30 ♂	0	7.4 (1.7–13.9)	18.0 (6.7–29.1)	6.5 (1.1–12.3)
	20–30 ♀	0	4.6 (1.1–9.2)	12.4 (4.0–23.2)	3.1 (0–4.1)
	30–40 ♂	0	5.4 (0.6–12.1)	15.2 (6.1–27.8)	6.2 (2.0–11.1)
	30–40 ♀	0	3.7 (0.4–10.1)	11.3 (4.2–19.8)	2.9 (0–7.5)
	40–60 ♂	0	4.6 (0.6–12.0)	12.7 (5.2–23.3)	5.5 (1.7–10.1)
	40–60 ♀	0	3.6 (0.2–9.1)	9.4 (2.4–18.0)	3.0 (0.1–6.5)
V$_3$	12–16	0.1 (0–1)	11.8 (2.0–33.0)	14.1 (3.0–34.0)	4.1 (0–13.0)
	16–20	0.1 (0–1)	8.5 (1.6–23.3)	10.7 (0.9–28.9)	5.1 (−3.7 to +13.5)
	20–30 ♂	0 (0–0.4)	11.6 (2.2–26.6)	10.6 (6.7–22.0)	6.5 (1.9–11.7)
	20–30 ♀	0 (0–0.4)	8.2 (2.3–17.5)	6.1 (4.0–14.2)	3.5 (0–8.6)
	30–40 ♂	0 (0–0.5)	9.4 (2.2–22.5)	10.0 (6.1–22.0)	6.3 (3.1–11.5)
	30–40 ♀	0 (0–0.5)	7.1 (0.8–23.3)	5.1 (4.2–11.9)	3.1 (0.5–7.7)
	40–60 ♂	0 (0–0.4)	8.4 (1.4–11.6)	9.8 (5.2–19.0)	6.0 (2.1–10.7)
	40–60 ♀	0 (0–0.4)	7.1 (1.0–17.7)	6.0 (2.4–13.5)	3.4 (0.1–7.4)
V$_4$	12–16	0.5 (0–3.0)	23.5 (5.0–51.0)	7.0 (1.0–30.0)	7.2 (0–17.2)
	16–20	0.1 (0–1.0)	12.7 (3.1–30.1)	6.3 (0.2–15.0)	4.7 (−3.6 to +12.6)
	20–30 ♂	0.3 (0–2.9)	16.6 (6.1–27.7)	6.1 (0–15.0)	5.6 (1.5–11.8)
	20–30 ♀	0.1 (0–0.7)	11.5 (5.0–19.6)	2.9 (0–8.5)	3.6 (1.0–7.8)
	30–40 ♂	0.2 (0–1.7)	14.8 (5.2–29.2)	5.7 (1.1–12.1)	5.4 (2.0–9.9)
	30–40 ♀	0.2 (0–1.4)	11.8 (4.1–25.9)	2.4 (0–7.8)	3.3 (0.8–7.0)
	40–60 ♂	0.1 (0–1.0)	14.2 (5.2–25.6)	6.3 (0.8–14.1)	5.4 (1.6–10.4)
	40–60 ♀	0.2 (0–1.3)	12.4 (3.7–23.6)	2.8 (0–7.7)	3.5 (1.0–6.3)
V$_5$	12–16	1.3 (0–4.0)	18.2 (5.0–35.0)	2.5 (0–12.0)	5.7 (0.5–11.5)
	16–20	0.5 (0–2.8)	11.4 (4.1–26.5)	2.2 (0–8.1)	3.8 (0.2–10.6)
	20–30 ♂	0.7 (0–3.1)	15.3 (5.9–24.0)	2.2 (0–6.4)	3.8 (0.8–8.1)
	20–30 ♀	0.3 (0–1.2)	11.5 (5.2–18.7)	1.0 (0–4.0)	3.0 (1.0–5.5)
	30–40 ♂	0.4 (0–2.0)	14.3 (8.1–24.8)	2.3 (0–6.7)	3.7 (1.3–7.0)
	30–40 ♀	0.3 (0–1.8)	11.8 (5.0–27.2)	0.8 (0–3.2)	2.9 (0.8–5.9)
	40–60 ♂	0.3 (0–1.6)	14.1 (5.9–25.0)	2.4 (1.0–6.9)	3.9 (1.3–7.8)
	40–60 ♀	0.3 (0–1.2)	12.4 (5.0–20.9)	1.0 (0–5.0)	2.9 (0.9–5.1)
V$_6$	12–16	1.3 (0–2.5)	12.5 (4.0–27.0)	1.0 (0–6.0)	4.0 (0.8–7.2)
	16–20	0.6 (0–4.2)	13.5 (7.0–21.0)	1.2 (0–5.0)	3.8 (0.8–7.1)
	20–30 ♂	0.7 (0–2.6)	11.6 (3.7–19.3)	0.9 (0–3.7)	2.6 (0.5–5.9)
	20–30 ♀	0.4 (0–1.8)	9.6 (5.2–16.3)	0.3 (0–1.8)	2.4 (0.9–5.0)
	30–40 ♂	0.5 (0–1.6)	10.9 (5.9–18.3)	0.8 (0–2.8)	2.5 (0.8–4.5)
	30–40 ♀	0.3 (0–1.5)	9.2 (4.0–20.2)	0.3 (0–1.7)	3.3 (0.6–4.7)
	40–60 ♂	0.4 (0–1.5)	10.5 (4.9–17.8)	0.7 (0–2.9)	2.6 (0.8–4.9)
	40–60 ♀	0.3 (0–1.4)	9.6 (3.6–16.8)	0.3 (0–2.6)	2.3 (0.7–4.6)

*Adapted from Lepeschkin E: *In* Altman PE, Dittmer DS (eds): Respiration and Circulation. Bethesda, Federation of American Societies for Experimental Biology, 1971, p 277, by permission of the author and the Federation of American Societies for Experimental Biology, Bethesda, Maryland.

reason, notching and slurring of the QRS complex may be seen in this lead without indicating abnormality (see Fig. 1–10). This also is true in the other inferior leads, but it occurs less frequently.

Q WAVE. A Q wave is inscribed in a lead when the initial QRS vectors are directed away from the positive electrode. The orientation of the initial forces that originate mostly from the excitation of the interventricular septum and apical anterior region of the ventricles are variable in the frontal plane. When the QRS axis is more vertical, Q waves are more likely to be seen in the inferior leads; when it is horizontal, in leads I and aVL. The Q wave is more common in one or more of the inferior leads (leads II, III, and aVF), occurring in more than half of normal adults. In leads I and aVL, it is present in less than half.[19,43] In lead aVR, the initial negativity usually is a part of the QS deflection.

The duration of the Q wave is of considerable importance in the diagnosis of myocardial infarction. With the exception of leads III and aVR, the Q waves in the limb leads normally do not exceed 0.03 second in duration.

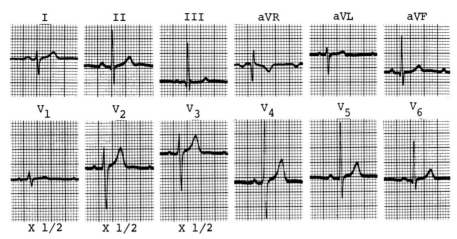

FIGURE 1-5. Normal ECG from a healthy 22-year-old man illustrating rightward QRS axis in the frontal plane. The R/S ratio in lead V_1 = 1.

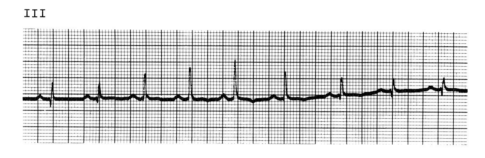

FIGURE 1-6. Respiratory variation in the morphology and amplitude of the QRS complexes in lead III.

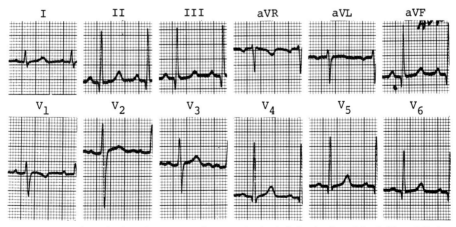

FIGURE 1-7. Relatively deep but narrow Q waves in the inferior leads and leads V_5 and V_6 in a healthy 23-year-old woman.

Indeed, less than 5 percent of the normal population have a Q wave greater than 0.02 second in these leads.[24] In lead III, the Q wave occasionally may have a width of 0.04 second but rarely 0.05 second. This is the lead from which most of the erroneous diagnoses of myocardial infarction are made.

The amplitude of the Q waves in the limb leads is small. It is less than 4 mm in all these leads except lead III, in which it may reach 5 mm.[24,43] The depth of the Q wave is less than 25 percent of the R wave in these leads, but lead III is the exception. Generally speaking, a normal Q wave tends to be more prominent in younger individuals (Fig. 1–7). For example, in lead I, it does not exceed 1.5 mm in adults except in those under 30 years of age.

R WAVE. As stated, the R wave amplitude in any lead depends on the direction of the maximum QRS vector. The lead whose axis is most parallel to and that has the same polarity as the maximum vector records the tallest R wave. The upper limit for the R wave in lead I is 15 mm; aVL, 10 mm; and II, III, and aVF, 19 mm. Larger amplitude occasionally may be seen in younger subjects.[23]

S WAVE. The S wave is most prominent in lead aVR. This lead has a polarity opposite to the general direction of the major QRS forces. An amplitude up to 16 mm may be seen in this lead in younger subjects. A relatively large S wave sometimes may be present in leads III and aVL, depending on the QRS axis. The magnitude usually does not exceed 9 mm. In leads I, II, and aVF, the S waves are less than 5 mm.[43]

If the amplitude of the entire QRS complex is less than 5 mm in all the limb leads, the voltage is considered abnormally low.

PRECORDIAL LEADS

The QRS complexes in the precordial leads represent the projections of the QRS vectors in the horizontal plane. Figure 1–8 illustrates the directions of the lead axes of V_1 through V_6. As the dominant left ventricular forces are directed leftward, the right precordial leads (V_1 and V_2) record predominantly negative deflections (S waves), and the left precordial leads (V_5 and V_6) record upright deflections (R waves). The early activation of the anterior wall and the late excitation of the posterior wall explain the initial positivity and terminal negativity of the complexes in the leads with an axis directed essentially anteriorly (e.g., V_1 through V_4). The R wave progressively increases in amplitude from lead V_1 toward leads V_5 and V_6, and the S wave decreases from the right toward the left precordial leads.

TRANSITIONAL ZONE. The transitional zone represents the location of the lead, having positive and negative deflections of the same magnitude. It is related to the direction of the QRS axis in the horizontal plane, which is not expressed in degrees in the routine interpretation of the ECG. As in the frontal plane, the QRS axis is perpendicular to the transitional lead. In normal adults, the transitional zone usually is located between leads V_2 and V_4, lead V_3 being the most common site. A slight notching of the complex occasionally may be observed in the transitional lead. A transitional zone located to the right of lead V_2 is referred to as *counterclockwise rotation*. If the transitional zone is displaced leftward and beyond lead V_5, *clockwise rotation* is present. An R/S ratio greater than 1 in lead V_1 generally is considered abnormal in adults. According to Lamb's data, however, 6.4 percent of normal men and 1.5 percent of normal women have an R/S ratio equal to 1 in V_1[24] (see Fig. 1–5). About 25 percent of men and 12 percent of women have a ratio of 1 in V_2. The tendency is toward leftward shift of the transitional zone in older individuals. An R/S ratio of less than 1 in V_5 and V_6 is usually abnormal, however, and less than 2.5 percent of Lamb's normal subjects had such a value.

Q WAVE. Small Q waves are present in the left precordial leads in more than 75 percent

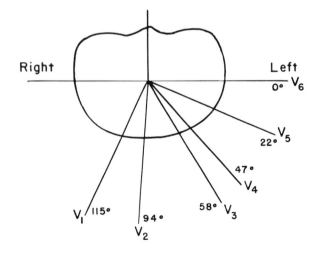

FIGURE 1–8. Directions of the lead axes of leads V_1 through V_6.

of normal subjects. They often are referred to as *septal* Q waves, suggesting that they are generated from the left-to-right septal activation. They are seen most frequently in lead V_6, less so in leads V_5 and V_4, and are rare in V_3. Q waves in these leads are present more often in younger subjects than in those above 40 years of age. There also is a relationship between the location of the transitional zone and the presence or absence of Q waves. Q waves are likely to be present in more leads when the transitional zone is located on the right side of the precordium. The duration of the Q waves is 0.03 second or less. Their amplitude usually is less than 2 mm, but it may reach 3 or even 4 mm. The deeper Q waves are seen more often in younger adults.[28] An amplitude of 4 mm or more may be encountered in teenagers.

R WAVE. The R wave increases in amplitude from the right toward the left precordium. In lead V_1, it may be absent, and a QS complex is recorded. QS deflection, however, is rare in lead V_2 in healthy subjects. The upper limit for the height of the R wave in V_1 is 6 mm but may be higher in younger adults.[28,43] The tallest R wave in the precordial leads is seen most commonly in lead V_4. Lead V_5 is the next most common lead, whereas lead V_6 generally has lower voltage than V_5. Echocardiographic studies suggest that proximity of the left ventricle to the chest wall is a major determinant of the R wave amplitude in leads V_5 and V_6 in normal subjects.[13] For the diagnosis of left ventricular hypertrophy, leads V_5 and V_6 are frequently used, and 25 mm generally is considered the upper normal limit of the R-wave amplitude in these two leads. Although this limit is applicable in older individuals, the amplitude in younger subjects may be greater than 30 mm.[26,30]

S WAVE. The S wave is deepest in the right precordial leads, usually lead V_2. It decreases in amplitude as the left precordium is approached. Although the upper limits of the S-wave amplitude in leads V_1, V_2, and V_3 have been given as 18, 26, and 21 mm, respectively,[43] an amplitude of 30 mm occasionally is recorded in healthy individuals.[26] An S wave often is absent in leads V_5 and V_6. On the other hand, in lead V_1, an S wave of less than 3 mm is considered abnormally small. Right ventricular hypertrophy or posterior myocardial infarction often is responsible for the decrease in the amplitude of the S wave in this lead.

INTRINSICOID DEFLECTION. The onset of the intrinsicoid deflection represents the moment when the epicardial muscle that lies under the electrode becomes depolarized. It is the beginning of the abrupt downstroke after the R wave reaches its peak. The time of the onset is measured from the beginning of the QRS complex to the point of the abrupt downstroke. In the right precordial leads, the upper limit of normal is 0.035 second. In the left precordial leads, it is 0.045 second. This interval is used mostly in the diagnosis of ventricular hypertrophy and bundle branch block when the onset of the intrinsicoid deflection is delayed.

THE ST SEGMENT

The ST segment is the segment between the end of the QRS complex (J point or ST junction) and the beginning of the T wave. It represents a state of unchanged polarization between the end of depolarization and the beginning of repolarization, or a stage when the terminal depolarization and the starting repolarization are superimposed and neutralize each other.

The most important information in regard to the ST segment is the presence or absence and degree of displacement from the isoelectric line. As a rule, the TP segment is used as the reference baseline. When the heart rate is rapid, however, the P wave of the succeeding beat may be superimposed on the later portion of the T wave, and the TP segment is no longer representative of the true baseline. In such cases, the PR segment is used. One of the arguments against using the PR segment is that it does not represent the isoelectric line because the atrial T (Ta) wave is being inscribed at the same time. In most instances, however, the duration of atrial repolarization is greater than 0.20 second. The Ta wave displaces not only the PR segment but also the early part of the ST segment. The inaccuracy inherent in using the PR segment as the baseline for determining ST displacement is therefore partially nullified. Because of the proximity of the PR and ST segments, it is technically easier to compare their levels. Indeed, for clinical purpose, it is more practical to use the PR segment rather than the TP segment to determine whether ST-segment displacement is present regardless of the heart rate. The problem of unstable baseline also is avoided.

In the limb leads, the ST segment is isoelectric in about 75 percent of normal adults.[19] ST-segment elevation or depression up to 1 mm generally is considered within normal limits.[23] ST-segment elevation is more common, however, and is usually present in the inferior leads. ST-segment depression seldom is seen in leads I, II, and aVF, because the ST vector in the frontal plane, if present, is directed inferiorly and usually leftward.

In the precordial leads, some ST-segment elevation is seen in more than 90 percent of normal subjects.[19] Men tend to have slightly higher degree of ST elevation than do women.[17] The elevation is most common and marked in leads V_2 and V_3, wherein the amplitude may reach 3 mm. In the left precordial leads, the elevation rarely exceeds 1 mm. The upward displacement is generally more pronounced in younger individuals. ST elevation of greater than 2 mm is uncommon in subjects over 40 years of age. Any ST-segment depression in the precordial leads is considered abnormal, since the normal ST vector in the horizontal plane is directed anteriorly and leftward.

T WAVE

The T wave represents the potential of ventricular repolarization. The ventricular recovery process proceeds in the general direction of ventricular excitation. The polarity of the resultant T vector is similar to that of the QRS vector. The reversal of the polarity of the forces associated with repolarization is counterbalanced by the epicardium-to-endocardium direction of the recovery process, which is the opposite of the direction of the excitation process.[14] In normal individuals, the orientation of the T vector is invariably leftward, inferior, and, in most adults, anterior. In children and young adults (especially females), it may be slightly posterior but becomes increasingly anterior with advancing age. Because the

T vector is directed leftward and inferiorly in the frontal plane the T waves are always upright in leads I and II and inverted in aVR. They may be upright or inverted in leads III and aVL, depending on whether the T vector is more vertical or horizontal. In lead aVF, the T wave usually is upright but occasionally may be flat or slightly inverted. In the horizontal plane, the T vector is directed leftward and usually anteriorly. Therefore, the T waves are always upright in the left precordial leads V_5 and V_6. In about 50 percent of women, the T wave is inverted in lead V_1.[19] An inverted, diphasic, or flat T wave is much less common in lead V_2 (less than 10 percent) and is seen only occasionally in V_3, mostly in younger patients. It rarely is present in V_4. In adult men, T-wave inversion in the right precordial leads is relatively uncommon. In Lamb's series, less than 1 percent of the adult men had inverted T waves in lead V_1.[24] When T-wave inversion is present in two or more of the right precordial leads in the normal adult, the phenomenon is called *persistent juvenile pattern* (Fig. 1–9). Some controversy exists as to whether this pattern is more common in blacks than in whites.

Amplitude

In the limb leads, the tallest T wave is seen most commonly in lead II. The T-wave amplitude is normally less than 6 mm in all the limb leads.[28] In leads I and II, where the T wave is normally upright, the amplitude should not be less than 0.5 mm. There is no significant difference in the amplitude in males and females. In the precordial leads, however, the amplitude is higher in males. The T waves in the precordial leads are tallest in leads V_2 and

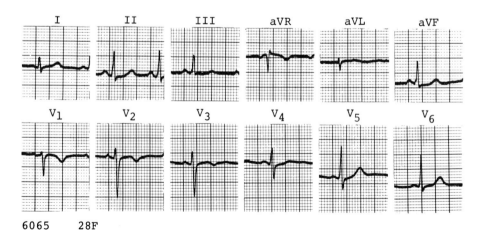

6065   28F

FIGURE 1–9. Persistent juvenile pattern in a healthy 28-year-old woman. There is T-wave inversion in leads V_1 through V_3.

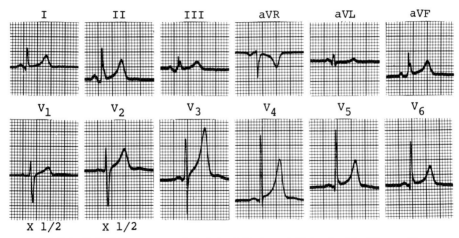

FIGURE 1–10. Tall T wave, especially in leads V_2 through V_4 in a healthy 22-year-old man.

V_3. In males, the amplitude in these leads has an average value of about 6 mm but may reach 12 mm or more (Fig. 1–10). It is significantly lower in men over the age of 40. In females, the amplitude is generally lower, with an average of 3 to 4 mm, and is seldom above 8 mm. Although Lepeschkin's data (see Table 1–1) show that the T-wave amplitude does not change appreciably with advancing age, others found a significant decrease.[17,20,43] In both sexes, the T waves in the left precordial leads generally are lower than those in the mid-precordial leads. They seldom are less than one tenth of the height of the R waves, however.

Morphology

The normal T wave is asymmetrical. Whether it is upright or inverted, the first half has a more gradual slope than the second half. The first portion has an upward concavity if the T wave is upright and a downward concavity if the T wave is inverted. In the right precordial leads, if the T wave is diphasic, the first portion is upright and the second portion inverted. A negative–positive diphasic T wave is abnormal, but a positive–negative T wave does not always indicate normality.

THE QT INTERVAL

The QT interval represents the duration of ventricular electrical systole. It is measured from the beginning of the QRS complex to the end of the T wave. The lead with a large T wave and a distinct termination is used. In practice, considerable difficulty often is encountered in obtaining an accurate measurement. The T wave may be low or its termination gradual. It may partly superimpose on a prominent U wave. When the heart rate is rapid, the T wave may overlap the P wave. Under such circumstances, the QT interval is estimated by extrapolating the downslope of the T wave. Leads V_2 and V_3 may be the best leads for measuring the QT interval.[10] The value so obtained usually approximates most closely the maximum QT interval determined from the 12 leads.

The QT interval varies with the heart rate (Table 1–2), lengthening as the heart rate decreases. Within the range of heart rate between 45 and 115 beats/min, the normal limits may vary between 0.46 and 0.30 second.[44] Women have longer QT intervals than do men and children, but the sex difference has been questioned.[44] The QT interval increases slightly with age.

There is also a diurnal variation of the QT interval corrected for the heart rate, being longer during sleep than during waking hours.[3] This diurnal variation is thought to be related to autonomic tone and concentrations of circulating catecholamines. Many formulas have been proposed to calculate the normal QT interval for a given heart rate. The most commonly used formula is that suggested by Bazett[2]: normal QT interval = K $\sqrt{RR}$, where K is a constant equal to 0.37 for men and children and 0.40 for women, and RR is the interval between two successive R waves. The QT interval corrected for heart rate, or QTc, may be obtained by dividing the measured QT interval by the square root of the RR. The upper limit of QTc is 0.39 second for men and 0.41 second for women.[28] Many clinical studies that involve the QT interval do not consider it

TABLE 1–2. Normal Limits for QT Interval*

| | Age (yr) | | | | | | | |
| | 18–29 | | 30–39 | | 40–49 | | 50–60 | |
Heart Rate	L	U	L	U	L	U	L	U
115–84	0.30	0.37	0.30	0.37	0.31	0.37	0.31	0.37
83–72	0.32	0.39	0.33	0.39	0.33	0.40	0.33	0.40
71–63	0.34	0.41	0.35	0.41	0.35	0.41	0.35	0.42
62–56	0.36	0.42	0.36	0.43	0.37	0.43	0.37	0.43
55–45	0.39	0.45	0.39	0.45	0.39	0.46	0.39	0.46

L = lower limit in seconds; U = upper limit in seconds.
*Adapted from Simonson E, Cady LD, Woodbury M: The normal Q-T interval. Am Heart J 63:747, 1962, by permission of CV Mosby.

abnormally long unless the QTc is greater than 0.44 second.

Because of the difficulties in obtaining exact measurement of the QT interval in many of the ECGs and because the normal limits given by various investigators vary, rigid adherence to a precise value for normality is not warranted. Minor deviation from the usual normal limits may not be clinically significant. In the routine interpretation of an ECG, I use 0.40 second as the normal upper limit of the QT interval for the heart rate of 70 beats/min. For every 10-beats/min increase or decrease of the rate, 0.02 second is deducted or added to the QT interval. The lower normal limits are 0.07 second less than the corresponding upper limits. Such a guideline avoids the necessity of calculation, and the values are close to those listed by Simonson and associates[44] within the rate of 45 to 115 beats/min.

THE U WAVE

The U wave is a small, low-frequency deflection that appears after the T wave. Its genesis is controversial. Two major hypotheses are favored. One of the proposed mechanisms is that the U wave represents the afterpotentials of the ventricular myocardium. The repolarization of the muscle at the end of the action potential proper is incomplete. The low-level potential that follows the action potential proper is called the *afterpotential.*[29] Another theory suggests that the U wave is the result of repolarization of the Purkinje fibers.[49] A good review of this subject was written by Lepeschkin.[29]

The vector of the normal U wave is directed leftward, inferiorly, and anteriorly. Therefore, the normal U wave is upright in the limb leads and precordial leads except in lead aVR. Its polarity is similar to that of the T wave, except that it is upright in the right precordial leads even though the T wave may be inverted as in the juvenile pattern. It is also upright in lead III in patients with normally inverted T waves in this lead. The amplitude of the normal U wave usually is proportional to that of the T wave, being about 5 to 25 percent of the latter's voltage. It is largest in leads V_2 and V_3,

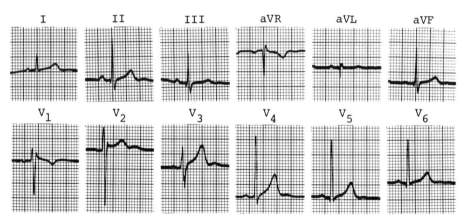

FIGURE 1–11. Normal U waves in a 22-year-old man. They are seen best in leads V_2 through V_4.

where it may reach 2.0 mm, but it has an average amplitude of 0.33 mm[27] (Fig. 1–11). It is prominent during slow heart rate and becomes difficult to identify at a rate above 90 beats/min, because it begins to superimpose on the succeeding P wave. The initial portion of the normal U wave has a steeper slope than the terminal portion. This is opposite to the morphology of the T wave, which has a steeper terminal portion.

It frequently is difficult to differentiate the U wave from the second peak of a notched T wave. Lepeschkin has prepared a nomogram that shows the predicted intervals between the onset of the Q wave to the apex of the T wave (aT) and U wave (aU) at different heart rates.[27] By measuring the intervals from the Q wave to the two peaks and comparing them with the predicted intervals on the nomogram, the distinction between a notched T or TU complex usually can be made. Furthermore, the apices of a notched T wave usually are less than 0.15 second apart, whereas the interval between the apices of the T and U waves are greater than 0.15 second.

NORMAL VARIANTS

$S_1S_2S_3$ Pattern

A terminal negative deflection is present in the QRS complex of all the standard limb leads in a significant number of normal individuals. The S waves are recorded when the terminal QRS vectors are originated from the outflow tract of the right ventricle or the posterobasal septum and are directed superiorly and rightward. In Hiss and colleagues' series of healthy adults, such an $S_1S_2S_3$ pattern was observed in over 20 percent.[19] The incidence of a true $S_1S_2S_3$ pattern, however, with the S wave's having an amplitude equal to or larger than the R wave in each of the three leads, is much lower. More commonly, the S waves in leads II and III are greater than the R waves, but the S_1 is smaller than R_1 (Fig. 1–12). We also include ECGs wherein the amplitudes of the S_1, S_2, and S_3 exceed the upper limits of normal for the various age groups, as defined by Simonson,[42] as having the $S_1S_2S_3$ pattern.* When the R/S ratio equals 1 in all three standard limb leads, the frontal plane mean QRS axis cannot be determined. Such a QRS axis is usually referred to as an *indeterminate* axis. The $S_1S_2S_3$ pattern should be distinguished from abnormal left axis deviation. In the latter case, the S_3 is larger than the S_2, whereas the reverse is true in the $S_1S_2S_3$ pattern.

An $S_1S_2S_3$ pattern also is seen in patients with right ventricular hypertrophy or pulmonary emphysema. In some healthy persons the $S_1S_2S_3$ pattern is associated with an rSr′ complex in lead V_1. This combination of findings closely mimics that seen in patients with right ventricular hypertrophy.

RSR′ Pattern in Lead V_1

An RSR′ (or rSr′) pattern in lead V_1 with a QRS duration of less than 0.12 second is found in 2.4 percent of healthy individuals[18] (Fig. 1–13). A higher incidence of this pattern is seen in leads V_{3R} and V_{4R}.[7] The secondary R wave

---

*Upper limits of the normal amplitude of the S waves in leads I, II, and III (modified from Simonson):
Age 20–29: S_1, 4 mm; S_2, 5 mm; S_3, 6 mm.
Age 30–39: S_1, 4 mm; S_2, 4 mm; S_3, 8 mm.
Age 40–49: S_1, 3 mm; S_2, 4 mm; S_3, 8 mm.

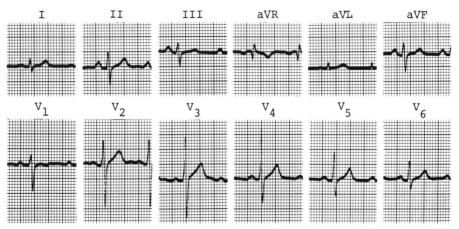

FIGURE 1–12. $S_1S_2S_3$ pattern in a healthy 20-year-old man. The amplitude of the S wave in lead II is greater than that in lead III.

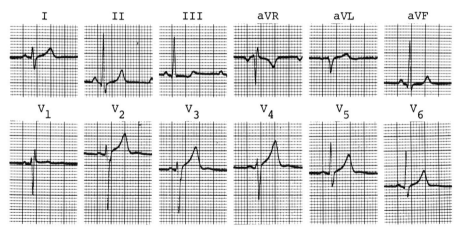

FIGURE 1–13. RSR' pattern in lead V_1 as a normal variant in a healthy 23-year-old man.

has been attributed to physiological late activation of the crista supraventricularis of the right ventricular outflow tract.

The RSR' pattern in lead V_1 also is seen in patients with organic heart disease, including those with right ventricular hypertrophy and other pathologic states. In healthy persons, the R' is usually smaller than the R wave. Its amplitude seldom exceeds 5 mm and is smaller than the S wave in the same lead. The primary R wave also has a normal amplitude that does not exceed 7 mm. When the right precordial leads are recorded at a lower intercostal space, the R' is likely to be absent.[46] A more detailed discussion of the differential diagnosis of the RSR' pattern in lead V_1 is given in Chapter 7.

Early Repolarization Syndrome (Normal Variant ST-Segment Elevation)

Some degree of ST-segment elevation, especially in the precordial leads, is present in most healthy individuals. In most people, the degree of elevation is minimal. Occasionally, however, the elevation may be more pronounced in some of the leads and may mimic the changes of myocardial injury or pericarditis (Figs. 1–14 and 1–15). This phenomenon has been attributed to early ventricular repolarization.[15,35] Wasserburger and colleagues described the following characteristic electrocardiographic findings in the early repolarization syndrome:[48] (1) an elevated takeoff of the ST segment at the J junction of the QRS complex, varying from 1 to 4 mm relative to the isoelectric line; (2) a distinct notch or slur on the downstroke of the R wave; (3) an upward concavity of the ST segment; and (4) symmetrically limbed T waves that are often of large amplitude. These findings have a distinct predilection for the precordial leads V_2 through V_5. A rightward displacement of the transitional zone of the QRS complexes (counterclockwise rotation) often is an associated finding. Although an early repolarization pattern was reported to be more common in young black adults, such a racial variation is not universally accepted. The ST-segment elevation may persist for decades, but the degree of elevation may vary from one recording to another.[21] In some individuals, the ST segment may be isoelectric in one or more of the follow-up tracings.[21] There is a tendency for the displacement to decrease with advancing age, however.

Poor R-Wave Progression in the Right Precordial Leads

In young adults, usually those under 30 years of age, small R waves may be present in leads V_1, V_2, and sometimes V_3 in the absence of cardiac or pulmonary disease. Little attention has been given to this finding in the recent literature.[1] In my experience, it is seen mostly in young women (Fig. 1–16).

THE ATHLETE HEART

The ECG of trained athletes often presents findings that are considered abnormal by the usual standards. The physiological adaptations of the heart to the prolonged and intensive training may result in functional and structural changes that mimic those seen in patients with organic heart disease.

One of the best known and most frequent physiological changes in athletes is the slowing of the heart rate. Sinus bradycardia with a

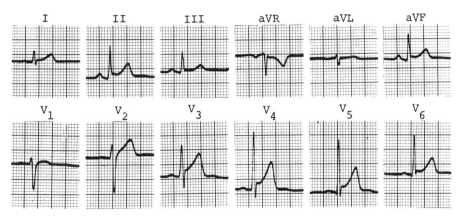

6043   26M

FIGURE 1-14. Diffuse ST-segment elevation especially in leads V_3 through V_5 as a normal variant in a healthy 26-year-old man.

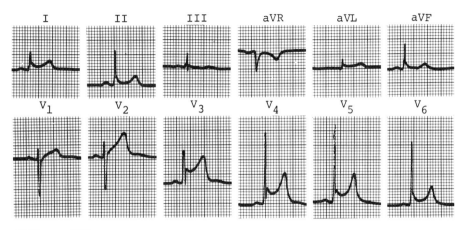

3231   18M

FIGURE 1-15. Marked ST-segment elevation in leads V_3 through V_5 as a normal variant in an 18-year-old man. Note the notching and slurring of the terminal part of the QRS complex.

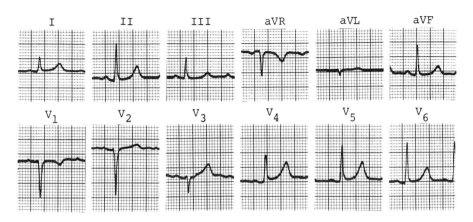

4492   27F

FIGURE 1-16. Poor progression of the R wave from leads V_1 through V_3 in a healthy 27-year-old woman.

heart rate between 30 and 40 beats/min at rest is not uncommon, especially in highly trained endurance athletes.[45,47] Sinus pauses of greater than 2 seconds are observed in the ambulatory ECG in more than one third of the athletes.[45,47] Prolongation of the PR interval that results in first-degree AV block is seen in a similar percentage of these athletes.[45] Second-degree AV block with Wenckebach phenomenon may occur.[33,45,47,50] Junctional escape beats or junctional escape rhythm may be present as a secondary phenomenon. The bradyarrhythmias and AV conduction delay are due mostly to an increase in vagal tone. They generally improve or disappear on cessation of training.[20,33]

Echocardiographic studies in athletes have demonstrated that there is often an increase in the left and right ventricular mass and cavity dimensions, increased left ventricular wall thickness, and left atrial enlargement.[31,41] Ventricular dilatation is seen mostly when the training is primarily isotonic rather than isometric. In the ECG, increased P wave amplitude and notching are noted occasionally. The QRS voltage is increased to suggest left or right ventricular hypertrophy. The reported incidence of left or right ventricular hypertrophy varies considerably depending on the criteria used for their diagnosis.[20,41] The increase in the QRS voltage may occur after only a few months of training, and the voltage decreases after deconditioning, although more slowly.[20]

ST-segment elevation, as part of the early repolarization syndrome described in the previous section, is seen more commonly in athletes. The T waves are often tall, especially in the precordial leads. These ST-segment and T-wave changes may decrease or "normalize" after cessation of training.[20] Inverted or biphasic T waves in the precordial or limb leads are well-known changes in athletes and simulate T-wave changes due to myocardial ischemia. Coronary arteriograms and thallium stress tests have been performed on some of these subjects and were normal.[37,38] These T-wave changes often are labile and may be normalized by physiologic and pharmacologic maneuvers.[51] Asymmetry of ventricular repolarization sequence has been suggested as a cause of these T-wave changes.[51]

In summary, the apparent abnormalities in the ECGs of well-trained athletes described here should be recognized as normal variants in these subjects. These findings are discussed further in the appropriate chapters in this text. Athletes can, however, have organic heart disease with similar ECG changes. Hypertrophic cardiomyopathy is one of the outstanding examples. Sudden death in competitive athletes is a subject of great concern.[32]

REFERENCES

1. Barker, JM: The Unipolar Electrocardiogram: A Clinical Interpretation. New York, Appleton-Century-Crofts, 1952, p 227
2. Bazett HC: An analysis of the time-relations of electrocardiograms. Heart 7:353, 1920
3. Bexton RS, Vallin HO, Camm AJ: Diurnal variation of the QR interval: Influence of the autonomic nervous system. Br Heart J 55:253, 1986
4. Boineau JP, Canavan TE, Schuessler RB, et al: Demonstration of a widely distributed atrial pacemaker complex in the human heart. Circulation 77:1221, 1988
5. Burger HC, van Milaan JB: Heart vector and leads. Br Heart J 10:229, 1948
6. Caceres CA, Kelser GA: Duration of the normal P wave. Am J Cardiol 3:449, 1959
7. Camerini F, Davies LG: Secondary R waves in right chest leads. Br Heart J 17:28, 1955
8. Castellanos A Jr, Castillo C, Agha A: Contribution of His bundle recording to the understanding of clinical arrhythmias. Am J Cardiol 28:499, 1971
9. Charles MA, Benziner TA, Glasser SP: Atrial injury current in pericarditis. Arch Intern Med 131:657, 1973
10. Cowan JC, Yosoff K. Moore M, et al: Importance of lead selection in QT interval measurement. Am J Cardiol 61:83, 1988
11. Dhingra RC, Rosen KM, Rahimtoola SH: Normal conduction intervals and responses in 61 patients using His bundle recording and atrial pacing. Chest 64:55, 1973
12. Durrer D, Van Dam RT, Freud GE, et al: Total excitation of the isolated human heart. Circulation 41:899, 1970
13. Feldman T, Childers RW, Borow KM, et al: Change in ventricular cavity size: Differential effects on QRS and T wave amplitude. Circulation 72:495, 1985
14. Franz MR, Bargheer K, Rafflebeul W, et al: Monophasic action potential mapping in human subjects with normal electrocardiograms: Direct evidence for the genesis of the T wave. Circulation 75:381, 1987
15. Goldman MJ: RS-T segment elevation in mid and left precordial leads as normal variant. Am Heart J 46:817, 1953
16. Gomes JA, Winter SL: The origins of the sinus node pacemaker complex in man: Demonstration of dominant and subsidiary foci. J Am Coll Cardiol 9:45, 1987
17. Green LS, Lux RL, Haws CW, et al: Effects of age, sex, and body habitus on QRS and ST-T potential maps of 1100 normal subjects. Circulation 71:244, 1985
18. Hiss RG, Lamb LE: Electrocardiographic findings in 122,043 individuals. Circulation 25:947, 1962
19. Hiss RG, Lamb LE, Allen MF: Electrocardiographic findings in 67,375 asymptomatic patients. Am J Cardiol 6:200, 1960
20. Huston TP, Puffer JC, Rodney WM: The athletic heart syndrome. N Engl J Med 313:24, 1985
21. Kambara H, Phillips J: Long-term evaluation of early repolarization syndrome (normal variant RS-T segment elevation). Am J Cardiol 38:157, 1976
22. Kilty SE, Lepeschkin E: Effect of body build on the QRS voltage of the electrocardiogram in normal men:

Its significance in the diagnosis of left ventricular hypertrophy. Circulation 31:77, 1965

23. Kossman CE: The normal electrocardiogram. Circulation 8:920, 1953
24. Lamb LE: Electrocardiography and Vectorcardiography. Philadelphia, WB Saunders, 1965
25. Langner PH: An octaxial reference system derived from a nonequilateral triangle for frontal plane vectorcardiography. Am Heart J 49:696, 1955
26. Leatham A: The chest lead electrocardiogram in health. Br Heart J 12:213, 1950
27. Lepeschkin E: The U wave of the electrocardiogram. Mod Concepts Cardiovasc Dis 38:39, 1969
28. Lepeschkin E: Duration of electrocardiographic deflections and intervals: Man. *In* Altman PE, Dittmer DS (eds): Respiration and Circulation. Chapter VI. Bethesda, Federation of American Societies for Experimental Biology, 1971, p 277
29. Lepeschkin E: Physiological basis of U wave. *In* Schlant RC, Hurst JW (eds): Advances in Electrocardiography. Volume 2, Chapter VII. New York, Grune & Stratton, 1976, p 353
30. Manning GW, Smiley JR: QRS-voltage criteria for left ventricular hypertrophy in a normal male population. Circulation 19:224, 1964
31. Maron BJ: Structural features of the athlete heart as defined by echocardiography. J Am Coll Cardiol 7:190, 1986
32. Maron BJ, Epstein SE, Roberts WC: Causes of sudden death in competitive athletes. J Am Coll Cardiol 7:204, 1986
33. Meytes I, Kaplinsky E, Yahini JH, et al: Wenckebach A-V block: A frequent feature following heavy physical training. Am Heart J 90:42, 1975
34. Morris JJ Jr, Estes EH Jr, Whalen RE, et al: P-wave analysis in valvular heart disease. Circulation 29:242, 1964
35. Myers GB, Klein HA, Stofer BE, et al: Normal variation in multiple precordial leads. Am Heart J 34:785, 1947
36. Narula OS, Scherlag RJ, Samet P, Javier RP: Atrioventricular block: Localization and classification by His bundle recordings. Am J Med 50:146, 1971
37. Nishimura T, Kambara H, Chen CH, et al: Noninvasive assessment of T-wave abnormalities in precordial electrocardiograms in middle-aged professional bicyclists. J Electrocardiol 14:357, 1981
38. Oakley DG, Oakley CM: Significance of abnormal electrocardiogram in highly trained athletes. Am J Cardiol 50:985, 1982
39. Okomoto N, Kaneko K. Simonson E, et al: Reliability of individual frontal plane axis determination. Circulation 44:213, 1971
40. Pipberger HV, Goldman MJ, Littman D, et al: Correlations of the orthogonal electrocardiogram and vectorcardiogram with constitutional variables in 518 normal men. Circulation 35:536, 1967
41. Roeske WR, O'Rourke RA, Klein A, et al: Noninvasive evaluation of ventricular hypertrophy in professional athletes. Circulation 53:286, 1976
42. Simonson E: Differentiation Between Normal and Abnormal in Electrocardiography. St Louis, CV Mosby, 1961
43. Simonson E: The effect of age on the electrocardiogram. Am J Cardiol 29:64, 1972
44. Simonson E, Cady LD, Woodbury M: The normal Q-T interval. Am Heart J 63:747, 1962
45. Talan DA, Bauernfeind RA, Ashley WW, et al: Twenty-four hour continuous ECG recordings in long-distance runners. Chest 82:19, 1982
46. Tapia FA, Proudfit WL: Secondary R waves in right precordial leads in normal persons and in patients with cardiac disease. Circulation 21:28, 1960
47. Viitasalo MT, Kala R, Eisalo A: Ambulatory electrocardiographic recording in endurance athletes. Br Heart J 47:213, 1982
48. Wasserburger RH, Alt WJ, Lloyd CJ: The normal RS-T segment elevation variant. Am J Cardiol 8:184, 1961
49. Watanabe Y: Purkinje repolarization as a possible cause of the U wave in the electrocardiogram. Circulation 51:1030, 1975
50. Zeppilli P, Fenici R, Sassara M, et al: Wenckebach second-degree A-V block in top-ranking athletes: An old problem revisited. Am Heart J 100:281, 1980
51. Zeppilli P, Pirrami MM, Sassara M, Fenici R: T wave abnormalities in top-ranking athletes: Effects of isoproterenol, atropine and physical exercise. Am Heart J 100:213, 1980
52. Zimmerman HA: The Auricular Electrocardiogram. Springfield, Ill, Charles C Thomas, 1968, p 19

Atrial Abnormalities

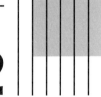

2

Many terms are used in the interpretation of P-wave abnormalities. The term *atrial enlargement* generally is used to imply the presence of atrial hypertrophy or dilatation or both. Some authors prefer the hemodynamic expressions of either *pressure* or *volume overloading.* As discussed later in this chapter, P-wave changes may not always be accompanied by any of these anatomic or hemodynamic states. Conduction defects and other factors may be present. It has therefore been suggested that a less specific term, such as *atrial abnormality* or *atrial involvement,* be used in the electrocardiographic (ECG) diagnosis of P-wave abnormalities.

Abnormal P waves may also be seen in patients with rhythm disturbances. This, however, is discussed in Part II of this book.

LEFT ATRIAL ENLARGEMENT

The left atrium normally is activated by impulses transmitted from the sinoatrial node through the right atrium. Its electrical potential is responsible for the inscription of the middle and late portions of the P wave. Because of the direction of spread of the depolarization process and the anatomic orientation of the left atrium, the left atrial forces are directed leftward and posteriorly. An increase in the left atrial forces may therefore exaggerate these normal characteristics of the late portion of the P wave. The duration of the atrial excitation may be prolonged, especially if left atrial conduction defect is also present. The various criteria for the diagnosis of left atrial enlargement are based essentially on these changes.

Diagnostic Criteria

1. The P terminal force in lead V_1 is equal to or more negative than -0.04 mm-sec. This measurement is the product of the depth of the terminal negative deflection (in millimeters) and its duration (in seconds)[23] (Figs. 2–1 and 2–2).

2. The P wave is notched with a duration of 0.12 second or more (the P mitrale)[35] (see Fig. 2–2).

3. A leftward shift of the P-wave axis in the frontal plane to $+15°$ or beyond or a leftward shift of the terminal P forces in the frontal plane (see Fig. 2–2).

Clinical and Anatomic Correlation

CRITERION 1: THE P TERMINAL
FORCE IN LEAD V_1

Morris and associates studied 100 normal subjects and 87 patients with aortic and mitral diseases.[23] They found that the product of the amplitude and duration of the negative component of the P wave in lead V_1, which they called the *P terminal force* at V_1, is more negative than -0.03 mm-sec in 2.5 percent of the normal population and in 92 percent of the patients with left-sided valvular disease. In actual practice, the P terminal force may be determined by simple visual inspection alone. A terminal portion of the P wave in lead V_1 that occupies one small box on the recording paper in depth $(-1.0$ mm) and duration (0.04 second) yields a P terminal force of -0.04. Any terminal negative component of the P wave in lead V_1 of this magnitude or greater is abnormal and suggests an increase in the posterior left atrial potential. In an evaluation of 62 patients with significant isolated mitral stenosis and left atrial enlargement proved at surgery,[32] the ECG met the Morris criterion in 68 percent of the cases. Similar results have been obtained from other studies.[8,18] It also has been shown that the P terminal force correlates more closely with left atrial volume than with left atrial pressure. This may be the reason that, in an anatomic correlation study,[28] only about half of the pa-

I II III V$_1$ V$_3$ V$_5$

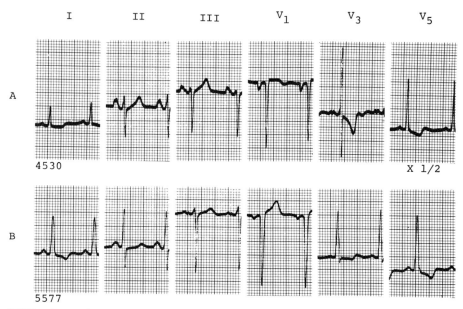

A

4530

X 1/2

B

5577

FIGURE 2–1. Left atrial enlargement in patients with aortic valve disease. (A) The patient is a 58-year-old man with aortic insufficiency and left ventricular failure. Abnormal P-terminal force is present in lead V$_1$. The P wave in lead II has an amplitude of 2.5 mm. The QRS and ST-T changes are suggestive of left ventricular hypertrophy. (B) The patient is a 45-year-old man with calcific aortic stenosis. A pressure gradient of 85 mm Hg across the aortic valve was demonstrated during cardiac catheterization. A prominent negative P wave in lead V$_1$ suggests left atrial enlargement. The QRS and ST-T changes are consistent with left ventricular hypertrophy.

tients with increased left atrial weight had an abnormal P terminal force in lead V$_1$.

A transient increase in the size of the negative component of the P wave in the right precordial leads is often seen in patients with left ventricular failure.[37] Romhilt and associates reported that signs of left atrial abnormality that satisfy the Morris criterion were present in 76 percent of the patients during an acute episode of pulmonary edema.[29] Half of the patients no longer exhibited these P-wave changes after 4 days (Fig. 2–3). An increase in the left atrial pressure and volume rather than in the atrial mass is apparently responsible for the P-wave changes.

In an evaluation of the specificity of the Morris criterion,[23] Kasser and Kennedy[18] observed a false-positive diagnosis of 6 percent in its prediction of increased left atrial volume and 24 percent in its prediction of increased left atrial pressure. In my experience, a false-positive diagnosis occurs most commonly in patients with chronic obstructive lung disease with or without cor pulmonale. In these patients, a prominent negative P wave may be seen in the right precordial leads without any evidence of left-sided heart disease (Fig. 2–4). Two factors probably are responsible for the negativity of the P wave in these

leads. The mean P vector in these patients is more vertical in its spatial orientation. Because of the lowering of the diaphragm, the usual electrode positions of leads V$_1$ and V$_2$ become abnormally high in relation to the anatomic position of the atria. Therefore, the mean P vector often projects on the negative side of the lead axes of V$_1$ and V$_2$, resulting in a negative P wave. A similar change occurs in patients with pectus excavatum.[7] I have also observed this finding in patients with the straight-back syndrome (Fig. 2–5). An erroneous diagnosis of organic heart disease may be made, especially because the chest radiograph often reveals a "pancake heart." Occasionally, a prominent negative component of the P wave may also be seen in a patient with a giant right atrium due to congenital heart disease. The markedly enlarged right atrium may present itself in both the anterior and posterior views of the heart and more or less envelop the left atrium. The posterior atrial forces are now generated from the right rather than the left atrium (Fig. 2–6).

Other criteria that use the prominent terminal posterior forces have been suggested. These include a P wave whose terminal negative deflection in lead V$_1$ is greater than 1 mm in depth or lasts more than 0.06 second.[2] The

I   II   III V_1 V_3 V_5

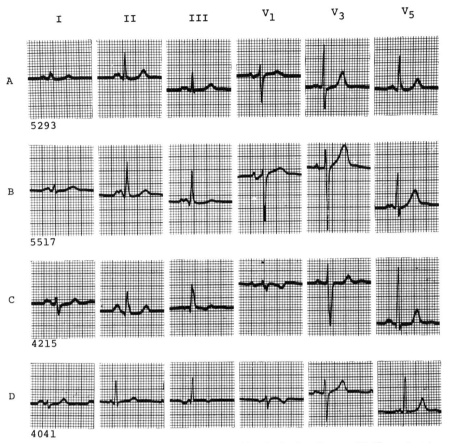

FIGURE 2–2. Left atrial enlargement in patients with mitral valve disease. (A) The patient is a 59-year-old woman with rheumatic heart disease and mitral stenosis. A mean diastolic pressure gradient of 7 mm Hg was demonstrated across the mitral valve at rest and 25 mm after exercise. The P wave is abnormally notched with a peak-to-peak interval of more than 0.04 second. (B) The patient is a 42-year-old man with rheumatic heart disease and mitral stenosis. Left atrial enlargement was confirmed by cardiac fluoroscopy and echocardiography. The P wave shows a P mitrale pattern. The P wave is abnormally wide and notched and is seen best in leads II, III, and V_5. Abnormal P terminal force is present in lead V_1. (C) The patient is a 31-year-old woman with rheumatic heart disease, mitral insufficiency, and P mitrale pattern. (D) The patient is a 31-year-old woman with rheumatic heart disease, mitral insufficiency, and mitral stenosis. Cardiac fluoroscopy demonstrated definite left atrial enlargement. The tracing demonstrates the P mitrale pattern as well as a leftward shift of the P-wave axis.

II V_1

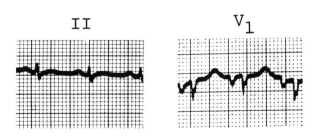

FIGURE 2–3. Left atrial enlargement during acute pulmonary edema. The tracing was recorded from a 27-year-old man with primary cardiomyopathy. The upper panels show the abnormal P terminal force in lead V_1 during the acute episode, which disappeared 4 days later as demonstrated in the lower panels. (Reproduced from Romhilt DW, Scott RC: Left atrial involvement in acute pulmonary edema. Am Heart J 83:328, 1972, by permission of C. V. Mosby Co.)

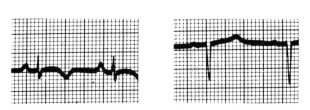

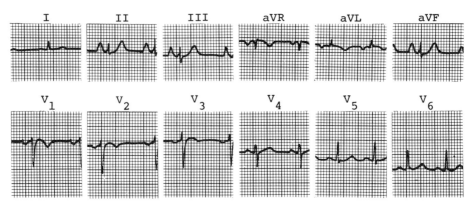

FIGURE 2–4. Abnormal P terminal force in the right precordial leads in pulmonary emphysema with chronic cor pulmonale. The patient is a 61-year-old man with chronic cor pulmonale. There is no clinical evidence of left-sided heart disease. The P wave shows a P pulmonale pattern with a vertical axis of nearly +90° in the frontal plane. The negative component of the P wave in leads V_1 through V_3 is abnormally large.

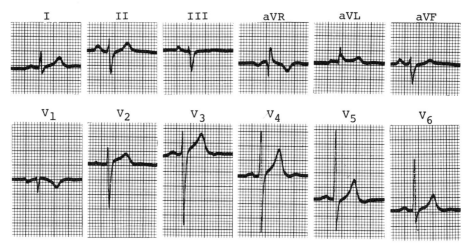

FIGURE 2–5. Abnormal P terminal force in lead V_1 that resembles left atrial enlargement in a 36-year-old man with the straight-back syndrome and "pancake heart."

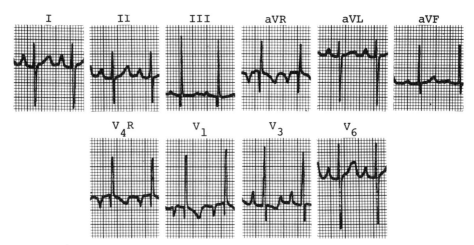

FIGURE 2–6. Right atrial enlargement with abnormal P terminal force in lead V_1 in congenital heart disease. The patient is a 49-month-old girl with total anomalous pulmonary venous return to a persistent left superior vena cava. Large right and small left atria were demonstrated by angiography. The prominent negative P wave in lead V_1 is replaced by a tall and peaked P wave in lead V_3. The limb leads show tall and peaked P waves with normal duration but the P-wave axis is +5°. The P-wave changes in the limb leads are consistent with the so-called P congenitale. The QRS and T-wave changes suggest right ventricular hypertrophy. (Courtesy of Dr. David Schwartz.)

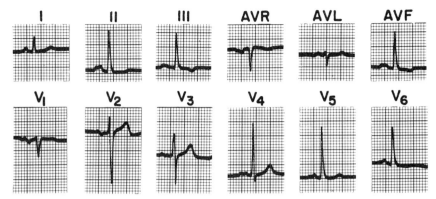

FIGURE 2–7. Abnormal notching and increased width of the P wave resembling P mitrale in a 58-year-old man with calcific constrictive pericarditis. The abnormal P wave is seen best in lead II.

reliability of these criteria has not been found to be superior to the criterion suggested by Morris.[22]

CRITERION 2: WIDE AND NOTCHED P WAVES

A prolongation of the P-wave duration to 0.12 second or more was found in about two thirds of patients with documented left atrial enlargement.[18,32] A significant positive relationship seems to exist between the duration of the P wave and the degree of left atrial dilatation.[8,27] The correlation between the P-wave duration and the left atrial volume is better than that with the left atrial pressure.[18] In autopsy studies, the P-wave duration also correlates better with the left atrial volume than with the weight.[12,22] Although the available data suggest that this criterion is specific, with false-positive diagnoses of only 6 percent,[18] this incidence probably is falsely low, because the criterion was tested in a group of normal subjects only.

Minor notching or slurring of the P wave is found in one or more leads in most normal ECGs. This is particularly true in the precordial leads. The bifid P wave has generally been attributed to the asynchronic activation of the right and left atria.[27] Definite notching with a peak-to-peak interval of greater than 0.04 second, however, is not usually found in normal subjects.[38] Thomas and DeJong observed a prolongation of the peak interval in most patients with mitral stenosis, especially when severe symptoms or marked cardiomegaly was present. Other investigators found abnormal notching in slightly less than half of patients with left-sided heart disease.[23] Abnormal bifid P waves, however, are also encountered in a

significant number of patients with constrictive pericarditis[6,38] (Fig. 2–7). In these patients, the P-wave duration may also be prolonged to mimic closely the P waves of patients with mitral disease. P-wave prolongation and notching are probably due to atrial involvement by the compression scar. Abnormal notching of the P wave may also occur when there is intraatrial conduction defect due to myocarditis, atrial ischemia, infarction, or fibrosis, which may also cause prolongation of the P wave.[1]

The term *P mitrale* has been used to describe a P wave that is abnormally notched and wide. This type of P wave is commonly seen, as the name implies, in patients with mitral valve disease, particularly mitral stenosis. The changes are most often present in leads I and II and the left precordial leads. The P mitrale pattern was observed in one third of the patients with isolated mitral stenosis proved at surgery.[32] As indicated previously, these changes are not always due to dilatation or hypertrophy of the left atrium. In fact, intraatrial conduction defect secondary to atrial myocardial damage may actually be responsible for the prolongation and notching of the P wave in patients with rheumatic mitral disease.[42]

CRITERION 3: LEFTWARD SHIFT OF THE P-WAVE AXIS

A leftward shift of the frontal plane P-wave axis to less than +30° or +15°[23,32] is observed in only 10 percent of patients with left atrial enlargement caused by left-sided valvular disease. This criterion gives a false-positive diagnosis in about 5 percent of the normal subjects. Conduction abnormalities in the atria or an ectopic atrial pacemaker may be responsible for some cases of abnormal leftward shift of the P vector. A leftward shift of the terminal P forces has also been used as a means of recognizing left atrial enlargement.[11] This is usually manifested by a late positive P deflection in lead aVL and a negative deflection limited to the terminal portion of the P wave in leads III and aVF. The sensitivity and specificity of this measurement have not been fully evaluated.

Tall P waves in the limb leads with an amplitude greater than 2.5 mm occasionally are seen in patients with left atrial enlargement due to left-sided valvular heart disease, espe-cially the mitral valve. About 5 to 10 percent of these patients display such abnormalities. They are more common in patients with hypertensive heart disease. When the duration of the P waves is not prolonged and the tall P waves are seen in the inferior leads II, III, and aVF, the changes closely mimic those of *P pulmonale*[4] (Fig. 2–8). An examination of the terminal forces in lead V_1 and the usually associated QRS and T changes of left ventricular hypertrophy may often, but not always, help in the differential diagnosis.

The *Macruz index* was used some years ago as one of the diagnostic criteria for left atrial enlargement.[21] It is determined by the ratio of

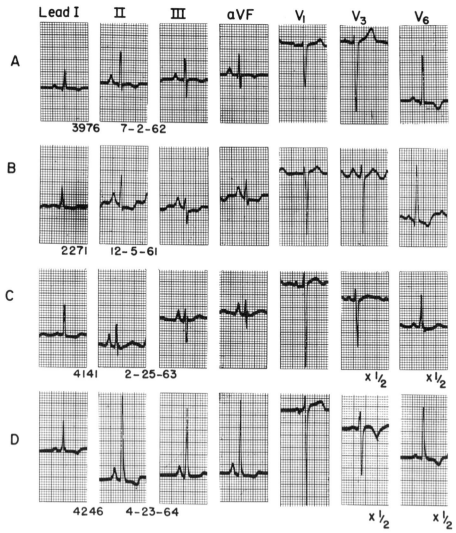

FIGURE 2–8. Tall P waves in the limb leads in patients with hypertensive heart disease mimicking the P pulmonale pattern. A and B were recorded from patients with hypertensive heart disease without heart failure. C and D were recorded from patients with hypertensive heart disease and early or questionable left ventricular failure. (Reproduced from Chou T-C, Helm RA: The pseudo P pulmonale. Circulation 32:96, 1965, by permission of the American Heart Association.)

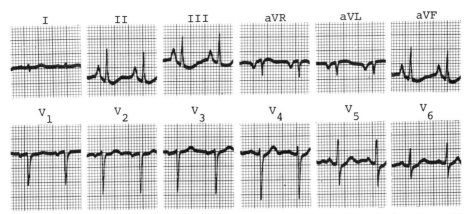

FIGURE 2–9. P pulmonale pattern in a 44-year-old woman with chronic obstructive lung disease. The frontal plane P axis is displaced toward the right (+85°). The ST-segment depression in leads II, III, and aVF is probably due to prominent atrial T waves. Negative P waves are visible in the right precordial leads.

the duration of the P wave to that of the PR segment. If the ratio is greater than 1.6, left atrial enlargement is believed to be present. Although this finding was seen in 52 to 72 percent of patients with proven mitral and aortic valve disease,[8,17,18,23,32] it was also observed in 24 to 56 percent of normal subjects.[18,32] The fact that the index is also affected by the atrioventricular conduction time is probably responsible for its low specificity. It is seldom used today.

RIGHT ATRIAL ENLARGEMENT

Because the right atrium is depolarized first, its potential is responsible for the inscription of the first portion of the P wave. The ana-

tomic location and the direction of the excitation of the right atrium are such that its forces are oriented inferiorly and anteriorly. They are slightly leftward but are more medial or vertical than the left atrial forces. An increase in the right atrial potential is therefore usually associated with a tall P wave in the inferior and anterior leads. Because the right atrial forces are responsible only for the early part of the P wave, any increase in the duration of right atrial activation usually will not prolong the total duration of the P wave.

Diagnostic Criteria

1. The P wave is tall and peaked, with a height of 2.5 mm or more in leads II, III, and

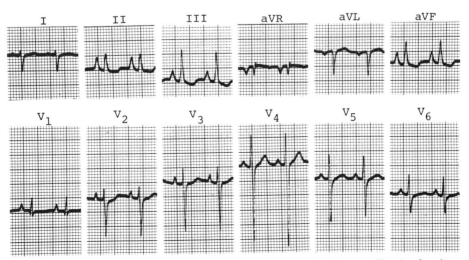

FIGURE 2–10. Right atrial enlargement in a 33-year-old man with pulmonary fibrosis, chronic cor pulmonale, and right ventricular failure. P pulmonale pattern is present in the limb leads with abnormally tall and peaked P waves also in leads V_1 through V_3.

aVF and has a normal duration—the P pulmonale (Figs. 2–9 and 2–10).

2. The P-wave axis in the frontal plane is +75° or greater (see Figs. 2–9 and 2–10).

3. The positive deflection of the P wave in lead V_1 or V_2 is greater than 1.5 mm (see Fig. 2–10).

Clinical and Anatomic Correlation

The ECG changes that are generally considered to be suggestive of right atrial hypertrophy or dilatation often correlate poorly with the clinical and anatomic findings. There is also a significant difference between the P-wave abnormalities seen in patients with right atrial enlargement secondary to chronic obstructive lung disease and those that result from congenital heart disease.

CRITERION 1: P PULMONALE

In patients with clinical evidence of chronic cor pulmonale, the pattern of P pulmonale is present in about 20 percent of the cases.[9,19] A similar incidence exists in the autopsy series.[10,26] The frequency of this finding is surprisingly low considering that patients with pulmonary emphysema without cor pulmonale may also have tall and peaked P waves in the inferior leads. Hemodynamic studies have failed to demonstrate any relationship between the height of the P wave and right atrial pressure in these patients.[43] Furthermore, the P pulmonade pattern is often unstable when multiple records are available.[10] The amplitude of the P wave may, in fact, even decrease as evidence of right ventricular hypertrophy progresses.[25]

In patients with congenital heart disease, such as pulmonic stenosis, tetralogy of Fallot, Eisenmenger physiology, and tricuspid atresia, as well as in patients with pulmonary hypertension not caused by chronic obstructive lung disease, the P pulmonale pattern is seen more frequently. It has been demonstrated that patients with both an increase in the right atrial pressure and arterial desaturation have the tallest P waves.[8] On the other hand, volume overload of the right atrium without an increase in pressure is often associated with a near-normal height of the P wave in the inferior leads, as in the case of atrial septal defect without pulmonary hypertension.[31]

As mentioned previously, chronic obstructive lung disease without cor pulmonale may also present a P pulmonale pattern. Although it is often difficult to exclude early chronic cor pulmonale in patients who have severe pulmonary emphysema, the P pulmonale pattern has been reported in up to 37 percent of patients with a mild degree of pulmonary function abnormality.[3] A lower incidence of the pattern, however, was reported by other observers.[36] Hyperinflation of the lungs with lowering of the diaphragm, which causes the heart to assume a more vertical position, as well as clockwise rotation of the heart along its long axis, probably is responsible for the increased amplitude of the P wave in the inferior leads in these patients.

Transient appearance of the P pulmonale pattern has been observed in patients with acute pulmonary embolism.[5] It is also seen in patients with bronchial asthma but mostly during the acute attack.[15] Arterial desaturation alone tends to increase the amplitude of the P wave and gives it a peaking appearance.[44]

A tall and peaked P wave may be seen in healthy subjects with asthenic body build and is probably related to the vertical position of the heart. The P-wave amplitude often increases with the standing position.[33] It may occur during expiratory effort against pressure.[13] It also occurs during tachycardia and exercise. Increased cardiac output and sympathetic stimulation may be responsible for the changes under these circumstances.[44]

The nonspecific nature of the P pulmonale pattern is further exemplified by a study I conducted.[4] In 100 consecutive patients whose ECGs showed the P pulmonale pattern, only 49 had diseases that could cause right atrial enlargement. Forty-six patients failed to reveal any clinical condition that would expose them to right atrial abnormalities. In 36 patients, the P pulmonale pattern probably represented left, rather than right, atrial enlargement. Figure 2–8 illustrates the *pseudo P pulmonale* pattern in patients with hypertensive heart disease with or without questionable left ventricular failure. Figure 2–11 depicts the proposed mechanism for the appearance of the P pulmonale pattern in patients with left atrial enlargement.

The P pulmonale pattern has also been described in patients with coronary artery disease and angina pectoris.[14] Hypoxemia of the atrial musculature and ischemic lesion of the left atrium are thought to cause the increase of voltage of the P wave as well as the rightward shift of the P-wave axis.[13]

The available anatomic studies also have failed to demonstrate any relationship between the P-wave amplitude and the right atrial weight.[12,22]

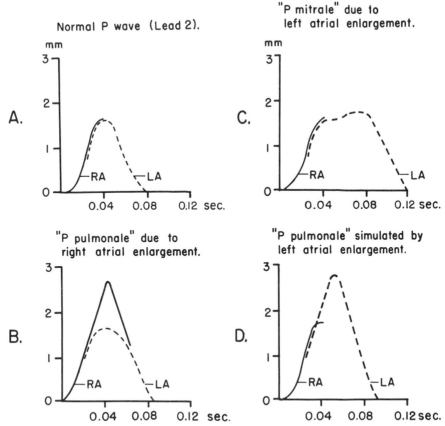

FIGURE 2–11. Proposed mechanism for the appearance of a P pulmonale pattern in patients with left atrial enlargement. (A) The right and left atrial components of a normal P wave. (B) P pulmonale pattern resulting from right atrial enlargement with an increase in the amplitude of the right atrial component of the P wave. (C) The P mitrale pattern associated with left atrial enlargement due to an increase in the left atrial component both in amplitude and duration. Some associated intra-atrial conduction defect may be responsible for the prolongation of the P-wave duration. (D) The pseudo P pulmonale pattern in left atrial enlargement. The amplitude of the left atrial component is increased without marked prolongation of the duration of left atrial depolarization. (Reproduced from Chou T-C, Helm RA: The pseudo P pulmonale. Circulation 32:96, 1965, by permission of the American Heart Association.)

A prominent atrial T (Ta) wave often accompanies a tall P wave.[41] The amplitude of the negative deflection in the inferior leads may exceed 1 mm. Because the duration of the atrial T wave may be as long as 0.45 second, the negative deflection in these leads may cause an apparent depression of the ST segment (see Fig. 2–9). It is important, therefore, to take this factor into consideration in the evaluation of ST-segment changes when a prominent P wave is present.

CRITERION 2: RIGHTWARD DEVIATION OF THE P-WAVE AXIS

A rightward or medial displacement of the P-wave axis in the frontal plane is found in a significant number of patients with right atrial

enlargement. The reported incidence is variable, since different values (+60° to +80°) have been used for the definition of rightward displacement. The upper limit of +75° is chosen here and is based on the large series of normal subjects studied by Hiss and associates.[16] The axis deviation is often, but not necessarily always, associated with a P pulmonale pattern. When the P axis is beyond +75°, the P wave becomes small in lead I and negative in lead aVL. It may become isoelectric in lead I if the axis is +90°. An axis greater than +90° is, however, uncommon. Therefore, a negative P wave in lead I is rarely seen, even in patients with marked right atrial enlargement. It is significant that right atrial enlargement secondary to chronic obstructive lung disease has a much greater incidence of rightward shift of the P-wave axis than that from other causes.[10] In fact, in patients with congenital heart disease, the P wave in lead I may be taller than that in lead III.[44] The term *P congenitale* has been used to describe this type of P wave (see Fig. 2–6).

As in the case of the P pulmonale pattern, the right axis deviation of the P wave is also not specific for right atrial enlargement. It is frequently present in patients with pulmonary emphysema without cor pulmonale and in other conditions described previously.

CRITERION 3: TALL P WAVE IN LEAD V_1 OR V_2

The initial positive deflection of the P wave in the right precordial leads is normally less than 1.5 mm in amplitude.[20] An abnormally tall P wave in leads V_1 and V_2 is seen in slightly more than 10 percent of patients with chronic cor pulmonale. As it was described previously, patients with pulmonary emphysema with or without cor pulmonale often have a large *negative* P wave in lead V_1, mimicking left atrial enlargement. In patients with cor pulmonale, a negative or biphasic P wave in V_1 may be accompanied by a tall and peaked P wave in lead V_2. This sudden transition is often helpful in leading one to suspect that the P-wave changes in V_1 result from right instead of left atrial involvement. Biatrial enlargement should also be considered, however. This phenomenon also occurs occasionally in patients with isolated right atrial enlargement due to congenital heart disease. In the latter condi-

tion, however, monophasic, abnormally tall P waves in leads V_1 and V_2 are encountered more frequently than in patients with chronic cor pulmonale.[8] In my experience, an abnormally tall P wave in the right precordial leads is a more specific finding for right atrial enlargement than the diagnostic criteria based on the limb leads.

A prolongation of the duration of the initial positive component of the P wave in lead V_1 to 0.04 second or more has also been suggested as an indication of right atrial enlargement.[9] This finding has not been used widely, and its reliability is not known.

BIATRIAL ENLARGEMENT

The presence of biatrial enlargement may be suspected when signs of both left and right atrial enlargement coexist. Because the two atria affect essentially different portions of the P wave, the recognition of biatrial enlargement is not as difficult as in the case of biventricular hypertrophy. ECG signs that satisfy both the diagnostic criteria for left and right atrial enlargement may be considered indicative of biatrial enlargement.

Diagnostic Criteria

1. The presence of a large diphasic P wave in lead V_1, with the initial positive component greater than 1.5 mm and the terminal negative component reaching 1 mm in amplitude and 0.04 second in duration ("abnormal P terminal force") (Figs. 2–12 and 2–13).

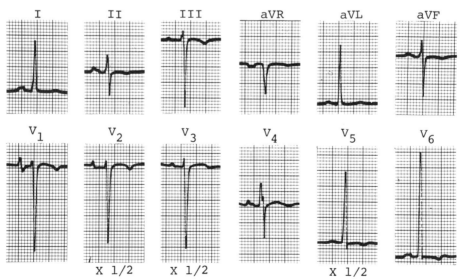

FIGURE 2–12. Biatrial enlargement in a patient with idiopathic cardiomyopathy proved at autopsy. A large biphasic P wave can be seen in lead V_1. The QRS changes suggest left ventricular hypertrophy.

2/14/69

V$_1$ V$_2$

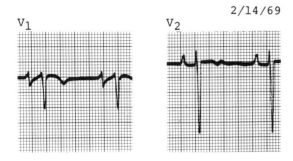

3/8/69

V$_1$

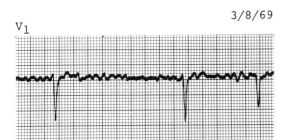

FIGURE 2–13. Coarse fibrillatory waves in a patient with atrial enlargement. The tracing was recorded from a 36-year-old man with advanced rheumatic heart disease and aortic and mitral valve disease proved at surgery. There was diffuse cardiomegaly. During sinus rhythm, the P waves in leads V$_1$ and V$_2$ suggested biatrial enlargement. Coarse fibrillatory waves appeared in lead V$_1$ when atrial fibrillation developed.

2. The presence of a tall, peaked P wave (more than 1.5 mm) in the right precordial lead and a wide, notched P wave in the limb leads or left precordial leads (V$_5$ and V$_6$) (Fig. 2–14).

3. An increase in both the amplitude (2.5 mm or greater) and duration (0.12 second or more) of the P wave in the limb leads.

Although many other combinations of signs of left and right atrial enlargement may occur, these criteria are most frequently encountered. In my experience, criterion 1 has been most useful. Systematic analysis of the reliability of these criteria is still lacking.

DIAGNOSIS OF ATRIAL ENLARGEMENT IN THE PRESENCE OF ATRIAL FIBRILLATION

Diagnostic Criterion

The amplitude of the fibrillatory waves in lead V$_1$ is 1 mm or greater (see Fig. 2–13).

In an analysis of 194 patients with atrial fibrillation, Thurmann and Janney demonstrated a significant relationship between the size of the fibrillatory waves and the origin of the heart disease.[40] Eighty-seven percent of the patients with coarse f waves in lead V$_1$ had rheumatic heart disease, and 88 percent of the patients with fine f waves in lead V$_1$ had arteriosclerotic heart disease. Thurmann and Janney defined coarse f waves as those fibrillatory waves measuring more than 0.5 mm in amplitude and fine f waves as measuring 0.5 mm or less. They also showed that coarse f waves in lead V$_1$ were associated with roentgenologic and anatomic evidence of left atrial enlargement or elevated left atrial pressure when these data were available.

The relationship between the size of the f waves in atrial fibrillation and the cause of the heart disease was also demonstrated in a larger series of patients studied by Skoulas and Horlick.[34] These investigators also noted changes in the pattern of the atrial fibrillation in about

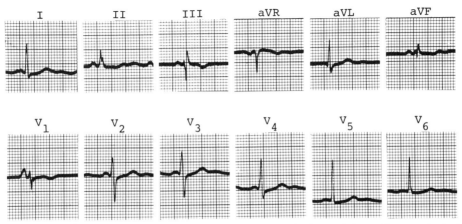

FIGURE 2–14. Biatrial enlargement in a 33-year-old woman with rheumatic heart disease and mitral and tricuspid stenosis proved at surgery. Lead I shows abnormal notching of the P wave, suggesting left atrial enlargement. Lead V$_1$ shows a tall P wave, suggesting right atrial enlargement.

16 percent of the patients. Coarse f waves might become fine f waves and vice versa. This occurred in patients with either arteriosclerotic or rheumatic heart disease. Patients with untreated congestive heart failure often presented coarse fibrillation, and the f waves became smaller with treatment. Atrial distention during failure was probably responsible for the increase in the size of the f waves. This phenomenon occurred more commonly in patients with arteriosclerotic heart disease.

A significant correlation has also been shown between the coarse fibrillatory waves and an abnormal P terminal force in lead V_1 during sinus rhythm as defined by Morris and colleagues.[23,24] (see Fig. 2–13). Fine f waves were usually associated with a normal P terminal force. Peter and associates suggested that the coarse fibrillatory waves should be considered signs of left atrial hypertrophy or "strain."[24] They used an amplitude of 1 mm or more, instead of more than 0.5 mm, as the criterion for a coarse f wave and found no significant difference in the results of the analysis. Because this amplitude is measured more easily, it has also been chosen by me as the value for the separation of fine and coarse fibrillatory waves.

Although the available studies imply the presence of *left* atrial enlargement when the fibrillatory waves are coarse, it is probable that right atrial enlargement may also be associated with coarse f waves. The rarity of atrial fibrillation in pure forms of right-sided heart disease is probably responsible for the infrequent observations. A few cases of coarse atrial fibrillation have been reported in patients with congenital heart disease and right atrial or biatrial enlargement.[39] Transient atrial fibrillation in patients with chronic cor pulmonale is often accompanied by large f waves in lead V_1. (Permanent atrial fibrillation is uncommon in patients with uncomplicated chronic cor pulmonale.)

DIAGNOSIS OF ATRIAL ENLARGEMENT IN THE PRESENCE OF ATRIAL FLUTTER

Limited available data have thus far failed to suggest any definite relationship between the size of the flutter wave in atrial flutter and atrial enlargement.[24] In a study of 312 patients with atrial flutter who were not receiving quinidine or procainamide, however, Rytand and associates demonstrated some correlation between the atrial rate and atrial size.[30] In patients without appreciable atrial enlargement, the mean atrial rate was 290 beats/min. In patients with moderate to massive atrial enlargement, the average atrial rate was 229 beats/min. An example of relatively slow atrial rate

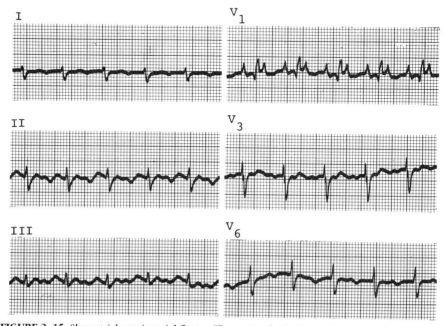

FIGURE 2–15. Slow atrial rate in atrial flutter. The patient had chronic obstructive lung disease with chronic cor pulmonale proved at autopsy. Right atrial enlargement and right ventricular hypertrophy were present. The atrial rate was 220 per minute. The patient was not receiving quinidine. The QRS changes were consistent with right ventricular hypertrophy.

in atrial flutter is given in Figure 2–15. The patient had chronic cor pulmonale with right atrial hypertrophy and dilation and right ventricular hypertrophy proved at autopsy.

REFERENCES

1. Abildskov JA: The atrial complex of the electrocardiogram. Am Heart J 57:930, 1959
2. Arevalo AC, Spagnuolo M, Feinstein AR: A simple electrocardiographic indication of left atrial enlargement: A study of young patients with rheumatic heart disease. JAMA 185:358, 1963
3. Calatayud JB, Abad JM, Khoi NB, et al: P-wave changes in chronic obstructive pulmonary disease. Am Heart J 79:444, 1970
4. Chou TC, Helm RA: The pseudo P pulmonale. Circulation 32:96, 1965
5. Cutforth RH, Oram S: The electrocardiogram in pulmonary embolism. Br Heart J 20:41, 1958
6. Dalton JC, Pearson RJ Jr, White PD: Constrictive pericarditis: A review and long-term follow-up of 78 cases. Ann Intern Med 45:445, 1956
7. DeOliveira JM, Sambhi MP, Zimmerman HA: The electrocardiogram in pectus excavatum. Br Heart J 20:495, 1958
8. DeOliveira JM, Zimmerman HA: Auricular overloadings: Electrocardiographic analysis of 193 cases. Am J Cardiol 3:453, 1959
9. Dines DE, Parkin TW: Some observations on the value of the electrocardiogram in patients with chronic cor pulmonale. Mayo Clin Proc 40:745, 1965
10. Fowler NO, Daniels C, Scott RC, et al: The electrocardiogram in cor pulmonale with and without emphysema. Am J Cardiol 16:500, 1965
11. Gooch AS, Calatayud JB, Gorman PA, et al: Leftward shift of the terminal P forces in the ECG associated with left atrial enlargement. Am Heart J 71:727, 1966
12. Gordon R, Neilson G, Silverstone H: Electrocardiographic P wave and atrial weights and volumes. Br Heart J 27:748, 1965
13. Gross D: Contributions to the functional morphology of the P wave. Am Heart J 61:436, 1961
14. Gross D: Electrocardiographic characteristics of P pulmonale waves of coronary origin. Am Heart J 73:453, 1967
15. Harkavy J, Romanoff A: Electrocardiographic changes in bronchial asthma and their significance. Am Heart J 23:692, 1942
16. Hiss RG, Lamb LE, Allen MF: Electrocardiographic findings in 67,375 asymptomatic subjects: X. Normal values. Am J Cardiol 6:200, 1960
17. Human GP, Snyman HW: The value of the Macruz index in the diagnosis of atrial enlargement. Circulation 27:935, 1963
18. Kasser I, Kennedy JW: The relationship of increased left atrial volume and pressure to abnormal P waves on the electrocardiogram. Circulation 39:339, 1969
19. Kilcoyne MM, Davis AL, Ferrer MI: A dynamic electrocardiographic concept useful in the diagnosis of cor pulmonale: Result of a survey of 200 patients with chronic obstructive pulmonary disease. Circulation 42:903, 1970
20. Leathan A: The chest lead electrocardiogram in health. Br Heart J 12:213, 1950
21. Macruz R, Perloff JK, Case RB: A method for the electrocardiographic recognition of atrial enlargment. Circulation 17:882, 1958
22. Mazzoleni A, Wolff R, Wolff L, et al: Correlation between component cardiac weights and electrocardiographic patterns in 185 cases. Circulation 30:808, 1964
23. Morris JJ Jr, Estes EH Jr, Whalen RE, et al: P-wave analysis in valvular heart disease. Circulation 29:242, 1964
24. Peter RH, Morris JJ Jr, McIntosh HD: Relationship of fibrillatory waves and P waves in the electrocardiogram. Circulation 33:599, 1966
25. Phillips JH, Burch GE: Problems in the diagnosis of cor pulmonale. Am Heart J 66:818, 1963
26. Phillips RW: The electrocardiogram in cor pulmonale secondary to pulmonary emphysema: A study of 18 cases proved by autopsy. Am Heart J 56:352, 1958
27. Reynolds G: The atrial electrogram in mitral stenosis. Br Heart J 15:250, 1953
28. Romhilt DW, Bove KE, Conradi S, et al: Morphologic significance of left atrial involvement. Am Heart J 83:322, 1972
29. Romhilt DW, Scott RC: Left atrial involvement in acute pulmonary edema. Am Heart J 83:328, 1972
30. Rytand DA, Onesti SJ Jr, Bruns DL: The atrial rate in patients with flutter: A relationship between atrial enlargement and slow rate. Stanford Med Bull 16:169, 1958
31. Sanchez-Cascos A, Deucher D: The P wave in atrial septal defect. Br Heart J 25:202, 1963
32. Saunders JL, Calatayud JB, Schulz KJ, et al: Evaluation of ECG criteria for P-wave abnormalities. Am Heart J 74:757, 1967
33. Shleser IH, Langendorf R: The significance of the so-called P-pulmonale pattern in the electrocardiogram. Am J Med Sci 204:725, 1942
34. Skoulas A, Horlick L: The atrial F wave in various types of heart disease and its response to treatment. Am J Cardiol 14:174, 1964
35. Sodi-Pollares D, Calder RM: New Bases of Electrocardiography. St Louis, CV Mosby, 1956
36. Spodick DH, Hauger-Klevene JH, Tyler JM, et al: The electrocardiogram in pulmonary emphysema: Relationship of characteristic electrocardiographic findings to severity of disease as measured by degree of airway obstruction. Am Rev Resp Dis 88:14, 1963
37. Sutnick AI, Soloff LA: Posterior rotation of the atrial vector: An electrocardiographic sign of left ventricular failure. Circulation 26:913, 1962
38. Thomas P, DeJong D: The P wave in the electrocardiogram in the diagnosis of heart disease. Br Heart J 16:241, 1954
39. Thurmann M: Coarse atrial fibrillation in congenital heart disease. Circulation 32:290, 1965
40. Thurmann M, Janney JG Jr: The diagnostic importance of fibrillatory wave size. Circulation 25:991, 1962
41. Wasserburger RH, Kelly JR, Rasmussen HK, et al: The electrocardiographic pentalogy of pulmonary emphysema: A correlation of roentgenographic findings and pulmonary function studies. Circulation 20:831, 1959
42. Wenger R, Hofmann-Credner D: Observations on the atria of the human heart by direct and semidirect electrocardiography. Circulation 5:870, 1952
43. Wood P: Electrocardiographic appearances in acute and chronic pulmonary heart disease. Br Heart J 10:87, 1947
44. Zimmerman HA, Bersano E, Dicosky C: The Auricular Electrocardiogram. Springfield, Ill, Charles C Thomas, 1968

Left Ventricular Hypertrophy

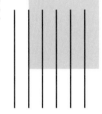

3

The electrocardiographic (ECG) diagnosis of left ventricular hypertrophy is based mainly on the increase of the QRS voltage generated from the left ventricle. The increase in the left ventricular muscle mass exaggerates the leftward and posterior QRS forces. The free wall of the hypertrophied left ventricle is brought closer to the chest wall and, therefore, to the precordial lead electrodes. When dilatation coexists, the area of the epicardial surface of the left ventricle in close contact with the chest wall further increases. These factors contribute further to the abnormally large amplitude of the QRS complexes in the precordial leads. The increase in the thickness of the left ventricular wall prolongs the ventricular activation time and may result in a delay of the onset of the intrinsicoid deflection in the left precordial leads as well as a lengthening of the total QRS duration.

Secondary changes of the ST segment and T wave often occur. Because of the delay in the completion of the endocardium-to-epicardium depolarization process, repolarization now may begin in the subendocardial instead of the subepicardial layer of the myocardium. The reversal of the direction of the recovery process is associated with a change in the direction of the ST and T vectors. Relative myocardial ischemia may be present because of the mismatch between the increased left ventricular mass and coronary blood flow even in the absence of coronary artery disease. In the typical cases of left ventricular hypertrophy, the ST and T vectors are opposite to the QRS forces.

DIAGNOSTIC CRITERIA

Numerous criteria have been proposed for the ECG diagnosis of left ventricular hypertrophy. Only the more generally used criteria are listed below. The others are included in Table 3–1.

Left ventricular hypertrophy is considered to be present if one or more of the following criteria are met. These criteria are based mainly on those suggested by Sokolow and Lyon.[52] They are applicable only if the duration of the QRS complex is less than 0.12 second.

Limb Leads

1. R wave in lead I + S wave in lead III > 25 mm.[19]
2. R wave in aVL > 11 mm.[52]
3. R wave in aVF > 20 mm.[52]
4. S wave in aVR > 14 mm.[46]

Precordial Leads

5. R wave in V_5 or V_6 > 26 mm.[52]
6. R wave in V_5 or V_6 + S wave in V_1 > 35 mm.[52]
7. Largest R wave + largest S wave in the precordial leads > 45 mm.[31]

Additional Supporting Criteria

8. Onset of the intrinsicoid deflection in V_5 or V_6 ≥ 0.05 second.[31]
9. ST-segment depression and T-wave inversion in the left precordial leads and in those limb leads whose major QRS deflection is upright in the presence of one or more of the above findings.

Romhilt and Estes[41] proposed a point-score system that uses a combination of the various findings listed in Table 3–2. Left ventricular hypertrophy is considered present if the total points are 5 or more and is probably present if the total points are 4.

More recently, Casale and associates suggested two sets of voltage criteria (Cornell voltage) for the diagnosis of left ventricular hypertrophy according to the sex of the patients.[13] Left ventricular hypertrophy is diagnosed if the R wave in lead aVL plus the S

TABLE 3–1. Sensitivity and Specificity of Other Criteria for the Diagnosis of Left Ventricular Hypertrophy

Criterion	Sensitivity (%)	Specificity (%) (False-Positives)
SV_1 or SV_2 + RV_5 $\geqslant$ 35	56	13
SV_1 + RV_5 or V_6 > 30	56	11
SV_1 or V_2 + RV_5 or V_6 > 35	56	12
SV_2 + RV_4 or RV_5 > 35	56	15
R + S > 40	55	14
SV_1 + RV_5 > 30	51	11
SV_2 + RV_5 > 35	50	11
RS > 35	41	9
SV_1 + RV_5 > 33 (females) / SV_1 + RV_5 > 36 (males)	39	7
RV_5 $\geqslant$ 20	38	9
SV_1 or SV_2 + RV_6 > 40	38	3
SV_2 + RV_5 or RV_6 > 45	34	3
LAD = −30° or greater	24	13
RaVL > 7.5	23	4
RV_6 > RV_5	23	11
RV_6 > 20	22	2
SV_1 $\geqslant$ 24	19	0
Lewis index* = +17 or greater	18	2
RaVL $\geqslant$ 11	13	1
R_1 > 13	11	0
RaVL > 12	9	0
R_1 > 15	8	0
RaVL > 13	8	0
RaVF > 19	1	1

*Lewis index = $(R_1 - R_3) + (S_3 - S_1)$.
Adapted from Romhilt DW, Bove KE, Norris RJ, et al: A critical appraisal of the ECG criteria for the diagnosis of left ventricular hypertrophy. Circulation 40:185, 1969, by permission of the American Heart Association, Inc.

wave in lead V_3 is greater than 28 mm in men and 20 mm in women. Roberts and Day[37] and Odom and associates[32] considered a total 12-lead QRS voltage exceeding 175 mm in persons over 40 years of age as an indication of left ventricular hypertrophy.

CLINICAL AND ANATOMIC CORRELATION

Many clinical, echocardiographic, and anatomic studies have been conducted to deter-mine the accuracy of the various ECG criteria for the diagnosis of left ventricular hypertro-phy. Because the anatomic studies are usually more dependable, they are emphasized in the following discussion.

Two different methods have been generally used to determine pathologically whether left ventricular hypertrophy is present. One method is based on the total heart weight and the thickness of the free wall of the left ven-tricle. The upper normal limit of the heart weight is determined by the patient's body

TABLE 3–2. Point-Score System

1. Amplitude . . . . 3 points
   Any of the following:
   a. Largest R or S wave in the limb leads $\geqslant$ 20 mm
   b. S wave in V_1 or V_2 $\geqslant$ 30 mm
   c. R wave in V_5 or V_6 $\geqslant$ 30 mm
2. ST-T–segment changes (typical pattern of left ventricular strain with the ST-T–segment vector shifted in direction opposite to the mean QRS vector)
   Without digitalis . . . . 3 points
   With digitalis . . . . 1 point
3. Left atrial involvement . . . . 3 points
   Terminal negativity of the P wave in V_1 is 1 mm or more in depth with a duration of 0.04 second or more
4. Left axis deviation −30° or more . . . . 2 points
5. QRS duration $\geqslant$ 0.09 second . . . . 1 point
6. Intrinsicoid deflection in V_5 and V_6 $\geqslant$ 0.05 second . . . . 1 point

length.[57] Left ventricular hypertrophy is considered to be present if the total heart weight is increased and the left ventricular wall thickness is 13 mm or more.[14,47,48] The other method, which is more accurate but tedious, is the chamber dissection technique. The epicardial fat is removed, and the left and right ventricles are weighed separately. Because it is difficult to separate the left and right septal masses, most studies included the entire interventricular septum as part of the left ventricle.[7,36] In our institution, Bove and co-workers considered left ventricular hypertrophy to be present if the left ventricle and septum weighed more than 200 g.[7] If the weight was in the normal range, a ratio of the left ventricle plus septum to the right ventricle of greater than 3.5 also suggested left ventricular hypertrophy.

In examining the reliability of the diagnostic criteria, the various studies tested them either individually or in combination.

Sensitivity and Specificity of the Combined Criteria

To evaluate the sensitivity of the combined criteria, Scott and associates studied 100 cases of isolated left ventricular hypertrophy with increased heart weight and left ventricular wall thickness at autopsy.[49] Using one or more of the criteria listed previously (except criterion 7), 85 percent of the cases were correctly diagnosed. In this study, however, ST-segment and T-wave changes alone were also considered as indicative of left ventricular hypertrophy. Later investigations by others gave similar as well as lower sensitivity (60 and 85 percent).[42,50] To test the specificity of these criteria, my colleagues and I reviewed the autopsy findings of 100 cases diagnosed as left

ventricular hypertrophy by ECG less than 3 months before death.[14] The tracings satisfied one or more of the listed criteria (except criterion 7). Cases with ST-segment and T-wave changes alone were not included. Forty-four cases had isolated left ventricular hypertrophy. Forty-five had combined ventricular hypertrophy. A false-positive diagnosis of left ventricular hypertrophy was made in 11 cases (i.e., 11 percent). Selzer and associates reported a slightly higher incidence (15 percent) of false-positive diagnosis.[50]

When two or three criteria are required for the diagnosis, it is reasonable to assume that the rate of recognition will decrease. Most of the studies did not report the results of such analysis. On the other hand, the specificity was definitely improved when multiple criteria were met. In Selzer and co-workers' series of 75 cases of anatomic left ventricular hypertrophy correctly diagnosed by ECG, 5 had high voltage alone.[50] When high voltage was accompanied by T-wave inversion, a false-positive diagnosis was seldom made.

The point-score system, tested in 360 autopsied hearts by the chamber dissection technique, gave a sensitivity of 54 percent, with only a 3 percent false-positive diagnosis.[41]

Sensitivity and Specificity of the Individual Criteria

Mazzoleni and co-workers examined the reliability of several of the individual criteria in the autopsied hearts with the chamber dissection technique.[29] In 185 unselected adult patients, anatomic left ventricular hypertrophy was recognized in 22 percent by the criterion RV_5 or $V_6 + SV_1 > 35$ and in 17 percent by the criterion RaVL > 10 mm. No false-positive diagnosis was encountered. A delay of the

TABLE 3–3. Sensitivity and Specificity of the Frequently Used Criteria for the Diagnosis of Left Ventricular Hypertrophy*

Criterion	Sensitivity (%)	Specificity (%) (False-Positives)
R + S > 45 mm	45	7
SV_1 + RV_5 or RV_6 > 35 mm	43	5
OID V_5 or V_6 = 0.05–0.07 second	29	1
RV_5 or RV_6 > 26 mm	25	2
RaVL > 11 mm	11	0
R_1 + S_3 > 25 mm	11	0
SaVR > 14 mm	7	0
RaVF > 20 mm	1	1

*OID = onset of intrinsicoid deflection.
Adapted from Romhilt DW, Bove KE, Norris RJ, et al: A critical appraisal of the ECG criteria for the diagnosis of left ventricular hypertrophy. Circulation 40:185, 1969, by permission of the American Heart Association, Inc.

intrinsicoid deflection in the left precordial leads was found to be an insensitive and non-specific sign of left ventricular hypertrophy.

The more recently proposed Cornell voltage criteria (RaVL + SV_3 > 28 mm in men and 20 mm in women) were tested in 135 patients at autopsy.[12] Increased left ventricular mass was present in 69 of the hearts. The criteria were found to have a sensitivity of 96 percent. Additional studies are needed to determine the accuracy of these criteria. The criteria that use the total 12-lead QRS voltage (greater than 175 mm) also require further evaluation.[32]

One of the most extensive anatomic correlation studies using the chamber dissection technique was conducted by Romhilt and associates.[40] Thirty-three different ECG criteria for left ventricular hypertrophy were evaluated. The sensitivity and specificity of the individual criteria are listed in Tables 3–1 and 3–3. The most frequently used criteria are included in Table 3–3. They are listed in the order of decreasing sensitivity.

VOLTAGE CRITERIA

In general, high voltage in the precordial leads was the most sensitive criterion for the diagnosis of left ventricular hypertrophy. A recognition rate of up to 56 percent may be achieved. However, it also was most frequently responsible for the false-positive diagnosis. Up to 15 percent of the normal hearts may be classified as having left ventricular hypertrophy by some of the criteria. As was expected, criteria that require lower voltage were more sensitive but less specific. The more popular criteria (i.e., SV_1 + RV_5 or V_6 > 35 mm or largest R + largest S wave in the precordial leads > 45 mm) had a sensitivity of 45 percent or less, but the false-positive diagnosis was also more acceptable, falling in the range of 7 percent or less.

High voltage in the limb leads occurred less frequently. Using the criteria of RaVL > 11 mm or R_1 + S_3 > 25 mm, only 11 percent of the hypertrophied hearts were recognized, but they were highly specific, with no false-positive diagnosis.

ONSET OF INTRINSICOID DEFLECTION

The delay of the onset of the intrinsicoid deflection in leads V_5 or V_6 to 0.05 second or greater appeared to be a relatively insensitive but highly specific criterion. This was in con-trast to the previous reports.[29,50] Selzer and associates had found an unacceptably high percentage (35 percent) of false-positive diagnosis.[50] In my experience, this criterion is quite specific, but other signs of left ventricular hypertrophy usually coexist when it is present.[14]

ABNORMAL LEFT AXIS DEVIATION

Abnormal left axis deviation of −30° or more was a rather poor sign of left ventricular hypertrophy when it was used alone. It was relatively insensitive and nonspecific. The result agreed with Grant's finding of a lack of correlation between the heart weight and left axis deviation.[17] Left ventricular fibrosis with left anterior hemiblock probably is responsible for the abnormal left axis deviation. Left ventricular hypertrophy may or may not coexist in patients with left ventricular fibrotic lesions.

OTHER ELECTROCARDIOGRAPHIC CHANGES IN LEFT VENTRICULAR HYPERTROPHY

Poor R-Wave Progression in the Precordial Leads

A leftward shift of the transitional zone in the precordial leads (i.e., R/S ratio < 1 in V_5) was said to be common in left ventricular hypertrophy,[4] but was not supported by anatomic correlation study.[29] Poor progression of the R wave in the right and mid-precordial leads is noted frequently, however. Occasionally, R waves are absent in leads V_1, V_2, and even V_3, resulting in a QS deflection in these leads to mimic anteroseptal myocardial infarction (Fig. 3–1).

Absent Q Wave in the Left Precordial Leads

In most normal persons, Q waves are recorded in the left precordial leads. This is particularly true in the younger population. In patients with left ventricular hypertrophy, Q waves often decrease in size or are no longer present (see Fig. 3–1). In autopsied hearts with left ventricular hypertrophy resulting from various causes, the Q wave was absent in about 50 percent (Chou TC, unpublished data, 1960). The absence of the Q wave in the left precordial leads is related to a leftward displacement of the initial QRS forces, which is also partly responsible for the decrease of the R wave in

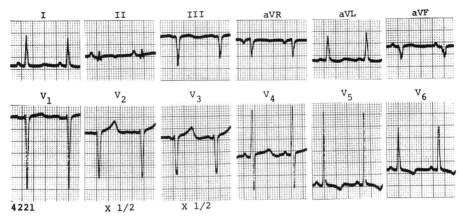

FIGURE 3–1. Coarctation of aorta. The patient was a 36-year-old man who died shortly after an unsuccessful correction of this congenital lesion. At autopsy, there was also evidence of healed dissecting aneurysm of the ascending aorta. The heart weighed 545 g with marked left ventricular hypertrophy and a moderate degree of dilatation. The left ventricular wall thickness was 25 mm. The coronary arteries revealed mild focal atherosclerosis with no significant narrowing of the lumen. The myocardium showed no evidence of fibrosis or infarction. The aortic valve was monocuspid with a centrally located orifice of approximately 7 mm in diameter. This ECG was recorded 1 day before surgery. It shows rather typical changes of left ventricular hypertrophy. The QS deflections in leads III and aVF suggest inferior wall myocardial damage and, in view of the autopsy findings, represent a pseudoinfarction pattern. The poor progression of the R waves in the precordial leads also suggests the possibility of anterior myocardial damage, which was not present.

the right precordial leads. Septal fibrosis or incomplete left bundle branch block has been suggested as the cause of the leftward deviation of the initial forces.

Abnormal Q Wave in the Inferior Leads

Occasionally, an abnormal Q wave may be recorded in leads III and aVF and, less often, in lead II to mimic inferior myocardial infarction. An example is given in Figure 3–1. The mechanism of this pseudoinfarction is not clear.

Notching and Prolongation of the QRS Complex

In some patients, there is a notching of the QRS complex, especially in the mid-precordial leads, although the duration of the QRS may or may not be within normal limits (Fig. 3–2). Intraventricular conduction defect is probably responsible. On the other hand, prolongation of the QRS duration to 0.11 second is often seen with, or in the absence of, the notching. Increased ventricular activation time or conduction abnormality or both may be the cause. Although it is a nonspecific finding, in my experience it is usually associated with larger hearts.

ST-Segment and T-Wave Changes

The classical ST and T-wave changes in left ventricular hypertrophy consist of ST-segment depression with upward convexity and T-wave inversion in the left precordial leads (Figs. 3–3 and 3–4). Reciprocal changes are present in the right precordial leads with ST-segment elevation and tall T wave. In the limb leads, the direction of the ST and T vectors is also away from the main QRS forces. Therefore, ST-segment depression and T-wave inversion are seen in leads I and aVL when there is a horizontal QRS axis and in leads II, III, and aVF when the QRS axis is vertical. These changes have been attributed to secondary repolarization abnormalities as well as to increased left ventricular tension and relative myocardial ischemia. The latter view has been responsible for the use of the term *ventricular strain*. These classical ST and T-wave changes are usually found in patients with fully developed left ventricular hypertrophy. Although they are nonspecific changes and may be caused by a great variety of pathologic and physiological abnormalities, they are valuable additional signs to support the diagnosis when other findings of left ventricular hypertrophy are also present. If both high QRS voltage and the classical "strain" pattern are present, a false-positive diagnosis of left ventricular hypertrophy is seldom made.[50] Less

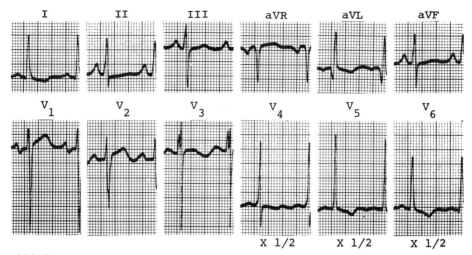

464 9

FIGURE 3–2. Left ventricular hypertrophy with inverted U waves. The patient is a 33-year-old man with severe hypertension, cardiomegaly, and congestive heart failure. The ECG shows high QRS voltage and notching of the R wave in lead V_3. With the addition of ST-segment and T-wave changes, the tracing is highly suggestive of left ventricular hypertrophy. The U waves are inverted in leads V_4 through V_6 and perhaps in leads V_2 and V_3. The P waves suggest left atrial enlargement.

typical changes such as slight ST-segment depression and/or flat T waves in the left precordial leads are also helpful, but to a lesser degree, in confirming the presence of anatomic left ventricular hypertrophy.

A common diagnostic problem encountered by clinicians is the interpretation of the left ventricular "strain" pattern in patients with high-voltage QRS complexes suggestive of left ventricular hypertrophy and chest pain suggestive of angina pectoris. It is often difficult to determine whether the ST-segment and T-wave changes represent repolarization abnormalities secondary to the hypertrophy or myocardial ischemia (anterolateral or inferolateral) due to coronary artery disease or both. If the ST-segment and T-wave changes are relatively recent, they may be caused by increased severity of the hypertrophy, increased left ventricular afterload, or obstructive coronary lesions.

By comparing patients with aortic stenosis and lateral myocardial infarction, Beach and associates suggested that the findings of J-

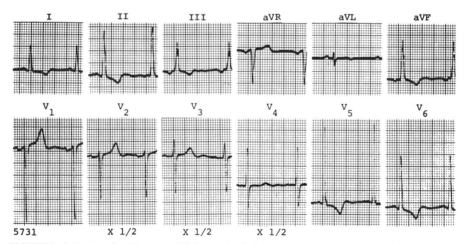

5731

FIGURE 3–3. Aortic valve disease with left ventricular hypertrophy. The patient is a 61-year-old man with aortic stenosis and insufficiency. A peak systolic pressure gradient of 88 mm Hg across the aortic valve was demonstrated during cardiac catheterization. Aortography revealed a 3 to 4+ aortic insufficiency. The coronary arteries were normal. The ECG shows high QRS voltage and the classic "strain pattern" of the ST segment and T waves. The P waves are suggestive of left atrial enlargement.

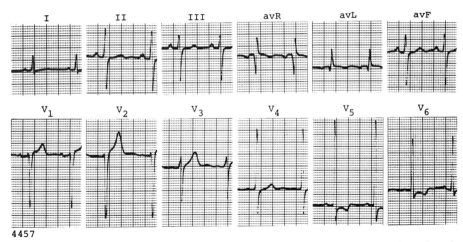

FIGURE 3–4. Congenital aortic valve disease. The patient is a 30-year-old man with moderately severe congenital aortic stenosis and insufficiency. The systolic pressure gradient across the aortic valve was 61 mm Hg, and there was 2.5+ aortic insufficiency demonstrated by aortogram. The ECG reveals typical changes of left ventricular hypertrophy. Abnormal left axis deviation is also present. The patient was not receiving digitalis at the time of the recording.

point depression, asymmetrical T-wave inversion, terminal positivity of the T wave, T-wave inversion in lead V_6 greater than 3 mm, and T-wave inversion greater in lead V_6 than in lead V_4 are in favor of the diagnosis of left ventricular strain.[5] The usefulness of these findings has not been substantiated in my experience. On the other hand, I have been impressed by the presence of marked ST-segment depression or deeply inverted T waves disproportional to the height of the R waves, ST and T-wave changes that involve also leads V_3 and V_4 in which the predominant deflections of the QRS complexes are negative (S waves), and rapid appearance or disappearance of these repolarization changes in patients with coexisting coronary artery disease. The reliability

of these findings has not been systematically tested, however.

U Wave

A prominent U wave is often seen in patients with left ventricular hypertrophy (Fig. 3–5). It is most noticeable in the right and mid-precordial leads. Lepeschkin reported a high incidence (62 percent) of inverted U waves in leads I, V_5, and V_6 in patients with left ventricular overload.[27] This finding may be transient and is more common in cases of diastolic overload than systolic overload. The T wave in the same lead may be either upright or inverted (Fig. 3–5). An inverted T wave is, however, more common[24] (see Fig. 3–2). In my expe-

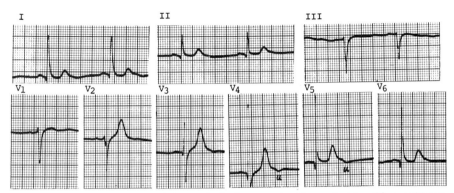

FIGURE 3–5. Inverted U waves in left ventricular hypertrophy. The patient is a 46-year-old man with a long history of hypertension and chronic renal failure. He had no symptoms suggestive of coronary artery disease. The chest roentgenogram showed cardiomegaly. In the ECG, QRS voltage criteria for left ventricular hypertrophy are met. The U waves are inverted in leads I and V_4 through V_6.

rience, the incidence of U-wave inversion in left ventricular hypertrophy is not nearly as high as that reported by Lepeschkin.[27]

LEFT VENTRICULAR HYPERTROPHY AND INCOMPLETE LEFT BUNDLE BRANCH BLOCK

When high QRS voltage and ST and T-wave changes in left ventricular hypertrophy are accompanied by increased QRS duration up to 0.11 second, absence of Q waves with a delay of the onset of intrinsicoid deflection in the left precordial leads, and sometimes notching of the QRS in the mid-precordial lead, the question of whether incomplete left bundle branch block coexists is often raised. Because of the lack of an adequate number of anatomic studies of the conduction system, a definitive answer is not available at this time. Because these changes are usually associated with hearts that are markedly hypertrophied it is reasonable to assume that some ventricular conduction abnormalities are present.

The relationship between left ventricular hypertrophy and complete left bundle branch block is discussed in Chapter 5.

Systolic and Diastolic Overload of the Left Ventricle

Cabrera and Monroy introduced the concept of systolic and diastolic overload of the left ventricle.[10] Later writers used the terms *pressure overload* and *volume overload*. The ECG pattern of left ventricular systolic overload includes high voltage of the R wave and

the classic ST-segment and T-wave changes in the left precordial leads (see Figs. 3–1 and 3–2). It occurs in such conditions as aortic stenosis, systemic hypertension, and coarctation of aorta in which there is an increase in the resistance of the left ventricular outflow. In diastolic overload of the left ventricle, which is seen in patients with aortic insufficiency, mitral insufficiency, and patent ductus arteriosus, the ECG usually presents high voltage of the R waves with prominent Q waves in the left precordial leads (Fig. 3–6). The ST segment is usually elevated, with a tall, peaked T wave.

Although the concept is theoretically attractive, its clinical application often has been disappointing, especially in patients with acquired heart disease. In either systolic or diastolic overload of the left ventricle, tall R waves in the left precordial leads may be the only abnormal finding, or the ST and T-wave changes may be minimal (Fig. 3–7). In the advanced stage of the disease, with severe dilatation and hypertrophy, both conditions may be associated with the classical ST and T-wave changes of the strain pattern in addition to the tall R waves in the left precordial leads. Although the overloading is of the diastolic type, the Q waves may be absent in these leads. In young patients with congenital heart disease, the correlation of the hemodynamic state and the ECG pattern usually is better. This is particularly true in patients with ventricular septal defect without pulmonary hypertension. A prominent Q wave followed by a tall R wave and an upright T wave is characteristic (Fig. 3–8).

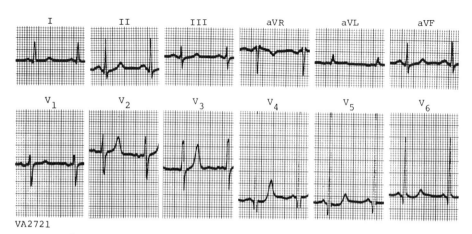

VA2721

FIGURE 3–6. Severe mitral insufficiency. The patient is a 52-year-old man with a 4+ mitral regurgitation demonstrated by left ventricular angiography. The ECG reveals deep Q waves and tall R waves in the left precordial leads. The ST-segments and T waves are within normal limits. The P-wave changes are suggestive of left atrial enlargement. This tracing illustrates the typical diastolic overload pattern of left ventricular hypertrophy.

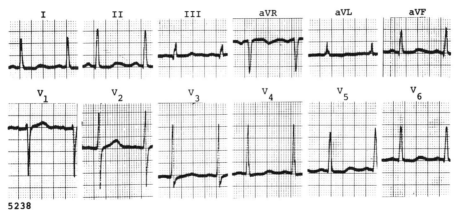

5238

FIGURE 3–7. Severe calcific aortic stenosis with minimal ST-segment and T-wave changes. The tracing was recorded from a 62-year-old woman with severe aortic stenosis and a peak systolic gradient of 130 mm Hg across the aortic valve. The right heart pressures were normal. The patient died of aortic valve surgery 4 weeks after the recording of the tracing. At autopsy, the heart weighed 510 g, with moderately severe hypertrophy and mild dilatation of the left ventricle and moderate hypertrophy of the right ventricle. The left ventricular wall thickness was 1.6 cm, and the right ventricular wall thickness was 0.4 cm. The coronary arteries were widely patent and showed only a mild degree of atherosclerosis. The myocardium showed no evidence of muscle damage. The ECG shows relatively high QRS voltage with $SV_1 + RV_5 > 35$ mm. Only minimal ST-segment and T-wave changes, however, are apparent in the left precordial leads, lead I, and lead aVL. The patient was not receiving digitalis at the time of the recording.

PHYSIOLOGICAL FACTORS THAT AFFECT THE RELIABILITY OF THE DIAGNOSTIC CRITERIA

Age

Age is one of the most important factors to be considered in the ECG diagnosis of left ventricular hypertrophy. Most of the voltage criteria were derived and tested against the older population. It is well known that adolescents and young adults have normally higher voltage of the QRS complex than do older individuals (Fig. 3–9). For example, from age 20 to 29 years, the normal 99th percentile for SV_1

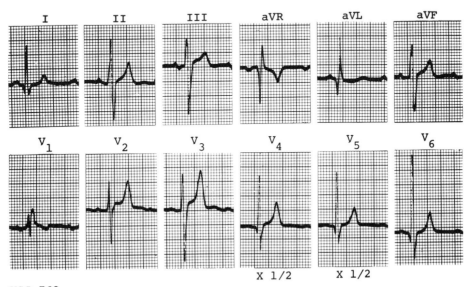

VCG 762

FIGURE 3–8. Ventricular septal defect. The patient is a 29-year-old man with ventricular septal defect proved by cardiac catheterization. The ECG shows deep Q waves in leads I, aVL, and V_4 through V_6. There are tall R waves in the left precordial leads. The ST segment is slightly elevated, and the T waves are tall and peaked in most of the precordial leads. The findings are consistent with diastolic overloading of the left ventricle. An R' is present in lead V_1, which suggests possible right ventricular hypertrophy or incomplete right bundle branch block.

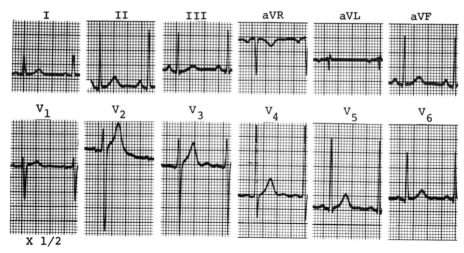

FIGURE 3–9. Normal young adult with high QRS voltage. The ECG was recorded from a healthy 22-year-old male medical student. $RV_5 + SV_1 = 46$ mm and $RV_5 + SV_2 = 49.5$ mm.

+ RV_5 or V_6 is 53 mm and the mean +2 standard deviation is 46 mm.[28] The voltage of SV_2 + RV_5 is greater than 35 mm in 32 percent of the normal men between 20 and 39 years of age (Chou TC, unpublished data, 1960). It has been estimated that the amplitude of the maximum spatial QRS vector decreases by 6.5 percent for each decade of life from age 20 to 78.[33]

DIAGNOSIS OF LEFT VENTRICULAR HYPERTROPHY IN YOUNG SUBJECTS

The normally higher amplitude of the complexes in children and young adults greatly impairs the usefulness of the voltage criteria for the diagnosis of left ventricular hypertrophy.[55] During routine interpretation of the ECG, it is my practice not to consider left ventricular hypertrophy seriously in patients under age 40 years if only the voltage criteria are met unless the amplitude is extremely high. Even the combination of high QRS voltage and ST and T-wave changes, which is reliable in older subjects, can no longer be applied with equal confidence. The ST and T-wave abnormalities may be due to other causes, and the high amplitude may reflect the patient's normal voltage. It is my practice to look for some other supporting evidence in the QRS complex before making a diagnosis of left ventricular hypertrophy. The presence of abnormal left axis deviation, a delay of the onset of the intrinsicoid deflection in leads V_5 and V_6, an increase of the QRS duration to 0.11 second, the presence of notching of the QRS complex in the mid-precordial leads, and

especially the poor progression of the R wave in the right and mid-precordial leads would give additional support to the diagnosis of left ventricular hypertrophy. Because most normal individuals have taller R waves in lead V_5 than in lead V_6, a reversal of this order also is suggestive of abnormality. When the patient is a child or a young adult, multiple abnormalities in addition to the high voltage are required before one can be confident in the ECG diagnosis of left ventricular hypertrophy.

Body Habitus

Kilty and Lepeschkin emphasized the effect of body build on the QRS voltage of the ECG.[23] Using the ponderal index (the height in inches divided by the cube root of the weight in pounds) as a measure of body build, they found a highly significant correlation between body build and the voltage of $R_1 + S_3$, largest R + S in the precordial leads, and largest R + S in a single precordial lead. The precordial lead criterion R + S > 45 mm underdiagnoses left ventricular hypertrophy in obese people and overdiagnoses it in thin people. Others have also noted that most false-positive diagnoses of left ventricular hypertrophy were made in emaciated individuals.[50] The amount of adipose or muscle tissue in the chest wall affects the distance between the precordial electrode and the heart, the resistance of the current flow, and therefore, the voltage recorded in the lead. An accumulation of adipose tissue around the heart of overweight persons may also be responsible in some cases. The term *little old lady syndrome* has been used to describe the high voltage seen in elderly individuals, usually women, who have lost considerable body weight but were found at autopsy to have either normal or small left ventricles.[48]

Sex and Race

Sex also has a significant effect on the amplitude of the QRS complex. Men have higher amplitude than women in both the limb leads and precordial leads, but especially in the latter.[51] In women, it is sometimes important to know whether lead V_4 was recorded with the electrode on or beneath the breast. A significant reduction of the voltage may occur if the electrode is placed on a large breast.

Black subjects are reported to have higher QRS voltage than white subjects.[33] The effects of race and sex on the QRS voltage may be illustrated by a study of 114 healthy adolescents.[3] The upper limit derived for the S wave amplitude in lead V_1 was 34 mm in black boys, 32 mm in white boys, 26 mm in black girls, and 16 mm in white girls. The corresponding values for the R wave in lead V_6 were 30, 24, 22, and 24 mm, respectively.

PATHOLOGIC STATES THAT AFFECT THE DIAGNOSIS OF LEFT VENTRICULAR HYPERTROPHY

The lung is a poor electrical conductor. In patients with chronic obstructive lung disease, the voltages of the QRS complex may be markedly reduced. The presence of left ventricular hypertrophy often is not recognized in such patients. Figure 3–10 represents an example of a patient with severe aortic insufficiency and pulmonary emphysema. The QRS voltage is within normal limits.

Pericardial effusion may likewise mask the left ventricular hypertrophy pattern because of the short-circuiting effect of the pericardial fluid. An example is given in Figure 3–11 in which the patient's earlier tracing showed a typical left ventricular hypertrophy pattern, but the later record no longer exhibited the high voltage when pericardial effusion developed. It is possible that the voltage changes in some patients with congestive heart failure are caused by the presence of pericardial fluid, which is common, or pulmonary edema, which also may reduce the body surface potential by its short-circuiting effect.[43] A reduction of the amplitude of the complexes is also seen in patients with pleural effusion, generalized anasarca, or pneumothorax.

Myocardial damage in patients with coronary artery disease, secondary myocardial disease such as amyloidosis, or scleroderma heart disease is often accompanied by a loss of QRS forces, which makes the diagnosis of left ventricular hypertrophy difficult. Although the presence of myocardial infarction did not affect the ECG recognition of left ventricular hypertrophy by the voltage criteria in an autopsy series,[48] it is a common clinical observation that large infarctions often significantly reduce the voltage, resulting in an abnormal small QRS complex in the area of damage.

When right ventricular hypertrophy coexists, the increased rightward forces may result in a decrease of the leftward potential. In most patients with right ventricular hypertrophy secondary to left ventricular disease, the effect is minimal and the diagnosis of left ventricular hypertrophy is not affected. When right ven-

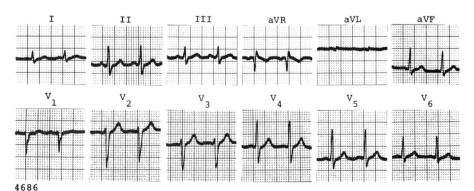

4686

FIGURE 3–10. Left ventricular hypertrophy in a patient with pulmonary emphysema. The patient is a 38-year-old man with pulmonary emphysema and severe aortic insufficiency with congestive heart failure caused by bacterial endocarditis. The diagnosis was confirmed by cardiac catheterization and at surgery. The coronary arteries were normal. The ECG is within normal limits. The relatively low voltage of the QRS complexes is probably the result of pulmonary emphysema.

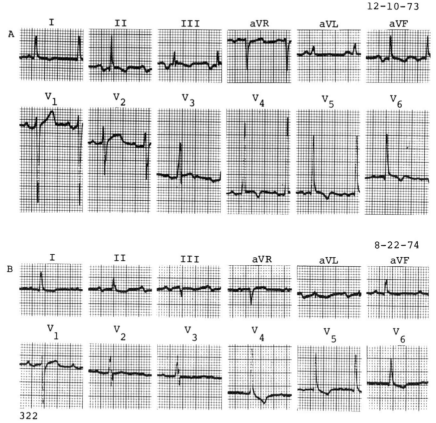

322

FIGURE 3-11. Effect of pericardial effusion on the ECG findings of left ventricular hypertrophy. The patient was a 68-year-old man who has rheumatic heart disease with aortic and mitral involvement. The chest roentgenogram reveals cardiomegaly. The tracing shown in A on 12-10-73 reveals abnormal P waves suggestive of left atrial enlargement. The QRS voltage in the precordial leads and the ST and T changes suggest left ventricular hypertrophy. The relatively short QT interval is probably due to digitalis effect. At the time of the recording of tracing B on 8-22-74, the patient had large pericardial effusion, supported by echocardiogram and pericardiocentesis. In this tracing, the voltage of the QRS complexes has markedly decreased, and the diagnosis of left ventricular hypertrophy can no longer be made. The ST and T changes persisted, however. After pericardiocentesis, the voltage of the QRS complexes returned toward its previous amplitude.

tricular hypertrophy is severe, however, the left ventricular hypertrophy pattern may not be apparent because of the cancelling effect of the rightward forces.

The effect of conduction abnormalities such as left and right bundle branch block on the diagnosis of left ventricular hypertrophy is discussed in Chapters 6 to 8 on conduction abnormalities.

ASSESSMENT OF THE SEVERITY OF VALVULAR LESIONS THAT CAUSES LEFT VENTRICULAR HYPERTROPHY

Most attempts to correlate the ECG with the severity of valvular lesion have been made in patients with valvular aortic stenosis. Abdin reported 53 patients with aortic stenosis, 19

of whom came to autopsy.[1] The depth of T-wave inversion in the left precordial leads bore a close relationship to the severity of the stenosis. The T-wave inversion was more frequent and more remarkable than in patients with systemic hypertension who had comparable degrees of left ventricular hypertrophy at autopsy. Hugenholtz and associates studied 95 patients with congenital aortic stenosis.[20] The age of the patients ranged from 6 weeks to 20 years. The aortic stenosis was considered severe if the pressure gradient across the aortic valve was 40 mm Hg or greater and mild if it was below 40 mm Hg. About three fourths of the patients with severe lesions revealed ECG evidence of left ventricular hypertrophy, and one fourth of those with mild lesions showed such evidence. When the ST and T-wave changes of ventricular strain pattern were evaluated alone, 30 percent of the patients with severe lesions failed to show the abnormalities, whereas 88 percent of the mild cases did not have these changes. In their series, abnormal left axis deviation was observed mostly in patients with severe stenosis. Braunwald and associates reported the hemodynamic and ECG findings in 100 patients with congenital aortic stenosis.[8] The age of the patients ranged from 2 to 51 years, with 36 patients under the age of 10. No single ECG change was found reliable in determining the severity of the obstruction. In patients under age 10 years, however, the ECG was more helpful than in older individuals. In this younger age group, severe obstruction was associated with a T-wave axis superior to $-40°$ and a QRS-T angle exceeding $100°$ in the frontal plane. When the R wave in lead V_5 is less than 20 mm, an S wave in lead V_1 less than 16 mm, or an R/S ratio in lead V_1 more than 0.40, the obstruction was relatively mild. In 65 cases of isolated congenital aortic stenosis under the age of 15, Fowler failed to find any relation between the degree of the stenosis and the voltage of the QRS complex.[16] The stenosis is usually severe, however, if the frontal axis of the T wave is superior to $+15°$ or an R/T ratio in lead V_5 or V_6 is greater than 10.

Patients with severe aortic stenosis may have normal ECGs. Figure 3–12 was recorded from a 49-year-old man with aortic stenosis and a systolic pressure gradient across the valve of 110 mm Hg. The tracing is within normal limits. In clinical practice, it is hazardous to rely on the ECG alone in assessing and managing patients with aortic stenosis. The echocardiogram is a superior noninvasive method for evaluating such patients. The ECG, however, is more reliable than the routine chest roentgenogram in diagnosing significant aortic stenosis as in the case of left ventricular hypertrophy in general.[42] It is also reasonable to assume that when high QRS voltage and the typical strain pattern of ST and T-wave changes are both present, the stenosis is severe.

In patients with chronic aortic insufficiency, the ECG may be useful in the estimation of the geometric and functional states of the left ventricle. Roman and associates correlated the ECG, echocardiographic, and radionuclide angiographic findings in 95 adults with severe, pure, chronic aortic insufficiency and no evidence of coronary artery disease.[39] Patients with left ventricular strain patterns in their ECGs had significantly greater left ventricular end-diastolic and end-systolic dimensions, left ventricular mass, and lower ejection fractions than did those patients with normal ST segments and T waves. Among the 73 asymptomatic patients who were followed for 28 months, symptoms developed in only 1 (3%) of the 37 patients with persistently normal ST and T waves but in 6 (24%) of the 25 patients who initially or later exhibited strain patterns. The correlation between the QRS voltage and the degree of left ventricular dilatation and dysfunction was, however, not strong.[39] Indeed, in patients with chronic aortic regurgitation and massive cardiomegaly (heart weighing 1 kg or more), the usual QRS criteria for left ventricular hypertrophy are

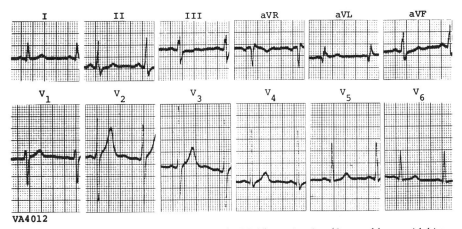

VA4012

FIGURE 3–12. Severe aortic stenosis with normal ECG. The patient is a 49-year-old man with history and physical findings consistent with severe aortic stenosis. A systolic pressure gradient across the aortic valve of 110 mm Hg was demonstrated during cardiac catheterization. The ECG is within normal limits.

often not present in the ECG.[38] The QRS voltage may be useful, however, in the follow-up of patients after aortic valve replacement for chronic aortic regurgitation. In the 21 patients reported on by Carroll and co-workers, postoperative reduction of the QRS voltage to normal was associated with complete regression of hypertrophy by echocardiography, whereas persistently increased voltage was indicative of incomplete regression.[11] The reduction in voltage generally occurred in the first 6 months after the valve replacement.[11]

In patients with mitral insufficiency, the correlation between the severity of the mitral lesion and the ECG changes is generally poor. In a series of 65 cases of dynamically significant mitral insufficiency without significant mitral stenosis confirmed at surgery or autopsy, the ventricular complex was normal in 50 percent and suggested left ventricular hypertrophy in 30 percent, right ventricular hypertrophy in 15 percent, and combined ventricular hypertrophy in 5 percent of the cases.[6] Figure 3–13 was recorded from a patient who had congestive heart failure and 3+ mitral insufficiency demonstrated by left ventriculogram. The ECG is within normal limits.

LEFT VENTRICULAR HYPERTROPHY IN SYSTEMIC HYPERTENSION

The findings on ECG were reported to be normal in almost half, borderline in one fifth, and definitely abnormal in one third of a group of 154 patients with the clinical diagnosis of hypertensive cardiovascular disease.[15] In an epidemiology study,[22] the incidence of ECG left ventricular hypertrophy pattern over a 14-year period of observation rose in proportion to the blood pressure in all age groups. About half the patients with systolic pressures above 200 mm Hg had or developed an ECG left ventricular hypertrophy pattern during the 14 years.

Ashizawa and associates reported a 26-year follow-up study of 601 patients with hypertension and ECG changes of left ventricular hypertrophy with both high QRS voltage and ST-segment and T-wave changes.[2] The patients were examined at 2-year intervals. In 60 subjects, the ECG signs of left ventricular hypertrophy developed during the observation period. In 37 of the subjects, high QRS voltage appeared first and was followed by ST and T-wave changes. In 10 patients, the ST and T-wave changes occurred first; in the other 13, the QRS and ST and T-wave changes appeared simultaneously. In 72 of the 601 subjects, regression of the ECG left ventricular hypertrophy was observed. The QRS voltage decreased to normal in 36, ST-T changes disappeared in 25, and both high QRS voltage and ST-T changes disappeared in 11 patients. In about half of these 72 subjects, the regression of the abnormal ECG findings, usually the QRS voltage, was associated with lowering of the blood pressure.

The predicted value of the ECG for the severity of the hypertension in the individual patient is limited, however. Nevertheless, a significant relationship has been observed between the ST-segment and T-wave changes and the level of the blood pressure. When both the ST-segment and T-wave changes and high QRS voltage are present, patients usually have a higher blood pressure than do those with high voltage of the QRS complex alone.[19,54] When the ECG is correlated with the systemic hemodynamic findings, the presence of T-wave changes also is likely to be associated with

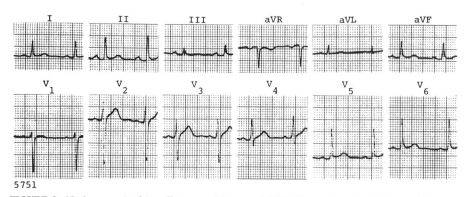

5751

FIGURE 3–13. Severe mitral insufficiency with normal ECG. The patient is a 35-year-old woman with slight cardiomegaly and a history of congestive heart failure; she was treated with digitalis and diuretics. Moderately severe (3+) mitral regurgitation was demonstrated by left ventriculogram. Both the left and right heart pressures were normal. The ECG is within normal limits.

higher systemic vascular resistance or intraarterial blood pressure at rest.[44]

Prognostic Value of the Electrocardiographic Changes

In patients with essential hypertension, Sokolow and Perloff reported a significant difference in the 5-year mortality between those with normal ECGs and those with left ventricular hypertrophy.[53] This was especially true when a diphasic or inverted T wave was present. In the Framingham epidemiology study, hypertensive patients with definite left ventricular hypertrophy pattern (tall R wave, ST-segment depression, flattened or inverted T wave, and increased ventricular activation time in the left precordial leads) had much higher mortality rates, even though the blood pressure level was the same.[21,22] In this study, there also was a threefold increased risk of clinically overt coronary artery disease in persons with such ECG left ventricular hypertrophy pattern independent of the effect of hypertension.

COMPARISON OF ELECTROCARDIOGRAM AND ECHOCARDIOGRAM IN THE DIAGNOSIS OF LEFT VENTRICULAR HYPERTROPHY

It is generally agreed that the echocardiogram is superior to the ECG in the detection of left ventricular hypertrophy and the M-mode is more accurate than the two-dimensional echocardiogram in the estimation of left ventricular mass.[26,35,45,56] In a study of 34 subjects, Reichek and Devereux found that the left ventricular mass calculated from the M-mode echocardiogram correlated well with the left ventricular weight at autopsy.[35] The echocardiogram diagnosed left ventricular hypertrophy with a sensitivity of 93 percent and a specificity of 95 percent.[35] In contrast, using the Romhilt-Estes[41] and Sokolow-Lyon[52] criteria, the ECG diagnosed the hypertrophy with a sensitivity of 50 and 21 percent, respectively.[35] The specificity of both criteria was 95 percent. In a similar study of 50 patients, Woythaler and associates found that these ECG criteria had a sensitivity and specificity of 54 and 86 percent, respectively.[56] The M-mode echocardiogram had a sensitivity of 88 percent and a specificity of 84 percent.[56]

In addition to the increased accuracy in the estimation of left ventricular weight, the echocardiogram is also able to determine whether the hypertrophy is concentric or eccentric and whether left ventricular dilatation is present. The echocardiogram is also superior to the ECG in the detection of left ventricular hypertrophy in the presence of ventricular conduction defect.[26]

REFERENCES

1. Abdin ZH: The electrocardiogram in aortic stenosis. Br Heart J 195:31, 1957
2. Ashizawa N, Seto S, Kitano K, et al: Effects of blood pressure changes on development and regression of electrocardiographic left ventricular hypertrophy: A 26-year longitudinal study. J Am Coll Cardiol 13:165, 1989
3. Bailey MA, Su JJ, Guller B: Racial and sexual differences in the standard electrocardiogram of black vs white adolescents. Chest 75:474, 1979
4. Barker JM: The Unipolar Electrocardiogram: A Clinical Interpretation. New York, Appleton-Century-Crofts, 1952, p 375
5. Beach C, Kenmure ACF, Short D: Electrocardiogram of pure left ventricular hypertrophy and its differentiation from lateral ischaemia. Br Heart J 46:285, 1981
6. Bentivoglio LG, Urricchio JF, Waldow A, et al: An electrocardiographic analysis of sixty-five cases of mitral regurgitation. Circulation 18:572, 1958
7. Bove KE, Rowlands DR, Scott RC: Observations on the assessment of cardiac hypertrophy utilizing a chamber partition technique. Circulation 33:558, 1966
8. Braunwald E, Goldblatt A, Aygen MM, et al: Congenital aortic stenosis: I. Clinical and hemodynamic findings in 100 patients. Circulation 27:426, 1963
9. Braverman IB, Gibson S: The outlook for children with congenital aortic stenosis. Am Heart J 53:487, 1957
10. Cabrera CE, Monroy JR: Systolic and diastolic loading of the heart: II. Electrocardiographic data. Am Heart J 43:669, 1952
11. Carroll JD, Gaasch WH, Naimi S, Levine HJ: Regression of myocardial hypertrophy: Electrocardiographic-echocardiographic correlations after aortic valve replacement in patients with chronic aortic regurgitation. Circulation 65:980, 1982
12. Casale PN, Devereux RB, Alonso DR, et al: Improved sex-specific criteria of left ventricular hypertrophy for clinical and computer interpretation of electrocardiograms: Validation with autopsy findings. Circulation 75:565, 1987
13. Casale PN, Devereux RB, Kligfield P, et al: Electrocardiographic detection of left ventricular hypertrophy: Development and prospective validation of improved criteria. J Am Coll Cardiol 6:572, 1985
14. Chou TC, Scott RC, Booth RW, et al: Specificity of the current electrocardiographic criteria in the diagnosis of left ventricular hypertrophy. Am Heart J 60:371, 1960
15. Dawber, TR, Kannel WB, Love DE, et al: The electrocardiogram in heart disease detection: A comparison of the multiple and single lead procedures. Circulation 5:559, 1952
16. Fowler RS: Ventricular repolarization in congenital aortic stenosis. Am Heart J 70:603, 1965
17. Grant RP: Left axis deviation. Circulation 14:233, 1956

18. Gubner R, Ungerleider HE: Electrocardiographic criteria of left ventricular hypertrophy. Arch Intern Med 72:196, 1943

19. Hamer J, Shinebourne E, James F: Significance of electrocardiographic changes in hypertension. Br Med J 1:79, 1969

20. Hugenholtz PG, Lees MM, Nadas AS: The scalar electrocardiogram, vectorcardiogram, and exercise electrocardiogram in the assessment of congenital aortic stenosis. Circulation 26:79, 1962

21. Kannel WB, Gordon T, Offutt D: Left ventricular hypertrophy by electrocardiogram: Prevalence, incidence, and mortality in the Framingham study. Ann Intern Med 71:89, 1969

22. Kannel WB, Margolis JR: Electrocardiographic left ventricular hypertrophy and risk of coronary heart disease: The Framingham study. Ann Intern Med 72:813, 1970

23. Kilty SE, Lepeschkin E: Effect of body build on the QRS voltage of the electrocardiogram in normal men: Its significance in the diagnosis of left ventricular hypertrophy. Circulation 31:77, 1965

24. Kishida H, Cole JS, Surawicz B: Negative U wave: A highly specific but poorly understood sign of heart disease. Am J Cardiol 49:2030, 1982

25. Klein RC, Vera Z, DeMaria AN, Mason DT: Electrocardiographic diagnosis of left ventricular hypertrophy in the presence of left bundle branch block. Am Heart J 108:502, 1984

26. Laird WP, Fixler DE: Left ventricular hypertrophy in adolescents with elevated blood pressure: Assessment by chest roentgenography, electrocardiography, and echocardiography. Pediatrics 67:255, 1981

27. Lepeschkin E: The U wave of the electrocardiogram. Mod Concepts Cardiovasc Dis 38:39, 1969

28. Manning GW, Smiley JR: QRS-voltage criteria for left ventricular hypertrophy in a normal male population. Circulation 29:224, 1964

29. Mazzoleni A, Wolff R, Wolff L et al: Correlation between component cardiac weighs and electrocardiographic patterns in 185 cases. Circulation 30:8008, 1964

30. McPhie J: Left ventricular hypertrophy: Electrocardiographic diagnosis. Australas Ann Med 7:317, 1958

31. Noth PH, Myers GB, Klein HA: The precordial electrocardiogram in left ventricular hypertrophy: A study of autopsied cases. J Lab Clin Med 32:1517, 1947

32. Odom H, Davis JL, Dinh HA, et al: QRS voltage measurements in autopsied men free of cardiopulmonary disease: A basis for evaluating total QRS voltage as an index of left ventricular hypertrophy. Am J Cardiol 58:801, 1986

33. Pipberger HV, Goldman MJ, Littman D et al: Correlations of the orthogonal electrocardiogram and vectorcardiogram with constitutional variables in 518 normal men. Circulation 35:536, 1967

34. Pringle SD, MacFarlane PW, McKillop JH, et al: Pathophysiologic assessment of left ventricular hypertrophy and strain in asymptomatic patients with essential hypertension. J Am Coll Cardiol 13:1377, 1989

35. Reichek N, Devereux RB: Left ventricular hypertrophy: Relationship of anatomic, echocardiographic and electrocardiographic findings. Circulation 63:1391, 1981

36. Reiner L, Mazzoleni A, Rodriguez FL, et al: Weight of the human heart. Arch Pathol (Chicago) 71:180, 1961

37. Roberts WC, Day PJ: Electrocardiographic observations in clinically isolated, pure, chronic, severe aortic regurgitation: Analysis of 30 necropsy patients aged 19 to 65 years. Am J Cardiol 55:431, 1985

38. Roberts WC, Podolak MJ: The king of hearts: Analysis of 23 patients with hearts weighing 1000 grams or more. Am J Cardiol 55:485, 1985

39. Roman MJ, Kligfield P, Devereux RB, et al: Geometric and functional correlates of electrocardiographic repolarization and voltage abnormalities in aortic regurgitation. J Am Coll Cardiol 9:500, 1987

40. Romhilt DW, Bove KE, Norris RJ, et al: A critical appraisal of the electrocardiographic criteria for the diagnosis of left ventricular hypertrophy. Circulation 40:185, 1969

41. Romhilt DW, Estes EH: Point-score system for the ECG diagnosis of left ventricular hypertrophy. Am Heart J 75:752, 1968

42. Rosenfeld I, Goodrich C, Kassebaum G, et al: The electrocardiographic recognition of left ventricular hypertrophy. Am Heart J 63:731, 1962

43. Rudy Y, Wood R, Plonsey R, Liebman J: The effect of high lung capacity on electrocardiographic potentials. Circulation 65:440, 1982

44. Sannerstedt R, Bjure J, Varnauskas E: Correlation between electrocardiographic changes and systemic hemodynamics in human arterial hypertension. Am J Cardiol 26:117, 1970

45. Savage DD, Drayer JIM, Henry WL, et al: Echocardiographic assessment of cardiac anatomy and function in hypertensive patients. Circulation 59:623, 1979

46. Schack JA, Rosenman RH, Katz LN: The AV limb leads in the diagnosis of left ventricular strain. Am Heart J 40:696, 1950

47. Scott RC: Correlation between the electrocardiographic patterns of ventricular hypertrophy and the anatomic findings. Circulation 21:256, 1960

48. Scott RC: Ventricular hypertrophy. Cardiovasc Clin 5:220, 1973

49. Scott RC, Seiwert VJ, Simon DL, et al: Left ventricular hypertrophy: Study of accuracy of current electrocardiographic criteria when compared with autopsy findings in one hundred cases. Circulation 11:89, 1955

50. Selzer A, Ebnother CL, Packard P, et al: Reliability of electrocardiographic diagnosis of left ventricular hypertrophy. Circulation 17:255, 1958

51. Simonson E: Differentiation Between Normal and Abnormal Electrocardiography. St Louis, CV Mosby, 1961

52. Sokolow M, Lyon TP: The ventricular complex in ventricular hypertrophy as obtained by unipolar precordial and limb leads. Am Heart J 37:161, 1949

53. Sokolow M, Perloff D: The prognosis of essential hypertension treated conservatively. Circulation 23:697, 1961

54. Sokolow M, Werdegar D, Kain HK, et al: Relationship between level of blood pressure measured casually and by portable recorders and severity of complications in essential hypertension. Circulation 34:279, 1966

55. Walker CHM, Rose RL: Importance of age, sex and body habitus in the diagnosis of left ventricular hypertrophy from the precordial electrocardiogram in childhood and adolescence. Pediatrics 28:705, 1961

56. Woythaler JN, Singer SL, Kwan OL, et al: Accuracy of echocardiography versus electrocardiography in detecting left ventricular hypertrophy: Comparison with postmortem mass measurements. J Am Coll Cardiol 2:305, 1983

57. Zeek PM: Heart weight: I. The weight of the normal human heart. Arch Pathol 34:820, 1942

Right Ventricular Hypertrophy

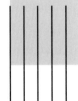

4

The right ventricular forces normally are directed anteriorly and rightward but are mostly masked by the dominant left ventricular potential. An increase in the right ventricular muscle mass modifies the resultant forces to a degree in proportion to the severity of the hypertrophy. In mild cases, no apparent change may be detected in the electrocardiogram (ECG). If the right ventricular hypertrophy is severe, the normally dominant left posterior QRS forces may be replaced by prominent right anterior forces, and the QRS patterns in the left and right precordial leads are reversed. Intermediate degrees of abnormality may be observed when the hypertrophy is moderate. Because lead V_1 is more proximal to the right ventricular mass, it is the most sensitive lead to record the changes. Taller R wave, smaller S wave, or a change in the R/S ratio may be observed. The onset of the intrinsicoid deflection in this lead may be delayed because of the prolongation of the right ventricular activation time and delayed activation of the right ventricular epicardium.[49] In some instances, the increased rightward forces are directed posteriorly instead of anteriorly. No apparent abnormality is seen in lead V_1, since it records more anterior than rightward forces. The left precordial leads may reveal deep S waves, however. In either case, the increased rightward forces may be recognized in the limb leads as right axis deviation.

Secondary changes of the ST segment and T wave often occur and are observed in the right precordial leads. A delay in the completion of the endocardium-to-epicardium depolarization may result in a relatively early onset of the repolarization of the endocardium. The reversal of the direction of recovery phase is accompanied by a change in the direction of the ST and T vectors, which become opposite to the QRS forces. Therefore, ST-segment depression and T-wave inversion are recorded in the right precordial leads. In some instances, the ST and T changes may be seen without apparent QRS abnormalities. Relative myocardial ischemia of the right ventricle or right ventricular "strain" may be responsible.

DIAGNOSTIC CRITERIA

Right ventricular hypertrophy is considered to be present if one or more of the following criteria are met, provided the QRS duration is less than 0.12 second. The criteria have been proposed mainly by Myers and associates[32] and by Sokolow and Lyon.[46]

More frequently used criteria:

1. Right axis deviation of $+110°$ or more.[32]
2. R/S ratio in V_1 (or V_{3R}) > 1.[32]
3. R wave in $V_1 \geq 7$ mm.[46]
4. S wave in $V_1 < 2$ mm.[46]
5. qR pattern in V_1 (or V_{3R}).[32]
6. R wave in V_1 + S wave in V_5 or $V_6 >$ 10.5 mm.[46]
7. R/S ratio in V_5 or $V_6 \leq 1$.[46]
8. Onset of intrinsicoid deflection in V_1 (or V_{3R}) = 0.035 to 0.055 second.[32]
9. rSR′ in V_1 with R′ ≥ 10 mm.[3]

Less frequently used criteria:

1. R wave in aVR ≥ 5 mm.[46]
2. R wave in V_5 or $V_6 < 5$ mm.[46]
3. S wave in V_5 or $V_6 \geq 7$ mm.[46]
4. $\dfrac{R/S \text{ in } V_5}{R/S \text{ in } V_1} \leq 0.4$.[46]
5. Drop of R/S ratio between two precordial leads to the right of transition.[35]

Supporting criterion:

ST depression and T-wave inversion in right precordial leads.[46]

CLINICAL AND ANATOMIC CORRELATION

The accuracy of the ECG criteria for the diagnosis of right ventricular hypertrophy has been evaluated by a number of hemodynamic and anatomic studies. In the autopsy series, two different methods have been used to determine whether right ventricular hypertrophy is present. One is based on the right ventricular wall thickness with or without an increase of the total heart weight. Right ventricular hypertrophy is considered present if the free wall of the right ventricle is 5 mm or more in thickness or 4 mm or more if right ventricular dilatation is present.[47] The other method uses the chamber dissection technique. The diagnosis of right ventricular hypertrophy is made if the right ventricular free wall weighs more than 70 or 75 g.[6,17] Relative right ventricular hypertrophy is considered present if the right ventricular weight is more than 30 percent of the total ventricular mass or if the ratio of the weight of the left ventricle plus septum to that of the right ventricle is less than 2.1.[6,17]

Sensitivity and Specificity of the Criteria

In contrast to the diagnosis of left ventricular hypertrophy, the reported sensitivity of the ECG criteria for right ventricular hypertrophy varies greatly. In the autopsy series in which the anatomic diagnosis was based mainly on the right ventricular wall thickness, the ECG met one or more of the criteria in 23 to 100 percent.[39] To test the specificity of the criteria, Roman and colleagues examined 118 hearts with the ECG diagnosis of right ventricular hypertrophy.[36] A false-positive diagnosis

was made in 60 percent of the cases. The criteria of R in V_1 + S in V_5 or V_6 > 10.5 mm and S in V_5 or V_6 > 7.0 mm were responsible for most of the erroneous diagnoses. Using the chamber dissection technique, Scott observed right ventricular hypertrophy pattern in 32 percent of 47 cases of isolated right ventricular hypertrophy.[40] I studied 97 patients in whom the presence of right ventricular hypertrophy was supported by hemodynamic data. The sensitivity of the ECG was 66 percent.[14]

The explanation for the marked differences in the results probably lies in the patient population sampled. The lower sensitivity was obtained mostly from unselected adult patients in a general hospital.[47] The development of right ventricular hypertrophy as a result of left ventricular disease is most common in these patients. The degree of hypertrophy usually is mild and likely to be masked by the dominant left ventricle on the surface ECG. The higher sensitivity values mostly came from centers with large numbers of congenital heart disease, a situation in which the degree of right ventricular hypertrophy tends to be severe.[51] The use of autopsy material by itself also may influence the results, because the hearts examined are most likely in the advanced stage of the disease. To a lesser extent, this may occur in patients who required cardiac catheterization.

One of the most extensive studies in the evaluation of the sensitivity and specificity of the *individual* ECG criterion in the diagnosis of right ventricular hypertrophy was per-

TABLE 4–1. Sensitivity, Specificity, and Correctness of Electrocardiographic Criteria for the Diagnosis of Right Ventricular Hypertrophy*

Criterion	Sensitivity (%)	Specificity (%) (False-Positives)	Correctness (%)
Right axis deviation ≥ 110°	12	4	78
R/S V_1 (or V_{3R}) > 1	6	2	78
RV_1 ≥ 7 mm	2	1	78
SV_1 < 2 mm	6	2	78
qR in V_1	5	1	79
RV_1 + SV_5 or V_6 > 10.5 mm	18	6	77
R/S V_5 or V_6 ≤ 1	16	7	77
OID in V_1 (or V_{3R}) = 0.035–0.055 sec	8	6	76
RSR' in V_1 with R' > 10 mm	0	0	78
RaV_R ≥ 11 5 mm	0	0	78
RV_5 (or RV_6) < 5 mm	13	13	71
SV_5 (or SV_6) ≥ 7 mm	26	10	76
$\frac{R/S\ V_5}{R/S\ V_1}$ ≥ 0.4	6	1	79
Drop of R/S ratio	28	24	65

OID = onset of intrinsicoid deflection.
*Adapted from Flowers NC, Horan LG: IV. Hypertrophy and infarction: Subtle signs of right ventricular enlargement and their relative importance. *In* Schlant RC, Hurst JW (eds): Advances in Electrocardiography. New York, Grune & Stratton, 1972, by permission.

formed by Flowers and Horan.[17] They used the chamber dissection technique to examine a total of 819 apparently unselected hearts, including 178 with right ventricular hypertrophy, to correlate them with the ECG. The sensitivity and specificity of the individual criteria are summarized in Table 4–1. The authors also calculated the percentage of correct diagnoses by dividing the true positives and true negatives by the total group studied.

The sensitivity of the individual criterion is low and is generally less than 20 percent. The more sensitive signs, such as those based on changes in the left precordial leads, usually are associated with higher number of false-positive diagnosis. By comparison, criteria based on abnormalities in lead V_1 are more specific but less sensitive. Flowers and Horan also evaluated the hearts with relative right ventricular hypertrophy (i.e., the weight of the free wall of the right ventricle is greater than 30 percent of the total heart weight). The results were similar to those listed in Table 4–1.

DIFFERENTIAL DIAGNOSIS

Abnormal Right Axis Deviation

Right axis deviation occurs normally in infants and children. The mean QRS axis in the first 4 weeks of life is +110° or greater.[26] After 1 month, the average axis is less than +90°, but a significant number of children still have a QRS axis of up to +110°. In the adult population, Hiss and colleagues reported that 2 percent of the normal subjects between 20 to 30 years of age have an axis of +105°.[25] Tall and slender subjects tend to have a rightward shift of the QRS axis. Axes of +110° or more in older individuals are uncommon, however, and usually suggest abnormality. Indeed, if the frontal plane QRS axis is +90° or greater in older patients, abnormal deviation of the axis should be suspected. This is especially true if it is accompanied by other abnormalities in the ECG (Fig. 4–1).

Other pathologic states also may be accompanied by abnormal right axis deviation. In patients with chronic obstructive lung disease, the frontal plane axis may be displaced to +90° or even +110° in the absence of pulmonary hypertension. The recognition or exclusion of right ventricular hypertrophy in these patients is difficult. In patients with chronic lung disease without right ventricular hypertrophy, the amplitude of the entire QRS complex in lead I tends to be small.

In patients with lateral wall myocardial infarction, the loss of leftward forces may result in a rightward shift of the QRS vector and dominate S waves in leads I and aVL. In these patients, however, the initial R wave in lead I is usually absent and a QS rather than an rS deflection is present. Abnormal Q waves are often observed also in the left precordial leads in these patients. Whereas the T waves may be inverted in leads I, aVL, V_5, and V_6 in patients with lateral myocardial infarction, this finding is uncommon in patients with right ventricular hypertrophy alone.

Abnormal right axis deviation also is seen in patients with left posterior hemiblock (Fig. 4–2). The delayed excitation of the postero-

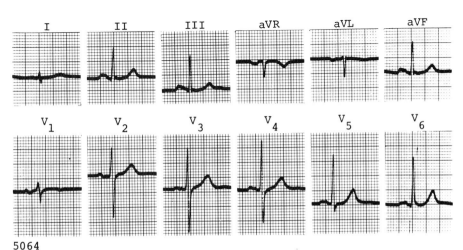

5064

FIGURE 4–1. Mitral stenosis. The patient is a 52-year-old woman with surgically proven mitral stenosis. In the ECG, the P waves are consistent with P mitrale. The frontal plane QRS axis is about 90°. The tracing is otherwise within normal limits.

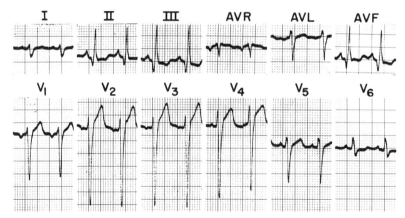

FIGURE 4–2. Abnormal right axis deviation due to left posterior hemiblock. The patient is a 52-year-old man wtih a history of myocardial infarction. Coronary arteriogram revealed a total occlusion of the right coronary artery at its proximal portion and 70 percent occlusion of the anterior descending branch of the left coronary artery. The ventriculogram showed akinesis of the inferior wall and apex. In the ECG, the frontal plane QRS axis is 110°. The QRS changes are consistent with inferior and possible anterior myocardial infarction. Note the deep S wave in lead V_5.

inferior part of the left ventricle displaces the late QRS vectors to the right. The frontal plane QRS axis typically is greater than +120°,[37] but a lesser degree of axis shift does occur.[12,37] Differentiation of abnormal right axis deviation due to right ventricular hypertrophy from that secondary to left posterior hemiblock often is not possible without clinical information. If the P waves are suggestive of right atrial enlargement, however, the presence of right ventricular hypertrophy may be inferred. Left posterior hemiblock is favored if signs of inferior or posterior myocardial infarction are evident.

Tall R Wave, Small S Wave, Increased R/S Ratio in Lead V_1

A tall R wave with or without a relatively small S wave in lead V_1 is a frequent finding in normal children. The average amplitude of the R wave in V_1 is greater than 7 mm in children under the age of 8 years.[52] The amplitude exceeds 7 mm in 20 percent of those between the ages of 8 and 12, and 11 percent of those between 12 and 16. A maximum height of 16 mm may be seen in normal adolescents. The R/S ratio in V_1 is greater than 1 in most of the children under 1 year of age,[52] but the ratio

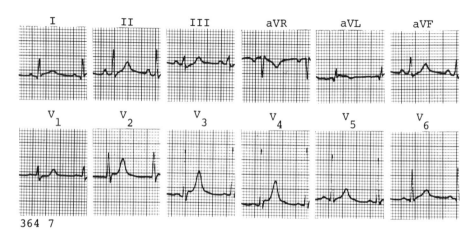

364 7

FIGURE 4–3. Tall R wave in lead V_1 due to posterior myocardial infarction. The patient is a 56-year-old woman. The diagnosis of myocardial infarction was supported by typical history and enzyme changes.

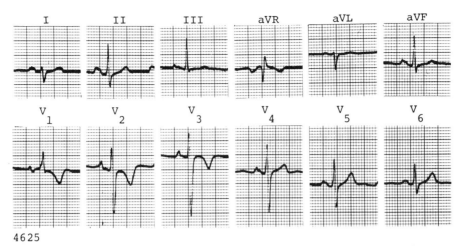

4625

FIGURE 4–4. Severe mitral stenosis. The patient is a 47-year-old man with severe mitral stenosis proved at surgery. In the ECG, the P waves are consistent with biatrial enlargement. The abnormal right axis deviation with an R/S ratio greater than 1 in lead V_1 and the T-wave inversion in the right precordial leads are consistent with right ventricular hypertrophy.

progressively decreases as the age increases. In the adult, an R/S ratio of 1 or more is seen in less than 1 percent of the normal population and is encountered mostly in individuals under the age of 30.[25] Such a ratio, however, is not uncommon in lead V_2, since it is observed in up to 10 percent of adults.[25]

In patients with true posterior myocardial infarction, the loss of the posterior QRS forces allows the anterior forces to dominate, resulting in a tall R or a small S wave in lead V_1 and an increase in the R/S ratio (Fig. 4–3). The polarity of the T wave in V_1 often is helpful in the differential diagnosis. Although exceptions do occur, an inverted T wave usually is seen in patients with right ventricular hypertrophy (Fig. 4–4), whereas an upright T wave in V_1 is likely to be associated with posterior myocardial infarction. The coexistence of ab-

normal right axis deviation in the frontal plane speaks in favor of right ventricular hypertrophy. Occasionally, however, this also may be observed in patients with posterior myocardial infarction when it is complicated by left posterior hemiblock. Because true posterior myocardial infarction often is accompanied by inferior wall damage, abnormal Q waves in the inferior leads suggest that the tall R wave in V_1 is secondary to myocardial infarction.

An R wave of 7 mm or more occasionally is seen in lead V_1 of patients with isolated left ventricular hypertrophy demonstrated at autopsy.[15] The S wave in lead V_1 usually is of large amplitude. The cause of the tall R wave is unclear. Patients with idiopathic hypertrophic subaortic stenosis often present a prominent R wave in the right precordial leads.[50]

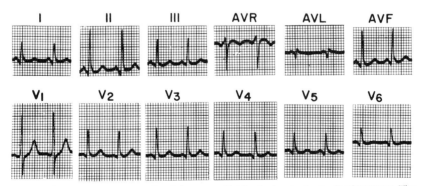

FIGURE 4–5. Tall R waves in the right precordial leads due to dextrodisplacement. The patient was a 28-year-old man with complete collapse of the right lung as a result of Hodgkin's disease. At autopsy, the heart weight was normal, and there was no evidence of ventricular hypertrophy or myocardial damage.

The S wave in lead V_1 may be small, resulting in an R/S ratio of less than 1. Deep Q waves are usually present in the left precordial leads as well as in leads II, III, and aVF. Marked hypertrophy of the interventricular septum is probably responsible for these abnormal forces.

Rightward displacement of the heart as a result of disease of the lung or pleura, such as massive pleural effusion or pneumothorax, may be accompanied by a tall R wave in lead V_1. (Fig. 4–5). Lead V_1 now may record left instead of right ventricular potential. In the absence of intrinsic organic heart disease, the T wave in V_1 is upright, whereas T-wave inversion often is observed in patients with right ventricular hypertrophy.

In type A Wolff-Parkinson-White syndrome, the area of preexcitation is in the posterior wall of the left ventricle. The initial ventricular activation proceeds anteriorly. Therefore, a prominent R wave is recorded in V_1. The differentiation from right ventricular hypertrophy is not difficult if the short PR interval and the initial slurring of the QRS complex (delta wave) are noted.

qR Pattern in Lead V_1

The qR complex in V_1 is one of the most specific signs of right ventricular hypertrophy (Fig. 4–6). It resembles the normal left precordial lead patterns and usually is associated with a severe degree of hypertrophy. Abnormal depolarization of the interventricular septum probably is responsible for the initial neg-

ativity of the complex.[20] It is possible that the right septal forces are now greater than the left, and the resultant vector is directed toward the left, which is opposite to the normal orientation. It has also been suggested that this complex is a manifestation of an enlarged right atrium that transmits to the right precordial leads the intracardiac potential from the right ventricle.[46] Others have ascribed this qR morphology to the extreme rotation of the heart so that the forces arising from the left ventricle are now recorded in the V_1 position.[29]

Some normal adults have a QS rather than an rS deflection in lead V_1. If such an individual develops right bundle branch block, a qR rather than an rSR' pattern will be recorded. If the QRS duration is 0.12 second or greater, the conduction defect usually can be readily recognized. If the bundle branch block is of the incomplete variety with QRS duration of 0.11 second or less, the differentiation becomes difficult. A similar problem exists in patients with anteroseptal myocardial infarction and right bundle branch block. The qR complex in these patients, however, usually is accompanied by abnormal Q waves in the adjacent precordial leads.

Deep S Wave, Small R Wave, R/S Ratio Less than 1 in Leads V_5 and V_6

One of the common causes of deep S waves in the left precordial leads, other than right ventricular hypertrophy, is left anterior hemiblock (Fig. 4–7). Whereas abnormal left axis

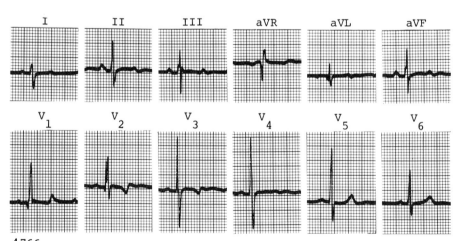

4766

FIGURE 4–6. Right ventricular hypertrophy caused by Eisenmenger's syndrome. The patient is a 24-year-old man with ventricular septal defect and severe pulmonary hypertension proved by cardiac catheterization. In the ECG, abnormal right axis deviation with a qR pattern is apparent in lead V_1 and T-wave changes are visible in the right precordial leads.

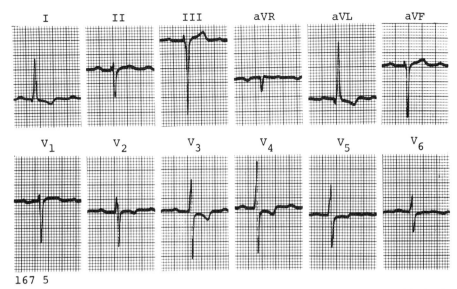

167 5

FIGURE 4–7. Deep S waves in the left precordial leads related to left anterior hemiblock. The patient is a 60-year-old man with hypertensive cardiovascular and coronary artery disease. The ECG reveals first-degree AV block, left anterior hemiblock, and left ventricular hypertrophy. The T-wave inversion in the precordial leads is consistent with anterior myocardial ischemia in view of the clinical information. The R/S ratio in V_{5-6} is less than 1.

deviation of the QRS complex in the frontal plane is the typical finding in this conduction abnormality, a leftward shift of the transitional zone in the precordial leads with deep S waves in leads V_5 and V_6 often occurs.[37] The R waves in these leads may be reduced in amplitude, and the R/S ratio is less than 1. The increased amplitude of the negative deflections in the left precordial leads is related to the fact that the lead axes of V_5 and V_6 are directed somewhat inferiorly. A marked superior displacement of the QRS axis results in its projection on the negative side of the lead axes and the appearance of S waves. If these leads are recorded at one interspace higher than the conventional level, the S waves decrease in size or disappear.

Left posterior hemiblock also may be accompanied by deep S waves in the left precordial leads (see Fig. 4–2). Abnormal right axis deviation is present in the limb leads, as has been described previously. It often is not possible to differentiate these two conditions electrocardiographically without clinical information.

In patients with chronic obstructive lung disease, the left precordial leads often display small R waves, deep S waves, and low R/S ratio. These changes may be observed in the absence of pulmonary hypertension or cor pulmonale. When the lung disease is not associated with right ventricular hypertrophy, however, the QRS complexes in the left pre-

cordial leads tend to be small, but the R/S ratio may be less than 1.

An rS pattern in leads V_5 and V_6 may be seen in patients with anterior myocardial infarction.[23] Abnormal Q waves or small r waves are likely to be present in other precordial leads. In the absence of complicating hemiblock the S waves in these leads usually are small.

rSR′ Pattern in Lead V_1

An rSR′ pattern in lead V_1 with the duration of the QRS complex less than 0.12 second is seen in normal individuals and in patients with incomplete right bundle branch block, acute right ventricular dilatation, right ventricular hypertrophy, and true posterior myocardial infarction. Occasionally, extracardiac abnormality such as pectus excavatum may be responsible for the changes. When the R′ is tall (e.g., greater than 10 mm) the presence of right ventricular hypertrophy is more likely.[5] Many patients with definite anatomic right ventricular hypertrophy, however, have an R′ of less than 10 mm (Fig. 4–8). Further discussion of the differential diagnosis of the rSR′ pattern is given in Chapter 7.

$S_1S_2S_3$ SYNDROME AS A MANIFESTATION OF RIGHT VENTRICULAR HYPERTROPHY

The $S_1S_2S_3$ syndrome is a frequently used descriptive term in electrocardiographic inter-

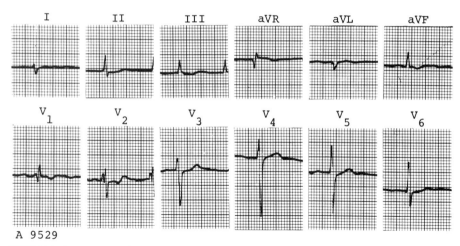

A 9529

FIGURE 4–8. Severe mitral stenosis. The patient was a 58-year-old man with severe mitral stenosis and right ventricular hypertrophy proved at autopsy. The ECG shows atrial fibrillation. There is abnormal right axis deviation with an RSR′ pattern in lead V_1 and an R/S ratio of less than 1 in V_5.

pretation. It is seen in normal individuals as well as in patients with pulmonary emphysema or right ventricular hypertrophy (see Figs. 4–6 and 4–9). A quantitative definition of the syndrome has not been suggested, however. We have elected to use the criterion of an R/S ratio equal to or less than 1 in leads I, II, and III or the S waves in these leads that exceed the upper limits of normal for the various age groups as defined by Simonson.[27a,44]* As a rule, smaller S-wave amplitudes are more likely to be seen in normal subjects, and deeper S waves, in patients with right ventricular hypertrophy. Adherence to the above criteria will probably exclude most of the normal individuals and some patients with right ventricular hypertrophy. It is appropriate to mention that in patients with right ventricular hypertrophy and the $S_1S_2S_3$ syndrome the prominent late QRS forces are directed rightward and superiorly. The S wave in lead II usually has a larger amplitude than that in lead III.

ST-SEGMENT AND T-WAVE CHANGES IN RIGHT VENTRICULAR HYPERTROPHY

In right ventricular hypertrophy, ST-segment depression and T-wave inversion are seen most commonly in the right precordial leads (see Figs. 4–4 and 4–6). These changes also

may be seen in leads II, III, and aVF (Fig. 4–10). In some instances, the ST-segment and T-wave abnormalities may be present without alteration of the QRS complex.

If the T waves are biphasic in the right precordial leads, it is useful to note whether the configuration is of the positive–negative or negative–positive type. A negative–positive biphasic T wave is abnormal and often is seen in patients with right ventricular hypertrophy[13,30] (Fig. 4–11), whereas the positive-negative configuration does not necessarily indicate abnormality.

SYSTOLIC AND DIASTOLIC OVERLOAD PATTERN

Cabrera and Monroy called attention to the different electrocardiographic changes in systolic and diastolic overloading of the right ventricle.[9] In systolic overloading, which also was called pressure overloading by later investigators, lead V_1 presents a tall monophasic R wave or a diphasic RS, Rs, or qR complex. The T wave usually is inverted in this lead. This pattern typically is seen in patients with pulmonary stenosis, tetralogy of Fallot, and pulmonary hypertension (see Figs. 4–6 and 4–11). In diastolic, or volume, overload of the right ventricle, lead V_1 usually shows an rSR′ pattern. This is the typical QRS complex in patients with atrial septal defects (Fig. 4–12), partial anomalous pulmonary venous return, and tricuspid insufficiency. The anatomic alteration consists mainly of dilatation of the right ventricle instead of hypertrophy as in the case of systolic overload.

The reliability of the clinical application of

---

*Upper limits of the normal amplitude of the S waves in leads I, II, and III:
Ages 20–29: S_1, 4 mm; S_2, 5 mm; S_3, 6 mm.
Ages 30–39: S_1, 4 mm; S_2, 4 mm; S_3, 8 mm.
Ages 40–49: S_1, 3 mm; S_2, 4 mm; S_3, 8 mm.

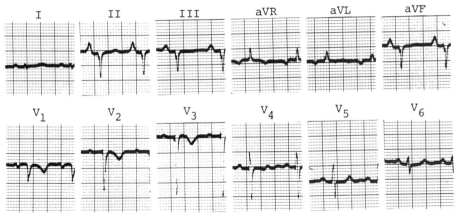

2816

FIGURE 4–9. Right ventricular hypertrophy resulting from chronic cor pulmonale. The patient was a 67-year-old man with severe pulmonary emphysema and chronic cor pulmonale proved at autopsy. There was severe right ventricular hypertrophy and dilatation. Mild atherosclerosis of the coronary arteries was present without evidence of myocardial fibrosis or infarction. In the ECG, the P wave is consistent with right atrial enlargement. There is an $S_1S_2S_3$ pattern with the QRS axis in the frontal plane directed rightward and superiorly. In the precordial leads, the QS deflection in the right precordial leads with T-wave inversion mimics anterior wall myocardial infarction. The R/S ratio in leads V_5 and V_6 is less than 1.

this concept has been questioned. The hemodynamic correlation of these two types of ECG overload patterns generally is more satisfactory in congenital heart disease, especially atrial septal defect. An rSR′ pattern in lead V_1 is not uncommon, however, in patients with pulmonary stenosis or tetralogy of Fallot.[43] This is especially true in mild and moderate pulmonary stenosis.[4] In acquired heart disease, this pattern occurs even more frequently (see Fig. 4–8). In a series of patients with mitral stenosis, such a complex was observed in 25 percent of cases.[21]

ELECTROCARDIOGRAPHIC CHANGES OF RIGHT VENTRICULAR HYPERTROPHY IN RELATION TO CAUSE OF HEART DISEASE

Mitral Stenosis

Fraser and Turner analyzed the ECGs of 177 patients with predominant mitral stenosis confirmed at operation.[4] ECGs were diagnostic of right ventricular hypertrophy in 115 (65 percent). Among these 115 patients, the R/S ratio in lead V_1 was greater than 1 in over

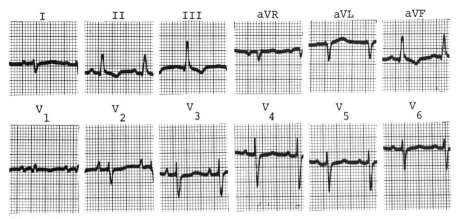

2871437

FIGURE 4–10. Pulmonary emphysema and chronic cor pulmonale. The patient is a 48-year-old man. Cardiac catheterization revealed a pulmonary arterial pressure of 71/38 mm Hg, with a mean value of 48 mm Hg. In the ECG, the tall P wave in lead V_2 suggests right atrial enlargement. T-wave changes are present in the inferior leads. Right ventricular hypertrophy is indicated by the abnormal right axis deviation, the QRS pattern in lead V_1, and the R/S ratio in the left precordial leads.

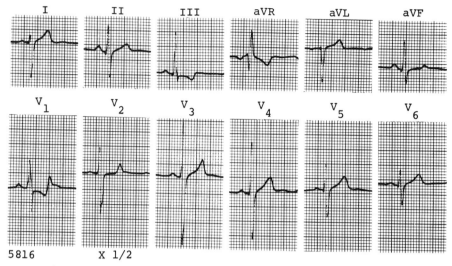

FIGURE 4–11. Pulmonary stenosis. The patient is a 19-year-old man with severe pulmonary stenosis. The right ventricular peak systolic pressure was 132 mm Hg. In the ECG, the findings suggestive of right ventricular hypertrophy are the abnormal right axis deviation and the R/S ratio in leads V_1, V_5, and V_6. The R wave in lead aVR is greater than 5 mm. Note the negative-positive biphasic T wave in lead V_1.

half of the cases. A delay in the onset of intrinsicoid deflection (> 0.03 second) was an equally sensitive criterion but was not seen in the absence of other positive signs. R wave in $V_1 > 7$ mm, an rSR′ pattern in V_1, and right axis deviation $> +100°$ were each seen in about one third of the patients. The R/S ratio was less than 1 in V_5 in 20 percent. T-wave inversion in leads V_1 through V_2 or V_3 was observed in more than 40 percent of patients and occasionally was the only abnormal finding in the tracing. Fraser and Turner also noted the value of leads V_{3R} and V_{4R} in the recognition of

right ventricular hypertrophy in mitral stenosis. The R/S ratio was greater than 1 in 80 percent of the cases in V_{3R} and in 96 percent in V_{4R}. These were the sole signs of right ventricular hypertrophy in 17 percent of the patients. The frequency of ECG right ventricular hypertrophy pattern in other series of significant mitral stenosis, including my own, was similar.[16,34] In my experience, the various criteria that are met in descending order of frequency are as follows: R/S ratio in $V_1 > 1$; a delay of onset of the intrinsicoid deflection in V_1; $RV_1 + SV_{5,6} > 10.5$ mm; S wave in $V_1 < 2$

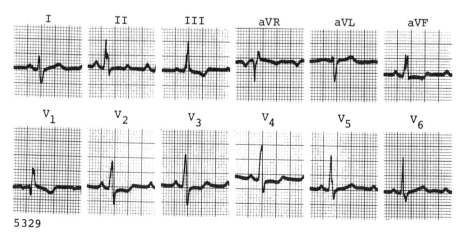

5329

FIGURE 4–12. Atrial septal defect. The patient is a 21-year-old woman with atrial septal defect proven by cardiac catheterization. The pulmonary arterial pressure was normal. The electrocardiogram shows a frontal plane QRS axis of 90° and a rSR′ pattern in lead V_1. These also are ST and T changes in the right and mid-precordial leads and inferior leads.

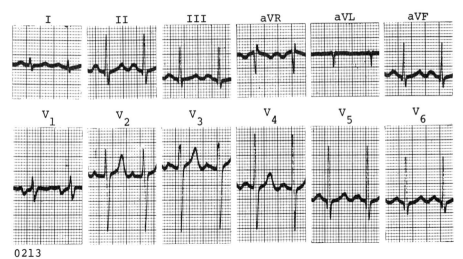

0213

FIGURE 4-13. Severe mitral stenosis. This ECG was recorded from a 42-year-old man who had a mean pulmonary arterial pressure of 60 mm Hg. The tracing suggests left atrial enlargement in lead V_1. The QRS complex shows no evidence of right ventricular hypertrophy except the R/S ratio in V_1 approaches to 1.

mm; R in $V_1 > 7$ mm; R/S ratio in V_5 or $V_6 \leqslant 1$; right axis deviation $\geqslant +110°$; rSR' in V_1; RaVR $\geqslant 5$ mm; qR in V_1. A significant number of patients with tight mitral stenosis may have normal or near-normal ECGs. This is illustrated in Figure 4-13.

Although exceptions often occur, there is a general relationship between the degrees of pulmonary hypertension in mitral stenosis and the appearance of right ventricular hypertrophy in the ECG. Fowler and associates[19] demonstrated that when the mean pulmonary arterial pressure was markedly elevated and over 42 mm Hg, nearly all the patients showed the hypertrophy pattern as indicated by an abnormal R/S ratio with delayed instrinsicoid deflection in lead V_1. Such evidence was not found in patients with a value under 28 mm Hg. Others have shown that when definitive evidence of right ventricular hypertrophy was found in the ECG, the mean pulmonary arterial pressure was uniformly 33 mm Hg or higher, and the total pulmonary vascular resistance exceeded 800 or 1000 dynes-sec/cm^{-5}.[41,42] The finding of a mean QRS axis that exceeded $+90°$ is thought by some to be a reliable indication of moderate or severe pulmonary hypertension,[42] whereas incomplete right bundle branch block or rSR' pattern gives poor quantitative estimation of the severity of the vascular obstruction. A monophasic R wave or qR complex in lead V_1 with T-

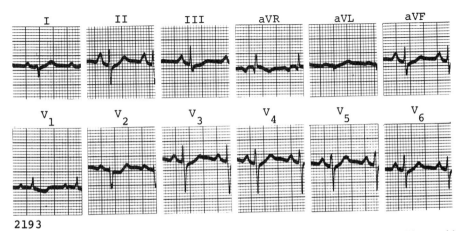

2193

FIGURE 4-14. Right ventricular hypertrophy due to mitral stenosis. The patient is a 38-year-old woman with severe mitral stenosis. The mean pulmonary arterial pressure is 53 mm Hg. In the ECG, the P wave is suggestive of right atrial enlargement. There is abnormal right axis deviation with a notched R wave in lead V_1 and an R/S ratio of less than 1 in leads V_5 and V_6.

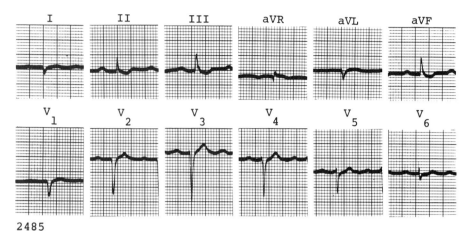

2485

FIGURE 4-15. Chronic cor pulmonale. The patient was a 63-year-old man with pulmonary emphysema and chronic cor pulmonale proved at autopsy. There was a moderate degree of right ventricular hypertrophy and dilatation. There also was a moderate degree of atherosclerosis of the coronary arteries, but the myocardium showed no evidence of fibrosis or infarction. In the ECG, there is a first-degree AV block. The QRS complex shows abnormal right axis deviation, with R/S ratio of less than 1 in leads V_5 and V_6. The QS deflections in leads 1, V_1, and V_2 with small R waves in leads V_3 through V_6 represent a pseudoinfarction pattern. The ST and T changes are consistent with digitalis effect.

wave inversion is uncommon in patients with mitral stenosis. When they are present, the disease is in its advanced stage (Fig. 4–14). Anatomically, the correlation between the right ventricular wall thickness and the height of R wave or R/S ratio in lead V_1 is poor.[21]

Chronic Cor Pulmonale

The sensitivity of the ECG in the diagnosis of right ventricular hypertrophy in patients with chronic cor pulmonale proved at autopsy is about 60 to 70 percent.[1,10,31,33] In clinical studies, however, the rate of recognition may be only 28 percent.[28] Although there are many exceptions, some correlation may be demonstrated between the ECG findings and the se-

verity of the disease. A normal or nondiagnostic ECG usually is associated with the least evidence of increased right ventricular weight or wall thickness. With moderate degree of right ventricular hypertrophy, the major QRS forces are displaced in the posterior and rightward direction. Right axis deviation appears in the limb leads. The precordial leads display deep S waves in lead V_5 and V_6, but the R waves in the right precordial leads are not prominent (see Figs. 4–9, 4–10, and 4–15). In the most severe cases of cor pulmonale, the QRS forces are oriented anteriorly and rightward. In addition to right axis deviation in the frontal plane, tall R waves appear in the right precordial leads (Fig. 4–16). In clinical practice, the deep S waves in V_5 and V_6 pattern is

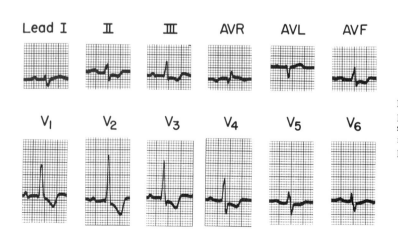

FIGURE 4-16. Severe chronic cor pulmonale with right heart failure secondary to pulmonary emphysema in a 54-year-old man. Note the qR pattern in lead V_1.

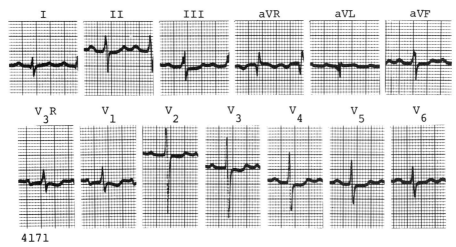

4171

FIGURE 4–17. Chronic cor pulmonale secondary to recurrent pulmonary embolism. The patient was a 56-year-old woman with a 6-year history of recurrent thrombophlebitis of the legs and pulmonary embolism. The diagnosis was verified at autopsy. The heart showed severe right ventricular hypertrophy and dilatation with marked right atrial hypertrophy. The ECG shows first-degree AV block. There is an $S_1S_2S_3$ pattern. The R/S ratio in lead V_1 is greater than 1. Deep S waves are present in the left precordial leads. ST and T changes are present in the right and mid-precordial leads. The patient was not receiving digitalis at the time.

seen most commonly. Patients with cor pulmonale secondary to pulmonary thromboembolism, idiopathic pulmonary hypertension, or obesity–hypoventilation syndrome, however, are more likely to have a taller R wave in V_1 than are those with pulmonary emphysema[8,18] (Figs. 4–17 and 4–18).

The relation between the ECG evidence of right ventricular hypertrophy and hemodynamic findings in patients with chronic cor

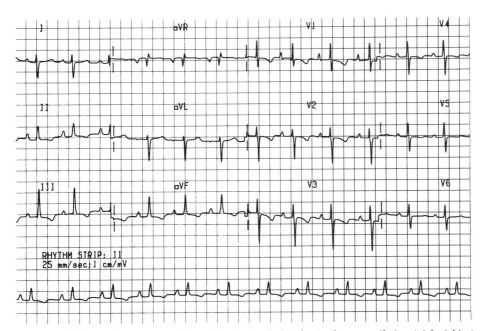

FIGURE 4–18. Chronic cor pulmonale in a patient with the obesity–hyperventilation (pickwickian) syndrome. The patient is a 37-year-old woman. Her body weight ranged between 250 and 300 pounds. She had a history of sleep apnea and syncope. There was clinical evidence of right ventricular failure. The pulmonary arterial pressure obtained during cardiac catheterization was at the systemic level. In the ECG, the P waves are tall and peaked in leads II, aVF, and V_1 through V_3 and are suggestive of right atrial enlargement. The presence of abnormal right axis deviation, an R/S ratio in lead V_1 greater than 1, and inverted T waves in leads V_1 through V_4 is highly suggestive of right ventricular hypertrophy. The T-wave inversion in the inferior leads also is related to right ventricular hypertrophy.

pulmonale has been studied by several investigators.[27,41] It was demonstrated that, if the ECG pattern of right ventricular hypertrophy was present, the mean pulmonary arterial pressure usually exceeded 30 mm Hg, but the reverse was not necessarily true. Figure 4–10 was recorded from a 48-year-old man with chronic obstructive lung disease and chronic cor pulmonale. The pulmonary arterial pressure was 71/38, with a mean value of 48 mm Hg. The ECG met several criteria for the diagnosis of right ventricular hypertrophy.

In an effort to detect early cor pulmonale, Kilcoyne and co-workers surveyed 200 patients with chronic obstructive lung disease.[28] They suggested one or more of the following fluctuations in the ECG as an indication of right ventricular abnormality or dilation: (1) a rightward shift of the mean QRS axis of $+30°$ or more; (2) T-wave abnormalities in right precordial leads; (3) ST-segment depression in leads II, III, and aVF; and (4) transitory right bundle branch block. These usually were associated with an arterial oxygen saturation of less than 85 percent and a mean pulmonary arterial pressure of 25 mm Hg or greater. Kilcoyne and associates maintained that right ventricular abnormality or dilatation, as an indication of early cor pulmonale, may not be accompanied by anatomic right ventricular hypertrophy.

Congenital Heart Disease

The accuracy of the ECG diagnosis of right ventricular hypertrophy in congenital heart disease is generally over 90 percent.[39] The higher rate of recognition in the congenital than in the acquired heart disease is due mainly to greater right ventricular systolic pressure, right ventricular thickness, and the frequent absence of left ventricular hypertrophy in the congenital group. The progression from physiological to pathologic right ventricular dominance without an intervening state of left ventricular dominance probably is partly responsible.[24]

As mentioned, the concept of systolic and diastolic overload is more useful when it is applied to right ventricular hypertrophy secondary to congenital heart disease. The classic examples are the tall R wave with T-wave inversion in V_1 seen in patients with pulmonary stenosis and the rSR′ pattern in V_1 in atrial septal defect, but there are many exceptions.

The relation between the ECG findings of right ventricular hypertrophy and the hemodynamic findings has been studied in patients with isolated pulmonary stenosis by several investigators.[4,7,12,22] According to Burch and DePasquale,[7] in patients with mild pulmonary stenosis and a peak right ventricular systolic pressure of less than 60 mm Hg, the ECG is normal in about 50 percent of the cases. When the elevation is moderate or severe, most showed changes of right ventricular hypertrophy.[7] A monophasic R wave or qR complex with T-wave inversion in V_1 usually is seen in patients with severe lesions, whereas the less typical rSR′ pattern is encountered more often in milder disease.[4,12] Based on 105 patients studied, Cayler and associates found that patients with R waves in lead V_1 of 20 mm or more almost always had systolic pressures in the right ventricle of at least 100 mm Hg.[12] Conversely, patients with R waves in V_1 of less than 20 mm rarely had pressures above 100 mm Hg. On the other hand, patients with pressures of 100 mm Hg or more almost always have either R waves in V_1 of 20 mm or taller, pure R or qR waves in V_1, or both. Although there is a general trend of taller R wave and increased R/S ratio in V_1 with higher right ventricular systolic pressure, it is generally agreed that the ECG cannot be relied on as an accurate means for the estimation of the severity of the lesion by itself (see Fig. 4–11).

The relation of the ECG and hemodynamic data in the other types of congenital defect is even less satisfactory.[7] In atrial septal defect, the basic pattern of rSR′ in lead V_1 is common in patients who have mean pulmonary arterial pressures less than 20 mm Hg, whereas most patients with a qR or rSR′S′ complex show higher pressures.[2] The overlap is considerable, however. Additional discussion of the ECG findings in atrial septal defect is included in Chapter 14.

REFERENCES

1. Armen RN, Kantor M, Weiser NJ: Pulmonary heart disease: With emphasis on electrocardiographic diagnosis. Circulation 17:164, 1958
2. Barboza ET, Brandenburg RO, Swan HJC: Atrial septal defect: The electrocardiogram and its hemodynamic correlation in 100 proved cases. Am J Cardiol 2:698, 1958
3. Barker JM, Valencia F: The precordial electrocardiogram in incomplete right bundle branch block. Am Heart J 38:376, 1949
4. Bassingthwaighte JB, Parkin TW, DuShane JW, et al: The electrocardiographic and hemodynamic findings in pulmonary stenosis with intact ventricular septum. Circulation 28:893, 1963
5. Booth RW, Chou TC, Scott RC: Electrocardiographic diagnosis of ventricular hypertrophy in the presence of right bundle branch block. Circulation 18:169, 1958

6. Bove KE, Rowlands DT, Scott RC: Observations on the assessment of cardiac hypertrophy utilizing a chamber partition technique. Circulation 33:558, 1966
7. Burch GE, DePasquale NP: Electrocardiography in the Diagnosis of Congenital Heart Disease. Philadelphia, Lea & Febiger, 1967, p 322
8. Burwell CS, Robin ED, Whaley RD, Bickelman AG: Extreme obesity associated with alveolar hypoventilation: A pickwickian syndrome. Am J Med 21:811, 1956
9. Cabrera E, Monroy JR: Systolic and diastolic loading of the heart: II. Electrocardiographic data. Am Heart J 43:669, 1952.
10. Caird FI, Wilcken DEL: The electrocardiogram in chronic bronchitis with generalized obstructive lung disease: Its relation to ventilatory function. Am J Cardiol 10:5, 1962
11. Camerini F, Goodwin JF, Zoob M: Lead V_{4R} in right ventricular hypertrophy. Br Heart J 18:13, 1956
12. Cayler GG, Ongley P, Nadas AS: Relation of systolic pressure in the right ventricle to the electrocardiogram: A study of patients with pulmonary stenosis and intact ventricular septum. N Engl J Med 258:979, 1958
13. Chou TC, Co P, Helm RA: Vectorcardiographic analysis of T-wave inversion in the right precordial leads. Am Heart J 78:75, 1969
14. Chou TC, Masangkay MP, Young R, et al: Simple quantitative vectorcardiographic criteria for the diagnosis of right ventricular hypertrophy. Circulation 48:1262, 1973
15. Chou TC, Scott RC, Booth RW, et al: Specificity of the current electrocardiographic criteria in the diagnosis of left ventricular hypertrophy. Am Heart J 60:371, 1960
16. Cosby RS, Levinson DC, Dimitroff SP, et al: The electrocardiogram in congenital heart disease and mitral stenosis: A correlation of electrocardiographic pattern with right ventricular pressure, flow and work. Am Heart J 46:670, 1953
17. Flowers NC, Horan LG: IV. Hypertrophy and infarction: Subtle signs of right ventricular enlargement and their relative importance. *In* Schlant RC, Hurst JW (eds): Advances in Electrocardiography. New York, Grune & Stratton, 1972.
18. Fowler NO, Daniels C, Scott RC, et al: The electrocardiogram in cor pulmonale with and without emphysema. Am J Cardiol 16:500, 1965
19. Fowler NO, Noble WJ, Giarratano SJ, et al: The clinical estimation of pulmonary hypertension accompanying mitral stenosis. Am Heart J 49:237, 1955
20. Fowler NO, Westcott RN, Scott RC: The Q wave in precordial electrocardiograms overlying the hypertrophied right ventricle: Intracavity leads. Circulation 5:441, 1952
21. Fraser HRL, Turner R: Electrocardiography in mitral valvular disease. Br Heart J 17:459, 1955
22. Gamboa R, Hugenholtz PG, Nadas AS: Corrected (Frank), uncorrected (cube), and standard electrocardiographic lead systems in recording augmented right ventricular forces in right ventricular hypertension. Br Heart J 28:62, 1966
23. Goodwin JF: The influence of ventricular hypertrophy upon the cardiogram of anterior cardiac infarction. Br Heart J 20:191, 1958
24. Goodwin JF, Abdin ZH: The cardiogram of congenital and acquired right ventricular hypertrophy. Br Heart J 21:523, 1959
25. Hiss RG, Lamb LE, Allen MF: Electrocardiographic findings in 67,375 asymptomatic subjects: X. Normal values. Am J Cardiol 6:200, 1960
26. James FW, Kaplan S: The normal electrocardiogram in the infant and child. Cardiovasc Clin 5:295, 1973
27. Johnson JB, Ferrer MI, West JR, et al: The relation between electrocardiographic evidence of right ventricular hypertrophy and pulmonary arterial pressure in patients with chronic pulmonary disease. Circulation 1:536, 1950
27a. Kamper D, Chou TC, Fowler NO, et al: The reliability of electrocardiographic criteria of chronic obstructive lung disease. Am Heart J 80:445, 1970
28. Kilcoyne MM, Davis AL, Ferrer MI: A dynamic electrocardiographic concept useful in the diagnosis of cor pulmonale: Result of a survey of 200 patients with chronic obstructive pulmonary disease. Circulation 32:903, 1970
29. Kossmann CE, Berger AR, Brumlik J, et al: An analysis of causes of right axis deviation based partly on endocardial potentials of the hypertrophied right ventricle. Am Heart J 35:309, 1948
30. McCaughan D, Primeau RE, Littmann D: The precordial T wave. Am J Cardiol 20:660, 1967
31. Millard FJC: The electrocardiogram in chronic lung disease. Br Heart J 29:43, 1967
32. Myers GB, Klein HA, Stofer BE: The electrocardiographic diagnosis of right ventricular hypertrophy. Am Heart J 35:1, 1948
33. Phillips RW: The electrocardiogram in cor pulmonale secondary to pulmonary emphysema: A study of 18 cases proved by autopsy. Am Heart J 56:352, 1958
34. Pruitt RD, Robinson JG: The electrocardiographic findings in patients undergoing surgical exploration of the mitral valve. Am Heart J 52:881, 1956
35. Ray CT, Horan LG, Flowers NC: An early sign of right ventricular enlargement. J Electrocardiol 3:57, 1970
36. Roman GT Jr, Walsh TJ, Massie E: Right ventricular hypertrophy: Correlation of electrocardiographic and anatomic findings. Am J Cardiol 7:481, 1961
37. Rosenbaum MB, Elizari MV, Lazzari JO: The Hemiblocks. Oldsmar, Fla, Tampa Tracings, 1970, p 94
38. Scott RC: The correlation between the electrocardiographic patterns of ventricular hypertrophy and the anatomic findings. Circulation 21:256, 1960
39. Scott, RC: The electrocardiographic diagnosis of right ventricular hypertrophy: Correlation with the anatomic findings. Am Heart J 60:659, 1960
40. Scott RC: The electrocardiographic diagnosis of right ventricular hypertrophy in the adult. Heart Bull 16:65, 1967
41. Scott RC, Kaplan S, Fowler NO, et al: The electrocardiographic pattern of right ventricular hypertrophy in chronic cor pulmonale. Circulation 11:927, 1955
42. Semler HJ, Pruitt RD: An electrocardiographic estimation of the pulmonary vascular obstruction in 80 patients with mitral stenosis. Am Heart J 59:541, 1960
43. Silver AM, Siderides LE, Antonius NA: The right precordial leads in congenital heart diseases manifesting right ventricular preponderance. Am J Cardiol 3:713, 1959
44. Simonson E: Differentiation Between Normal and Abnormal in Electrocardiography. St Louis, CV Mosby, 1961
45. Sodi-Pallares D: A New Basis of Electrocardiography. St Louis, CV Mosby, 1956, p 49
46. Sokolow M, Lyon TP: The ventricular complex in

right ventricular hypertrophy as obtained by unipolar precordial and limb leads. Am Heart J 38:273, 1949

47. Walker IC, Helm RA, Scott RC: Right ventricular hypertrophy: I. Correlation of isolated right ventricular hypertrophy at autopsy with the electrocardiographic findings. Circulation 11:215, 1955

48. Waler IC, Scott RC, Helm RA: Right ventricular hypertrophy: II. Correlation of electrocardiographic right ventricular hypertrophy with the anatomic findings. Circulation 11:223, 1955

49. Wallace AG, Spach MS, Estes EH, et al: Activation of the normal and hypertrophied human right ventricle. Am Heart J 75:728, 1968

50. Wigle ED, Baron RH: The electrocardiogram in muscular subaortic stenosis: Effect of a left septal incision and right bundle-branch block. Circulation 34:585, 1966

51. Woods A: The electrocardiogram in the tetralogy of Fallot. Br Heart J 14:193, 1952

52. Ziegler RF: Electrocardiographic Studies in Normal Infants and Children. Springfield, Ill, Charles C Thomas, 1951

Combined Ventricular Hypertrophy

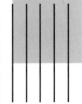

5

In combined ventricular hypertrophy, the increased left and right ventricular forces may counterbalance each other, and no evidence of hypertrophy is detectable in the electrocardiogram (ECG). If the hypertrophy of one ventricle is proportionally greater than that of the other, the ECG findings may be indicative of the dominant ventricle alone. It is only in the minority of the cases that the signs of both left and right ventricular hypertrophy are present in the ECG.

DIAGNOSTIC CRITERIA

The diagnosis of combined ventricular hypertrophy may be made if one of the following criteria is met:

1. The ECG meets one or more of the diagnostic criteria for isolated left and right ventricular hypertrophy.
2. The precordial leads show signs of left ventricular hypertrophy, but the QRS axis in the frontal plane is greater than $+90°$.[7]
3. The R wave is greater than the Q wave in lead aVR and the S wave is greater than the R wave in lead V_5, with T-wave inversion in lead V_1 in conjunction with signs of left ventricular hypertrophy.[6]

CLINICAL AND ANATOMIC CORRELATION

The ECG is an insensitive tool for the recognition of combined ventricular hypertrophy. In a total of 172 cases with anatomic combined ventricular hypertrophy studied by four groups of investigators, the ECG was diagnostic in only 17 percent of cases.[2,4–6] It showed signs of isolated left or right ventricular hypertrophy each in 28 percent of the cases. Most of the patients presented only nonspecific findings. In my own experience, ECG left

ventricular hypertrophy pattern is seen more commonly in patients with anatomic combined hypertrophy than the right ventricular hypertrophy pattern. The secondary right ventricular hypertrophy in patients with hypertensive cardiovascular disease or other types of left-sided heart disease usually is masked by the dominant left ventricular hypertrophy (see Fig. 5–3). The anatomic left ventricular hypertrophy often seen in patients with chronic cor pulmonale, on the other hand, usually is not detectable in the ECG (see Fig. 5–4).

The specificity of the ECG diagnosis of combined ventricular hypertrophy has not been well studied. In an early series, 81 percent of the cases so diagnosed were substantiated by clinical or autopsy findings. The ECG criteria, used, however, were not defined quantitatively.[3] In a small autopsy series I examined, only 10 of 22 cases (45 percent) had anatomic combined ventricular hypertrophy, the remainder showing isolated left ventricular hypertrophy. The criteria most commonly responsible for the false-positive diagnosis of coexisting right ventricular hypertrophy were an R wave in $V_1 > 7$ mm and R in V_1 + S in $V_5V_6 > 10.5$ mm.[1]

Figures 5–1 through 5–7, on pages 70 to 72, illustrate the spectrum of the ECG changes seen in patients with anatomic combined ventricular hypertrophy.

REFERENCES

1. Chou TC, Scott RC, Booth RW, et al: Specificity of the current electrocardiographic criteria in the diagnosis of left ventricular hypertrophy. Am Heart J 60:371, 1960
2. Fraser HRL, Turner R: Electrocardiography in mitral valvular disease. Br Heart J 17:459, 1955
3. Langendorf R, Hurwitz M, Katz LN: Electrocardiographic patterns of combined ventricular strain. Br Heart J 5:27, 1943
4. Levine HD, Phillips E: An appraisal of the newer elec-

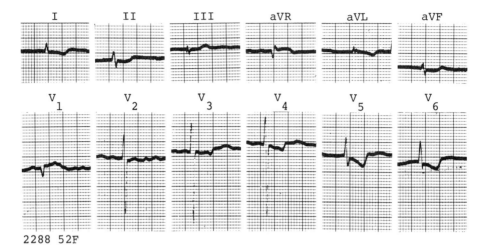

2288 52F

FIGURE 5–1. Combined ventricular hypertrophy with nondiagnostic ECG. The patient was a 52-year-old woman with rheumatic heart disease and severe mitral stenosis, mitral insufficiency, aortic stenosis, and aortic insufficiency. At autopsy, the heart weighed 400 g, with left and right ventricular hypertrophy and left atrial dilatation. The left ventricular wall measured 19 mm in thickness, and the right ventricular wall, 7 to 9 mm. The coronary arteries were widely patent, and there was no evidence of myocardial infarction. The ECG shows atrial fibrillation and low amplitude of the QRS complexes in the limb leads. There are abnormal ST-segment and T-wave changes. There is no evidence, however, of combined ventricular hypertrophy.

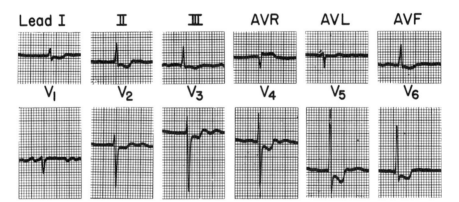

FIGURE 5–2. Combined ventricular hypertrophy with nondiagnostic ECG. The patient was a 56-year-old man with rheumatic heart disease, aortic stenosis and insufficiency, mitral stenosis and insufficiency, and tricuspid insufficiency. At autopsy, the heart weighed 680 g. There were marked dilatation and hypertrophy of the right atrium and right ventricle and mild hypertrophy of the left ventricle. The right ventricular wall measured 6 to 8 mm in thickness, and the left ventricular wall, 15 mm. The ECG shows atrial fibrillation and ST and T-wave abnormalities. The QRS complex shows no definite evidence of either left or right ventricular hypertrophy.

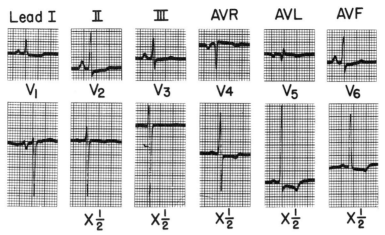

FIGURE 5–3. Anatomic combined ventricular hypertrophy with a left ventricular hypertrophy pattern on ECG. The patient was a 40-year-old man with advanced hypertensive cardiovascular disease and severe congestive heart failure. At autopsy, the heart weighed 550 g, with marked hypertrophy and dilatation of all the heart chambers. The ECG shows left atrial enlargement and left ventricular hypertrophy. No evidence is seen, however, of right ventricular hypertrophy.

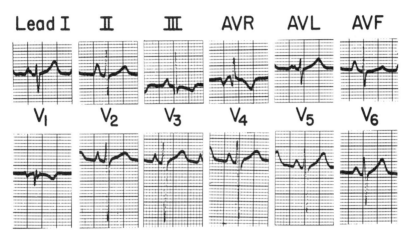

FIGURE 5–4. Combined ventricular hypertrophy with a right ventricular hypertrophy pattern on ECG. The patient was a 25-year-old extremely obese woman (400 pounds). She was believed to have the pickwickian syndrome with chronic cor pulmonale and recurrent pulmonary embolism. At autopsy, the heart weighed 615 g, with marked right ventricular hypertrophy and moderate left ventricular hypertrophy. The right ventricular wall measured 9 mm in thickness, and the left ventricular wall, 19 mm. There also was marked right atrial hypertrophy and dilatation. In the ECG, the P waves are consistent with right atrial enlargement. An abnormal right axis deviation with deep S waves in the left precordial leads suggests right ventricular hypertrophy. There is no evidence to suggest coexisting left ventricular hypertrophy, however.

FIGURE 5–5. Idiopathic dilated cardiomyopathy. The patient was a 45-year-old woman with autopsy-proven idiopathic dilated cardiomyopathy and combined ventricular hypertrophy. The ECG shows evidence of left ventricular hypertrophy. The presence of P waves suggestive of right atrial enlargement and an S wave in lead I suggests coexisting right ventricular hypertrophy, even though definite signs are not observed.

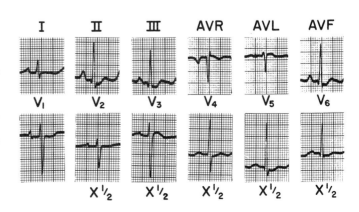

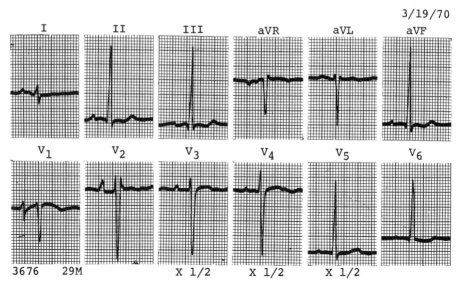

FIGURE 5–6. Rheumatic heart disease with combined ventricular hypertrophy. The patient is a 29-year-old man with severe aortic and mitral valve disease proved at cardiac catheterization and surgery. In the ECG, the P waves are consistent with biatrial enlargement. The frontal plane QRS axis is +90°. This finding, in the presence of signs of left ventricular hypertrophy, suggests coexisting right ventricular hypertrophy.

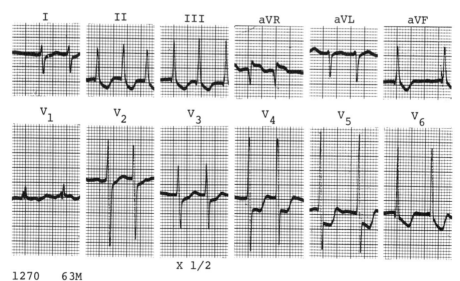

FIGURE 5–7. Combined ventricular hypertrophy demonstrated in the ECG. The patient was a 63-year-old man with severe mitral and aortic stenosis and mild aortic insufficiency. At autopsy, the heart weighed 850 g, with hypertrophy and dilatation of all chambers. The left ventricular wall measured 20 mm in thickness, and the right ventricular wall, 9 mm. The coronary arteries were patent, and there was no evidence of myocardial infarction. The ECG shows atrial fibrillation. The abnormal right axis deviation and the RSR′ pattern in lead V_1 suggest right ventricular hypertrophy. The voltage of the R waves and ST and T-wave changes in the left precordial leads suggest left ventricular hypertrophy. Some of the ST and T changes are the result of digitalis effect.

trocardiography: Correlations in one hundred and fifty consecutive autopsied cases. N Engl J Med 245:833, 1951

5. Lipsett MB, Zinn WJ: Anatomic and electrocardiographic correlation in combined ventricular hypertrophy. Am Heart J 45:86, 1953

6. Pagnoni A, Goodwin JF: The cardiographic diagnosis of combined ventricular hypertrophy. Br Heart J 14:451, 1952

7. Soulie P, Laham J, Papanicolis I, Voci G: Les principaux types electrocardiographiques de surcharge ventriculaire combinee. Arch Mal Coeur 42:791, 1949

Left Bundle Branch Block

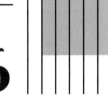

6

The interruption of the impulse conduction through the left bundle branch results in the initiation of ventricular activation at the base of the anterior papillary muscle of the right ventricle through the right bundle branch. The early ventricular excitation involves the right septum, apex, and ventricular free wall. Because the electrical forces from the right septum and the free wall are opposite in direction, they are mostly cancelled by each other. The manifested early forces originate from the endocardium-to-epicardium depolarization of the right ventricular apex. The initial QRS vectors are therefore directed leftward, anteriorly, and inferiorly. The leftward orientation of the initial forces explains the absence of the normal "septal" Q wave in lead I and in the left precordial leads, since these forces now point toward the positive end of these leads. As the right-to-left septal activation continues and involves the left septum, the forces generated are oriented leftward, posteriorly, and inferiorly. The leftward direction of the ventricular forces remains as the activation process proceeds in the free wall of the left ventricle. As a result, leads I, V_5, and V_6 continue to inscribe an upward deflection. Because the conduction pathway is abnormal and does not follow the Purkinje network, slurring and notching of the R wave occur. The increase in the time required for the completion of the activation process prolongs the QRS duration to 0.12 second or more.

Abnormal ventricular depolarization in left bundle branch block is associated with secondary alteration of the recovery process. The repolarization also proceeds in a generally right-to-left direction. Because the electrical forces that result from repolarization are opposite in polarity to those generated from depolarization when the process advances in the same direction, the ST and T vectors are therefore discordant to the QRS. ST-segment depression and T-wave inversion are observed in leads I, V_5, and V_6, where the major deflection of the QRS complex is upright.

DIAGNOSTIC CRITERIA FOR COMPLETE LEFT BUNDLE BRANCH BLOCK[10,54]

1. QRS duration of 0.12 second or greater.
2. Presence of a broad monophasic R wave in leads I, V_5, and V_6, which is usually notched or slurred.
3. Absence of Q waves in leads I, V_5, and V_6.
4. Delay of onset of the intrinsicoid deflection (the R peak time) in leads V_5 and V_6.
5. Displacement of ST segment and T wave in a direction opposite to the major deflection of the QRS complex.

OTHER ELECTROCARDIOGRAPHIC FINDINGS IN COMPLETE LEFT BUNDLE BRANCH BLOCK

1. Poor progression of the R wave in the right and mid-precordial leads (Fig. 6–1). Because most of the QRS forces are directed leftward and posteriorly in complete left bundle branch block, the R wave in the right and mid-precordial leads usually is small. One may occasionally observe a decrease in the amplitude of the R wave from lead V_1 through V_3 or V_4 in uncomplicated left bundle branch block. The S waves in these leads are broad and often slurred and notched. A QS deflection also may be recorded in these leads without the presence of myocardial infarction. Because the ST segment usually is elevated in the right precordial leads, an erroneous diagnosis of acute myocardial infarction may be made.
2. RS complex in the left precordial leads. Although leads V_5 and V_6 typically present a nonphasic R wave, an RS deflection occasionally may be seen. This usually is observed in patients with massively enlarged hearts. A monophasic R wave usually is demonstrated if

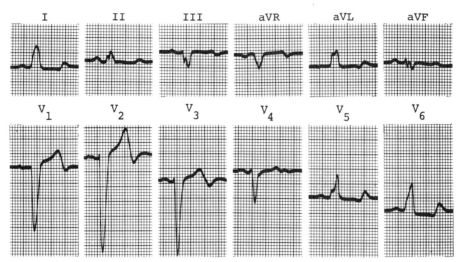

FIGURE 6–1. Benign left bundle branch block. The patient is a 29-year-old, otherwise healthy athlete. No other clinical evidence of heart disease was found.

leads V_7 and V_8 are recorded. In patients who also have abnormal left axis deviation, the superiorly directed QRS forces may project on the negative side of the lead axes of V_5 and V_6, which are directed slightly inferiorly as well as leftward. Consequently, RS complexes rather than monophasic R waves are recorded in these leads.

3. Abnormal left axis deviation. It has been reported that left bundle branch block does not significantly change the QRS axis in the frontal plane,[21] and some investigators believe that most patients with left bundle branch block and left axis deviation have left anterior hemiblock separately.[31] In a study of 98 cases of intermittent left bundle branch block, however, Rosenbaum and associates found that a marked shift of the QRS axis may occur from left bundle branch block alone.[37] In about 70 percent of the cases, a leftward displacement of the axis was observed. The average degree of change was 40° with a range of 2° to 160°. In the remainder, a rightward shift or no shift had occurred. In patients with QRS axes superior to −45° during left bundle branch block, only 30 percent showed the abnormal left axis in the absence of the bundle branch block. Therefore, the bundle branch block is responsible for the marked left axis deviation in most. This conclusion also is supported by an analysis of 231 cases of intermittent left bundle branch block performed by Swiryn and associates.[47] Figure 6–2 illustrates the left displacement of the QRS axis as a result of left bundle branch block. The patient had hypertensive cardiovascular and coronary artery disease with myocardial infarction proved at au-

topsy. In leads I and II, the intraventricular conduction becomes more normal in the beats after the postextrasystolic pauses. The QRS axis of these beats is normal.

The axis shift in left bundle branch block may be explained by the manner or the earliest site that the activation front arrives. If the right-to-left transeptal activation arrives at the Purkinje network of the posterior division of the left bundle first, the delay of excitation of the anterior and lateral wall of the left ventricle results in a leftward shift of the QRS axis. If it arrives at the anterior division first, or reaches both divisions simultaneously, the axis is shifted rightward or remains normal.

4. QS deflection in the inferior leads, which may be present without anatomic demonstration of inferior myocardial infarction. In patients with intermittent left bundle branch block, Q waves in the inferior leads often disappear when the ventricular conduction becomes normal.[1,48]

CLINICAL AND PATHOLOGIC CORRELATION

Clinical Significance

Coronary artery disease and hypertensive heart disease, or a combination of the two, are the most common causes of left bundle branch block (see Figs. 6–2 and 6–3). In an early study of a group of 555 patients with this conduction defect, Johnson and associates found that hypertension was the most common cause.[20] Later reports, however, sug-

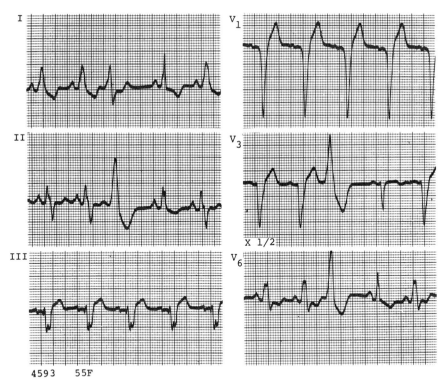

FIGURE 6–2. Complete left bundle branch block in a 55-year-old man with hypertensive and coronary heart disease. The cardiac diagnosis was supported by clinical and pathologic findings. An area of myocardial infarction involving the apex of the left ventricle was found at autopsy. The heart weighed 525 g, with marked left ventricular hypertrophy and moderate right ventricular hypertrophy. In the ECG, the basic complexes show typical complete left bundle branch block pattern. The frontal plane QRS axis is about −30°. A partial normalization of the QRS complex occurs in the postventricular extrasystolic beats. The QRS axis in these beats is normal.

gested that most patients (about 70 percent) had evidence of ischemic heart disease.[5,43] In the Framingham study, Schneider and associates reported the appearance of new left bundle branch block in 55 of the 5209 people followed for 18 years.[41] The conduction defect occurred mostly in subjects with antecedent hypertension, cardiomegaly, coronary heart disease, or a combination of these. Because the left bundle branch receives blood from both the anterior descending branch of the left coronary artery and the right coronary artery, complete interruption of the bundle branch usually implies involvement of both vessels.[19] The lesion usually is severe.[17] Left bundle branch block is observed in 2 to 4 percent of patients with acute myocardial infarction, about 1 percent of the cases being caused by the acute event.[35,40] Most of the infarctions are anterior in location.[35]

Other types of heart disease often associated with left bundle branch block include primary and secondary cardiomyopathy, rheumatic heart disease, calcific aortic stenosis, and luetic heart disease. About 15 percent of patients with primary myocardial disease manifest this conduction defect.[32] Wood reported an incidence of left bundle branch block of 14 percent in 250 patients with aortic stenosis.[55] Sclerosis and calcification of the left side of the cardiac skeleton, or Lev disease, occasionally may be the cause of this conduction defect in elderly subjects[29] (Fig. 6–4).

Left bundle branch block occasionally is seen in the absence of overt heart disease. In some of the patients, it is caused by primary degenerative disease of the conduction system.[12,26] Others may have benign left bundle branch block (see Fig. 6–1). In the 10 patients reported on by Beach and associates, cardiac catheterization and coronary arteriography showed no significant abnormalities.[8] It was suggested that the continued minimal hemodynamic trauma to the origin of the left bundle branch may be responsible for the conduction defect in these individuals.

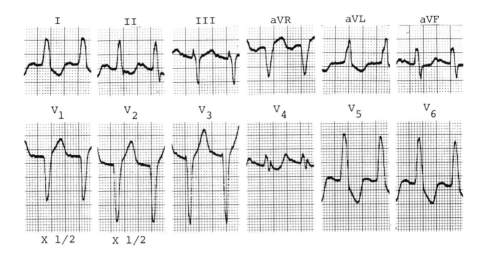

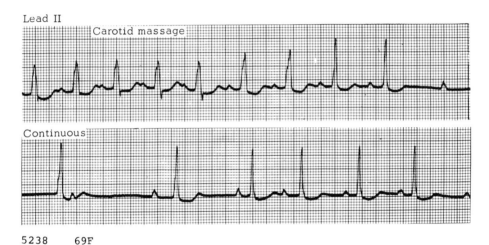

5238   69F

FIGURE 6–3. Complete left bundle branch block with normal intraventricular conduction during carotid sinus massage. The patient is a 69-year-old woman with diabetes mellitus, hypertension, coronary artery disease, and congestive heart failure. The 12-lead tracing shows complete left bundle branch block. With carotid sinus massage, a slowing of the heart rate occurred, with normalization of intraventricular conduction. Transient AV block was induced during the massage.

Pathologic Correlation

In a study of the anatomic basis of left bundle branch block in 25 patients, Lenegre found total destruction of the left bundle branch in 9 and subtotal destruction in 9.[27] There were partial lesions in 5 and no lesion in 2 of the patients. In a later report from the same institution summarizing the examination of 48 cases of complete left bundle block branch, significant lesions in the left bundle were found in 44 patients.[3] One patient had only partial lesion, and 3 patients had no lesion in the left bundle branch.

In eight cases examined by Lev and associates,[28] serial sections of the conduction system revealed marked involvement of the main left bundle in all. The region affected was the junction point between the bundle of His and the main left bundle. They also found that there was no difference in the pathologic findings in the left bundle branch between patients with left axis deviation and those with a normal QRS axis. They suggested that sclerosis of the left side of the cardiac skeleton, including the summit of the ventricular septum, may be partially responsible for the development of the bundle branch block in some patients. Figure 6–4 gives an example of this entity.

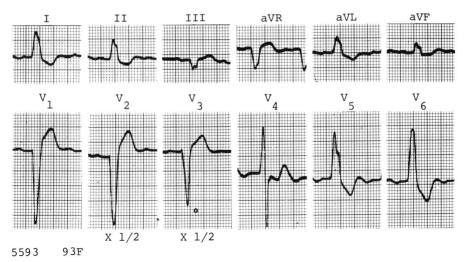

5593   93F

FIGURE 6–4. Left bundle branch block resulting from sclerosis of the left side of the cardiac skeleton or Lev's disease. The patient was a 93-year-old woman with severe calcification and stenosis of the aortic and mitral valves. There also was calcification of the mitral annulus and base of the aorta. The pathologic findings were believed to represent the result of sclerosis of the left side of the cardiac skeleton. There was cardiomegaly with left ventricular hypertrophy. Only mild atherosclerosis of the coronary arteries was found, with no evidence of myocardial infarction.

Prognosis

The prognosis of patients with left bundle branch block varies considerably, depending largely on the cause and other associated clinical findings. In the absence of other demonstrable evidence of heart disease, the prognosis is generally favorable.[23,36,38] Many such patients continue to live normal lives with no restrictions of physical activity. Rotman and Triebwasser reported a clinical and follow-up study of left bundle branch block in 121 Air Force flying personnel and applicants.[38] The mean age of the subject was 40 ± 7 years, with a range of 20 to 56 years at the time of diagnosis. One hundred and eight (89 percent) of the subjects had no evidence of cardiovascular disease at the time of initial examination. Eleven (9 percent) and 8 (7 percent) of those studied had coronary heart disease and hypertension, respectively. In a mean follow-up period of 8.8 ± 4.8 years of 114 subjects, coronary artery disease and hypertension developed in 6 (5 percent) and 9 (8 percent), respectively. Nine subjects (8 percent) died.

In a representative sample of adult population included in the Framingham study, Schneider and associates reported the development of left bundle branch block in 55 subjects during 18 years of observation.[41] Forty-nine (89 percent) of those subjects had clinically apparent cardiovascular abnormalities before, coincident with, or after the onset of left bundle branch block. Fifty percent of the patients died from cardiovascular disease within 10 years of the onset of left bundle branch block. These investigators also found that patients who had no evidence of left atrial abnormalities, QRS axes of 0° or greater, or normal electrocardiograms (ECGs) before the appearance of left bundle branch block were more likely to remain free of clinical cardiovascular disease than those with one or more of these abnormalities.[42] In hospital-based studies, the average survival time of patients with left bundle branch block was reported to be about 3 years,[20,45] but the survival time in the individual patients depends largely on the type and severity of the underlying heart disease. In 60 patients with chronic left bundle branch block followed prospectively by Denes and co-workers, 21 (35 percent) died suddenly within 3 years.[11] The number of non-sudden deaths directly related to cardiovascular disease was much smaller, but a specific figure was not given. Ventricular fibrillation but not bradyarrhythmias appeared to be the mechanism of sudden death in most of those patients. McAnulty and associates studied 104 patients with chronic left bundle branch block prospectively.[34] Twenty-one percent of the patients died in 2 years, and 11 percent died suddenly. These authors also noted that complete AV block was an uncommon cause of sudden death in these patients. Freedman and associates reviewed the clinical data of 250 patients with left bundle branch block with coronary artery disease included in the Coronary Artery Surgery Study (CASS).[15] They found that patients with left bundle branch block had a higher incidence of congestive heart failure, worse left ventricular function, and more extensive coronary artery disease than those without the conduction defect. The presence of left bundle branch block also contributed to increased risk of death independent of the extent of left ventricular dysfunction and coronary artery disease. The mechanism by which left bundle branch block independently contributes to mortality could not be determined, however. Patients with acute myocardial infarction and left bundle branch block carry a poor prognosis. Mortality in these patients is high, varying between 22 and 65 percent.[1,18,35,40] Among the 163 patients with acute myocardial infarction and left bundle branch block reported by Hindman and associates, the hospital mortality was 24 percent and 1-year follow-up mortality was 32 percent, with a total mortality of 48 percent.[18] High-degree AV block was a major contributing factor for the increased hospital mortality.

DIVISIONAL VERSUS PREDIVSISIONAL LEFT BUNDLE BRANCH BLOCK

By convention, left bundle branch block implies the interruption of conduction in the main left bundle branch. This is supported by the demonstration of pathologic lesions in most cases. The same ECG pattern also may be observed, however, when lesions exist simultaneously in both the anterior and posterior divisions of the left bundle branch. The term *divisional left bundle branch block* is used when left anterior and left posterior hemiblocks coexist.[37] Although the assumption appears to be reasonable, histologic studies to support this variety of left bundle branch block are lacking.

TRANSIENT AND INTERMITTENT LEFT BUNDLE BRANCH BLOCK

In transient left bundle branch block, normal intraventricular conduction subsequently returns, if only temporarily[7] (Fig. 6–5). The condition also has been called *paroxysmal,*

unstable, or *temporary* left bundle branch block. Its origin is similar to that of the stable variety, with most patients having ischemic or hypertensive heart disease or both. Transient bundle branch block may complicate acute myocardial infarction or may occur during attacks of angina. It may appear during an episode of congestive heart failure and disappear with improvement of the cardiac status. Most patients eventually have permanent block. Occasionally, however, the patient may revert to normal conduction even years after consistently demonstrating the block.

Intermittent left bundle branch block is distinguished from transient left bundle branch block by the presence of complexes that show the block and normal conduction in a single ECG recording or within a short period while the patient's clinical status is unchanged (Fig. 6–6). The underlying heart diseases, however, are similar to those of the transient or permanent form of block. It is also seen in apparently healthy individuals.[23] It may appear allorhythmically. An example of alternating 2:1 left bundle branch block is given in Figure 6–7.

In both transient and intermittent left bundle branch block, the appearance and disappearance of the conduction defect often is related to the heart rate (see Figs. 6–3 and 6–5). There frequently is a critical heart rate above which left bundle branch block appears and below which normal conduction returns.[6,53] Prolongation of the refractory period of the left bundle branch as a result of an anatomic or functional lesion is responsible for its failure of conduction at higher rate. Various maneuvers, such as deep inspiration, carotid sinus stimulation, and pharmacologic agents, have been used to slow the heart rate and normalize the conduction.[48] Rarely, the heart rate has a paradoxical effect. Bundle branch block occurs when the rate is slower.[13,33,52] Figure 6–8 gives an example of such bradycardia-dependent left bundle branch block. This phenomenon has been attributed to the spontaneous depolarization during diastole (phase 4 depolarization) of the bundle branch at slower heart rate and thus becomes refractory to the next arriving impulse.[28]

In many patients, the unstable intraventricular conduction defect has no relationship to the heart rate (see Fig. 6–6). Hemodynamic factors may play a major role in some of the patients, whereas no apparent cause can be found in the others.

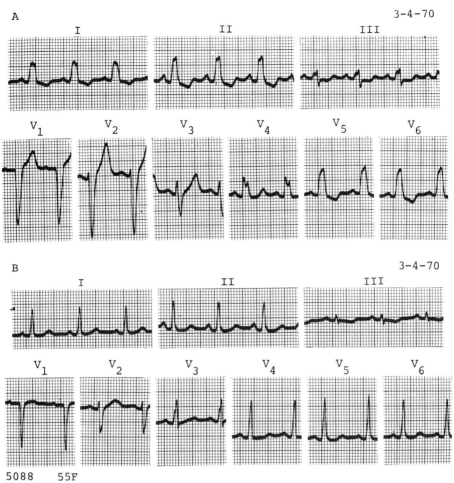

A   3-4-70

B   3-4-70

5088   55F

FIGURE 6–5. Transient left bundle branch block. The patient was a 55-year-old woman with a history of chest pain but with a normal coronary arteriogram. (A) Complete left bundle branch block pattern. Tracing taken later on the same day when the heart rate was slower showed normal intraventricular conduction (B). The relation between the heart rate and left bundle branch block was demonstrated repeatedly.

INCOMPLETE LEFT BUNDLE BRANCH BLOCK

The ECG diagnosis of incomplete left bundle branch block has been a controversial subject. Using intracavitory recordings in humans with apparently incomplete left bundle branch block, Sodi-Pallares and associates demonstrated a reversal of the direction of septal activation in patients with incomplete left bundle branch block that was similar to that found in patients with complete left bundle branch block.[46] They proposed that the presence of initial slurring of the R waves in leads I, aVL, V_5, and V_6 and the absence of Q waves in these leads (even though this is not necessary) were indications of this conduction defect. The duration of the QRS may be less than 0.10 sec-

ond. Later study by others did not confirm their findings,[25] but many clinical observations do support the existence of such an entity.[4,16,39] Figure 6–8 illustrates the various degrees of incomplete left bundle branch block in addition to complete left bundle branch block in a patient with coronary artery disease. Similar examples were given by Fisch and Miles.[13]

Diagnostic Criteria

The following criteria are adapted from those used by Unger and co-workers,[51] except that a QRS duration of 0.10 to 0.11 second instead of 0.10 to 0.12 second is used. At least three of the four criteria have to be met for the di-

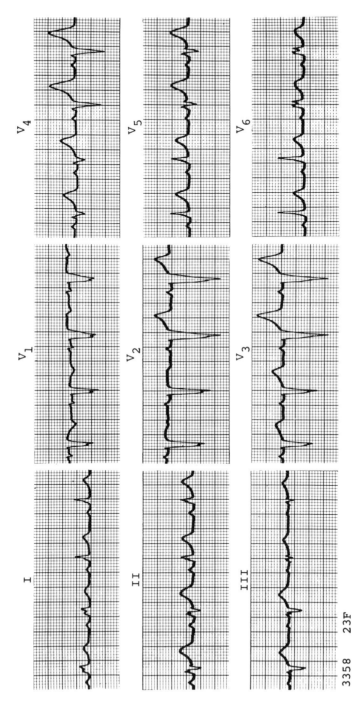

3358   23F

FIGURE 6–6. Intermittent left bundle branch block unrelated to heart rate. The patient was a 23-year-old woman with cardiomegaly, probably caused by cardiomyopathy. The ECG reveals intermittent patterns of complete and incomplete left bundle branch block. The change in the intraventricular conduction is not related to heart rate. Cardiac catheterization, including left ventriculogram performed 2 years later when the patient's clinical condition was considerably improved, revealed no abnormal findings.

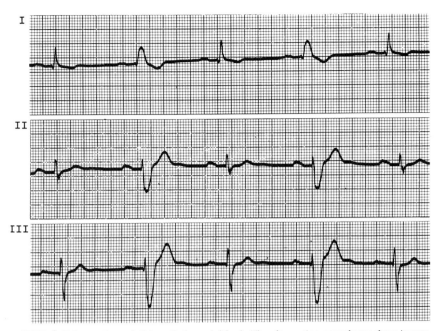

FIGURE 6-7. Intermittent left bundle branch block. The alternating complexes show incomplete and complete left bundle branch block. There also is a first-degree AV block. The P waves are suggestive of left atrial enlargement.

agnosis of incomplete left bundle branch block to be made (see Figs. 6-6 and 6-9).

1. A QRS duration of 0.10 to 0.11 second.
2. Prolongation of the time of onset of the intrinsicoid deflection to at least 0.06 second in the left precordial leads.
3. Absence of a Q wave in the left precordial leads.
4. Notching or slurring of the ascending limb of the R wave in the left precordial leads.

Unger and co-workers performed comprehensive pathologic studies of the conduction system and myocardium in four patients that met these criteria.[51] A close correlation was found between the assumed block from the ECG findings and the lesions of the left bundle branch.

It is a common clinical observation that the ECGs of many patients with left ventricular hypertrophy present the findings of incomplete left bundle branch block (see Fig. 6-9). The question often is raised whether this conduction defect coexists with left ventricular hypertrophy or the changes are secondary to left ventricular hypertrophy alone. Because of the limited number of hearts that have been examined in detail in regard to the conduction system, this question remains unanswered.

DIAGNOSIS OF VENTRICULAR HYPERTROPHY IN THE PRESENCE OF LEFT BUNDLE BRANCH BLOCK

Left Ventricular Hypertrophy

Because of the abnormal sequence of ventricular activation in left bundle branch block, the resultant electrical forces are altered both in amplitude and direction. The usual voltage criteria for the diagnosis of ventricular hypertrophy are no longer applicable. Scott and Norris correlated the ECG and the pathologic findings in 29 cases of complete left bundle branch block.[44] Anatomic left ventricular hypertrophy was found in all, but the ECGs fulfilled the usual criteria for left ventricular hypertrophy in only 17 patients (60 percent). Zmyslinski and associates found anatomic left ventricular hypertrophy at autopsy in all but 2 of 43 cases of complete left bundle branch block.[56] In those patients in whom the ECGs before the development of left bundle branch block were also available for study, the abnormally high QRS voltage tended to fall after the conduction defect appeared. Thus, most patients with the pattern of complete bundle branch block have anatomic left ventricular hypertrophy, but the diagnosis can be made only by inference in many cases. Because most patients with left bundle branch block have

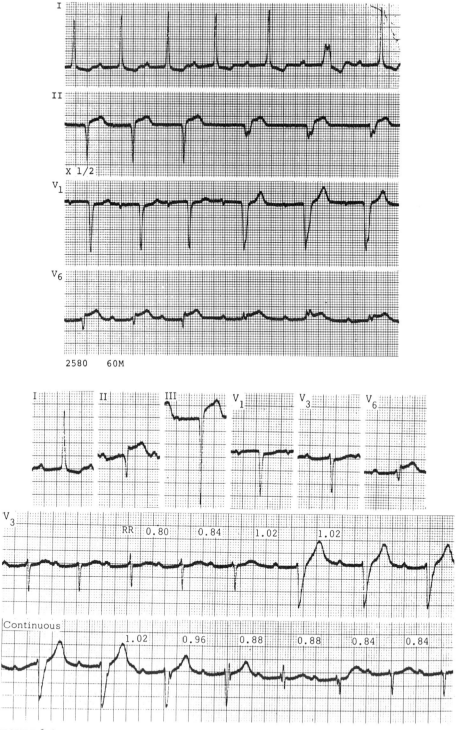

FIGURE 6–8. Bradycardia-dependent bundle branch block. The patient is a 60-year-old man with coronary artery disease and inferior and anterior myocardial infarction. The tracing illustrates the appearance of incomplete and complete left bundle branch block when the heart rate is slower.

organic heart disease, however, ventricular hypertrophy is likely to be present when the patients come to autopsy. The close correlation between left bundle branch block and anatomic left ventricular hypertrophy demonstrated at autopsy may not be true in clinical practice. Klein and colleagues used echocardiography to separate patients with left bundle branch block with or without left ventricular hypertrophy.[22] They reported a sensitivity

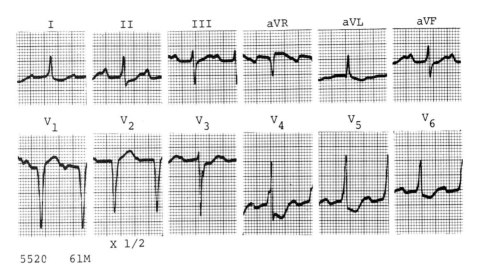

FIGURE 6–9. Incomplete left bundle branch block. The patient was a 61-year-old man who had aortic valve perforations due to bacterial endocarditis and severe triple vessel coronary artery disease, with anteroseptal myocardial infarction proved at autopsy. The tracing was recorded 3 days before death. The heart weighed 550 g, with biventricular hypertrophy. The ECG shows first-degree AV block, left ventricular hypertrophy, and possible previous anteroseptal myocardial infarction. The QRS duration is 0.10 second. There is no Q wave, but there is slurring of the initial part of the R wave in leads I and V_4 through V_6. Notching of the QRS complex is present in leads V_3 and V_4. The time of onset of the intrinsicoid deflection in V_6 is 0.06 second.

of 86 percent and a specificity of 100 percent using the criterion of $SV_2 + RV_6 > 45$ mm for the diagnosis of left ventricular hypertrophy. A QRS duration greater than 160 msec plus left atrial enlargement also strongly supported the diagnosis. The reliability of these criteria was not verified, however, by autopsy study.[14]

Right Ventricular Hypertrophy

The recognition of right ventricular hypertrophy in the presence of left bundle branch block generally has been considered untenable. In a vectorcardiographic study, however, Chou and Helm reported on five cases of atypical left bundle branch block with anatomic or hemodynamic evidence of right ventricular hypertrophy.[9] The QRS loop resembled that of the classical left bundle branch block except that it was displaced rightward. In the conventional ECG, an S wave was present in lead I and sometimes also in leads V_5 and V_6 (Fig. 6–10). Similar cases also were reported by Tranchesi and co-workers.[50] The precordial leads

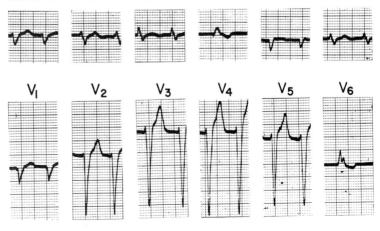

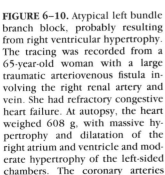

FIGURE 6–10. Atypical left bundle branch block, probably resulting from right ventricular hypertrophy. The tracing was recorded from a 65-year-old woman with a large traumatic arteriovenous fistula involving the right renal artery and vein. She had refractory congestive heart failure. At autopsy, the heart weighed 608 g, with massive hypertrophy and dilatation of the right atrium and ventricle and moderate hypertrophy of the left-sided chambers. The coronary arteries were normal. Multiple pulmonary emboli, both recent and old, were observed. The ECG shows atrial fibrillation. The precordial leads are consistent with left bundle branch block. The limb leads show right axis deviation with a prominent S wave in lead I.

were consistent with left bundle branch block, but the limb leads revealed abnormal right axis deviation. From the clinical data, the authors proposed that right ventricular hypertrophy may be one of the factors responsible for the abnormal right axis deviation.

REFERENCES

1. Abben R, Denes P, Rosen KM: Evaluation of criteria for diagnosis of myocardial infarction: Study of 256 patients with intermittent left bundle branch block. Chest 75:575, 1979
2. Atkins JM, Leshin SJ, Blomqvist G, et al: Ventricular conduction blocks and sudden death in acute myocardial infarction: Potential indications for pacing. N Engl J Med 288:281, 1973
3. Baragan J, Maurice P, Lenegre J: Block complet de la branche gauche at infarctus du myocarde. Arch Mal Coeur 56:445, 1963
4. Barold SS, Linart JW, Hildner FJ, et al: Incomplete left bundle-branch block: A definite electrocardiographic entity. Circulation 38:702, 1968
5. Bauer GE: Bundle branch block: Some usual and some unusual features. Austarlas Ann Med 13:62, 1964
6. Bauer GE: Bundle branch block under voluntary control. Br Heart J 26:167, 1964
7. Bauer GE: Transient bundle-branch block. Circulation 29:730, 1964
8. Beach TB, Gracey JG, Peter RH, et al: Benign left bundle branch block. Ann Intern Med 70:269, 1969
9. Chou TC, Helm RA: The diagnosis of right ventricular hypertrophy in the presence of left bundle branch block. *In* Hoffman I (ed): Vectorcardiography 2: Proceedings of the XIth International Symposium on Vectorcardiography. New York, North-Holland, 1971
10. Criteria Committee of the New York Heart Association: Diseases of the Heart and Blood Vessels, Nomenclature and Criteria for Diagnosis. Boston, Little, Brown, 1969
11. Denes P, Dhingra RC, Wu D, et al: Sudden death in patients with chronic bifascicular block. Arch Intern Med 137:1005, 1977
12. Dhingra RC, Amat-Y-Leon F, Wyndham C, et al: Significance of left axis deviation in patients with chronic left bundle branch block. Am J Cardiol 42:551, 1978
13. Fisch C, Miles WM: Deceleration-dependent left bundle branch block: A spectrum of bundle branch conduction delay. Circulation 65:1029, 1982
14. Flowers NC: Left bundle branch block: A continuously evolving concept. J Am Coll Cardiol 9:684, 1987
15. Freedman RA, Alderman EL, Sheffield LT, et al: Bundle branch block in patients with chronic coronary artery disease: Angiographic correlates and prognostic significance. J Am Coll Cardiol 10:73, 1987
16. Gardberg M, Rosen IL: Electrocardiogram and vectorcardiogram in various degrees of left bundle branch block. Am J Cardiol 1:592, 1958
17. Haft JI, Herman MV, Gorlin R: Left bundle branch block: Etiologic, hemodynamic, and ventriculographic considerations. Circulation 43:279, 1971
18. Hindman MC, Wagner GS, JaRo M, et al: The clinical significance of bundle branch block complicating acute myocardial infarction: I. Clinical characteris-

tics, hospital mortality, and one-year follow-up. Circulation 58:679, 1978
19. James TN, Burch GE: Blood supply of the human interventricular septum. Circulation 17:391, 1958
20. Johnson RP, Messer L, Shreenivas, et al: Prognosis in bundle branch block: II. Factors influencing the survival period in left bundle branch block. Am Heart J 41:225, 1951
21. Jones AN, Feil H: Axis deviation in human bundle branch block. Am Heart J 36:98, 1948
22. Klein RC, Vera Z, DeMaria JA, et al: Electrocardiographic diagnosis of left ventricular hypertrophy in the presence of left bundle branch block. Am Heart J 108:502, 1984
23. Krikler DM, Lefevre A: Intermittent left bundle-branch block without obvious heart disease. Lancet 1:498, 1970
24. Lamb LE: Electrocardiography and Vectorcardiography: Instrumentation, Fundamentals and Clinical Applications. Philadelphia, WB Saunders, 1965, p 306
25. Leighton RF, Ryan JM, Goodwin RS, et al: Incomplete left bundle-branch block: The view from transseptal intraventricular leads. Circulation 36:261, 1967
26. Lenegre J: Etiology and pathology of bilateral bundle branch block in relation to heart block. Prog Cardiovasc Dis 6:409, 1964
27. Lenegre J: Contribution à l'Étude des Blocs de Branche. Paris, JB Bailliere et Fils, 1958
28. Lev M, Unger PN, Rosen KM, et al: The anatomic substrate of complete left bundle branch block. Circulation 50:479, 1974
29. Lev M: Anatomic basis for atrioventricular block. Am J Med 37:742, 1964
30. Lewis CM, Dagenais GR, Friesinger GC, et al: Coronary arteriographic appearances in patients with left bundle branch block. Circulation 41:299, 1970
31. Lichstein E, Mahapatra R, Gupta PK, et al: Significance of complete left bundle branch block with left axis deviation. Am J Cardiol 44:243, 1979
32. Marriott HJL: Electrocardiographic abnormalities, conduction disorders and arrhythmias in primary myocardial disease. Prog Cardiovasc Dis 7:99, 1964
33. Massumi RA: Bradycardio-dependent bundle-branch block: A critique and proposed criteria. Circulation 38:1066, 1968
34. McAnulty JH, Rahimtoola SH, Murphy ES, et al: A prospective study of sudden death in "high risk" bundle-branch block. N Engl J Med 299:209, 1978
35. Nimetz AA, Shubrooks SJ, Hutter AM, et al: The significance of bundle branch block during acute myocardial infarction. Am Heart J 90:439, 1975
36. Rodstein M, Gubner R, Mills JP, et al: A mortality study in bundle branch block. Arch Interm Med 87:663, 1951
37. Rosenbaum MB, Elizari MV, Lazzari JO: The Hemiblocks. Oldsmar, Fla, Tampa Tracings, 1970
38. Rotman M, Triebwasser JH: A clinical and follow-up study of right and left bundle branch block. Circulation 51:477, 1975
39. Schamroth L, Bradlow BA: Incomplete left bundle branch block. Br Heart J 26:285, 1964
40. Scheidt S, Killip T: Bundle-branch block complicating acute myocardial infarction. JAMA 222:919, 1972
41. Schneider JF, Thomas HE, Kreger BE, et al: Newly acquired left bundle-branch block: The Framingham study. Ann Intern Med 90:303, 1979
42. Schneider JF, Thomas HE, McNamara PM, Kannel WB: Clinical–electrocardiographic correlates of newly acquired left bundle branch block: The Framingham study. Am J Cardiol 55:1332, 1985

43. Scott RC: Left bundle branch block: A clinical assessment: Part I. Am Heart J 70:535, 1965

44. Scott RC, Norris RJ: Electrocardiographic–pathologic correlation study of left ventricular hypertrophy in the presence of left bundle-branch block. Circulation 20:766, 1959

45. Smith A, Hayes WL: The prognosis of complete left bundle branch block. Am Heart J 70:157, 1965

46. Sodi-Pallares D, Estandia A, Soberson J, et al: Left intraventricular potential of the human heart: II. Criteria for diagnosis of incomplete bundle branch block. Am Heart J 40:655, 1950

47. Swiryn S, Abben R, Denes P, et al: Electrocardiographic determinants of axis during left bundle branch block: Study in patients with intermittent left bundle branch block. Am J Cardiol 46:46, 1980

48. Tavazzi L, Salerno JA, Chimienti M, et al: Tachycardia-dependent and bradycardia-dependent intraventricular conduction defects in acute myocardial infarction: Electrocardiographic, electrophysiologic, and clinical correlates. Am Heart J 102:675, 1981

49. Timmis GC, Gangadharan V, Ramos RG, Gordon S: Reassessment of Q waves in left bundle branch block. J Electrocardiol 9:109, 1976

50. Tranchesi J, Moffa P, Ebaid M: Right axis deviation in left bundle branch block: An electrovectorcardiographic study. *In* Hoffman I (ed): Vectorcardiography 2: Proceedings of the XIth International Symposium on Vectorcardiography. New York, North-Holland, 1971

51. Unger PN, Greenblatt M, Lev M: The anatomic basis of the electrocardiographic abnormality in incomplete left bundle branch block. Am Heart J 76:486, 1968

52. Vesell H, Lowen G: Bundle branch block on cardiac slowing at a critical slow heart rate. Am Heart J 66:329, 1963

53. Vesell H: Critical rates in ventricular conduction: Unstable bundle branch block. Am J Med Sci 202:198, 1941

54. Willems JL, Robles deMedina EO, Bernard R, et al: Criteria for intraventricular conduction disturbances and pre-excitation. J Am Coll Cardiol 5:1261, 1985

55. Wood P: Aortic stenosis. Am J Cardiol 1:553, 1958

56. Zmyslinski RW, Richeson JF, Akiyama T: Left ventricular hypertrophy in presence of complete left bundle-branch block. Br Heart J 43:170, 1980

Right Bundle Branch Block

7

In right bundle branch block, the interruption of impulse conduction in the right bundle branch delays the activation of the right ventricle. The left ventricle is depolarized in a normal fashion by the intact left bundle branch, but right ventricular activation is altered, since it now depends on impulse propagated from the left ventricle. The left and right ventricles are depolarized sequentially rather than simultaneously. The time required for the completion of ventricular excitation or the QRS duration is prolonged to 0.12 second or more.

Normally, the morphology of the QRS complex recorded from the body surface is determined mainly by the dominant left ventricular potential. In right bundle branch block, because the left ventricular activation proceeds normally, the early part of the QRS complex (usually 0.03 to 0.04 second) remains essentially unchanged. As the left ventricular excitation is near completion and the delayed abnormal activation of the right ventricular septum and free wall begins, changes of the QRS complex occur. The left-to-right activation of the right ventricle is associated with QRS forces directed anteriorly and rightward. Because these late forces are no longer opposed by the left ventricular potential, prominent positive deflection (R′) is recorded in the right precordial leads. The left precordial leads V_5 and V_6, as well as lead I, record a terminal S wave. Because the spread of impulse is abnormal and proceeds mainly by the slower muscle-to-muscle conduction, these terminal deflections are wide and slurred.

The abnormal sequence of ventricular activation is accompanied by a change in the course of repolarization. The latter also proceeds in a generally left-to-right direction. The ST and T vectors are therefore directed leftward and opposite to the terminal part of the QRS complex.

DIAGNOSTIC CRITERIA

The diagnosis of complete right bundle branch block is made when the following criteria are met[46]:

1. Prolongation of QRS duration to 0.12 second or greater.
2. A secondary R wave (R′) in the right precordial leads, with the R′ greater than the initial R wave (i.e., rsR′ or rSR′).
3. A delay in the onset of the intrinsicoid deflection in the right precordial leads greater than 0.05 second.
4. A wide S wave in leads I, V_5, and V_6.

OTHER ELECTROCARDIOGRAPHIC FINDINGS IN RIGHT BUNDLE BRANCH BLOCK

The QRS complex in complete right bundle branch block may be divided into two parts. The first portion is sometimes called the unblocked part, which is slender and normally inscribed and occupies the first 0.06 to 0.08 second of the QRS interval. The development of right bundle branch block does not alter the initial components (usually 0.03 to 0.04 second) of this normally inscribed portion of the QRS complex. Therefore, in uncomplicated cases, the early QRS forces are normal. To determine the mean QRS axis in the frontal plane, the unblocked portion or the first half of the QRS complex is used.[33] This value represents essentially the average QRS forces of left ventricular activation.

The second portion of the QRS complex is slurred and slowly inscribed. It has a duration of 0.04 second or longer. It corresponds to the wide S waves seen in leads I, V_5, and V_6 and R′ in lead V_1. The terminal deflection may be upright or downward in the inferior leads but is always upright in lead aVR and downward in lead aVL.

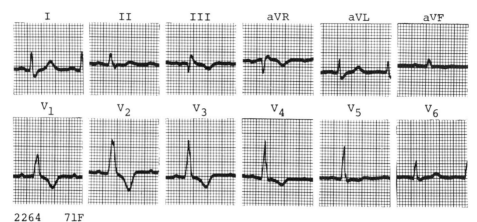

2264   71F

FIGURE 7–1. Complete right bundle branch block. The tracing was recorded from a 71-year-old woman with coronary artery disease. At autopsy, there was about 50 percent narrowing of the three major coronary arteries. Mild myocardial fibrosis without infarction or ventricular hypertrophy also was noted.

In lead V_1, which is the most important lead for the diagnosis of right bundle branch block, the typical finding is the rSR′ pattern. Many variations exist, however. The S wave may be small or absent, and a notched R or rR′ complex is seen (Fig. 7–1). The initial R wave may be absent in V_1, resulting in a qR pattern. The R′ may be smaller than the initial R wave but remains wide.

In uncomplicated right bundle branch block, there usually is little ST-segment displacement. The T wave is opposite to the terminal, slowly inscribed deflection of the QRS complex. It is upright in leads I, V_5, and V_6 and inverted in the right precordial leads. Therefore, the T-wave polarity may appear normal. Some patients, however, may have di-

phasic T waves in the right precordial leads. The initial component is negative and the terminal component positive, which is an abnormal finding (Fig. 7–2).

CLINICAL AND ANATOMIC CORRELATION

Clinical Significance

Most patients with right bundle branch block have organic heart disease, with coronary artery disease as the most common cause. In patients with acute myocardial infarction, complete right bundle branch block is present in 3 to 7 percent of the cases.[37] In such cases, it often is accompanied by left anterior hemi-

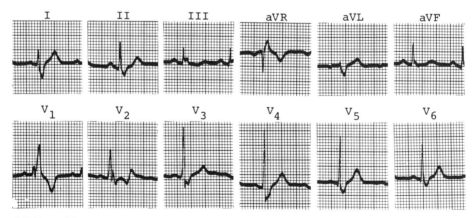

4655   30M

FIGURE 7–2. Complete right bundle branch block in a healthy individual. The tracing was recorded from a 30-year-old physician. The right bundle branch block was known to be present for 7 years. He has no symptoms or other evidence of cardiovascular abnormality.

block and is the result of an anterior myocardial infarction.[30] This conduction defect also may be due to hypertension, rheumatic heart disease, acute and chronic cor pulmonale, myocarditis (Fig. 7–3), cardiomyopathy, sclerosis of the left side of the cardiac skeleton, and degenerative disease of the conduction system. Transient right bundle branch block also may be the result of trauma inflicted during right-sided heart catheterization. It also has been reported after steering wheel injuries to the chest.[20] Right bundle branch block is a frequent finding in patients who have undergone cardiac transplantation (see Chapter 26). In patients who underwent coronary bypass surgery, right bundle branch block is the most common perioperative ventricular conduction defect.[6] In 913 patients with perioperative ventricular conduction abnormalities reported by Chu and colleagues, 156 (17 percent) had transient and 126 (14 percent) had persistent changes. Complete right bundle branch block was found in 93 (60 percent) of the patients with transient changes and in 36 (29 percent) of those with persistent changes.[6] Left anterior hemiblock was the next most frequent conduction defect, followed by incomplete right bundle branch block. They found that the development of new perioperative ventricular conduction abnormalities did not worsen the survival rate in

patients followed for up to 3 years after surgery. Among the congenital heart diseases, it may be seen in Ebstein's anomaly and in a small percentage of patients with atrial septal defect. The most common cause of right bundle branch block in children, however, is open heart surgery for the correction of tetralogy of Fallot or ventricular septal defect (Fig. 7–4).

Many subjects with right bundle branch block have no evidence of underlying heart disease (see Fig. 7–2). Such isolated right bundle branch block occurs more commonly than does isolated left bundle branch block. In a study of more than 122,000 apparently normal male Air Force personnel and applicants between the ages of 16 and 55, Hiss and Lamb found an incidence of right bundle branch block of 1.8 per 1000.[18] There was an increase in the incidence with age. Below the age of 30, the incidence was 1.3 or less per 1000. Between the ages of 30 and 44, it ranged between 2.0 and 2.9 per 1000. Seven years later, most of these individuals revealed no significant increase over the normal population in the development of cardiovascular disease.[22]

In another report from the same institution, the results of a clinical and follow-up study of 394 subjects with right bundle branch block were given.[35] The age range of the subjects at

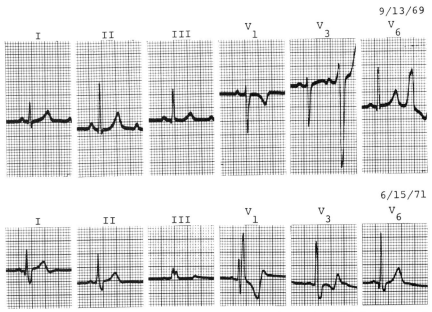

FIGURE 7–3. Complete right bundle branch block due to rheumatic carditis in a 12-year-old boy. Both records were taken during acute rheumatic fever. The tracing from 1969 shows occasional premature atrial beats with aberrancy but is otherwise normal. The tracing from 1971 reveals right bundle branch block. Follow-up cardiovascular examinations revealed normal findings except for the conduction abnormality.

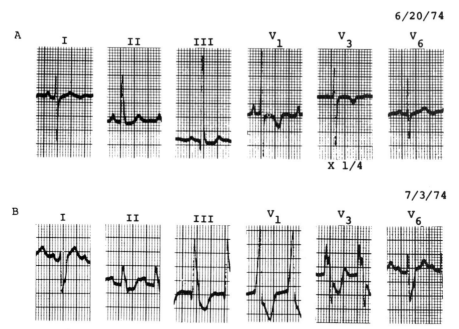

FIGURE 7-4. Surgically induced right bundle branch block. The patient was a 9-year-old boy with tetralogy of Fallot. (A) The preoperative tracing shows right atrial enlargement and right ventricular hypertrophy. (B) The postoperative ECG reveals complete right bundle branch block. The first half of the QRS complex still demonstrates marked right axis deviation.

the time of the diagnosis was 17 to 58 years, with a mean age of 36 ± 9 years. Of the 372 individuals who had complete clinical evaluations, normal cardiovascular findings (other than the conduction defect) were present in 348, 10 of the group had coronary artery disease, and 9 had hypertensive cardiovascular disease. The remainder had congenital heart disease, rheumatic heart disease, or myocarditis. Three hundred and seventy-two of the subjects were followed for a mean period of 10.8 ± 4.7 years. Coronary heart disease or hypertension each developed in an additional 21 (6 percent) of these patients. Fourteen (4 percent) patients died. In only 3 was the cause of death cardiac in origin.

Many other groups of otherwise healthy young individuals with right bundle branch block have been reported, some of which were studied by cardiac catheterization and coronary arteriography.[42,43] Although a change from a normal pattern to bundle branch block is a strong indication of organic heart disease,[39] no evidence of such is demonstrable in many of the patients who have no symptoms.[43] The cause of right bundle branch block in these otherwise healthy individuals remains uncertain. Mild and clinically unrecognized myocarditis has been suggested to account for some of the cases.[45] Because of the long, slen-

der structure of the right bundle branch, it is vulnerable to even a localized lesion. Others have attributed the conduction defect to a congenital deformity of the right bundle branch system.[12]

As in left bundle branch block, the prognosis of patients with right bundle branch block varies greatly and depends on the presence or absence and the type of associated heart disease. Those without other evidence of heart disease are likely to have a benign course, and their survival time is not greatly different from that of the general population.[13,34,35] In the Framingham epidemiology study, Schneider and associates followed 70 persons who had right bundle branch block during 18 years of observation.[39] Only 15 (21 percent) of these subjects remained free from clinically apparent cardiovascular abnormalities. The incidence of cardiovascular disease mortality in these 70 subjects was almost three times greater than that in an age-matched sample of population-at-large. Freedman and colleagues evaluated 272 patients with chronic coronary artery disease and right bundle branch block from the Coronary Artery Surgery Study (CASS).[15] These patients had more extensive coronary artery disease and worse left ventricular function and congestive heart failure than those without any ventricular conduction defect, but the anatomic and function abnormalities were less severe than those seen in patients with left bundle branch block. The mortality rate in patients with bundle branch block was lower in patients with right bundle branch block than left. It is about two times instead of five times that of patients without bundle branch block. In contrast to patients with left bundle branch block and coronary artery disease, right bundle branch block is not an independent predictor of the mortality rate. As in patients with left bundle branch block, most patients with right bundle branch block did not have a responsible lesion in the left anterior descending artery as expected in acute infarction. On the other hand, when right bundle branch block is associated with acute myocardial infarction, a mortality of 36 to 61 percent has been reported.[37] Hindman and associates reported an in-hospital mortality of 24 percent and a total 1-year mortality of 48 percent in patients with acute myocardial infarction and right bundle branch block.[17] The time of onset of the block in relation to the infarction was uncertain in many of the cases. They believed that the increased mortality is due mostly to the development of high-degree AV block.

Anatomic Correlation

Good correlation has been demonstrated between the electrocardiographic (ECG) findings of right bundle branch block and the histopathologic changes of the bundle branch.[23,24] Lev and associates performed detailed pathologic examination of the conduction system and the entire heart in eight cases of coronary artery disease and in one case of myocarditis with right bundle branch block.[24] Significant lesion of the right bundle branch was found in all. In most cases, the lesions were incomplete. They emphasized that the ECG pattern of complete bundle branch block does not necessarily imply a complete anatomic disruption of the continuity of the bundle branch. A unilateral delay of impulse conduction through a functionally altered portion of a bundle branch could produce the ECG pattern of complete bundle branch block if this delay exceeds the time required for the spread of impulses from the contralateral ventricle through the ventricular septum.

Observations made during open heart surgery for the correction of congenital heart defects suggest additional mechanism of production of right bundle branch block. It is known that right bundle branch block may occur after the repair of ventricular septal defect through the tricuspid valve and is caused by injury to the proximal right bundle branch during the procedure.[31] It is also well known, however, that right bundle branch block is a common complication after right ventriculotomy. Krongrad and associates noted that there was no relation between the length of the ventricular incision and the QRS duration, but the pattern appeared with an incision of 1 cm or less at a specific site.[21] They suggested that the disruption of a distal branch or branches of the right bundle was responsible. Therefore, the ECG pattern of right bundle branch block may be the result of involvement of either the main bundle itself or its distal branches. Others believe that damage of the more peripheral right ventricular Purkinje network also may be a responsible mechanism.[31] The findings from electrophysiological studies performed in postoperative patients gave additional support to the concept that ECG changes of right bundle branch block may be due to lesions at any of three levels: proximal branch, distal branches, and peripheral ramifications.[19]

TRANSIENT AND INTERMITTENT RIGHT BUNDLE BRANCH BLOCK

As in the case of left bundle branch block, right bundle branch block may be transient or intermittent (see Chapter 6). Both conditions are commonly rate related, the conduction defect appearing during the faster rate (Fig. 7–5). Rarely, the opposite may occur, and the bundle branch block is bradycardia dependent.[27] Other cases have no apparent relation to the rate. The clinical significance of the unstable form of right bundle block generally is the same as that of the stable form. Transient right bundle branch often is seen during an acute event such as acute myocardial infarction, congestive heart failure, myocarditis, pulmonary embolism, and right-sided heart catheterization.

A related phenomenon is the appearance of aberrant ventricular conduction associated with premature atrial contractions or supraventricular tachycardia. It also is called functional bundle branch block.[16] The aberrantly conducted beats often present a right bundle branch block pattern.[7] The right bundle branch is more susceptible to transmission failure probably because its fibers have longer action potential and refractory period compared with those of the left bundle branch.[36]

ABERRENT VENTRICULAR CONDUCTION

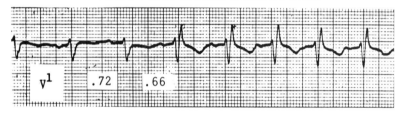

Continuous

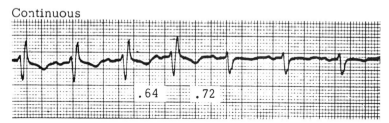

FIGURE 7–5. Rate-related right bundle branch block. The right bundle branch block appears when the RR interval is less than 0.72 second. (Courtesy of Dr. Kenneth Gimbel.)

INCOMPLETE RIGHT BUNDLE BRANCH BLOCK

The diagnosis of incomplete right bundle branch block is suggested when the morphology of the QRS complex is similar to the complete variety but the QRS duration is between 0.08 and 0.11 second.[1,45] This entity caused considerable controversy. Some investigators doubted its existence and attributed the ECG pattern to right ventricular hypertrophy rather than to a delay in the impulse conduction. Massing and James[26] cited the work by Lenegre,[23] who noted that the right bundle branch was histologically normal in 25 (76 percent) of 33 patients with the incomplete right bundle branch block pattern and that 31 (94 percent) of them had right ventricular hypertrophy. Moore and associates performed electrophysiological studies in dogs with the incomplete right bundle branch pattern and found that the conduction time of the right bundle branch and the right ventricular Purkinje system was normal.[29] They attributed the ECG changes to focal hypertrophy of the right ventricle.

In right bundle branch block induced experimentally in humans during right-sided heart catheterization, however, minor or intermediate degrees of right bundle branch block were observed when pressure was applied to the right septal surface.[32] A QRS morphology similar to incomplete right bundle branch block also has been noted during right ventriculotomy, suggesting a more distal origin of the conduction abnormality.[21] The existence of this conduction defect is no longer questioned.[45]

It appears that the ECG pattern of incomplete right bundle branch block is most likely caused by more than one mechanism. In addition to its recognition, its separation from other pathologic conditions that are associated with similar ECG changes is important. In some cases, both conduction defect and right ventricular hypertrophy are present. The conduction defect, whether within the right bundle branch or in its subendocardial Purkinje network, may have a functional rather than an organic basis. Right ventricular dilatation or increased right ventricular intracavitory pressure seen in patients with right ventricular hypertrophy also may affect the conduction time.

Liao and associates followed 1960 white men, 222 of whom had incomplete right bundle branch block, to evaluate their clinical course and prognosis.[25] The men with incomplete right bundle branch block were found to be at greater risk of developing left axis deviation and complete right bundle branch block. The likelihood that these men would develop complete right bundle branch block in 11 years was 5.1 percent, compared with 0.7 percent for those without such defect. There was no demonstrable increased risk of death from cardiovascular disease in 20 years. The authors suggested that such block is frequently a manifestation of primary abnormality of the cardiac conduction system in middle-aged men.

DIFFERENTIAL DIAGNOSIS OF THE RSR' PATTERN IN LEAD V₁

An RSR' pattern in lead V_1, with a QRS duration of *less* than 0.12 second may be seen in the following conditions.

A Normal Variant

An RSR' pattern with a duration less than 0.12 second is found in lead V_1 in 2.4 percent of healthy individuals.[18] A higher incidence is observed when additional right precordial leads (V_{3R}, V_{4R}) are recorded.[3] The secondary R wave has been attributed to physiological late activation of the outflow tract of the right ventricle or, specifically, the crista supraventricularis. The R' usually is smaller than the R wave (Fig. 7–6). It is likely to be absent when the right precordial leads are recorded at a lower intercostal space.[44]

To separate the normal from the abnormal RSR' pattern, Tapia and Proudfit suggested the following criteria for normality[44]:

1. A primary R wave in lead V_1 of less than 8 mm
2. An R' of less than 6 mm
3. An R'/S ratio of less than 1.0

In their study, nearly all the normal subjects met these criteria. Eighty percent of patients with congenital heart disease and 46 percent of patients with acquired heart disease had values that exceeded these limits.

Changes in the limb leads and other precordial leads are often helpful in deciding the normality of the RSR' in lead V_1 pattern. Although a normal finding does not exclude organic heart disease, the presence of abnormal P waves or QRS complex in the other leads greatly favors an abnormal origin of the RSR' pattern.

Right Ventricular Hypertrophy

In patients with congenital heart disease, the RSR' pattern in lead V_1 usually is associated with a relatively mild degree of right ventricular hypertrophy. Typically, it is seen in diastolic or volume overload of the right ventricle, such as atrial septal defect (see Fig. 4–12). It also is observed in patients with ventricular septal defect (see Fig. 3–8) and biventricular hypertrophy. The pattern occasionally is encountered in coarctation of the aorta beyond the age of infancy and has been related to involution of preexisting right ventricular hypertrophy.[47]

In acquired heart disease, the pattern is seen in about one third of patients with mitral stenosis.[14] (see Fig. 4–8). Correlation between the severity of the valve lesion and this ECG pattern is poor.[41] In chronic cor pulmonale, however, it usually is associated with a more advanced degree of right ventricular hypertrophy.

Incomplete Right Bundle Branch Block

As discussed previously, it is difficult to separate incomplete right bundle branch block from the other causes of the RSR' pattern. The diagnosis often depends on the exclusion of the other possibilities from both the ECG changes and the clinical data (Figs. 7–7 and

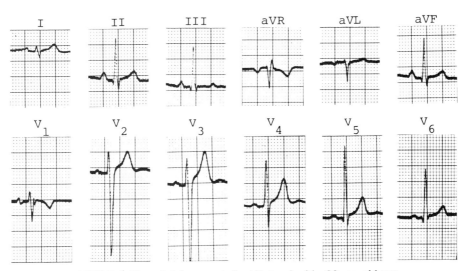

FIGURE 7–6. Normal rSr' pattern in lead V_1 in a healthy 22-year-old man.

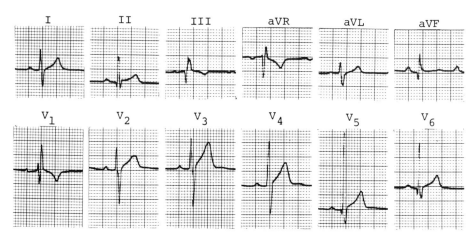

FIGURE 7–7. An rSR' pattern in lead V_1 due to incomplete right bundle branch block in a healthy 23-year-old man.

7–8). In the ECG, when the R' is tall (> 10 mm), it is unlikely that the RSR' is caused by incomplete right bundle branch block alone, and therefore right ventricular hypertrophy is probably present. This is also true if the frontal plane shows abnormal right axis deviation. On the other hand, a small but wide and slurred R' is more suggestive of incomplete right bundle branch block. Abnormal P waves suggestive of atrial enlargement also indicate that the right ventricular hypertrophy is responsible for the RSR' pattern by inference.

Acute Right Ventricular Dilatation

In acute pulmonary embolism, the acute right ventricular dilatation may be associated with

the appearance of an rSr' pattern in lead V_1. Right ventricular conduction defect is probably the responsible mechanism. The secondary R wave usually is small and transient, but a broad R' due to complete right bundle branch block may be seen. The development of an S_1Q_3, P pulmonale pattern and T-wave inversion in the right precordial leads gives further support to the diagnosis. The most important diagnostic feature is the transient nature of these changes.

True Posterior Myocardial Infarction

Although true posterior myocardial infarction usually is associated with a tall R wave in lead V_1, an rSr' pattern occasionally may be ob-

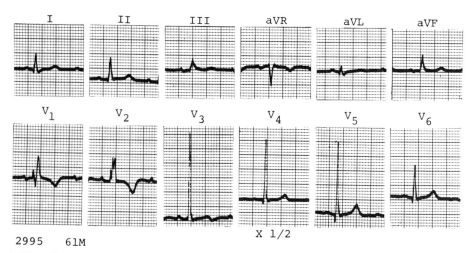

2995   61M

X 1/2

FIGURE 7–8. Incomplete right bundle branch block. The tracing was recorded from a 61-year-old man with chronic myelogenous leukemia. At autopsy, mild atherosclerosis of the coronary arteries was noted. There was no ventricular hypertrophy, myocardial infarction, or significant fibrosis.

served. In contrast to right ventricular hypertrophy or incomplete right bundle branch block, the T wave in this lead is more likely to be upright than inverted. An inverted T wave in lead V_1 is seen only during the early phase of an acute posterior infarction. Abnormal Q waves in the inferior leads suggestive of inferior myocardial infarction also support the diagnosis of posterior wall myocardial damage.

Pectus Excavatum and the Straight Back Syndrome

An rSr' pattern in lead V_1 often is recorded in these skeletal deformities (Fig. 7–9). The r' usually is small. A change in the position of the heart as a result of the decrease in the anteroposterior diameter is believed to cause the ECG changes.[8–11] The P wave in lead V_1 may be inverted to resemble left atrial enlargement.

Recording Artifacts

Incorrect lead placement frequently is responsible for the appearance of an rSr' in V_1 pattern. This occurs commonly when the lead V_1 electrode is placed in the third instead of the fourth intercostal space. A clue to the high electrode location is that the P, QRS, and T waves resemble those in lead aVR, since the electrode is closer to the right shoulder. The findings are somewhat similar to those associated with the skeletal deformities described earlier.

DIAGNOSIS OF VENTRICULAR HYPERTROPHY IN THE PRESENCE OF RIGHT BUNDLE BRANCH BLOCK

Right Ventricular Hypertrophy

Barker and Valencia suggested that if the R' in lead V_1 is greater than 15 mm in complete right bundle branch block, right ventricular hypertrophy is present (Fig. 7–10).[1] In a small number of the autopsy cases examined by Booth and associates, two of three cases that met this criterion had anatomic right ventricular hypertrophy, but seven cases with anatomic combined ventricular hypertrophy did not meet this criterion.[2]

In patients with transient right bundle branch block, or when ECGs before and after the development of the conduction defect are available, an R' greater than 15 mm may be observed during block even though the control tracing shows no evidence of right ventricular hypertrophy.[10,38,40] Therefore, it is generally agreed that the amplitude of the R' in lead V_1 is not a reliable sign of right ventricular hypertrophy in complete right bundle branch block.

Chou and associates analyzed the vectorcardiograms and ECGs of patients who developed right bundle branch block after surgical correction of tetralogy of Fallot.[5] The findings suggested that the diagnosis of right ventricular hypertrophy may be made from the first portion of the QRS loop. By analogy, abnormal right axis deviation of the unblocked portion of the QRS complex in the conventional ECG may have a similar implication (see Figs. 7–4

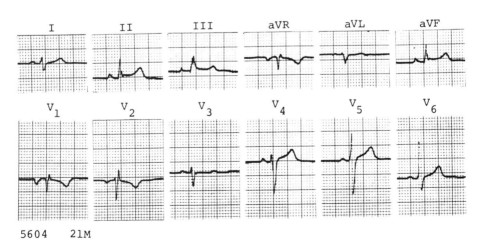

5604   21M

FIGURE 7–9. Pectus excavatum in a 21-year-old man. R' is present in the right precordial leads. Note the prominent negative P wave in lead V_1.

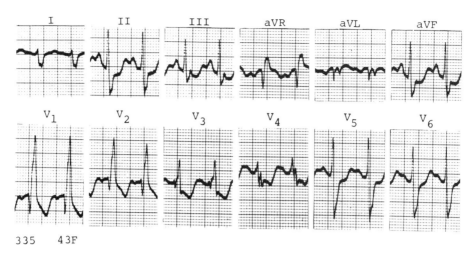

335   43F

FIGURE 7–10. Right bundle branch block with right ventricular hypertrophy. The patient was a 43-year-old woman with chronic cor pulmonale due to chronic obstructive lung disease. At autopsy, there was marked right atrial and ventricular hypertrophy and dilatation. The free wall of the right ventricle measured 1 cm in thickness. There also was mild left ventricular hypertrophy. Coronary atherosclerosis was minimal, and there was no evidence of myocardial infarction. In the ECG, there is marked right axis deviation of the first half of the QRS complex in the frontal plane. The R' in lead V₁ is tall and exceeds 15 mm.

and 7–10). A systematic examination of the reliability of this finding is needed.

In incomplete right bundle branch block, Barker and Valencia considered right ventricular hypertrophy to be present if the R' in V₁ is greater than 10 mm.[1] Milnor suggested the criterion of (1) a rightward mean frontal plane QRS axis of +110° to +270° or (2) an R/S or R'/S ratio in lead V₁ greater than 1.0, provided that the R or R' wave in V₁ is greater than 5 mm.[28] In 28 autopsied cases analyzed in our institution,[28] the specificity of either Barker and Valencia[1] or Milnor's[28] criteria was about 60 percent. Carouso and associates found that only 3 of 24 cases of right ventricular hypertrophy confirmed postmortem had an R' in V₁ greater than 10 mm.[4] Therefore, these criteria give a significant number of false-positive diagnoses and are particularly low in sensitivity.

Left Ventricular Hypertrophy

The ECG findings of left ventricular hypertrophy often are obscured by the presence of right bundle branch block. In 37 autopsied cases that had hypertrophied left ventricle and ECG changes of complete or incomplete right bundle branch block, only 1 case met the usual ECG criteria for left ventricular hypertrophy.[2] In patients with intermittent or transient right bundle branch block, the amplitude of the R wave in the left precordial leads is reduced in most instances when the block

develops (Chou TC, unpublished data). Therefore, the sensitivity of the conventional voltage criteria is impaired. On the other hand, when these criteria are met, the incidence of a false-positive diagnosis is decreased.

INTRAVENTRICULAR CONDUCTION DEFECT

In many ECGs, the QRS duration may be prolonged to 0.11 second or more but the QRS morphology does not satisfy the criteria for either left or right bundle branch block (Figs. 7–11 and 7–12). The terms *nonspecific* and *diffuse* intraventricular conduction defect have been used to describe this type of change. It is assumed that the conduction delay occurs in the more peripheral part of the intraventricular conduction system. In most instances, the QRS changes resemble closely those seen in left bundle branch block. Abnormal notching or slurring may or may not be present.

Prolongation of the QRS duration may be seen in healthy individuals and probably represents a normal variant. A duration of 0.12 second or more was reported in 0.4 percent of such a population.[16] In patients with organic heart disease, this type of intraventricular conduction defect often is observed in association with a large heart (see Fig. 7–11). The cause of the heart disease is variable. Other causes of wide QRS complexes include

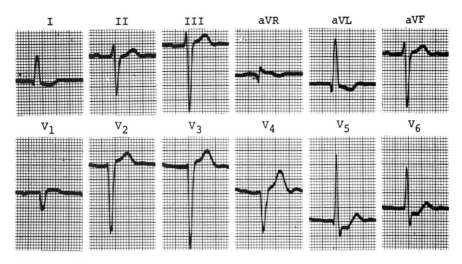

1159   71M

FIGURE 7–11. Intraventricular conduction defect. The patient had rheumatic heart disease with severe mitral insufficiency. At autopsy, the heart weighed 565 g, with moderate dilatation of both ventricles and left atrium and left ventricular hypertrophy. There was a moderate degree of coronary atherosclerosis but no evidence of myocardial infarction. The ECG shows first-degree AV block, abnormal P waves, left anterior hemiblock, left ventricular hypertrophy, and digitalis effect. There is poor progression of the R wave in leads V_1 through V_4. The QRS duration is 0.13 second, which cannot be explained by the hemiblock and ventricular hypertrophy alone.

drugs such as quinidine, procainamide, encainide, flecainide, and tricyclic antidepressants, as well as hyperkalemia and hypothermia.

The term *intraventricular conduction defect* also is used frequently when there is an abnormal notching of the QRS complex, even though the duration is within normal limits. The pathogenesis and clinical significance of such a finding is unclear in most instances. Notching of the QRS complex often occurs in the inferior leads, especially in lead III, in normal individuals.

REFERENCES

1. Barker JM, Valencia F: The precordial electrocardiogram in incomplete right bundle branch block. Am Heart J 38:376, 1949
2. Booth RW, Chou TC, Scott RC: Electrocardiographic diagnosis of ventricular hypertrophy in the presence of right bundle branch block. Circulation 18:169, 1958

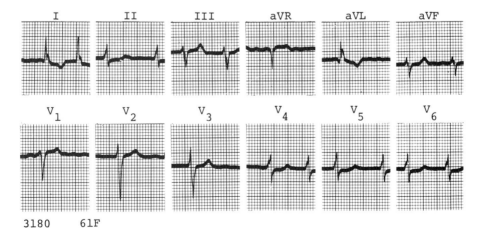

3180   61F

FIGURE 7–12. Intraventricular conduction defect. The patient had hypertension and coronary artery disease. Autopsy revealed dilatation and hypertrophy of the atria and ventricles and old inferior and lateral myocardial infarction. The ECG shows atrial fibrillation, notching of the QRS complex in many of the leads, and ST and T-wave changes.

3. Camerini F, Davies LG: Secondary R waves in right chest leads. Br Heart J 17:28, 1955
4. Carouso G, Maurice P, Scebat L, et al: L'electrocardiogramme de l'hypertrophie ventriculaire droite. Arch Mal Coeur 44:769, 1951
5. Chou TC, Schwartz D, Kaplan S: Vectorcardiographic diagnosis of right ventricular hypertrophy in the presence of right bundle branch block. *In* Hoffman I, Hamby RI (eds): Vectorcardiography 3, Amsterdam, North-Holland, 1976, p 21
6. Chu A, Califf RM, Pryor DB, et al: Prognostic effect of bundle branch block related to coronary artery bypass grafting. Am J Cardiol 59:798, 1987
7. Cohen SI, Lau SH, Stein E, et al: Variations of aberrant ventricular conduction in man: Evidence of isolated and combined block within the specialized conduction system. Circulation 38:988, 1968
8. deLeon AC, Perloff JK, Twigg H, et al: The straight back syndrome: Clinical cardiovascular manifestations. Circulation 32:193, 1965
9. deOliveira JM, Sambhi MP, Zimmerman HA: The electrocardiogram in pectus excavatum. Br Heart J 20:495, 1958
10. Dodge HT, Grant RP: Mechanisms of QRS complex prolongation in man: Right ventricular conduction defects. Am J Med 21:534, 1956
11. Elisberg EI: Electrocardiographic changes associated with pectus excavatum. Ann Intern Med 49:130, 1958
12. Fisch C: Bundle branch block of the broad S type: Report of 11 cases without any evidence of heart disease, with one instance showing partial and transient block. J Indiana Med Assoc 40:1128, 1947
13. Fleg JL, Das DN, Lakatta EG: Right bundle branch block: Long-term prognosis in apparently healthy men. J Am Coll Cardiol 1:887, 1983
14. Fraser HRL, Turner R: Electrocardiography in mitral valvular disease. Br Heart J 17:459, 1955
15. Freedman RA, Alderman EL, Sheffield LT, et al: Bundle branch block in patients with chronic coronary artery disease: Angiographic correlates and prognostic significance. J Am Coll Cardiol 10:73, 1987
16. Hecht HH, Kossmann CE: Atrioventricular and intraventricular conduction. Am J Cardiol 31:232, 1973
17. Hindman MC, Wagner GS, JaRo M, et al: The clinical significance of bundle branch block complicating acute myocardial infarction: I. Clinic characteristics, hospital mortality, and one-year follow-up. Circulation 58:679, 1978
18. Hiss RG, Lamb LE: Electrocardiographic findings in 122,043 individuals. Circulation 25:947, 1962
19. Horowitz LN, Alexander JA, Edmunds LH: Postoperative right bundle branch block: Identification of three levels of block. Circulation 62:319, 1980
20. Jackson DH: Transient post-traumatic right bundle branch block. Am J Cardiol 23:877, 1969
21. Krongrad E, Hefler SE, Bowman FO, et al: Further observations on the etiology of the right bundle branch block pattern following right ventriculotomy. Circulation 50:1105, 1974
22. Lamb LE: Electrocardiography and vectorcardiography: Instrumentation, fundamentals and clinical applications. Philadelphia, WB Saunders, 1965, p 286
23. Lenegre J: Contribution à l'etude des blocs de branche. Paris, JB Bailliere et Fils, 1958
24. Lev M, Unger PN, Lesser ME, et al: Pathology of the conduction system in acquired heart disease: Complete right bundle branch block. Am Heart J 61:593, 1961
25. Liao Y, Emidy LA, Dyer A, et al: Characteristics and prognosis of incomplete right bundle branch block:

An epidemiologic study. J Am Coll Cardiol 7:492, 1986
26. Massing GK, James TN: Conduction and block in the right bundle branch: Real and imagined. Circulation 45:1, 1972
27. Massumi RA: Bradycardia-dependent bundle-branch block: A critique and proposed criteria. Circulation 38:1066, 1968
28. Milnor WR: The electrocardiogram and vectorcardiogram in right ventricular hypertrophy and right bundle branch block. Circulation 16:348, 1957
29. Moore EN, Boineau JP, Patterson DF: Incomplete right bundle-branch block: An electrocardiographic enigma and possible misnomer. Circulation 44:678, 1971
30. Nimetz AA, Shubrooks SJ, Hutter AM, et al: The significance of bundle branch block during acute myocardial infarction. Am Heart J 90:439, 1975
31. Okoroma EO, Guller B, Maloney JD, et al: Etiology of right bundle-branch block pattern after surgical closure of ventricular septal defects. Am Heart J 90:14, 1975
32. Penaloza D, Gamboa R, Sime F: Experimental right bundle branch block in the normal human heart: Electrocardiographic, vectorcardiographic and hemodynamic observations. Am J Cardiol 8:767, 1961
33. Pryor R, Blount SG: The clinical significance of true left axis deviation: Left intraventricular blocks. Am Heart J 72:391, 1966
34. Rodstein M, Gubner R, Mills JP, et al: A mortality study in bundle branch block. Arch Intern Med 87:663, 1951
35. Rotman M, Triebwasser JH: A clinical and follow-up study of right and left bundle branch block. Circulation 51:477, 1975
36. Schamroth L: The Disorders of Cardiac Rhythm. Oxford and Edinburgh, Blackwell Scientific Publications, 1971, p 202
37. Scheidt S, Killip T: Bundle-branch block complicating acute myocardial infarction. JAMA 222:919, 1972
38. Scherlis L, Lee YC: Transient right bundle branch block: An electrocardiographic and vectorcardiographic study. Am J Cardiol 11:173, 1963
39. Schneider JF, Thomas HE, Kreger BE, et al: Newly acquired right bundle-branch block: The Framingham study. Ann Intern Med 92:37, 1980
40. Scott RC: The correlation between the electrocardiographic patterns of ventricular hypertrophy and the anatomic findings. Circulation 21:256, 1960
41. Semler HJ, Pruitt RD: An electrocardiographic estimation of the pulmonary vascular obstruction in 80 patients with mitral stenosis. Am Heart J 59:541, 1960
42. Shaffer AB, Reiser I: Right bundle branch system block in healthy young people. Am Heart J 62:487, 1961
43. Smith RF, Jackson DH, Harthorne JW, et al: Acquired bundle branch block in a healthy population. Am Heart J 80:746, 1970
44. Tapia FA, Proudfit WL: Secondary R waves in right precordial leads in normal persons and in patients with cardiac disease. Circulation 21:28, 1960
45. Vazifdar JP, Levine SA: Benign bundle branch block. Arch Intern Med 89:568, 1952
46. Willems JL, Robles de Medina EO, Bernard R, et al: Criteria for intraventricular conduction disturbances and pre-excitation. J Am Coll Cardiol 5:1261, 1985
47. Ziegler RF, Lam CR: Indications for the surgical correction of coarctation of the aorta in infancy. Am J Cardiol 12:60, 1963

Hemiblocks, Bifascicular and Trifascicular Blocks

8

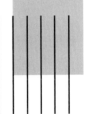

Shortly after its departure from the His bundle, the left bundle branch divides into two divisions or fascicles, the anterior (or superior) division and the posterior (or inferior) division. The anterior division supplies Purkinje fibers to the anterior and lateral walls of the left ventricle, and the posterior division supplies the inferior and the posterior walls. The two divisions anastomose with each other through the Purkinje system.

Normally, the left ventricle is activated by impulse conducted simultaneously through the two divisions of the left bundle branch. A delay or interruption of the impulse conduction in one of the divisions results in asynchronous activation of the left ventricle. In left anterior hemiblock (or fascicular block), the impulse spreads inferiorly through the posterior division. The excitation of the anterior and lateral wall is, however, delayed. It depends on the impulse arriving retrograde from the posterior division. Therefore, the late QRS vectors are displaced in the leftward and superior direction. These late forces become prominent, probably because they are mostly unopposed. Consequently the mean QRS axis is shifted leftward and superiorly, resulting in abnormal left axis deviation. Because the initial forces from the septum and inferior wall are directed rightward and inferiorly, an initial q wave is recorded in lead I, with an r wave in the inferior leads. Therefore, in left anterior hemiblock, lead I usually presents a qR complex, and the inferior leads record rS complexes.

In left posterior hemiblock (or fascicular block), the opposite sequence of events occurs. The activation of the inferior and posterior wall of the left ventricle is delayed and depends on the impulse coming from the anterolateral wall of the left ventricle. The late QRS vectors are directed inferiorly and rightward. These mostly unopposed forces result in a rightward displacement of the mean QRS axis, or abnormal right axis deviation. The early activation of the anterolateral wall is ac-

companied by left superior QRS vectors that manifest as an initial R wave in lead I and as q waves in the inferior leads. Therefore, lead I displays an rS complex, and the inferior leads record qR deflections.

LEFT ANTERIOR HEMIBLOCK (LEFT ANTERIOR FASCICULAR BLOCK)

Diagnostic Criteria

1. Displacement of the mean QRS axis in the frontal plane to between $-30°$ and $-90°$ (abnormal left axis deviation).
2. A qR complex (or an R wave) in leads I and aVL; an rS complex in leads II, III, and aVF.
3. Normal or slightly prolonged QRS duration.

ABNORMAL LEFT AXIS DEVIATION

Left axis deviation is the major criterion for the diagnosis of left anterior hemiblock (Figs. 8–1 through 8–3). There are some differences in opinion as to the degree of axis shift required for the diagnosis. Many years ago, Grant considered a QRS axis superior to $-30°$ as indicative of left ventricular "parietal block" resulting from conduction defect in the fibers of the anterior division of the left bundle.[27,28] Later, Pryor and Blount used the same value for "true left axis deviation" or left anterior fascicular block.[43] Rosenbaum, who has contributed much to the renewed and deserved attention to the various intraventricular conduction abnormalities, suggested $-45°$ as the lower limit of the QRS axis for the diagnosis of left anterior hemiblock.[50] He stated that this limit is an arbitrary choice and believed that a QRS axis of $-30°$ probably represents "incomplete" left anterior hemiblock. Because most of the reported clinical and pathologic studies relating to this subject used $-30°$ as the lower limit, I use it also.

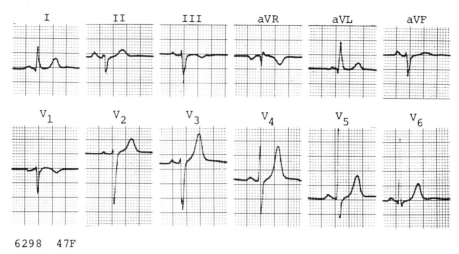

6298   47F

FIGURE 8–1. Left anterior hemiblock in a 47-year-old woman with mild hypertension.

MORPHOLOGY OF THE QRS-T COMPLEX IN THE LIMB LEADS

The leftward shift of the QRS axis results in a tall R wave in leads I and aVL, since the major forces are directed toward the left arm. The large amplitude of the R wave in lead aVL may cause a false-positive diagnosis of left ventricular hypertrophy (see Fig. 8–3). For the same reason, $R_1 + S_3$ may exceed 25 mm in the absence of left ventricular hypertrophy.

Although a small q wave usually is present in leads I and aVL, its absence does not exclude the diagnosis. In left anterior hemiblock that developed during selective coronary arteriogram, the initial QRS vectors were not significantly modified.[23] In 222 newly developed cases of marked left axis deviation without apparent heart disease, Rabkin and associates found that Q waves remained absent or unchanged from the previous tracings in leads I and aVL in most (81 percent).[44]

In the uncomplicated cases of left anterior hemiblock, an rS complex is recorded in the inferior leads. The S wave in lead III is larger than that in lead II, since the mean QRS axis is more parallel to the negative side of the lead III axis. If S_2 is greater than S_3, the mean QRS axis is in the right superior quadrant of the frontal plane, and extreme right axis deviation is present.

Patients with inferior myocardial infarction may show a QS or Qr deflection in the inferior leads. If the Q wave is deep, the calculated mean QRS axis may be superior to $-30°$. Such a finding, however, does not represent left anterior hemiblock, even though the QRS axis is shifted leftward, because the initial, rather than the terminal, forces are displaced superiorly. When QS complexes are present in the

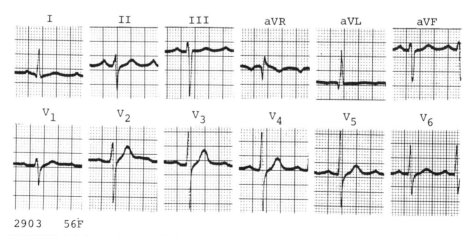

2903   56F

FIGURE 8–2. Left anterior hemiblock in a woman with chronic renal disease. Deep S waves are seen in the left precordial leads.

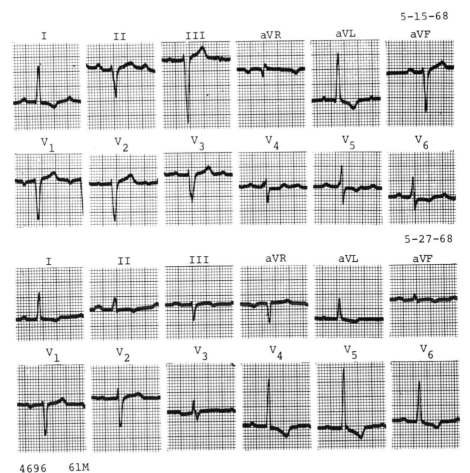

5-15-68

I II III aVR aVL aVF

V_1 V_2 V_3 V_4 V_5 V_6

5-27-68

I II III aVR aVL aVF

V_1 V_2 V_3 V_4 V_5 V_6

4696 61M

FIGURE 8–3. Intermittent left anterior hemiblock. The tracings were recorded from a 61-year-old man with coronary artery disease. The change in the QRS axis was observed on many occasions. There is an increase of the QRS duration from 0.08 to 0.10 second during left anterior hemiblock (5-15-68). The R-wave amplitude increases in leads I and aVL and decreases in leads V_4 through V_6 with the appearance of deep S waves in leads V_4 through V_6 during hemiblock.

inferior leads, left anterior hemiblock may coexist with the infarction.

In the absence of coexisting repolarization abnormalities, the ST segment and T waves are not significantly different from those of the normal individuals.

QRS PROLONGATION

In uncomplicated cases of left anterior hemiblock, the QRS duration may be normal or slightly prolonged. In patients with intermittent left anterior hemiblock, the widening of the QRS usually is less than 0.02 second when the hemiblock pattern appears[53] (see Fig. 8–3). Das reported an average increase of 0.025 second in 63 subjects who had abnormal left axis deviation of −30° or more.[12] The degree of prolongation appeared to be in proportion to the degree of axis shift.

Changes in the Precordial Leads

DEEP S WAVE IN THE LEFT PRECORDIAL LEADS
(see Figs. 8–2 and 8–3)

In left anterior hemiblock, the transitional zone in the precordial leads may be displaced to the left, with a decrease in the amplitude of the R waves and an increase of the depth of the S waves in the left precordial leads. These changes are related to the superior displacement of the QRS forces. The lead axes of V_5 and V_6 are directed not only leftward but also slightly downward. A superior displacement of the QRS vectors results in a smaller projection on the lead axes and therefore a smaller R wave in these leads. If the late QRS forces are markedly superior, they may project on the negative side of the lead axes, and rather deep S waves are recorded.

qrS PATTERN IN THE RIGHT PRECORDIAL LEADS

A less common but clinically important finding in left anterior hemiblock is the appearance of a small q wave in the right precordial leads to suggest anterior myocardial infarction. This is due to a change in the orientation of the initial QRS forces. They are directed inferiorly and may project on the negative side of the lead axes of these leads. This explanation is supported by the fact that q waves are not recorded when these precordial leads are recorded one intercostal space below their routine locations.[37,50]

Figure 8–3 gives an example of intermittent left anterior hemiblock and illustrates many of the changes associated with the development of this conduction defect.

Clinical and Pathologic Correlation

Because marked left axis deviation usually is caused by left anterior hemiblock, these two terms are commonly used interchangeably. Although no rigid distinction is made between them in the following review of the literature, it should be mentioned that marked left superior displacement of the mean QRS axis may occur occasionally with inferior myocardial infarction and other pathologic processes in the absence of left anterior hemiblock.

Abnormal left axis deviation is one of the most common abnormal electrocardiographic (ECG) findings. In 67,375 Air Force men without symptoms, Hiss and associates found a frontal plane QRS axis between $-30°$ and $-90°$ in 128 (1.9 percent).[30] In the Tecumseh epidemiologic study of 4678 persons past the age of 20, abnormal left axis deviation was found in 248 (5 percent).[40] It was more prevalent in men than in women, and the frequency increased with age among both sexes. Fifty-nine percent of the individuals with left axis deviation had other findings suggestive of heart disease. The remainder had no other evidence of cardiac abnormalities.

Eliot and associates examined 195 apparently healthy men with a mean age of 41 years who had marked left axis deviation but no other ECG abnormality.[22] During the initial investigation and the follow-up period up to 22 months, 113 (58 percent) subjects were found to have cardiovascular disease or diabetes mellitus. Sixty-six (34 percent) had evidence of coronary artery disease; 28 (14 percent) had hypertension; and 13 (7 percent) had subclinical diabetes mellitus. Among the

363 male insurance applicants age 30 years and over with left anterior hemiblock examined by Corne and associates, 194 (53 percent) were not associated with cardiovascular abnormalities.[10] There was no significant difference in the occurrence of heart disease between the group of subjects with a QRS axis of $-31°$ to $-59°$ and the group with an axis of $-60°$ to $-90°$.

In most of the clinical and pathologic series, coronary artery disease with or without myocardial infarction was by far the most common cause of abnormal left axis deviation.[3,27] In acute myocardial infarction, isolated left anterior hemiblock occurs in about 4 percent of the patients.[2,39,57,68] Another 5 percent of the patients have left anterior hemiblock in conjunction with right bundle branch block.[2,57,68] The location of the infarction usually is anteroseptal or anterolateral (Fig. 8–4). The left anterior descending artery usually is the vessel involved. Left anterior hemiblock also is seen in patients with acute inferior myocardial infarction, however.[7] One explanation is that the His bundle receives a dual blood supply from the septal branch of the left anterior descending artery and the AV nodal artery. There is a longitudinal dissociation of the conduction of the His bundle. Ischemia of the His bundle due to AV nodal artery disease may affect only that part of the His bundle that consists of the left anterior fascicle, resulting in left anterior hemiblock.[7] Hypertensive heart disease, aortic valve disease, and primary and secondary cardiomyopathy are the other common causes. Among patients without apparent heart disease, left anterior hemiblock may be caused by degenerative disease of the conduction tissue[33] or sclerosis of the left side of the cardiac skeleton.[35]

Pathologically, myocardial fibrosis has been demonstrated in most patients with marked left axis deviation when gross myocardial infarction is absent.[11,27] This relationship was shown by Grant's classical study on this subject.[27] He also pointed out the lack of direct relation between left axis deviation and left ventricular hypertrophy per se. Demoulin and associates performed histopathologic studies on 10 cases of chronic anterior hemiblock.[14] Fibrotic lesions that involved predominantly the anterior fascicle of the left bundle branch were found in 5 hearts. In the other 5, disseminated changes were seen in all parts of the left bundle branch. The results of later studies by the same group of investigators and by Rossi gave further support to the view that left anterior hemiblock is a reliable sign of left

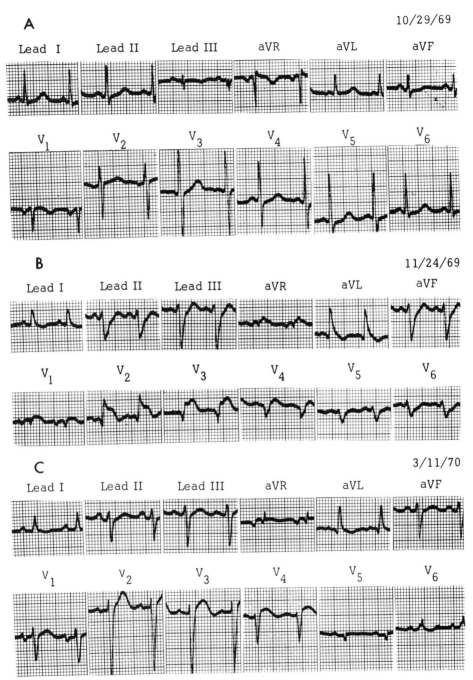

FIGURE 8–4. Left anterior hemiblock due to anterior myocardial infarction. (A) Routine electrocardiogram recorded before hysterectomy. The tracing is within normal limits except for prominent negative P wave in lead V_1, which suggests left atrial enlargement. (B) Acute anteroseptal myocardial infarction developed after surgery. There is a marked leftward shift of the QRS axis to −60° consistent with left anterior hemiblock. The QRS duration increases from 0.07 to 0.12 second. Additional intraventricular conduction defect is present. (C) Follow-up tracing recorded 3½ months later. The QRS duration is 0.08 second. The QRS axis remains at −60°. The precordial leads reveal signs of old anterior myocardial infarction with persistent ST-segment elevation in leads V_2 through V_4.

bundle branch disease but the underlying lesions are more widely distributed than the ECG terminology implies.[15,54]

Pulmonary emphysema has frequently been described as a cause of abnormal left axis deviation. The terminal QRS forces in these patients are directed superiorly but rightward. Although deep S waves are present in the inferior leads, a small S wave also is recorded in lead I. These changes are regarded as a pseudo–left axis deviation pattern.[43] Hyperkalemia may cause a reversible form of left axis deviation.[4,43]

Among acyanotic congenital heart diseases, abnormal left axis deviation is seen most commonly in patients with endocardial cushion defects, which include atrial septal defect of the primum type, atrioventricular canal, and common atrium. The mechanism of left axis deviation in these patients probably is related to early activation of the posterobasal left ventricular wall rather than left anterior hemiblock.[41] In isolated ventricular septal defect, left axis deviation occurs in about 4 percent of the cases. In cyanotic congenital heart disease, left axis deviation typically is seen in patients with tricuspid atresia. About one third of the patients with a single ventricle have this conduction defect.[43] Abnormal left axis deviation also is occasionally seen in patients with transposition of the great vessels and double-outlet right ventricle.[59] Isolated congenital left axis deviation without evidence of heart disease also has been reported.[29]

Diagnosis of Left Ventricular Hypertrophy in the Presence of Left Anterior Hemiblock

As it was mentioned and demonstrated in the early part of this chapter, left anterior hemiblock may cause a false-positive diagnosis of left ventricular hypertrophy by increasing the R-wave amplitude in leads I and aVL (see Fig. 8–3). Abnormal left axis deviation is included, however, in the Romhilt–Estes criteria for the recognition of left ventricular hypertrophy.[47] Based on an echocardiographic study, Gertsch and associates proposed that, if the voltage of the S wave in lead II plus that of the largest RS complex in the precordial leads is equal to or greater than 30 mm, left ventricular hypertrophy is present.[25] In 50 patients with left anterior hemiblock, 26 with and 24 without left ventricular hypertrophy, the specificity of their criterion was 87 percent and sensitivity was 96 percent. The reliability of this criterion requires further testing. In my practice, ST-segment and T-wave changes consistent with strain pattern are required for the diagnosis of left ventricular hypertrophy if the increased QRS voltage is limited to the limb leads and left anterior hemiblock is present.

LEFT POSTERIOR HEMIBLOCK (LEFT POSTERIOR FASCICULAR BLOCK)

Diagnostic Criteria

1. A frontal plane QRS axis of +90° to +180°.
2. An S_1Q_3 pattern.
3. Normal or slightly prolonged QRS duration.

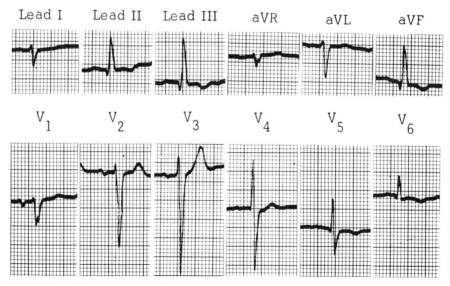

FIGURE 8–5. Left posterior hemiblock in a patient with apical myocardial infarction (due to periarteritis nodosa involving the coronary artery) proved at autopsy. The frontal plane QRS axis is +115°.

ABNORMAL RIGHT AXIS DEVIATION

Rosenbaum and co-workers suggested a QRS axis of +120° as a criterion for the diagnosis of left posterior hemiblock, but they stated that the diagnosis may perhaps be considered with an axis of +90° or even +70°.[50] They indicated that the latter probably represents an incomplete form of left posterior hemiblock. Others are less precise with the definition. Pryor emphasized the terminal QRS vector, which is directed inferiorly at +90° to +110° in left posterior fascicular block.[42] In an illustrated case with histologic evidence of fibrosis that involved the posterior division, the QRS axis was less than +90°.[43] The experimental work by Watt and Pruitt in primate hearts also suggested that left posterior hemiblock need not be accompanied by an extreme right axis deviation.[67] Because few cases were correlated with histologic examination of the conduction system, the criterion is rather arbitrary.[43,46]

Figure 8–5 gives an example of left posterior hemiblock with a QRS axis of +115°. Figure 8–6 illustrates a case of intermittent left posterior hemiblock with an axis of +80° during the block. The conduction defect occurred during an anginal episode and was observed again on another occasion. Figure 8–7 shows the development of left posterior hemiblock during acute inferior myocardial infarction. Another example is shown in Figure 8–8. Left posterior hemiblock, complete left bundle branch block, and complete AV block were observed in a 24-year-old man with Marfan's syndrome and aortic aneurysm.

It is important to exclude other causes of abnormal right axis deviation before the diagnosis of left posterior hemiblock is made. Right ventricular hypertrophy, vertical heart, pulmonary emphysema, and extensive lateral

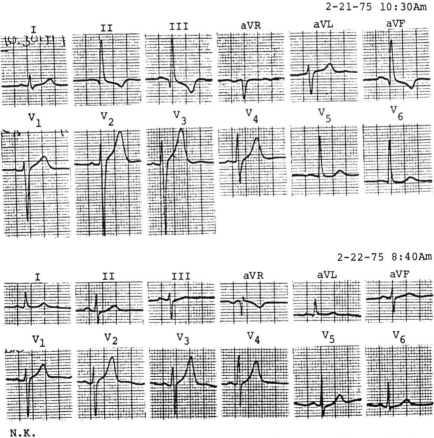

FIGURE 8–6. Intermittent left posterior hemiblock. The patient had unstable angina. The bottom tracing (2-22-75) is representative of ECGs taken when the patient was free of symptoms. The top tracing (2-21-75) was recorded during an anginal attack at rest. The QRS axis was displaced from −20° to +80° with the appearance of S wave in lead I and q waves in leads II, III, and aVF during pain. The tracing returned to his normal pattern after the pain subsided. A similar episode with identical ECG changes was observed again later. Although the QRS axis was only +80° during left posterior hemiblock, a shift of the axis of +100° occurred. The QRS duration increased from 0.07 to 0.10 second during the block. (Courtesy of Dr. Vijay Sanghvi.)

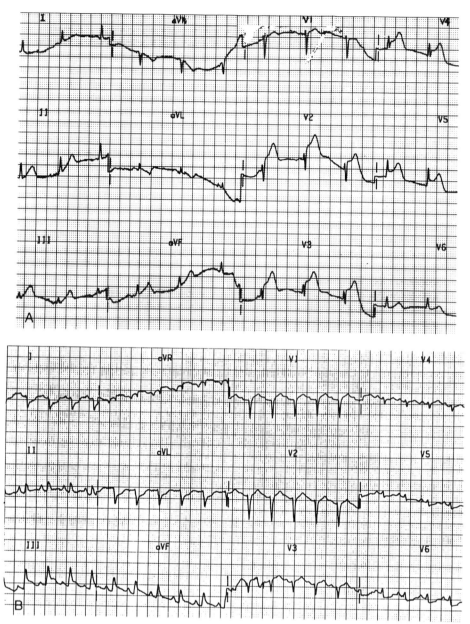

FIGURE 8–7. Left posterior hemiblock developed during acute myocardial infarction. The patient was a 49-year-old woman with severe chest pain of 2 hours' duration. The ECG recorded on her arrival at the hospital (A) shows marked ST-segment elevation in leads V_1 through V_5, consistent with acute anterior myocardial injury. One hundred milligrams of tissue plasminogen activator was administered intravenously over a 60-minute period. Chest pain was markedly improved in 10 minutes but recurred after 4 hours and was accompanied by severe hypotension. The ECG recorded at that time (B) shows sinus tachycardia, a marked rightward shift of the QRS axis from +45° (as shown in A) to +120°. ST-segment elevation is seen in leads II, III, and aVF. The previous ST-segment elevation in the precordial leads is no longer present. The acute onset of the abnormal right axis deviation can be contributed to left posterior hemiblock. At autopsy, the heart was normal in weight. There was almost complete occlusion of the proximal left anterior descending and right coronary arteries. An extensive myocardial infarction that involved the anterior wall, interventricular septum, and inferior wall was found.

wall myocardial infarction also may be accompanied by abnormal right axis deviation.

In right ventricular hypertrophy, a tall R wave or an RSR′ pattern with T-wave inversion may be present in the right precordial leads. Such a finding is uncommon in left posterior hemiblock unless true posterior myocardial infarction or right bundle branch block coex-

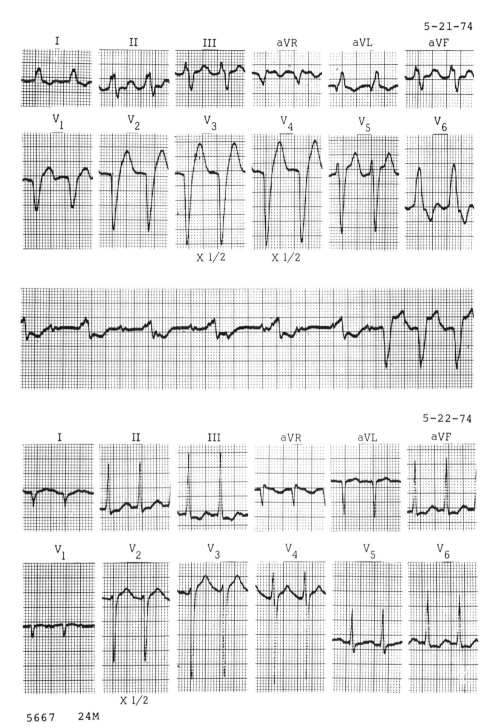

FIGURE 8–8. Various conduction abnormalities observed in a 24-year-old man with Marfan's syndrome and aortic aneurysm demonstrated by aortogram. The tracing on 5-21-74 shows complete left bundle branch block. The rhythm strip (MCL₁ lead) reveals transient complete AV block with idioventricular rhythm. The bottom tracing (5-22-74) is consistent with left ventricular hypertrophy. The marked right axis deviation without clinical evidence of right ventricular hypertrophy suggests left posterior hemiblock. The occurrence of left bundle branch block and complete AV block may be the result of additional intermittent block in the anterior division of the left bundle branch or in both of the two remaining fascicles. The appearance of the QRS complexes during complete AV block supports the diagnosis of trifascicular block.

ists. If the P wave is suggestive of right atrial enlargement, the abnormal right axis deviation is most likely indicative of right ventricular hypertrophy by inference. In pulmonary emphysema, the low amplitude of the QRS complex in the limb leads and left precordial leads and the P pulmonale pattern often are helpful in suggesting the correct interpretation. In lateral wall myocardial infarction, a QS rather than an rS complex is recorded in leads I and aVL to account for the abnormal right axis deviation. The T waves in these leads often are inverted, which is uncommon in uncomplicated left posterior hemiblock. The coexistence of lateral wall myocardial infarction and left posterior hemiblock, however, has been reported.

In many instances, the differentiation of left posterior hemiblock from the other entities cannot be accomplished by the ECG alone. Other clinical data are required. When abnormal right axis deviation is observed in a patient with left ventricular disease and there is no clinical evidence of right-sided heart involvement, the diagnosis of left posterior hemiblock is strongly suggested (see Fig. 8–8).

S_1Q_3 PATTERN

The early activation of the anterolateral wall of the left ventricle in left posterior hemiblock displaces the initial QRS forces leftward and superiorly.[50] Therefore, lead I records an initial R wave, and leads II, III, and aVF record Q waves. Such a shift of the initial vectors has been observed in patients with transient left posterior hemiblock[6] and is demonstrated in Figure 8–6. Some investigators, however, did not observe a significant change in the direction of these forces.[23] The relatively deep S wave in lead I is a consistent finding as the terminal QRS forces are invariably directed rightward.

QRS PROLONGATION

The development of left posterior hemiblock usually is accompanied by a prolongation of the QRS duration of no more than 0.02 second.[6,50] The QRS interval may therefore remain within the normal limits. However, a duration of up to 0.12 second from left posterior hemiblock alone has been reported.[23] In the patient with intermittent block illustrated in Figure 8–6, the increase of QRS duration was 0.03 second.

Changes in the Precordial Leads

Although the most essential findings of left posterior hemiblock are observed in the limb leads, significant changes also are present in the precordial leads. The transitional zone often is displaced leftward.[6] The smaller R waves and deeper S waves in the left precordial leads resemble those seen in right ventricular hypertrophy, causing further difficulties in the differentiation of the two conditions (see Fig. 8–5). If Q waves are present in the left precordial leads before the block develops, the leftward shift of the initial QRS forces with the hemiblock may cause them to disappear.[65]

Clinical and Pathologic Correlation

In contrast to left anterior hemiblock, left posterior hemiblock, especially in the isolated form, is considered rare. Rosenbaum and colleagues attributed the low incidence to the following characteristics of the posterior division of the left bundle branch[50]: (1) It is short and thick. (2) It has a dual blood supply from the anterior and posterior descending coronary arteries. (3) It belongs to the less turbulent left ventricular inflow tract. (4) It is the first group of fibers to depart from the bundle of His.

Coronary artery disease is the most common cause of left posterior hemiblock. Hypertension, cardiomyopathy, and aortic valve disease also may be responsible. It also has been described in patients who have heavy calcifications of the left side of the cardiac skeleton.[13] Theoretically, its cause should be similar to that of left anterior hemiblock, even though our knowledge in regard to this ECG entity is still limited.[5,46,50]

Its incidence in acute myocardial infarction is by far the lowest of all the intraventricular conduction defects, varying from 0.2 to 0.4 percent among the larger reported series.[9,46,57] The prognosis of these patients is poor because of the severity of the myocardial damage.[46] An example of such a relation is given in Figure 8–7. Transient left posterior hemiblock has been observed during selective coronary arteriography when the contrast material was injected into the right coronary artery.[23]

Left posterior hemiblock was suggested by Gaum and associated as the mechanism for the right axis deviation in some patients with supravalvular aortic stenosis and coarctation of the aorta.[24] It also was described in a case of dissecting aneurysm.[58]

As mentioned earlier, few cases of left posterior hemiblock have been studied pathologically. Pryor and Blount described two cases with careful histologic examination.[43] Significant fibrosis that involved the inferior division of the left bundle was found in both. Rizzon and associates reported on two patients with acute myocardial infarction and isolated left posterior hemiblock.[46] Acute histologic changes that affected the conduction fibers of the posterior septal area were observed. In four hearts of patients with isolated left posterior hemiblock examined by Demoulin and associates, maximal interruptive lesions were found in the posterior division fibers or posterior portion of the main left bundle branch.[13]

BIFASCICULAR, TRIFASCICULAR, AND BILATERAL BUNDLE BRANCH BLOCK

The intraventricular conduction system may be considered as a trifascicular system consisting of the right bundle branch and the two divisions of the left bundle branch. A third division, namely the medial or septal fascicle of the left bundle, also has been described.[63] In most of the literature, however, the three-division concept has not been applied. The possible types of block involving more than one fascicle are as follows.

1. Right bundle branch block with left anterior hemiblock.
2. Right bundle branch block with left posterior hemiblock.
3. Divisional left bundle branch block or simultaneous block in both divisions of the left bundle branch.
4. Bilateral bundle branch block or simultaneous block in the two main bundle branches.
5. Trifascicular block, or simultaneous block in the right bundle branch and the two divisions of the left bundle branch.

For the sake of simplicity, simultaneous block of the main left bundle branch and one of its divisions is not included in the list. Simultaneous block in both divisions of the left bundle branch has the same ECG changes as a block at the level of the main bundle. Figure 8–8 is probably an example of such a combination. It also should be mentioned that some authors described right bundle branch block with left anterior or posterior hemiblock as a form of partial or incomplete bilateral bundle branch block.[34,56] In this text, such blocks are referred to as *bifascicilar block,* and the term *bilateral bundle branch block* is reserved for involvement of the two main bundle branches. As in the case of monofascicular block, the block in one of the fascicles may be intermittent or transient.[51]

Right Bundle Branch Block with Left Anterior Hemiblock

Right bundle branch block with left anterior hemiblock is the most common type of bifascicular block. It was called the "variant," "classic," or "uncommon" type of right bundle branch block in the past. The so-called left bundle branch block masquerading as right bundle branch block described previously belongs to this type of conduction abnormality.[45,64]

When the impulse conduction is interrupted or delayed in the right bundle branch and anterior division of the left bundle branch, ventricular activation begins in the area supplied by the posterior division of the left bundle branch. The excitation of the anterolateral wall of the left ventricle is slightly delayed, since it now depends on impulse arriving retrograde from the posterior division. Right ventricular depolarization follows as the impulse propagates transseptally from the left septum toward the right. The first portion of the QRS complex therefore has the characteristics of isolated left anterior hemiblock, and the last portion has those of right bundle branch block (Fig. 8–9).

DIAGNOSTIC CRITERIA

1. Prolongation of the QRS duration to 0.12 second or longer.
2. An RSR' pattern in lead V_1, with the R' being broad and slurred.
3. Wide and slurred S waves in leads I, V_5, and V_6.
4. The first half or 0.06 second of the QRS complex having a frontal plane axis of $-30°$ to $-90°$.
5. An initial r wave in the inferior leads.

Some confusion exists as to how the QRS axis is determined when right bundle branch block is present. This is best done by using the unblocked portion of the QRS complex. The first portion (usually the first half or 0.06 second) of the complex is rapidly inscribed. In

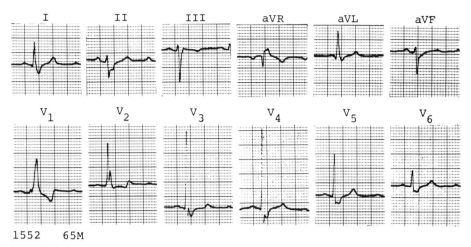

1552   65M

FIGURE 8–9. Right bundle branch block with left anterior hemiblock. The QRS duration is 0.13 second. An rR′ complex is seen in lead V_1 and a wide S wave in leads I, V_5, and V_6 consistent with complete right bundle branch block. In the limb leads, the first 0.06-second QRS forces are inscribed rapidly and have a mean axis of −45°, suggesting left anterior hemiblock.

most instances, it is not difficult to detect the onset of the slurred portion that is related to right bundle branch block. As in the case of monofascicular block, the conduction defect may be transient or intermittent. The unstable pattern may involve either the right bundle branch or the left anterior division.

CLINICAL SIGNIFICANCE AND ANATOMIC CORRELATION

Right bundle branch block with left anterior hemiblock is common. Its incidence in the hospital population is about 1 percent.[32,66] The common types of heart disease that cause this conduction defect are the following:

1. Coronary artery disease
2. Hypertensive heart disease
3. Aortic valve disease
4. Cardiomyopathy
5. Lenegre's disease
6. Lev's disease
7. Congenital heart disease
8. Surgical trauma
9. Cardiac transplantation

Coronary artery disease is the most common cause of this bifascicular block. In the larger series, it is responsible for 41 to 61 percent of the cases.[32,55] In patients with acute myocardial infarction, it occurs in about 4.8 to 7 percent.[2,9,38,57,68] The location of the infarction usually is anterior. This can be explained by the fact that the anterior division of the left bundle branch and the right bundle branch

run in close proximity in the anterior part of the interventricular septum. Both fascicles share a common blood supply via the septal branches of the left anterior descending coronary artery. This relationship also explains the frequency with which the two fascicles are involved together.

To correlate the ECG with the pathologic findings, Lenegre examined 12 cases of right bundle branch block and left anterior hemiblock with serial histologic sections.[33] Myocardial infarction with either complete or partial destruction of the right and left bundle branch was found in all.

Hypertensive heart disease is the next most common underlying cause and accounts for about 20 to 25 percent of the cases.[32,55] Many of the patients had clinical evidence of both coronary artery disease and hypertension.

Aortic valve disease, especially aortic stenosis, is responsible for a significant percentage of this conduction abnormality.[62] Both fascicles may be involved by an extension of the fibrocalcific process of the aortic valve at the level of the pseudobifurcation (i.e., the point at which the right bundle branch separates from the most anterior fibers of the left bundle branch). Cardiomyopathy, either idiopathic or secondary to a systemic disease, is another causative factor. Myocardial fibrosis or an infiltrative process that involves the conduction system is responsible.

One group of patients has no apparent associated heart disease. Such patients have no symptoms and have normal-sized hearts. They may, however, develop complete heart block and Stokes-Adams seizures. Histologic examination reveals a sclerodegenerative process limited to the conduction tissue. Rosenbaum and co-workers[50] called this entity Lenegre's disease in recognition of the French author who was the first to describe it.[33]

Lev described an intraventricular conduction defect caused by sclerosis of the left side of the cardiac skeleton. He stated that, with advancing age, there is normally a progressive fibrosis and calcification of the mitral annulus, the central fibrous body, the pars membranacea, the base of the aorta, and the summit of the muscular septum. Because the conduction system is adjacent to some of this structure, a fibrotic process at the summit of the muscular septum may injure the right bundle branch and anterior division of the left bundle branch. This conduction defect usually is seen in elderly individuals. No other evidence of heart disease may be present.[35,60] Lev disease and Lenegre disease often are grouped together under the entity label *primary conduction disease*. In Dhingra and associates' series of 452 patients with chronic bifascicular block, 86 (19 percent) had primary conduction disease.[18] Three hundred thirty-nine of the patients had right bundle branch block and left hemiblock, and 113 had left bundle branch block. The incidence of primary conduction disease was 23 percent in the former and 7 percent in the latter.

Hyperkalemia has been reported to cause transient block in these two fascicles.[4]

Among the congenital heart diseases, right bundle branch block and left anterior hemiblock occur mainly in endocardial cushion defects. The mechanism by which the abnormal left axis deviation is produced is still open to question, however. From electrophysiologic observations in patients with ostium primum atrial septal defect during open heart surgery, it has been suggested the changes are due to premature activation of the posterobasal portion of the left ventricle rather than to the delayed excitation of the anterolateral wall.[21]

Right bundle branch block and left anterior hemiblock may be the result of surgical trauma. In a series of 200 patients who underwent coronary bypass graft surgery, this bifascicular block developed in 7 (4 percent).[69] At the Cincinnati Children's Hospital, it was found in about 6 percent of patients with ventricular septal defect and in 11 percent with tetralogy of Fallot who underwent corrective surgery.[20] This conduction defect also has been observed after tricuspid valve replacement.[1]

Right bundle branch block is a very common postoperative finding in patients who undergo cardiac transplantation. Occasionally, left anterior hemiblock also develops in these patients (see Chapter 27).

RELATION OF RIGHT BUNDLE BRANCH BLOCK AND LEFT ANTERIOR HEMIBLOCK TO COMPLETE AV BLOCK

In patients with right bundle branch block and left anterior hemiblock, the development of incomplete or complete AV block may be the result of additional damage to the posterior division of the left bundle branch, the main left bundle branch itself, the His bundle, or the AV node (Fig. 8–10). Lasser and associates reported the progression to complete AV block in 10 percent of patients with chronic form of bifascicular block.[32] Scanlon and associates found an incidence of progression to complete AV block in 14.4 percent of patients in an average follow-up of 2 years.[55] On the other hand, in patients who have transient or permanent complete heart block, 59 percent were shown to have the bifascicular block pattern before the development of the complete heart block.

In an editorial that discussed the prognosis of patients with chronic bifascicular block, Surawicz summarized the data from five prospective studies involving 950 patients.[61] Most of the patients had right bundle branch block and left anterior hemiblock. The average duration of the follow-up ranged from 1 to 3 years. Sudden death occurred in 82 patients. The presence of complete AV block immediately before death was documented in only 6 and suspected in 31 patients. In the 452 patients with chronic bifascicular block (277 of them were included in one of the previously mentioned five prospective studies) reported by Dhingra and co-workers, the cumulative incidence of AV block at 5 years was 11 percent, with 7 percent reflecting AV block developed spontaneously without an apparent precipitating cause.[18] The site of the AV block varied and was trifascicular in fewer than half of the patients. The same group of investigators also reported a high risk of developing trifascicular block in those patients with chronic bifascicular block if the His bundle recording showed a prolonged rather than

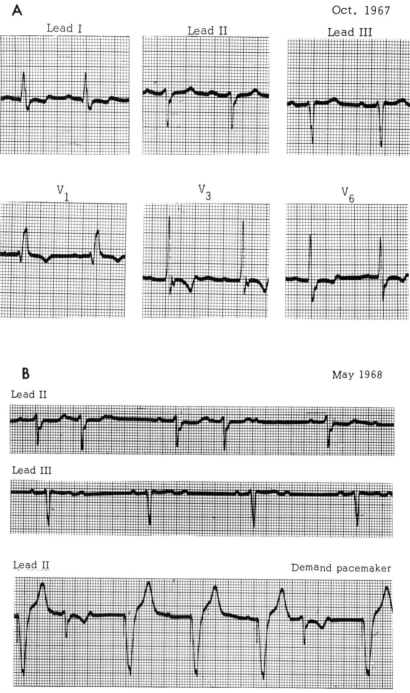

FIGURE 8–10. (A) Right bundle branch block with left anterior hemiblock and first-degree AV block (October 1967) followed by (B) Mobitz type II second-degree AV block (May 1968) in a 62-year-old man with hypertensive heart disease, luetic aortic insufficiency, and syncope. The bottom strip shows a functioning ventricular demand pacemaker.

normal HV interval.[17] Patients with primary conduction disease had a significantly lower incidence of spontaneous AV block as well as cardiovascular and sudden death mortality than those with organic heart disease.[19]

In patients with acute myocardial infarction and this variety of bifascicular block, complete heart block develops more frequently. The reported incidence varies between 24 and 43 percent.[2,56] The mortality in these patients even without AV block is high, varying between 36 and 59 percent.[26,39,56,57]

Right Bundle Branch Block with Left Posterior Hemiblock

In right bundle branch block with left posterior hemiblock, ventricular activation begins in the anterior and lateral wall of the left ventricle through the anterior division of the left bundle branch. This is followed by the excitation of the inferoposterior wall by retrograde conduction of the impulse from the anterior to the posterior division. The activation of the right ventricle is further delayed and depends on the impulse advancing transseptally from the left side.

In the ECG, the first portion, usually 0.06 second of the QRS complex, displays the characteristics of the left posterior hemiblock, and the last portion shows the right bundle branch block (Figs. 8–11B and 8–12).

DIAGNOSTIC CRITERIA

1. Prolongation of the QRS to 0.12 second or longer.

2. An RSR' pattern in lead V_1, with the R' being broad and slurred.

3. Wide and slurred S waves in leads I, V_5, and V_6.

4. The first half or 0.06 second of the QRS having a frontal plane axis of +90° or farther to the right, with an rS deflection in lead I and qR waves in leads II, III, and aVF.

As in the case of isolated left posterior hemiblock, the presence of right ventricular hypertrophy, pulmonary emphysema, vertical heart, and lateral myocardial infarction should be excluded before the diagnosis is made.

CLINICAL AND ANATOMIC CORRELATION

Right bundle branch block and left posterior hemiblock is an uncommon form of bifascicular block. This is related to the rarity of left posterior hemiblock, which was explained previously. In fact, this bifascicular block occurs more commonly than does iso-

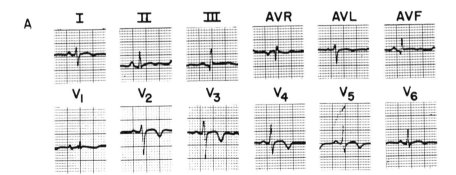

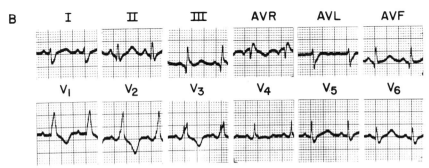

FIGURE 8–11. (A) Left posterior hemiblock associated with true posterior myocardial infarction. The tracing was obtained from a 51-year-old woman with severe coronary artery disease. Coronary arteriogram demonstrated 90 percent obstruction of the right coronary artery near its origin and 50 percent narrowing of the anterior descending artery and the left circumflex artery distal to a large marginal branch. In the ECG, the frontal plane QRS axis is +110°. Lead V_1 shows an rsr's' pattern. T-wave inversion is present in many of the leads. (B) Probable posterior and inferior myocardial infarction with right bundle branch block and left posterior hemiblock from the same patient 10 months after A was recorded. There is an increase of the amplitude of the Q waves in the inferior leads since the previous tracing. Right bundle branch block is present in addition to left posterior hemiblock.

2/25/70

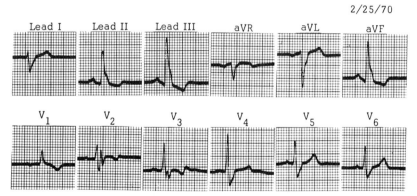

FIGURE 8–12. Right bundle branch block with left posterior hemiblock in a 77-year-old man with no other clinical evidence of heart disease.

lated left posterior hemiblock. When the disease process is extensive enough to cause left posterior hemiblock, involvement of the other fascicles is likely.

The cause of this conduction defect is similar to the causes of right bundle branch block with left anterior hemiblock, coronary artery disease being the most common[50,56] (see Fig. 8–11). In patients with acute myocardial infarction, it occurs in less than 0.8 percent of the cases.[2,46,57,68] Postmortem examination in some of these cases[46] revealed infarction that involved either the entire intraventricular septum or a large portion of it. Severe atherosclerosis was present in all three main coronary vessels or in the left anterior descending and right coronary arteries. Histologically, lesions were found in both bundle branches in the cases examined.

RELATION OF RIGHT BUNDLE BRANCH BLOCK WITH LEFT POSTERIOR HEMIBLOCK TO COMPLETE AV BLOCK

The reported incidence of progression of chronic right bundle branch block and left posterior hemiblock to advanced AV block varies. In Rosenbaum's 30 cases, complete or high-grade AV block developed in 19 patients (60 percent) and Stokes-Adams seizures developed in 18 (60 percent).[49] Other investigators have also described the frequent progression to complete AV block.[8,31] Scanlon and associates observed such a development in 8 of 49 patients followed for an average of 2 years.[55] An even lower incidence was reported by Dhingra and colleagues.[16] Only 2 of 21 patients had documented progression of the conduction defect in an average 2-year follow-

up period. It may be significant, however, that in their series the PR interval in the initial ECG was normal in most of the patients.

Trifascicular Block

A complete trifascicular block results in complete AV block. The idioventricular escape rhythm has a slower rate and a wide QRS complex because the pacemaker is located at the peripheral part of the conduction system distal to the sites of the block. Such a rhythm may be difficult to differentiate from bifascicular or bundle branch block combined with complete block at a higher level such as the AV node or His bundle. Besides a slower ventricular rate, a change in the morphology of the QRS complex from a previous known bifascicular pattern is strongly suggestive of a trifascicular origin of the complete AV block. A His bundle recording is required for a definitive diagnosis, however.

If the block in one of the three fascicles is incomplete, the ECG displays a bifascicular block with first- or second-degree AV block. Therefore, the possible manifestations are right bundle branch block with left anterior hemiblock or left posterior hemiblock, divisional left bundle branch block and PR prolongation, or second-degree AV block. As mentioned previously, however, such an ECG finding may not always indicate that the PR prolongation is due to the involvement of the third fascicle. The conduction delay may also be at the level of the AV node or bundle of His. To evaluate the significance of the PR prolongation in bifascicular block, Levitas and Haft reviewed the results of His bundle recording in 89 patients and compared them with those of 172 patients with bifascicular block but normal PR intervals.[36] In patients with right bundle branch block, left anterior hemiblock, and PR prolongation, the HV interval was prolonged to suggest a diseased third fascicle in 68 percent of 40 cases. Thirty percent of 102 patients without PR prolongation also had abnormally long HV intervals. In patients with right bundle branch block, the HV interval was prolonged in over 50 percent of the cases regardless of the PR interval. The difference in the HV interval between the groups with or without first-degree AV block was not statistically significant. The authors concluded that it is difficult to determine whether trifascicular block is present in the individual patient from the body surface ECG.

Trifascicular block may be suspected if there is a permanent block in one fascicle and an intermittent block of the other two fasci-

cles. For example, if a patient with a stable right bundle branch block shows left anterior hemiblock and left posterior hemiblock on different occasions, the presence of disease of all three fascicles is implied. Depending on which fascicular block is permanent, three possible combinations exist. It also is possible that the block in all three fascicles is intermittent. Refer to the articles by Rosenbaum and associates for more detailed discussion.[48,51,52]

Figure 8–13 is an example of trifascicular block. There is a Mobitz type II second-degree AV block. The QRS complexes show the alternating patterns of left anterior hemiblock, right bundle branch block with left anterior hemiblock, and left bundle branch block. A His bundle recording revealed that the AV block was distal to the His bundle.

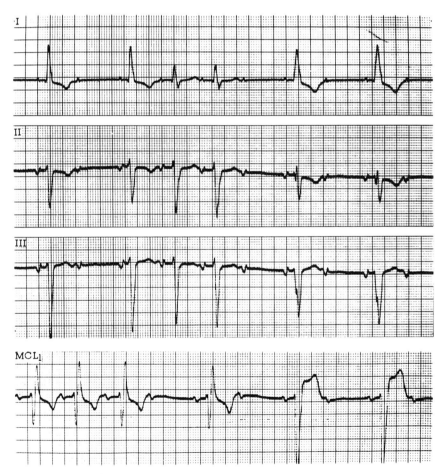

FIGURE 8–13. Trifascicular block. Leads I, II, and III were recorded simultaneously. There is a Mobitz type II second-degree AV block. The first two QRS complexes show left anterior hemiblock, the third and fourth show left anterior hemiblock with right bundle branch block, and the last two show left bundle branch block. The MCL$_1$ lead recorded at about the same time reveals alternating right and left bundle branch block patterns with Mobitz type II second-degree AV block. A His bundle recording demonstrated that the AV block was distal to the His bundle.

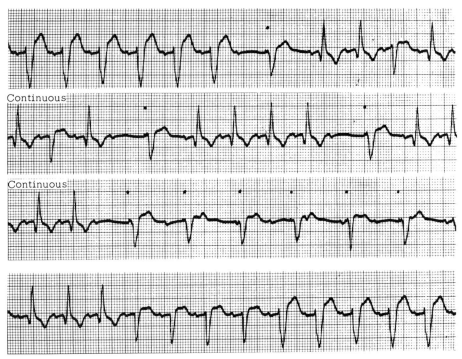

FIGURE 8–14. Bilateral bundle branch block. The rhythm strips were recorded from a patient with acute myocardial infarction. An MCL₁ monitor lead was used. The bottom strip shows the pattern of right bundle branch block, normal conduction, and left bundle branch block. The top three strips demonstrate the varying ventricular conduction defect and high-degree AV block. An electronic ventricular demand pacemaker is functioning. The paced beats are marked by a dot. The pacemaker spikes are small.

Bilateral Bundle Branch Block

In this text, the term *bilateral bundle branch block* is used to indicate impairment of impulse conduction at the level of the main bundle branches. A complete interruption of conduction in both bundles results in complete AV block. The rhythm usually cannot be distinguished from complete trifascicular block. Occasionally, if there is alternating intermittent block of the two bundles, the presence of bilateral bundle branch block can be assumed (Fig. 8–14). If the block in one of the bundles is incomplete, first- or second-degree AV block plus unilateral bundle branch block is observed. Such a condition, however, cannot be differentiated from a partial block at the level of the AV node or His bundle in addition to left or right bundle branch block without a His bundle recording. If the block in both bundles is incomplete but the delay of conduction is equal bilaterally, the QRS complex may be normal, because both ventricles are depolarized simultaneously as in the normal process. The PR interval is prolonged. Incomplete bundle branch block patterns are ob-

served if the delay of conduction on both sides is unequal.[34]

REFERENCES

1. Aravindakshan V, Elizari MV, Rosenbaum MB: Right bundle-branch block and left anterior fascicular block (left anterior hemiblock) following tricuspid valve replacement. Circulation 42:895, 1970
2. Atkins JM, Leshin SJ, Blomqvist G, et al: Ventricular conduction blocks and sudden death in acute myocardial infarction: Potential indications for pacing. N Engl J Med 288:281, 1973
3. Bahl OP, Walsh TJ, Massie E: Left axis deviation: An electrocardiographic study with post-mortem correlation. Br Heart J 31:451, 1969
4. Bashour T, Hsu I, Gorfinkel HJ, et al: Atrioventricular and intraventricular conduction in hyperkalemia. Am J Cardiol 35:199, 1975
5. Benchimol A, Desser KB: The Frank vectorcardiogram in left posterior hemiblock. J Electrocardiol 4:129, 1971
6. Bobba P, Salerno JA, Casari A: Transient left posterior hemiblock: Report of four cases induced by exercise test. Circulation 46:931, 1972
7. Bosch X, Theroux P, Roy D, et al: Coronary angiographic significance of left anterior fascicular block during acute myocardial infarction. J Am Coll Cardiol 5:9, 1985

8. Castellanos A, Maytin O, Arcebal AG, et al: Significance of complete right bundle-branch block with right axis deviation in absence of right ventricle hypertrophy. Br Heart J 32:85, 1970

9. Col JJ, Weinberg SL: The incidence and mortality of intraventricular conduction defects in acute myocardial infarction. Am J Cardiol 29:344, 1972

10. Corne RA, Beamish RE, Rollwagen RL: Significance of left anterior hemiblock. Br Heart J 40:552, 1978

11. Corne RA, Parkin TW, Bradenburg RO, et al: Significance of marked left axis deviation: Electrocardiographic-pathologic correlative study. Am J Cardiol 15:605, 1965

12. Das G: Left axis deviation: A spectrum of intraventricular conduction block. Circulation 53:917, 1976

13. Demoulin JC, Kulbertus HE: Histopathologic correlates of left posterior fascicular block. Am J Cardiol 44:1083, 1979

14. Demoulin JC, Kulbertus HE: Histopathological examination of concept of left hemiblock. Br Heart J 34:807, 1972

15. Demoulin JC, Simar LJ, Kulbertus HE: Quantitative study of left bundle branch fibrosis in left anterior hemiblock: A stereologic approach. Am J Cardiol 36:751, 1975

16. Dhingra RC, Denes P, Wu D, et al: Chronic right bundle branch block and left posterior hemiblock: Clinical, electrophysiologic and prognostic observations. Am J Cardiol 36:867, 1975

17. Dhingra RC, Paliteo E, Strasberg B: Significance of the HV interval in 517 patients with chronic bifascicular block. Circulation 64: 1265, 1981

18. Dhingra RC, Wyndham C, Amat-Y-Leon F, et al: Incidence and site of atrioventricular block in patients with chronic bifascicular block. Circulation 59:238, 1979

19. Dhingra RC, Wyndham C, Bauernfeind R, et al: Significance of chronic bifascicular block without apparent organic heart disease. Circulation 60:33, 1979

20. Downing JW, Kaplan S, Bove KE: Postsurgical left anterior hemiblock and right bundle-branch block. Br Heart J 34:263, 1972

21. Durrer D, Roos JP, Van Dam RT: The genesis of the electrocardiogram of patients with ostium primum defects (ventral atrial septal defects). Am Heart J 71:642, 1966

22. Eliot RS, Millhon WA, Millhon J: The clinical significance of uncomplicated marked left axis deviation in men without known disease. Am J Cardiol 12:767, 1963

23. Fernandez F, Scebat L, Lenegre J: Electrocardiographic study of left intraventricular hemiblock in man during selective coronary arteriography. Am J Cardiol 26:1, 1970

24. Gaum WE, Chou TC, Kaplan S: The vectorcardiogram in supravalvular aortic stenosis and coarctation of the aorta. Am Heart J 84:5, 1972

25. Gertsch M, Theler A, Foglia E: Electrocardiographic detection of left ventricular hypertrophy in the presence of left anterior fascicular block. Am J Cardiol 61:1098, 1988

26. Godman MJ, Lassers BW, Julian DG: Complete bundle-branch block complicating acute myocardial infarction. N Engl J Med 282:237, 1970

27. Grant RP: Left axis deviation. An electrocardiographic–pathologic correlation study. Circulation 14:233, 1956

28. Grant RP: Left axis deviation. Mod Concepts Cardiovasc Dis 27:437, 1958

29. Gup AM, Granklin RB, Hill HE: The vectorcardiogram in children with left axis deviation and no apparent heart disease. Am Heart J 69:619, 1965

30. Hiss RG, Lamb LE, Allen MF: Electrocardiographic findings in 67,375 asymptomatic subjects. Am J Cardiol 6:200, 1960

31. Kulbertus H, Collignon P: Association of right bundle-branch block with left superior or inferior intraventricular block: Its relation to complete heart block and Adams-Stokes syndrome. Br Heart J 31:435, 1969

32. Lasser RP, Haft JI, Friedberg CK: Relationship of right bundle-branch block and marked left axis deviation (with left parietal or peri-infarction block) to complete heart block and syncope. Circulation 37:429, 1968

33. Lenegre J: Etiology and pathology of bilateral bundle branch block in relation to complete heart block. Prog Cardiovasc Dis 6:409, 1964

34. Lepeschkin E: The electrocardiographic diagnosis of bilateral bundle branch block in relation to heart block. Prog Cardiovasc Dis 6:445, 1964

35. Lev M: Anatomic basis for atrioventricular block. Am J Med 37:742, 1964

36. Levitas R, Haft JI: Significance of first degree heart block (prolonged PR interval) in bifascicular block. Am J Cardiol 34:259, 1974

37. McHenry PL, Phillips JF, Fisch C, et al: Right precordial qrS pattern due to left anterior hemiblock. Am Heart J 81:498, 1971

38. Nimetz AA, Shubrooks SJ, Hutter AM, et al: The significance of bundle branch block during acute myocardial infarction. Am Heart J 90:439, 1975

39. Norris RM, Croxson MS: Bundle branch block in acute myocardial infarction. Am Heart J 79:728, 1970

40. Ostrander LD: Left axis deviation: Prevalence, associated conditions and prognosis. Ann Intern Med 75:23, 1971

41. Perloff JK, Roberts NK, Cabeen WR: Left axis deviation: A reassessment. Circulation 60:12, 1979

42. Pryor R: Fascicular blocks and the bilateral bundle branch syndrome. Am Heart J 83:441, 1972

43. Pryor R, Blount SG Jr: The clinical significance of true left axis deviation. Am Heart J 72:391, 1966

44. Rabkin SW, Mathewson FAL, Tate RB: Natural history of marked left axis deviation (left anterior hemiblock). Am J Cardiol 43:605, 1979

45. Richman JL, Wolff L: Left bundle branch block masquerading as right bundle branch block. Am Heart J 47:383, 1954

46. Rizzon P, Rossi L, Baissus C, et al: Left posterior hemiblock in acute myocardial infarction. Br Heart J 37:711, 1975

47. Romhilt DW, Estes EH: Point-score system for the ECG diagnosis of left ventricular hypertrophy. Am Heart J 75:752, 1968

48. Rosenbaum MB: Types of right bundle branch block and their clinical significance. J Electrocardiol 1:221, 1968

49. Rosenbaum MB: The hemiblocks: Diagnostic criteria and clinical significance. Mod Concepts Cardiovasc Dis 39:141, 1970

50. Rosenbaum MB, Elizari MV, Lazzari JO: The Hemiblocks. Oldsmar, Fla, Tampa Tracings, 1970

51. Rosenbaum MB, Elizari MV, Lazzari JO, et al: Intraventricular trifascicular blocks: The syndrome of right bundle branch block with intermittent left anterior and posterior hemiblock. Am Heart J 78:306, 1969

52. Rosenbaum MB, Elizari MV, Lazzari JO, et al: Intraventricular trifascicular blocks. Review of the literature and classification. Am Heart J 78:450, 1969

53. Rosenbaum MB, Elizari MV, Levi RJ, et al: Five cases of intermittent left anterior hemiblock. Am J Cardiol 24:1, 1969

54. Rossi L: Histopathology of conducting system in left anterior hemiblock. Br Heart J 38:1304, 1976

55. Scanlon PJ, Pryor R, Blount SG: Right bundle-branch block associated with left superior or inferior intraventricular block: Clinical setting, prognosis and relation to complete heart block. Circulation 42:1123, 1970

56. Scanlon PJ, Pryor R, Blount SG: Right bundle-branch block associated with left superior or inferior intraventricular block: Associated with acute myocardial infarction. Circulation 42:1135, 1970

57. Scheinman M, Brenman BA: Clinical and anatomic implications of intraventricular conduction blocks in acute myocardial infarction. Circulation 46:753, 1972

58. Scott RC, Manitsas GT, Kim, OJ, et al: Left posterior hemiblock: A new diagnostic sign in dissecting aneurysm? J Electrocardiol 4:261, 1971

59. Shaher RM: Left ventricular preponderance and left axis deviation in congenital heart disease. Br Heart J 25:726, 1963

60. Sugiura M, Okada R, Keisuke H, et al: Histological studies on the conduction system in 14 cases of right bundle branch block associated with left axis deviation. Jpn Heart J 10:121, 1969

61. Surawicz B: Prognosis of patients with chronic bifascicular block. Circulation 60:40, 1979

62. Thompson R, Mitchell A, Ahmed M, et al: Conduction defects in aortic valve disease. Am Heart J 98:3, 1979

63. Uhley HN: Some controversy regarding the peripheral distribution of the conduction system. Editorial. Am J Cardiol 30:919, 1972

64. Unger PN, Lesser ME, Kugel VH, et al: The concept of "masquerading" bundle branch block: An electrocardiographic–pathologic correlation. Circulation 17:397, 1968

65. Wagner R, Rosenbaum MB: Transient left posterior hemiblock: Association with acute lateral myocardial infarction. Am J Cardol 29:558, 1972

66. Watt TB, Pruitt RD: Character, cause and consequence of combined left axis deviation and right bundle branch block in human electrocardiograms. Am Heart J 77:460, 1969

67. Watt TB, Pruitt RD: Left posterior fascicular block in canine and primate hearts. Circulation 40:677, 1969

68. Waugh RA, Wagner GS, Haney TL, et al: Immediate and remote prognostic significance of fascicular block during acute myocardial infarction. Circulation 47:765, 1973

69. Zeldis SM, Morganroth J, Horowitz LN: Fascicular conduction disturbances after coronary bypass surgery. Am J Cardiol 41:860, 1978

Myocardial Infarction, Myocardial Injury, and Myocardial Ischemia

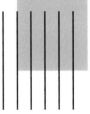

9

The normal QRS complex represents the resultant of the electrical forces generated from the various portions of the myocardium during ventricular depolarization. In myocardial infarction, the zone of necrosis becomes electrically silent. The balance of the vectoral forces tends to point away from this area as the opposing potential becomes dominant. If the displacement of the resultant vectors is marked, an electrode facing the infarcted myocardium records an abnormal negative deflection during depolarization (Fig. 9–1). If this part of the myocardium normally is depolarized early in the sequence of activation, an initial negativity or abnormal Q wave is recorded and the infarction is called *Q-wave infarction.* Therefore, in anterior Q-wave myocardial infarction, abnormal Q waves are seen in the precordial leads. In inferior Q-wave myocardial infarction, abnormal initial deflections are present in leads II, III, and aVF. As the posterobasal portion of the left ventricle is depolarized late, the changes of posterior left ventricular infarction are seen in the later portion of the QRS complex. If an electrode is placed on the dorsal aspect of the chest, a large negative deflection is recorded either as an exaggeration of the normal Q wave or as a second downward deflection. Because posterior chest leads are not taken in the routine electrocardiogram (ECG), the reciprocal changes in the anterior precordial leads are used to recognize posterior infarction. They are usually displayed in lead V_1 as a tall R wave or, less commonly, as an rR′ or rSR′ pattern.

In many cases of myocardial infarction, abnormal Q waves are not observed in the ECG. This type of infarction is described as non–Q-wave myocardial infarction. The reason for the absence of abnormal Q waves often is not apparent. In some instances, the necrotic area may be small or subendocardial, or the infarcted tissue may be scattered and separated by viable myocardium. The displacement of the initial QRS forces due to the infarcted area

or areas may not be in the same direction. Consequently, the electrodes overlying the necrotic zone may not record a negative deflection, and only ST-segment and T-wave changes are observed. Although non–Q-wave infarction often is referred to as subendocardial infarction and Q-wave infarction as transmural, the implied ECG and anatomic association cannot be verified by autopsy findings in a large number of cases.

In myocardial injury, the involved area is depolarized incompletely. It remains electrically more positive than the uninjured area at the end of the depolarization. If an exploring electrode is placed in this region, the relatively positive potential causes an elevation of the ST segment. Conversely, if the electrode is located over the uninjured myocardium opposite the injured area, it faces the negative end of the ST vector. ST-segment depression is recorded. Similarly, if the injury is limited to the subendocardial layer of the ventricular wall, the exploring electrode is separated from the injured area by the normal epicardial layer of the myocardium. The latter becomes electrically more negative than the injured endocardium at the end of depolarization. The ST vector therefore points away from the adjacent electrode, resulting in ST-segment depression. (In this discussion, the theory of "blocking of depolarization" is used to explain the ST changes of myocardial injury. The "current of injury" theory also has been proposed but is not described here for the sake of simplicity.)

Myocardial ischemia delays the repolarization process. Consequently, the ischemic zone is electrically more negative than the unaffected area during the recovery phase, and the T vector points away from it. An exploring electrode overlying the ischemic area records a negative T wave. If the ischemia is subendocardial rather than transmural, the delay in repolarization does not alter the direction of the recovery process, since repolarization nor-

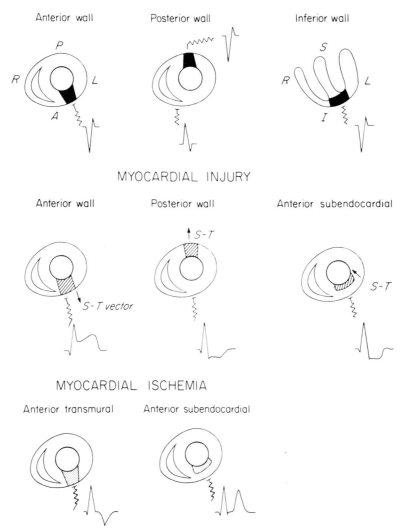

FIGURE 9–1. Diagrams depicting the ECG changes in Q-wave myocardial infarction, myocardial injury, and myocardial ischemia.

mally proceeds from the epicardium toward the endocardium. Therefore, an electrode that faces that area of the ventricle records an upright T wave. Because the electrical potential generated by the delayed repolarization in the subendocardium is unopposed, the T waves become abnormally tall.

In acute Q-wave myocardial infarction, the area of necrosis is surrounded by a zone of injury and a zone of ischemia. Therefore, ST-segment elevation and T-wave changes are recorded in the leads displaying the abnormal Q waves as well as in the leads adjacent to the infarcted area. As stated previously, only ST-segment and T-wave changes are seen in the non–Q-wave myocardial infarction.

DIAGNOSTIC CRITERIA OF LEFT VENTRICULAR Q-WAVE INFARCTION

Anteroseptal myocardial infarction (Fig. 9–2):
QS deflections in leads V_1, V_2, V_3, and sometimes V_4.

Anterior myocardial infarction (Fig. 9–3):
An rS deflection in V_1 followed by abnormal Q waves in leads V_2 through V_4.

Anterolateral myocardial infarction (Fig. 9–4):
Abnormal Q waves in leads V_4 through V_6, I, and aVL.

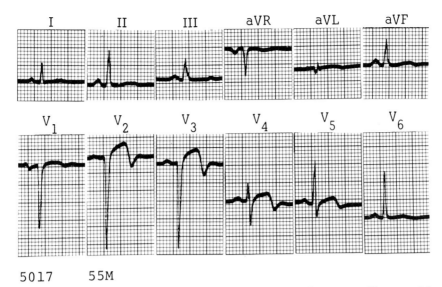

5017   55M

FIGURE 9-2. Recent anteroseptal myocardial infarction proved at autopsy. There was 95 percent narrowing of the left anterior descending coronary artery. The infarction was transmural. Mild left ventricular hypertrophy also was present.

Extensive anterior myocardial infarction Fig. 9–5):
QS deflections in all or nearly all the precordial leads with or without abnormal Q waves in leads I and aVL.

Lateral or high lateral myocardial infarction (Fig. 9–6):
Abnormal Q waves in leads I and aVL.

Inferior myocardial infarction (Figs. 9–7 and 9–8):
Q waves in leads II, III, and aVF, the Q wave in aVF being abnormal.

Inferolateral myocardial infarction (Fig. 9–9):
Q waves in leads II, III, and aVF that met the criteria for inferior infarction, plus abnormal Q waves in leads V_5 and V_6.

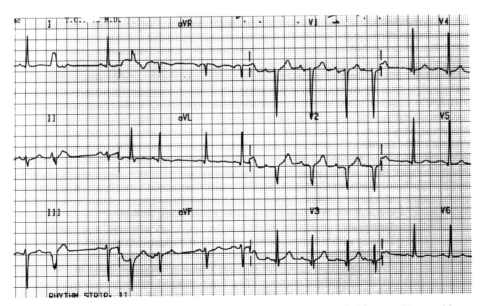

FIGURE 9-3. Old anterior myocardial infarction. The tracing was recorded from an 81-year-old man who had a documented anterior myocardial infarction 2 years ago. Note the QS deflection in lead V_2 and abnormal Q wave in lead V_3. A small R wave is present in lead V_1. Premature ventricular beats, voltage criteria for left ventricular hypertrophy, left anterior hemiblock, and minor T-wave changes also are seen in the tracing.

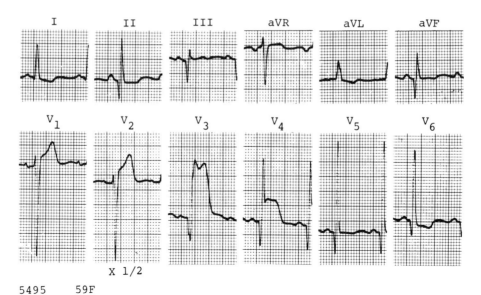

5495   59F

FIGURE 9–4. Acute anterolateral and old inferior myocardial infarction proved by autopsy. This ECG was recorded from a 59-year-old woman 1 hour after the onset of severe substernal pain. An inferior myocardial infarction occurred 2 years previously. The ECGs made before this tracing showed abnormal Q waves only in leads II, III, and aVF. Marked ST-segment elevation is seen in leads V_3 and V_4. New Q waves have appeared in leads V_3 through V_6. The tracing also suggests left ventricular hypertrophy.

True posterior myocardial infarction (Figs. 9–10 through 9–12):
Initial R waves in leads V_1 and V_2 that have a duration of 0.04 second or longer, with an R/S ratio equal to or greater than 1[213] (in patients over 30 years of age without right ventricular hypertrophy).

An abnormal Q wave generally is defined as a Q wave that has a duration of 0.04 second or longer.[13,107,192,193] Some authors consider a Q-wave duration of longer than 0.03 second[132] or an amplitude of the Q wave that is greater than 25 percent of the following R wave as abnormal.[13,107] These definitions do

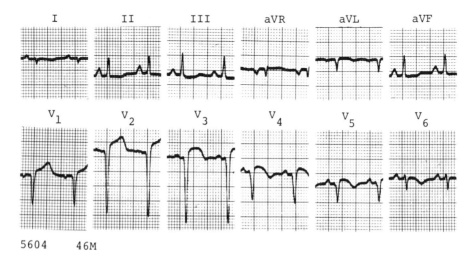

5604   46M

FIGURE 9–5. Extensive acute anterior myocardial infarction proved by autopsy. The ECG shows the loss of anterior QRS forces throughout the entire precordial leads with ST-segment elevation and T-wave inversion. QS deflections also are present in leads I and aVL. This tracing was recorded 1 week after the onset of chest pain. The patient died of cardiogenic shock. At autopsy, there was severe atherosclerosis involving all three major coronary arteries. There was an extensive recent transmural myocardial infarction that involved the anterior portion of the interventricular septum and the anterior and lateral wall of the left ventricle. An inferior wall subendocardial infarction also was present. It was estimated that the infarction involved about half of the left ventricle.

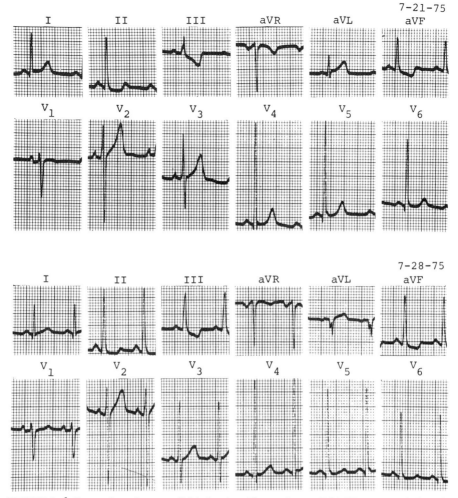

FIGURE 9–6. Recent lateral myocardial infarction. The tracing on 7-21-75 was recorded on the day of onset of chest pain. It shows slight ST-segment elevation in leads I and aVL. The voltage criteria for left ventricular hypertrophy are met in the precordial leads. In the follow-up tracing on 7-28-75, QS deflections develop in lead aVL. The ST segment becomes less elevated in leads I and aVL. Serial cardiac enzyme levels were consistent with myocardial necrosis.

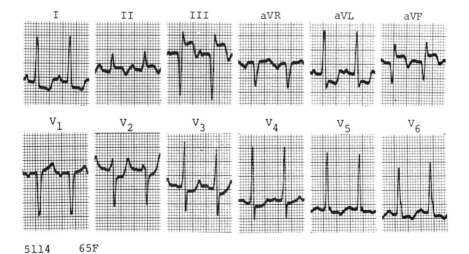

5114   65F

FIGURE 9–7. Acute inferior myocardial infarction proved by autopsy. In the ECG, the P wave in lead V_1 is suggestive of left atrial enlargement. The abnormal Q waves in leads III and aVF with ST elevation and T-wave inversion in leads II, III, and aVF are consistent with acute inferior myocardial infarction. There is reciprocal ST-segment depression in leads I, aVL, and the precordial leads, especially leads V_2 through V_4. The high voltage of the R wave in lead aVL strongly suggests left ventricular hypertrophy.

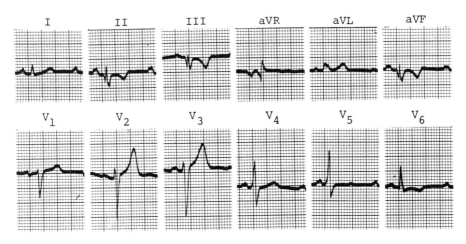

2892   45M

FIGURE 9-8. Old inferior myocardial infarction proved by autopsy. This ECG was recorded 9 months after the acute event. Abnormal left axis deviation also is present.

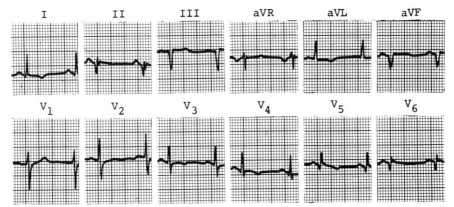

FIGURE 9-9. Inferolateral myocardial infarction of undetermined age. Abnormal Q waves are present in leads II, III, aVF, V₅, and V₆. There is a slight ST-segment elevation in leads II, III, and aVF. T-wave abnormalities are present in many of the leads. Because the cardiac enzymes were not elevated and the follow-up tracings showed no significant change, the age of the infarction cannot be determined.

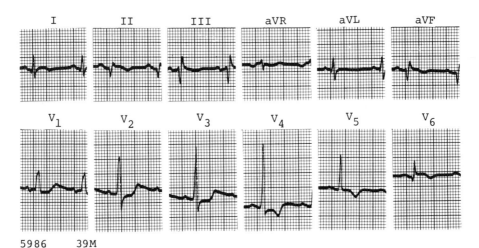

5986   39M

FIGURE 9-10. Recent inferoposterolateral myocardial infarction. The patient had an acute myocardial infarction supported by serial ECG and cardiac enzyme changes 12 days before this tracing was recorded. A Qr deflection is present in lead II and an rSR′ pattern in leads III and aVF. A qR complex is present in lead V₆. ST-segment elevation and T-wave inversion are present in the inferolateral leads. A monophasic R wave is present in lead V₁, and the R wave in lead V₂ is tall. ST-segment depression and upright T waves are present in the right precordial leads. These findings are consistent with infarction of the inferoposterior and lateral wall of the left ventricle.

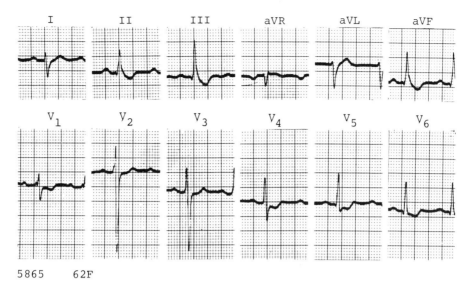

5865   62F

FIGURE 9–11. Old, true posterior myocardial infarction proved by autopsy. In the ECG, there is an rR'S pattern in lead V_1. The initial positive deflections have a duration of 0.06 second. The frontal plane QRS axis is about +110° and is consistent with left posterior hemiblock. Additional ST and T-wave abnormalities are present, some of which are probably related to digitalis effect.

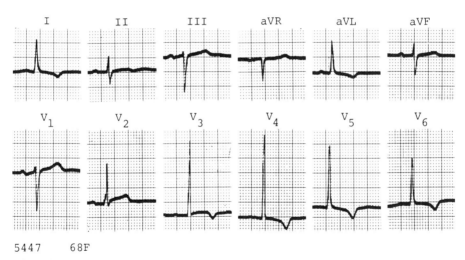

5447   68F

FIGURE 9–12. True posterior and anterior myocardial infarction demonstrated by autopsy. This tracing was recorded in a patient with a 3-year history of angina pectoris. A tall R wave is present in lead V_2 but not in V_1. The T-wave inversion in leads V_3 through V_6 may be due to anterior (non–Q-wave) infarction. The tracing also is consistent with left ventricular hypertrophy, which was confirmed anatomically.

not apply to lead III, aVR, and V_1, in which the Q waves are often wide and deep in normal subjects. In lead aVL, the Q wave is considered abnormal only when it has a duration of 0.04 second or longer or an amplitude of greater than 50 percent of the following R wave in the presence of an upright P wave.[107]

Although these criteria for the localization of infarction are generally accepted guidelines, there is considerable variation in the number and location of the leads that display the abnormal findings. This is illustrated by

the accompanying examples. Furthermore, these criteria do not include the ST-segment and T-wave abnormalities that are useful both in confirming the diagnosis and, by their serial changes, in determining the stage of the infarction.

EVOLUTIONARY CHANGES IN ACUTE Q-WAVE MYOCARDIAL INFARCTION

In most instances, the first indication of an acute Q-wave myocardial infarction is ST-segment elevation in leads that face the area of infarction, with reciprocal ST-segment depression in the opposite leads. As a rule, the ST-segment elevation is recorded in a larger area than the developing abnormal Q waves. The degree of elevation varies greatly. In some cases, it is less than 1 or 2 mm and may be considered normal unless a previous or later tracing is available for comparison (see Fig. 9–6). Others reveal striking elevation of 5 mm or more, often obscuring the downstroke of the R wave (see Figs. 9–4 and 9–13). The initial ST-segment elevation decreases significantly in the first 7 to 12 hours after the onset of chest pain.[83,290] The total duration of the ST-segment elevation also is variable. It may last for only hours, but most subside in a few days. Mills and associates found that the ST-segment elevation after acute myocardial infarction resolved within 2 weeks in 90 percent of inferior infarctions but in only 40 percent of anterior infarctions.[182] If the elevation persisted for more than 2 weeks, it did not resolve during a follow-up period of 1 to 6 months. I have not noted such a high incidence of persistent ST-segment elevation in anterior infarction in my experience. As discussed later, the possibility of ventricular aneurysm should be considered in these individuals.

There has been considerable controversy in recent years about the clinical implications of the reciprocal ST-segment depression in acute Q-wave myocardial infarction. Reciprocal ST-segment depression is seen in up to 82 percent of patients with acute myocardial infarction.[37] It is most marked in the early hours of infarction and is resolved within 24 hours in more than half of the patients.[37,185] The degree of the reciprocal ST-segment depression tends to be, but is not always, more pronounced when the ST elevation in the infarction zone is higher. The reciprocal depression also is more likely to be greater in inferior than in anterior myocardial infarction.[37,67] The conventional explanation for such ST-segment depression is that it represents a simple electrical phenomenon. The positive potential recorded by the electrodes that face the area of acute injury projects as negative deflections in the opposite leads. Angiographic and radionuclide studies in patients with acute inferior myocardial infarction suggest, however, that this reciprocal ST-segment depression in the precordial leads may be the result of concomitant disease of the left anterior descending artery and anterior wall ischemia.[241,248] Others found that such ST-segment depression was related to more extensive inferior or in-

ferolateral wall infarction or involvement of the adjacent posterolateral wall rather than anterior ischemia.[102,104] Similar results also were observed in patients with acute anterior myocardial infarction in that reciprocal ST-segment depression in the inferior leads was found mostly in patients with more extensive anterior myocardial infarction.[123] Croft and associates were not able to relate the reciprocal ST-segment depression to additional ischemia in the remote area or more extensive myocardial damage.[67] Fuchs and co-workers studied the ECG findings in patients with myocardial ischemia and infarction and one-vessel disease.[94] Of the 57 patients in whom ST elevation was recorded during the course of myocardial infarction, 31 (54 percent) had ST segment depression in other leads on the same tracing.

Norell and colleagues studied the ST-segment changes in the inferior leads during angioplasty of the left anterior descending artery.[199] Among the 18 patients who had ST-segment elevation in the anterior leads during balloon inflation, ST-segment depression appeared in the inferior leads in 13. The magnitude of the ST-segment elevation was higher in those patients with reciprocal ST-segment depression than in those without such depression. No concurrent inferior wall motion abnormalities were seen in the patients with reciprocal ST-segment depression in the inferior leads. Lew and associates, based on angiographic findings, suggested that the absence of inferior ST-segment depression during acute anterior myocardial infarction either is due to occlusion of a left anterior descending artery that also supplies the inferior wall or is the source of collateral circulation to a previously occluded posterior descending artery in patients with prior inferior infarction.[156] In acute inferior myocardial infarction, they found that the degree of the reciprocal ST-segment depression in the precordial leads is proportional to that of the ST-segment elevation in the inferior leads, unless there is concomitant right ventricular or lateral left ventricular wall involvement.[188] From the available data, most of the results appear to support the original concept that the reciprocal ST-segment depression in patients with acute myocardial infarction is mostly, if not entirely, due to reciprocal electrical alteration. It may be seen most frequently when the infarction is extensive.

Abnormal Q waves usually appear within several hours or days after the onset of the clinical manifestations of the acute infarction (see Fig. 9–13). Most commonly, they develop while the ST segment is still elevated and persist indefinitely. In a significant number of patients, however, they do not persist (see Fig. 9–14). The reported incidence of nondiagnostic ECGs in patients with previously documented myocardial infarction varies between 12 and 20 percent.[6,65,143,144,272] In 251 men who survived the first 8 weeks after a Q-wave myocardial infarction, Kaplan and Berkson reported the persistence of diagnostic Q waves in 70 percent of the patients after 3.5 years.[144] The Q waves became nondiagnostic, but still suspicious, in 15 percent. No significant Q waves could be seen in the other 15 percent. The average length of time for the complete disappearance of the abnormal Q waves was 1.5 years. In 6 percent of the patients, the ECG became entirely normal. In the 775 patients followed by Kalbfleisch and associates for 1 month to 10 years after myocardial infarction, 6.7 percent showed disappearance of the abnormal Q waves, and 5.2 percent showed only equivocal Q waves.[143] In a small number of patients, the pathologic Q waves regressed within 1 month of the acute event. Most of the reversion occurred in 2 years, and none occurred after 6 years.[143] In the 313 consecutive patients with Q-wave infarction followed for an average of 65 months by Coll and associates, 34 (11 percent) lost

their Q waves.[59] Congestive heart failure was more common among patients with persistent Q waves. The authors suggested that the loss of Q waves after acute myocardial infarction may be related to smaller infarct size.

Tall and often peaked T waves may be the earliest sign of acute myocardial infarction[76,271] (see Figs. 9–13 and 9–15). They are seen in the diagnostic leads within minutes or hours after the onset of chest pain and are believed to be due to subendocardial ischemia. They are transient, however, and most tracings fail to record such changes. The elevated ST segment usually is the dominant finding in the early phase of acute infarction. As the ST segment begins to return to the isoelectric line, symmetrical inversion of the T waves appears. The inverted T waves become progressively deeper as the ST-segment deviation subsides.[208] It is common to see a negative T wave preceded by an almost isoelectric ST segment that has an upward convexity. This rather characteristic waveform has been named *coronary T wave*[207] and *cove-plane T wave*.[204] As in the case of ST-segment elevation, the T-wave changes also are seen in more leads than are the abnormal Q waves. They are attributed to myocardial ischemia.

The symmetrical T-wave inversion may disappear within months or years or may persist indefinitely. The characteristic "ischemic" T-

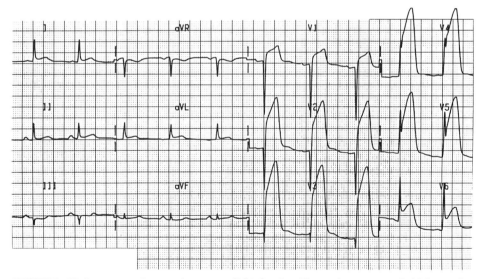

FIGURE 9–13. Acute extensive anterior myocardial infarction. The tracing was recorded 2 hours after the onset of chest pain. There is marked ST-segment elevation in the entire precordial leads, obscuring the downstroke of the R wave in lead V_3. The T waves in leads V_2 through V_5 are abnormally tall. Q waves already have appeared in leads V_1 through V_3. Coronary arteriogram performed 1 week later revealed 80 percent occlusion of the proximal portion of the left anterior descending artery. The absence of reciprocal ST-segment depression in the inferior leads of this tracing may be explained by extension of the injury to the apical inferior part of the left ventricle, which also is supplied by the left anterior descending artery.

9/26/60

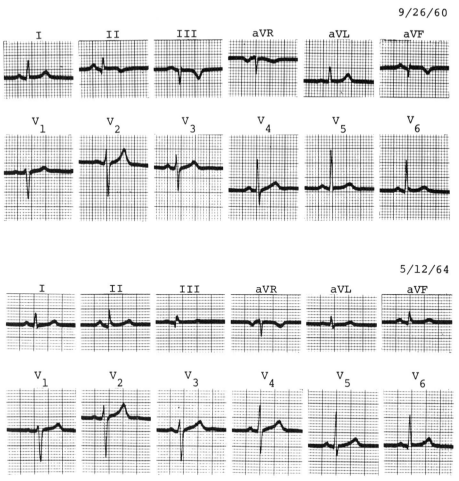

5/12/64

FIGURE 9–14. Normalization of the ECG after myocardial infarction. The patient was a 40-year-old man who had an acute inferior Q-wave myocardial infarction in 1960, which is illustrated in the top tracing. Four years later, the ECG was normal except for borderline low voltage of the QRS complex in the limb leads.

wave morphology often gradually changes to nonspecific types of abnormalities. The T waves are flat or slightly inverted, asymmetrical and may or may not be accompanied by slight ST segment depression.

To describe the various stages of myocardial infarction, the terms *acute, subacute, recent, remote, previous,* or *old* have been used by different interpreters. Although no precise definitions have been proposed, the term *acute* is used when the ST segment elevation is still present, and *subacute* is used when the ST segment has returned to the isoelectric line. The term *recent* usually means subacute. Unless the ST elevation is marked, the staging of the infarction without previous ECGs for comparison is difficult, since ST elevation may be seen many months or years after the acute event. Similarly, the diagnosis of subacute or recent myocardial infarction depends on the

availability of clinical information and serial tracings. Abnormal Q waves with symmetrical T-wave inversion are encountered in infarction of days, months, or years in duration. My practice is to define the infarction as old if it is known to exist for at least 2 months. Pathologically, most infarctions are healed after this interval.

NON–Q-WAVE MYOCARDIAL INFARCTION

Until recent years, non–Q-wave myocardial infarction was called subendocardial or nontransmural infarction, and Q-wave infarction was called transmural infarction. Subendocardial infarction generally has been defined as infarction that involves no more than the inner half of the total thickness of the ventricular wall, and nontransmural infarction is de-

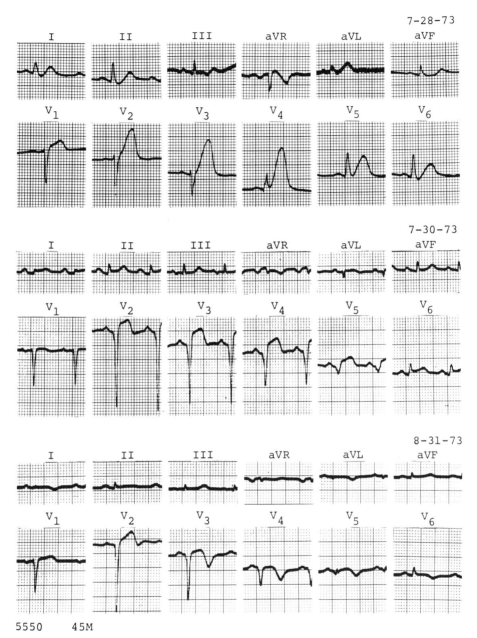

FIGURE 9–15. Evolutionary changes of acute Q-wave myocardial infarction. The tracing on 7-28-73 was recorded shortly after the onset of chest pain. Tall and broad T waves are present in the precordial leads. There is a slight ST-segment elevation in lead V_4. Two days later, the tracing shows typical changes of an extensive anterior myocardial infarction. There is also a reduction of the QRS voltage in most of the limb leads. Further evolutionary changes are demonstrated in the tracing recorded on 8-31-73.

fined as that involving more than the inner half but less than 75 percent of the ventricular wall.[61,92,100] The pitfalls of using the presence or absence of abnormal Q waves to separate transmural from nontransmural infarction were discussed by Spodick[255] and Phibbs.[215] Many autopsy studies showed that abnormal Q waves were often recorded in patients with subendocardial or nontransmural infarction, whereas patients with transmural infarction may not display pathologic Q waves.[61,92,195,230,244,258,287] The long-held concept that the subendocardium is electrically silent as far as the QRS complex is concerned is apparently incorrect.[215,220] Savage and colleagues demonstrated that even very small subendocardial infarcts with only 10 to 20 percent of ventricular wall thickness involved can cause abnormal Q waves.[244] Raunio and associates reported the findings in the ECGs taken 48 hours before death in 80 patients with myocardial infarction.[230] Abnormal Q waves were seen in 8 (53 percent) of 15 patients with subendocardial infarction and in 42 (65 percent) of 65 patients with transmural infarction. Similar findings were reported by Antaloczy and co-workers after they correlated the ECG and pathologic data from 100 patients with myocardial infarction.[7] Because of the different clinical course that patients with and without abnormal Q waves may exhibit, classification of myocardial infarction based on the QRS morphology appears more meaningful and is generally adopted.

The prevalence of non–Q-wave infarction among patients with acute myocardial infarction was reported to range between 16 and 40 percent.[102,135,153,165,168,238,256,281] Most cardiologists classify the infarction as non–Q-wave even if there are QRS changes but the conventional criteria for abnormal Q waves are not met.[75,105,153,201] Some investigators, however, consider cases with marked reduction of the R wave amplitude or the development of new small Q waves as Q-wave infarction.[102,258] This difference in the definition of non–Q-wave

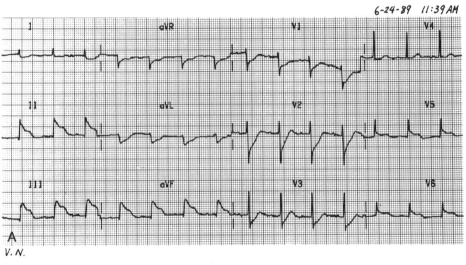

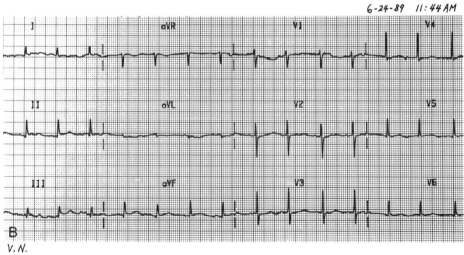

FIGURE 9–16. Acute non–Q-wave inferolateral myocardial infarction. The patient was a 69-year-old woman who complained of chest pain when tracing A was obtained. It shows ST-segment elevation in leads II, III, aVF, V_5, and V_6, with reciprocal ST-segment depression in leads I, aVL, and V_1 through V_3. Five minutes later, a repeat tracing (B) shows almost total resolution of the ST-segment displacement. Serial cardiac enzymes confirmed the diagnosis of acute myocardial infarction. The follow-up tracings are similar to tracing B without the development of abnormal Q waves. The rapid spontaneous resolution of the ST-segment changes in this patient with acute infarction is unusual.

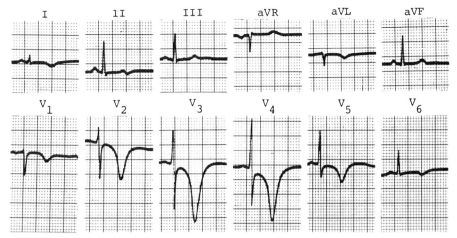

FIGURE 9–17. Non–Q-wave infarction. The patient is a 44-year-old man who had substernal chest pain 1 day before this ECG was recorded. Serial cardiac enzyme determinations revealed changes consistent with myocardial necrosis. The striking ST and T-wave changes in the ECG persisted, but the T-wave inversion in the precordial leads was less pronounced 5 days later.

myocardial infarction may account for some of the different results obtained in the ECG and anatomic correlation studies. In either case, the characteristic ECG changes of non–Q-wave infarction are in the ST segment and T waves (Figs. 9–16 through 9–19). In the acute phase, the ST segment may be elevated or depressed in the leads that face the epicar-dial surface of the infarcted area. The relative frequency of the displacement in either direction varies among the reported series that provide such information. In the 93 cases of non–Q-wave infarction studied by Ogawa and associates, 35 (38 percent) had ST-segment elevation, 49 (52 percent) had ST-segment depression, and 9 (10 percent) had T-wave

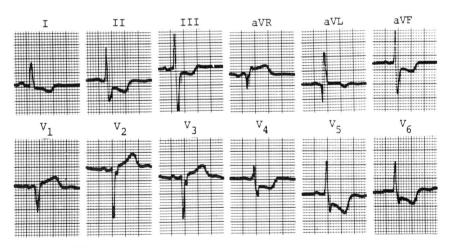

1911   69F

FIGURE 9–18. Old anterolateral transmural myocardial infarction and recent inferior suben-docardial infarction demonstrated at autopsy. The anterolateral myocardial infarction was extensive, involving about 40 percent of the left ventricular free wall. The subendocardial infarction was recent, and the posterior part of the ventricular septum also was involved. Ninety-five percent narrowing of the lumen was present in all three major coronary arteries. In the ECG, there is poor progression of the R wave in the right precordial leads and abnormal Q wave is recorded in lead aVL. Marked ST-segment depression with T-wave inversion is present in the inferior and left precordial leads. Although anterolateral transmural infarction is present anatomically, the ECG does not show abnormal Q waves in the corresponding leads. The ST and T-wave changes without abnormal Q waves in the inferior leads correlate with the pathologic findings of inferior subendocardial infarction. Anatomic left ventricular hypertrophy also was present, but the QRS voltage in the ECG does not suggest such a diagnosis.

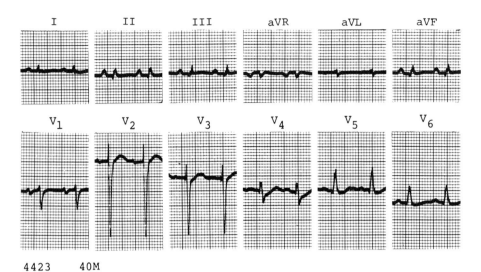

4423   40M

FIGURE 9–19. Non–Q-wave myocardial infarction.The patient was a 40-year-old man with severe coronary atherosclerosis that involved the left anterior descending and circumflex arteries. At autopsy, there was an extensive old subendocardial infarction that involved about one third to one half of the inner portion of the myocardium of the apical two thirds of the left ventricle. This ECG was recorded 2 months before death. The limb leads show low voltage of the QRS complexes. Small q waves and a decrease in R-wave amplitude are seen in leads V_3 and V_4. Some of the ST and T changes are probably related to digitalis effect.

changes alone.[200] In patients included in the Multicenter Investigation of the Limitation of Infarct Size (MILLIS) study, Willich and associates found ST-segment elevation in the initial ECG in 207 (61 percent) and ST segment depression in 97 (29 percent) of 340 patients with non–Q-wave infarction.[281] Other than the direction of the ST-segment displacement, the degree of the segment shift and the number of leads involved may differ among patients. Generally speaking, however, the extent of the ST elevation in patients with non–Q-wave infarction is less than that in those with Q wave infarction.[135]

The direction of the ST segment shifts in the initial ECG is a poor predictor of subsequent development of Q waves. In 439 patients with the admission diagnosis of non–Q-wave myocardial infarction, Boden and colleagues found ST-segment elevation in 187 (43 percent) and ST-segment depression or T-wave inversion or both in 252 (57 percent).[20] Twenty percent of the patients with initial ST-segment elevation and 15 percent of those with ST-segment depression or T-wave inversion eventually developed Q waves during the hospital course.

In non–Q-wave infarction, inverted T waves usually evolve in the leads with either ST-segment elevation or depression. The T-wave inversion is often deep (see Fig. 9–17). Indeed, newly developed and persistent marked ST-segment depression with deeply inverted T waves is highly suggestive of acute myocardial infarction. Because myocardial injury or ischemia without infarction and other nonischemic states also may be accompanied by the ST and T-wave changes seen in non–Q-wave infarction, however, the latter diagnosis usually cannot be made by the ECG alone. A diagnosis of non–Q-wave infarction may be made only if the ST-segment and T-wave changes are accompanied by elevation of cardiac enzyme levels indicative of myocardial necrosis.

RIGHT VENTRICULAR INFARCTION

Myocardial infarction that involves the free wall of the right ventricle rarely occurs in isolated form.[4,89] Most pathologic studies revealed that it is present in 14 to 36 percent of patients with left ventricular inferior Q-wave infarction but is not seen in hearts with isolated anterior myocardial infarction.[140,229,269] A more recent prospective autopsy study of 107 patients by Andersen and co-workers, however, revealed that right ventricular involvement was found with equal frequency in anterior and inferior (posterior) left ventricular infarction.[4] The size of the anterior right ventricular infarcts was small and was estimated to be about 1 percent of the right ventricle. They were located primarily near the apex of the heart. Cabin and associates found anterior right ventricular infarction in 13 (13 percent) of 97 hearts with anterior left ventricular myocardial infarction.[35] The right ventricular infarcts involved from 10 to 50 percent of the circumference of the right ventricular free wall from base to apex. The left ventricular infarcts were all anteroseptal and large. Although the association between anterior left ventricular infarcts and right ventricular infarcts needs to be examined further, it appears that those right ventricular infarcts associated with inferior left ventricular infarction are clinically more important.

ELECTROCARDIOGRAPHIC CRITERIA FOR THE DIAGNOSIS OF ACUTE RIGHT VENTRICULAR INFARCTION

1. Signs of acute inferior or inferoposterior myocardial infarction; *and*
2. ST-segment elevation of 1 mm or more in one or more of the right precordial leads.[50,52,81,164]

The conventional 12-lead ECG may reveal the ST-segment elevation in lead V_1 and, in some instances, also in leads V_2 and V_3 (Figs. 9–20 and 9–21), and, occasionally, in leads V_1 through V_5.[50,96] The right-sided chest leads

5-25-79

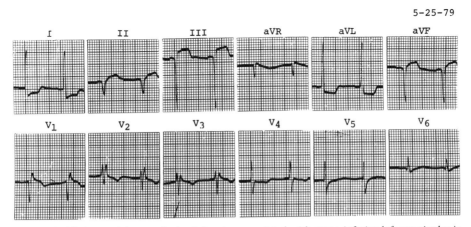

FIGURE 9–20. Acute right ventricular infarction associated with acute inferior left ventricular infarction proved at autopsy. The tracing shows acute Q-wave inferior myocardial infarction, left ventricular hypertrophy, and incomplete right bundle branch block. The ST-segment elevation in lead V_1 suggests right ventricular infarction.

7-1-79

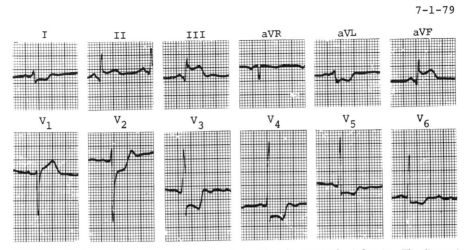

FIGURE 9–21. Acute inferior myocardial infarction with right ventricular infarction. The diagnosis of right ventricular infarction is supported by hemodynamic data. The ECG shows small Q waves with marked ST-segment elevation in leads II, III, and aVF. There is reciprocal ST-segment depression in leads I, aVL, and V_2 through V_6. The ST segment in lead V_1 is, however, elevated. The follow-up tracings revealed evolutionary changes of acute inferior Q-wave infarction, and the ST-segment elevation in lead V_1 subsided.

V_{3R} through V_{6R} are, however, more sensitive for the recognition of acute right ventricular infarction.[25,38,67] (Fig. 9–22) This is especially true with lead V_{4R}.[163] Braat and associates noted that the ST-segment elevation in the right precordial leads was short-lived, disappearing within 10 hours after the onset of chest pain in half of their patients.[25] Thus, in patients with acute inferior left ventricular infarction, it is important that the right-sided chest leads V_{3R} through V_{5R} be routinely added to the 12-lead ECG, especially in the initial recordings.

Although abnormal Q waves with ST and T-wave changes suggestive of acute inferior myocardial infarction usually alert one to look for signs of right ventricular infarction, QRS changes specific for acute right ventricular infarction have not been described. Cardenas and associates observed a loss of anterior QRS forces in some of the right precordial leads in patients with right ventricular infarction.[39] We noted the development of abnormal Q waves in the right precordial leads and right bundle branch block in right ventricular infarction induced experimentally in dogs.[48] Subsequent to the animal study, I analyzed 11 consecutive cases of well documented acute right ventricular infarction (unpublished data, 1987). Four of the 11 patients displayed QS complexes in leads V_1 through V_3 (Figs. 9–23, and 9–24). Three of the patients also showed ST-segment elevation in these leads. These findings suggest acute anteroseptal left ventricular infarction, but the coronary arte-

riograms in all of the four patients revealed no significant lesion in the left anterior descending artery. The right coronary artery was completely occluded at its proximal portion in all these patients. The fact that acute right ventricular infarction may mimic acute anterior infarction is not only clinically important but also raises a basic question about the genesis of R waves in the right precordial leads in the normal ECG.

The experimental finding of right bundle branch block in association with right ventricular infarction was encountered clinically in two of our patients (see Fig. 9–20). Because right bundle branch block may develop in patients with acute anterior myocardial infarction, but rarely in those with inferior myocardial infarction, its appearance in association with the latter may imply right ventricular involvement.

Because of the lack of specific QRS changes and the transient nature of the ST-segment elevation, *old* right ventricular infarcts cannot be diagnosed by the ECG.

PATHOLOGIC CORRELATION: SENSITIVITY AND SPECIFICITY OF THE ELECTROCARDIOGRAM

The classical studies by Myers and associates demonstrated the relation between the ECG and pathologic findings of myocardial infarction at various locations.[188–194] It was appreciated then and was substantiated by later experience, however, that there is considerable

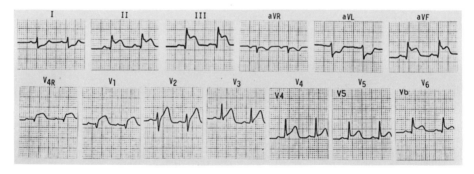

FIGURE 9–22. Acute inferoposterior myocardial infarction with right ventricular infarction in a 37-year-old man. The tracing was obtained on the day of onset of chest pain, and the diagnosis of acute myocardial infarction was supported by serial cardiac enzyme changes. Radionuclide angiocardiography revealed akinetic inferior and posterior wall of the left ventricle and severe hypokinesis of the right ventricle. The left ventricular ejection fraction was 48 percent and the right 11 percent. Physical examination revealed marked jugular venous distention. The ECG shows small Q waves with marked ST-segment elevation in leads II, III, and aVF. Reciprocal ST-segment depression is present in leads I and aVL. Some ST-segment elevation is present in the left precordial leads. Its cause is uncertain. Marked ST-segment elevation in leads V_1 and V_{4R} is suggestive of right ventricular infarction. The ST-segment elevation in all of the precordial leads subsided on the next day.

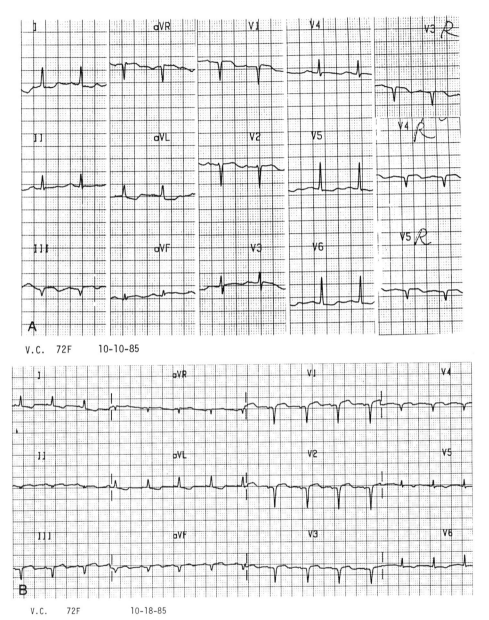

V.C.   72F   10-10-85

V.C.   72F   10-18-85

FIGURE 9–23. Acute right ventricular infarction mimicking acute anteroseptal myocardial infarction. The patient was a 72-year-old woman with onset of severe chest pain on 10-9-85. The ECG on 10-10-85 (A) shows a QS deflection in lead III, with ST-segment elevation in leads III, aVF, V_1, and V_{3R} through V_{5R} that is suggestive of inferior and right ventricular injury. Reciprocal ST-segment depression is present in leads I, aVL, V_5, and V_6. Serial cardiac enzymes were consistent with acute myocardial infarction. Subsequent records revealed the development of inferior wall Q-wave infarction with loss of R waves in leads V_1 through V_4 (B). The QS complexes with ST-segment elevation in leads V_1 through V_4 suggest acute anteroseptal myocardial infarction. Coronary arteriogram on 10-16-85 showed complete occlusion of the right coronary artery at its proximal portion, but the left anterior descending artery was normal. There was a 60 percent stenotic lesion of the distal part of the left circumflex artery. The echocardiogram and radionuclide ventriculogram showed minimal inferior wall motion abnormalities, with normal left ventricular ejection fraction. The right ventricle was dilated and akinetic. The right ventricular ejection fraction estimated from the radionuclide ventriculogram was 19 percent.

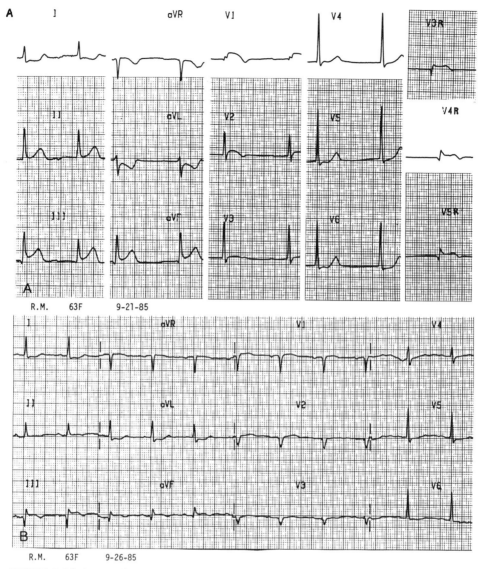

FIGURE 9–24. Acute right ventricular infarction mimicking anteroseptal myocardial infarction. (A) Tracing on 9-21-85 shows first-degree AV block, abnormal P waves, and inferior and right ventricular injury. The absence of S wave in lead V_1 and the presence of a tall R wave in lead V_2 suggest true posterior myocardial infarction. Follow-up ECGs reveal the development of acute inferior myocardial infarction and pattern of anteroseptal myocardial infarction, as illustrated by the tracing on 9-26-85 (B). Coronary arteriogram showed complete occlusion of the right coronary artery at its origin, but both the left anterior descending and left circumflex arteries were normal. The right ventricular ejection fraction determined by radionuclide ventriculogram was 16 percent, and the left ventricular ejection fraction was 75 percent.

limitation in the diagnostic capability of the ECG in myocardial infarction. This is true also in the case of non–Q-wave infarction.

Many factors influence the accuracy of the ECG diagnosis of myocardial infarction. They include (1) the size of circumferential dimension of the infarct; (2) the age of the infarct (i.e., whether it is acute or old); (3) the thickness of the ventricular wall involved (i.e., whether it is transmural or subendocardial);

(4) the location of the infarct (i.e., whether it is in the anterior, inferior, posterior, or lateral wall of the left ventricle); (5) the presence or absence of multiple infarcts; (6) the presence or absence of ventricular hypertrophy; (7) the presence or absence of ventricular conduction abnormality; and (8) the availability of adequate number of records, including those before infarction occurs. Because it is well known that some ventricular conduction de-

fects have a profound effect on the accuracy of the diagnosis, the following discussion is limited to those cases without abnormal prolongation of the QRS duration. The diagnosis of myocardial infarction in the presence of ventricular conduction defect is dealt with in a separate section.

In the absence of intraventricular conduction defect, the reported overall sensitivity of the ECG in the recognition of myocardial infarction based on autopsy cases varies from 48 to 82 percent.[31,117,132,258,277,284] In the earlier series, the criteria used were not precisely defined. In more recent studies,[117,132] which used criteria similar to those listed in this chapter, 55 to 61 percent of the proven cases of infarcts were recognized. If the infarction is acute, the incidence of false-negative diagnoses is low, varying from 6 to 25 percent.[154,211,284] Conversely, old myocardial infarctions are more likely to be missed. In one series, 80 percent of patients with old infarction failed to reveal definite ECG signs.[154] Anterior infarctions are generally more easily recognized than inferior or true posterior infarction.[32] (Fig. 9–25). Those limited to the lateral wall are even more difficult to diagnose even if they are in the acute stage.[79,132,258] The prediction of the exact location of the infarct often is inaccurate.[117] The extension of an old infarct often is difficult to detect, and a second infarction at another location may obliterate the signs of the first infarct[258] (Figs. 9–26 and 9–27). The presence of anatomic left ventricular hypertrophy often masks (and mimics) the ECG signs of myocardial infarction. In one series, left ventricular hypertrophy was found in half of the cases with infarction that was not diagnosed by the ECG.[154] Because the diagnosis of myocardial infarction in these studies was based on the presence of abnormal Q waves, it is to be expected that non–Q-wave infarcts are responsible for the false-negative cases.

In clinical practice, the diagnosis of myocardial infarction often is made without abnormal Q waves or QS deflection. If there are ST-segment and T-wave changes suggestive of myocardial injury and ischemia, acute myocardial infarction may be suspected even if the changes of the QRS complex are not typical. For example, an anterior wall myocardial infarction is probably present if there is a poor progression or a decrease in the amplitude of the R wave in leads V_1 through V_4 associated with serial ST and T changes. If a previous tracing is available, the demonstration of a reduction of the R wave accompanied by the ST and T-wave changes is a strong indication of acute myocardial damage (Fig. 9–28). The appearance of a new Q wave, even though less than 0.04 second in duration, also is highly significant. This occurs often in patients with inferior myocardial infarction but may be easily overlooked if a careful comparison is not made with the previous ECGs. In inferior

1/2/70

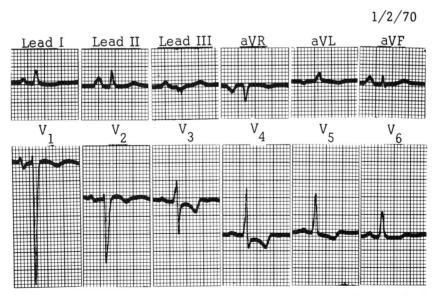

FIGURE 9–25. Old inferior myocardial infarction demonstrated anatomically but not by the ECG. Severe coronary atherosclerosis that involved all major branches was present. There also was anatomic evidence of left ventricular hypertrophy, which is shown in the ECG. The T-wave inversion in leads V_1 through V_3 is consistent with anterior myocardial ischemia.

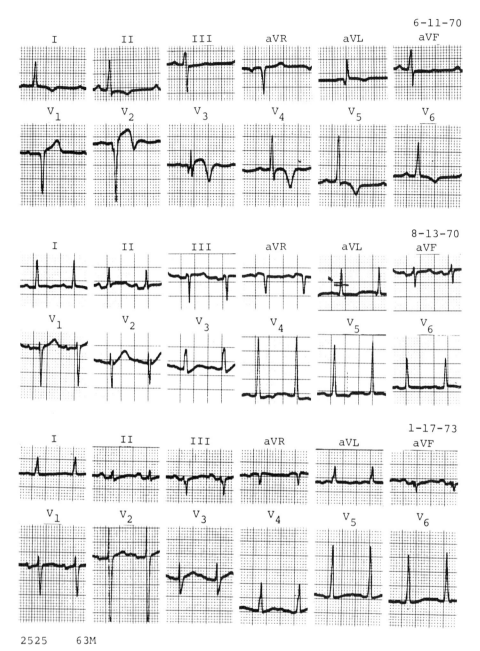

2525   6 3M

FIGURE 9–26. Multiple infarctions. The tracing on 6-11-70 shows changes suggestive of a recent anteroseptal myocardial infarction and anterolateral ischemia. Two months later, the patient had clinical evidence of acute myocardial infarction that probably involved the inferior wall because the tracing on 8-13-70 shows ST-segment elevation in leads II, III, and a aVF. Atrial infarction may be present, as there is depression of the PR segment in the inferior leads. The R waves in the right precordial leads have returned. The tracing on 1-17-73 reveals no evidence of anterior myocardial infarction. The changes in the inferior leads are not typical of inferior myocardial infarction, but the notching of the early part of the QRS complex makes one suspect it. The patient died on 1-19-73. At autopsy, the heart weighed 620 g with biventricular hypertrophy. There was severe coronary atherosclerosis. Old myocardial infarction that involved the anterior part of the interventricular septum and posterolateral wall of the left ventricle was found. The atria were not examined carefully for old atrial infarction. This case is an example of the masking of one infarction by a second one at another location.

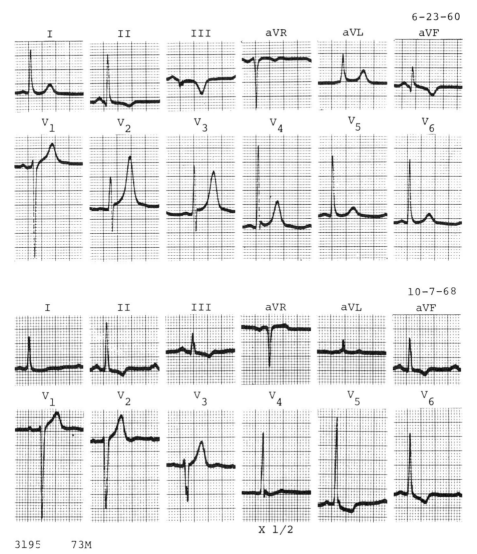

6-23-60

10-7-68

X 1/2

3195   73M

FIGURE 9–27. Posterior, anteroseptal, and anterolateral myocardial infarction demonstrated by autopsy. The patient was a 73-year-old man with hypertension. He had an acute myocardial infarction in 1960. *Serial* ECGs recorded during that episode suggest inferoposterior myocardial infarction, but the usual criteria for such a diagnosis are not met in the individual tracings. One of the tracings is illustrated in the top panel. The voltage of the QRS complexes is consistent with left ventricular hypertrophy. In the ensuing 8 years, the patient gave no history suggestive of recurrent myocardial infarction. The tracing on 10-7-68 suggests left ventricular hypertrophy and digitalis effect. No signs of myocardial infarction are evident. At autopsy, there was a total occlusion of the distal part of the right coronary artery, the marginal branch of the left circumflex, and the left anterior descending artery. The myocardium showed old true posterior, anteroseptal, and anterolateral myocardial infarction. Marked left ventricular hypertrophy and dilatation were present.

myocardial infarction, a minute R wave may remain in leads II, III, and aVF and is followed by a downward deflection that is notched or slurred.

When the criteria used are less stringent, the increase in the diagnostic sensitivity is likely to be accompanied by a decrease in the specificity. The terms *probable* and *possible* usually are used when the diagnosis of infarction is based on less typical changes.

The usefulness of the ECG in the diagnosis of right ventricular infarction was not recognized until recently. Anatomic correlation studies to determine its diagnostic reliability are few in number. Based on available clinical and pathologic data, ST-segment elevation of 1.0 mm or more in lead V_{4R} (the most reliable lead) has a sensitivity of 70 to 93 percent and a specificity of 77 to 100 percent.[157] The variation in the reported diagnostic accuracy

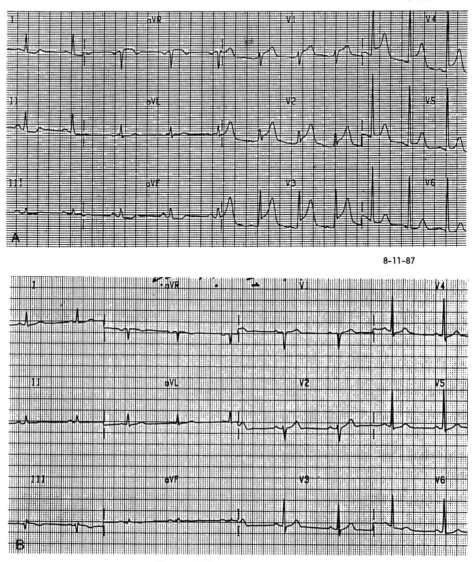

Figure 9-28. *Legend on next page.*

probably is due to the criteria used to confirm the presence of right ventricular infarction and the time relationship between the ECG recording and onset of the acute infarction. Old right ventricular infarction cannot be recognized by the ECG because of the absence of specific QRS changes associated with right ventricular infarction in general.

The ECG not only fails to recognize myocardial infarction in a large number of cases but it also often gives a false-positive diagnosis. In the autopsy series reported by Gunnar and associates, the overall incidence of false-positive diagnoses was 31 percent.[117] Horan and co-workers analyzed the ECGs of 768 patients with no anatomic evidence of myocar-

dial infarction.[132] Eleven percent showed abnormal Q waves with a duration greater than 0.03 second. When the abnormal Q waves were limited to the anteroseptal (V_1 through V_4) or inferior leads (II, III, aVF) alone, the percentage of false-positive diagnoses was high (46 percent). If the abnormal Q waves were located in the anterolateral zone (V_5 through V_6), however, or if they were present in more than one location, a false prediction of infarction was seldom made (4 percent). Their results in inferior infarctions were somewhat different from those reported by Pearce and Chapman,[212] who found a false-positive diagnosis in only 2 of 17 patients with a Q wave in lead aVF of 0.04 second or

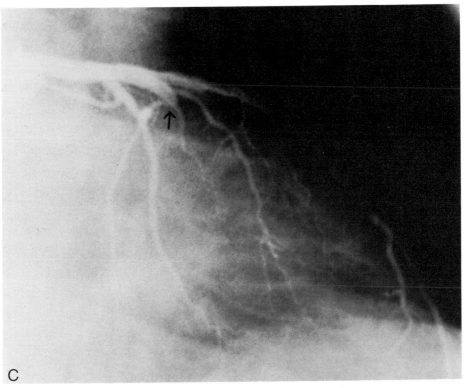

FIGURE 9–28. Acute myocardial infarction with minimal residual ECG abnormalities. The patient was a 60-year-old man with acute anterior myocardial infarction diagnosed by history, elevation of cardiac enzymes, and ST-segment elevation in leads V_1 through V_4 (A). Coronary arteriogram revealed total occlusion of the left anterior descending artery just distal to the origin of its first diagonal branch (C). Four days later, the ECG (B) showed minimal ST-segment and T-wave changes. In comparison with the tracing in A, the tracing in B shows a reduction of the R-wave amplitude in leads V_1 and V_2. The patient did not receive any thrombolytic agent.

more. When the criterion of QaVF greater than 25 percent of RaVF was used, however, 10 of 29 cases failed to show infarction at autopsy examination.

CORRELATION WITH CORONARY ARTERIOGRAM AND VENTRICULOGRAM

The correlation of the ECG findings with angiographic evidence of coronary obstruction and ventricular asynergy is of considerable clinical importance. The pathologic studies by James[142] have contributed much to our knowledge about the arterial blood supply to the various areas of the myocardium. The anterior descending artery travels in the anterior interventricular sulcus and supplies branches to most of the interventricular septum and the adjacent wall of the left ventricle. It then curves about the apex to ascend in the posterior interventricular sulcus for a variable distance that is inversely proportional to the length of the posterior descending artery.

Therefore, anteroseptal and anterior myocardial infarctions are nearly always the consequence of occlusion of the left anterior descending artery, which often is also responsible for infarction of the apex. The left circumflex artery supplies the lateral wall of the left ventricle, and its occlusion will result in lateral infarctions (anterolateral, inferolateral, or high lateral). In about 10 percent of human hearts, the left circumflex artery crosses the crux of the heart and supplies the posterior descending artery. Its occlusion is accompanied by infarction of the inferior and true posterior walls, as well as the lateral wall of the left ventricle. In 90 percent of the human hearts, however, the right coronary artery is dominant and supplies the posterior descending artery. It is the vessel most responsible for true posterior, inferior, and right ventricular myocardial infarctions.

It is generally known that the resting ECG may be completely normal in the presence of significant coronary artery disease. Benchimol and associates reported normal ECGs in 16 percent of patients with significant triple-vessel disease, some of whom had complete obstruction of one of the vessels.[16] On the other hand, in patients with 100 percent obstruction in one or more of the coronary arteries, 71 percent had abnormal Q waves suggestive of myocardial infarction. In 480 consecutive coronary arteriograms, Martinez-Rios and associates found 21 cases with normal ECGs but complete or nearly complete occlusion of one or more of the three major coronary branches.[174] Significant collateral circulation was demonstrated in most of these cases, which the authors believed to be responsible for the absence of ECG abnormalities. Fig. 9–28 is an example of a nearly normal ECG 4 days after an acute anterior myocardial infarction due to total occlusion of the left anterior descending artery.

Normal ECGs also have been recorded in patients with significant coronary artery disease (75 percent or more obstruction of at least one major vessel) and ventricular asynergy.[113] Nearly 40 percent of patients with significant coronary artery disease and asynergy of the anterior and apical segments of the left ventricle did not have abnormal Q waves in the precordial leads.[286] Because ventricular asynergy is not necessarily accompanied by an infarction, these results cannot be considered a true indication of the sensitivity of the ECG in the diagnosis of myocardial infarction.

Fuchs and associates correlated the ECG and angiographic findings in patients with myocardial infarction and one-vessel coronary artery disease.[94] Sixty patients had abnormal Q waves. With two exceptions, the presence of abnormal Q waves in leads I, aVL, and V_1 through V_4 was associated with disease of the left anterior descending artery, and their presence in leads II, III, and aVF was associated with the left circumflex or right coronary artery. According to these authors, the ECG was unable to distinguish right coronary from left circumflex artery disease.

Blanke and co-workers performed coronary arteriograms in 152 patients within 6.3 ± 6.0 hours from the onset of acute myocardial infarction and correlated the findings with the ECGs.[18] A typical ECG pattern of acute anteroseptal myocardial infarction was found to be highly reliable in predicting left anterior descending artery as the infarct-related vessel with a sensitivity of 90 percent and a specificity of 95 percent. A typical pattern of acute inferior myocardial infarction correctly identified right coronary or left circumflex artery as the infarct-related vessel in 94 percent of

the cases. When the ECG showed changes of true posterior or isolated lateral wall infarction but no typical findings of acute infarction in the inferior leads, the infarct-related artery was most likely left circumflex. On the other hand, the presence of typical findings of infarction in the inferior leads without changes suggestive of true posterior or lateral wall infarction was highly specific for right coronary artery disease. Fifty-six percent of patients with left circumflex artery as the infarct-related vessel presented nondiagnostic ECG abnormalities. In all the patient subgroups, no apparent differences were noted in the ECG findings between those with subtotal and those with total occlusions of the vessels. Figure 9–29 illustrates the nonspecific findings in a patient with total occlusion of the left circumflex artery at its midportion.

Huey and colleagues compared the ECGs of 40 consecutive patients with acute myocardial infarction due to left circumflex artery occlusion with those of 107 patients with occlusion of the right coronary artery.[134] Acute ST-segment elevation was present in only 48 percent of patients with occlusion of the circumflex artery versus 71 percent of patients with occlusion of the right coronary artery. Thirty-eight percent of patients with circumflex artery-related infarct had no significant ST-segment elevation or depression. In patients with inferior myocardial infarction, the presence of ST-segment elevation in one or more of the lateral leads (leads I, aVL, V_5, and V_6) was highly suggestive of occlusion of the circumflex artery. Abnormal R wave in lead V_1 consistent with true posterior myocardial infarction was a highly specific marker for circumflex artery occlusion. In addition, this finding was invariably associated with multivessel disease and larger infarction. This relation between abnormal R wave in lead V_1 and circumflex artery occlusion and multi-vessel disease also was demonstrated in the study by Bough and Korr.[24] The usefulness of ST-segment elevation in the lateral leads for identifying circumflex artery occlusion as the cause of inferior myocardial infarction also is shown in the report by Bairey and associates.[11]

In patients with right ventricular infarction, the infarct-related vessel is, as expected, the right coronary artery. In my own experience in patients with acute inferior and right ventricular infarction and *impaired* right ventricular function, the right coronary artery was occluded, or nearly occluded, at its proximal portion in nearly all cases (see Figs. 9–23 and 9–24). In cases of right ventricular infarction

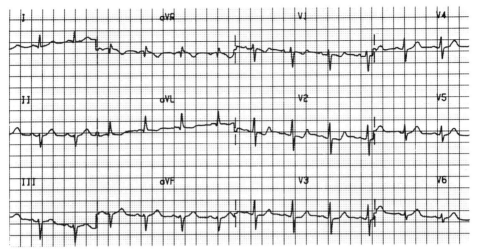

FIGURE 9–29. Acute occlusion of left circumflex artery with minimal T-wave changes. The tracing was recorded after percutaneous transluminal coronary angioplasty of a 90 percent obstructive lesion in the mid–left circumflex artery. The patient had chest pain after the procedure, and biphasic T waves appeared in leads V_1 and V_2 of the ECG. Repeat arteriogram showed total occluson of the left circumflex artery at its midportion. The T wave changes that mimic anterior myocardial ischemia subsided after the artery was redilated. The other coronary arteries were normal. The tracing also shows left anterior hemiblock, which is a stable pattern. Cardiac enzymes were consistent with acute myocardial infarction.

associated with occlusion of the right coronary artery at its midportion, there often was no evidence of right ventricular dysfunction even though the infarction was diagnosed by ECG. Weinshel and associates evaluated the coronary arteriograms of 23 patients with acute left ventricular inferior myocardial infarction.[276] In 6 patients, the right coronary occlusion occurred proximal to all of the free wall branches and all 6 patients had right ventricular infarction documented by hemodynamic data. In contrast, of 9 patients in whom the obstruction occurred distal to all of the free wall branches, none had right ventricular infarction.

In recent years, the practice in some institutions of performing coronary arteriograms on patients soon after the onset of acute myocardial infarction has added new information about the status of the infarct-related vessel. DeWood and associates studied the degree of coronary obstruction in 322 patients admitted within 24 hours of Q-wave infarction.[74] Total coronary occlusion was observed in 87 percent of 126 patients who were evaluated within 4 hours of the onset of symptoms and 65 percent of 57 patients from 12 to 24 hours after the onset of symptoms. The decrease in the frequency of total coronary occlusion within the initial 24 hours of a Q-wave infarction led the investigators to believe that coronary spasm, thrombus formation with subse-

quent recanalization, or both may be important in the evolution of infarction. A group of investigators from the same institution later reported a similar study in 341 patients within 1 week of non–Q-wave myocardial infarction.[75] Total occlusion of the infarct-related vessel was found in 26 percent (49 of 192), 37 percent (35 of 94), and 42 percent (23 of 55) of the patients studied within 24 hours, within 24 to 72 hours, and within 72 hours to 1 week, respectively. Thus, in contrast to Q-wave infarction, total coronary occlusion of the infarct-related vessel is infrequently observed in the early hours of non–Q-wave infarction, but the frequency increases moderately over the next few days. The authors suggested that some degree of perfusion, either antegrade or by means of collateral vessels, is present soon after non–Q-wave infarction, but it is not sufficient to prevent the initial necrosis. Significantly higher incidence of occlusive thrombi in Q-wave than in non–Q-wave infarction also is found by other investigators, even though the coronary arteriogram was not performed in the early hours of the infarction.[30,71]

In patients with significant coronary artery disease but without other types of heart disease, intraventricular conduction defect, or ventricular hypertrophy, the ECG findings in Q-wave myocardial infarction accurately predict the presence and site of ventricular asynergy. Ventricular asynergy was demonstrated in 80 to 95 percent of such patients.[12,21,181,280] Abnormal Q waves in the precordial leads almost invariably are accompanied by asynergy of the anterior segment of the left ventricle, whereas the incidence of asynergy of the inferior wall is slightly lower in patients with abnormal Q waves in the inferior leads. Generally speaking, when abnormal Q waves are present in a large number of precordial leads, the degree of abnormal ventricular wall motion is more severe. The presence of ST-segment elevation with T-wave inversion in an old myocardial infarction also indicates a greater degree of ventricular asynergy and more extensive area of involvement.[12,181] When pathologic Q waves are absent in patients with significant major vessel disease, the incidence of ventricular asynergy was reported to be about 25 to 50 percent.[21,181] The abnormality of wall motion was of milder form.

ELECTROCARDIOGRAPHIC CHANGES IN ACUTE MYOCARDIAL INFARCTION AFTER CORONARY REPERFUSION

Thrombolytic agents such as tissue plasminogen activator and streptokinase often are adminstered in the early hours of acute myocardial infarction in an attempt to restore blood flow in the infarct-related artery, to relieve myocardial ischemia, and to limit infarct size. Coronary reperfusion may be signified clinically by the relief of chest pain, early rapid rise and peaking in creatine kinase activity, and ECG changes. It occurs in about 80 percent of the patients with coronary occlusion if the thrombolytic agent is administered less than 4 hours after the onset of chest pain.[5,111] The ECG changes of reperfusion consist of an acceleration of the evolution of the acute infarction pattern and the development of cardiac arrhythmias.

Rapid reduction in the ST-segment elevation is the most common and useful electrocardiographic sign of reperfusion.[5,19,95,232,266] A decrease in the ST-segment elevation of 2 mm or more may be observed within 30 minutes after the beginning of the thrombolytic therapy[232] (Fig. 9–30). The rapid reduction in the ST-segment elevation with reperfusion may continue for 3 to 6 hours.[5] Loss of R-wave amplitude or the development of Q waves also is accelerated in the early hours of reperfusion[5,27,266] (Fig. 9–31). After 12 hours

or more, however, the opposite may be true. The Q waves may be smaller or seen in fewer leads and the reduction of the R-wave amplitude is less in patients with reperfusion than those without.[5,9]

Premature ventricular beats, accelerated idioventricular rhythm, ventricular tachycardia, sinus bradycardia, and AV block may develop during reperfusion. Although ventricular premature beats are invariably present, the most characteristic reperfusion arrhythmia is accelerated idioventricular rhythm[40,111] (Fig. 9–32). Using 24-hour Holter monitoring, Cercek and associates found that 90 percent of patients had runs of accelerated idioventricular rhythm and 23 percent had ventricular tachycardia during the first 24 hours after reperfusion.[40] The frequency of arrhythmias began to decrease 8 to 12 hours after reperfusion. Accelerated idioventricular rhythm was observed by Gorgels and colleagues in 26 (45 percent) of 58 patients who had angiographic evidence of reperfusion and in only 1 of the 14 patients whose infarct-related artery remained occluded.[111] The authors also found that the morphology of the QRS complexes during accelerated idioventricular rhythm was somewhat related to the coronary artery reperfused. Reperfusion of the left anterior descending artery was associated with a variety of QRS configurations but the QRS duration was relatively short. Reperfusion of the left circumflex artery was never accompanied by a left bundle branch block QRS morphology, whereas that of the right coronary artery always had a superior axis. These investigators believed that the QRS morphology during the arrhythmia may be useful in identifying the area of myocardial necrosis and the infarct-related vessel.

Bradyarrhythmias, such as sinus bradycardia and second- and third-degree AV block, also have been observed during coronary reperfusion. They are associated mostly with restoration of flow in arteries supplying the inferoposterior left ventricle.[106]

Although the ECG changes, especially the ST-segment shifts and the development of accelerated idioventricular rhythm, are useful signs of reperfusion in patients with acute myocardial infarction who are receiving thrombolytic agents, there are considerable limitations in their use in the prediction of recanalization of the infarct-related artery. Reperfusion may have occurred without significant decrease in the ST-segment elevation, and the reverse is also true. Kircher and associates

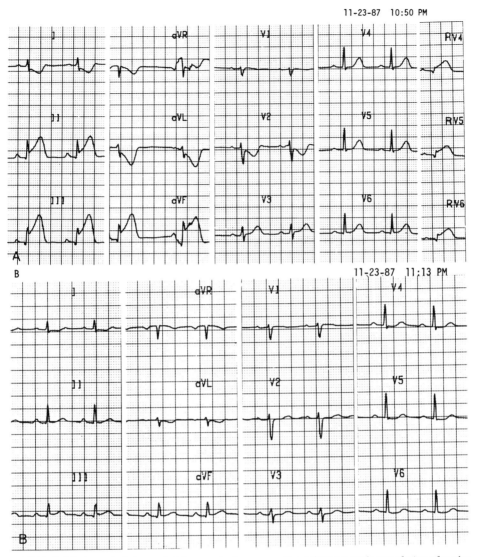

FIGURE 9–30. Acute inferior and right ventricular myocardial infarction with reperfusion after the administration of thrombolytic agent. The patient was a 54-year-old woman who had severe chest pain for 2 hours when the tracing in A was recorded. The tracing shows marked ST-segment elevation in leads II, III, aVF, and V_{4R} through V_{6R}, with reciprocal ST-segment depression and T-wave inversion in leads I, aVL, and V_2. Tissue plasminogen activator was administered intravenously. Twenty-three minutes later, the chest pain subsided and the ECG (B) shows that the ST segment has returned almost to the isoelectric line. Three hours later, the chest pain recurred and coronary arteriogram revealed a dominant right coronary artery with 90 percent stenosis in its midportion at the origin of the second right ventricular free wall branch. The other coronary arteries were normal. A successful percutaneous transluminal coronary angioplasty was performed. The serum creatinine kinase level reached its peak 12 hours after the onset of chest pain. Radionuclide ventriculogram revealed a left ventricular ejection fraction of 48 percent, with inferior wall akinesis and a right ventricular ejection fraction of 58 percent.

analyzed their data from 56 consecutive patients with acute myocardial infarction 90 minutes after they received thrombolytic therapy.[148] Rapid decrease of ST segment alone as an indicator of reperfusion had a sensitivity of 52 percent, a specificity of 88 percent, and a predictive value of 88 percent. The development of reperfusion arrhythmia had a sensitivity of 37 percent, a specificity of 84 percent, and a predictive value of 82 percent. In 5 patients who experienced relief of chest pain, rapid ST-segment changes, and reperfusion

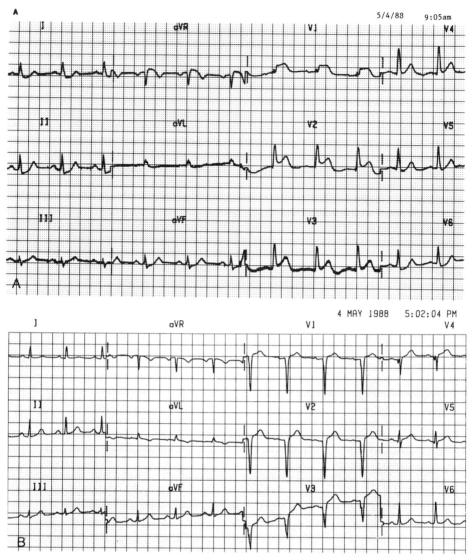

FIGURE 9–31. Accelerated Q-wave development with coronary reperfusion. The patient was a 57-year-old man who had severe chest pain 75 minutes before the tracing in A was recorded. The ECG shows counterclockwise rotation, marked ST-segment elevation in leads V_1 and V_2, and reciprocal ST-segment depression in the anterolateral and inferior leads. Tissue plasminogen activator was administered intravenously. Acute myocardial infarction was confirmed by elevated cardiac enzyme levels. Eight hours later, the tracing in B shows the appearance of QS deflection with slight ST elevation in leads V_1 through V_4. Coronary arteriogram revealed an 80 percent stenotic lesion of the proximal left anterior descending artery.

arrhythmias, the predictive value of recanalization of the artery was 100 percent.

PROGNOSTIC VALUE OF THE ELECTROCARDIOGRAM IN MYOCARDIAL INFARCTION

The prognosis of patients with acute myocardial infarction depends on many factors. The importance of the infarct size, the degree of impairment of ventricular function, and the presence or absence of ventricular conduction defect and major cardiac arrhythmias is well known. To a certain degree the resting 12-lead ECG also may be useful in the prediction of the future clinical course of the patient.

As discussed previously, the presence of abnormal Q waves correlates well with the presence and location of ventricular dyskinesis.[181] The greater number of leads with abnormal Q waves, the wider and deeper Q waves, and

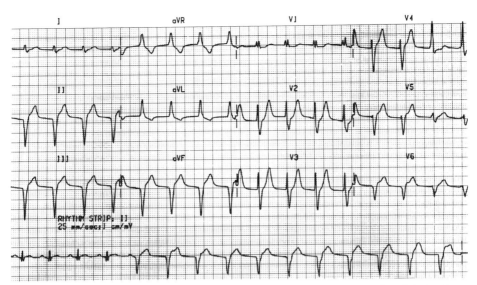

FIGURE 9–32. Reperfusion arrhythmia. Accelerated idioventricular rhythm developed during thrombolytic therapy in a 55-year-old man with acute inferior myocardial infarction. The ventricular rate is 92 beats per minute. Four normal sinus beats are present in the rhythm strip. Two fusion beats are present in the left precordial leads. The QRS axis is −90°.

larger decrease of the R-wave amplitude are associated with more severe impairment of left ventricular ejection fraction.[205]

It generally is agreed that anterior myocardial infarction carries a poorer prognosis than inferior myocardial infarction, even if the infarct size is comparable.[121,257] Hands and coworkers analyzed 789 consecutive patients who had suffered their first myocardial infarction.[121] Of these patients, 398 had anterior myocardial infarctions and 391 had inferior myocardial infarctions. The patients were matched for infarct size determined by the peak creatine kinase levels. Both the early mortality (days 1 to 28 after myocardial infarction) and 1-year mortality were higher among those with anterior (10 and 18.3 percent) than those with inferior myocardial infarction (6.4 and 10.5 percent). In 471 patients with a first myocardial infarction analyzed by Stone and associates, they found that patients with anterior infarction had a lower left ventricular ejection fraction, higher incidence of congestive heart failure, and higher cumulative cardiac mortality than did patients with inferior infarction, even after adjustment for infarction size.[257] This is true whether the infarction was Q-wave or non–Q-wave in type.

Although inferior myocardial infarction generally has a less complicated clinical course than does anterior myocardial infarction, this may not be true in the case of inferior myocardial infarction with extensive right ventricular involvement. Of 25 patients with severe right ventricular infarction reported by Rodrigues and associates, 6 died in the late hospital period.[235] In 11 consecutive patients with right ventricular infarction I reviewed recently, 5 had ventricular tachycardia/ventricular fibrillation, 5 had complete AV block, and 1 died while in the hospital.

The clinical outcome of Q-wave versus non–Q-wave infarction has been the subject of considerable interest in recent years. Q-wave infarcts usually are larger than non–Q-wave infarcts.[153,257] The mortality of patients with Q-wave infarction is higher than those with non–Q-wave infarction in the early phase of the acute event.[172,187] The rate of recurrent infarction in the late in-hospital period is, however, much higher in patients with non–Q-wave infarct.[172,187] Recurrent infarction in patients with non–Q-wave infarct is associated with a high mortality.[169,171,188] As a result, the long-term prognoses of these two types of infarction are not significantly different. Klein and Helfant have written a useful summary comparing the various aspects of Q-wave and non–Q-wave infarction.[150]

MYOCARDIAL INFARCTION IN THE ABSENCE OF CORONARY ATHEROSCLEROSIS

Although myocardial infarction most often is the result of coronary atherosclerosis and thrombosis, it occasionally is associated with other types of pathologic states that reduce the coronary artery blood supply. The arterial lumen may be narrowed by other types of disease of the arterial wall or obstructed by embolus. There may be disproportion between myocardial oxygen demand and blood supply even though the coronary artery itself is normal. The role of coronary spasm has been brought forth in recent years. Finally, in infants and children, congenital anomalies of the coronary artery may be responsible.

Myocardial infarction may be seen in patients with tertiary syphilis that involves the coronary ostia and the proximal portions of the coronary arteries.[126] Such a cause for coronary occlusion is rare, especially in recent years. A similar process is seen in Takayasu's disease.[44] Various forms of connective tissue diseases have been reported to cause acute myocardial infarction by involving the coro-

nary arteries. This is most common in polyarteritis nodosa[118,225] (Fig. 8–5) but also has been reported in systemic lupus erythematosus,[22,31] rheumatoid arthritis,[145] rheumatic fever,[23] and ankylosing spondylitis.[242] Coronary artery aneurysms and thrombosis are common in children with the mucocutaneous lymph node syndrome (Kawasaki disease)[149,285] (Fig. 9–33). In pseudoxanthoma elasticum, the coronary artery may be involved with fragmentation of the tunica elastica and medial calcification, which may predispose the coronary artery to premature development of atherosclerosis and myocardial infarction.[88] The deposition of mucopolysaccharides in the arterial wall in Hurler's disease may narrow the lumen and result in myocardial infarction.[245] Coronary arterial occlusion also has been seen in patients with homocystinuria.[246]

Myocardial infarction may occur as a result

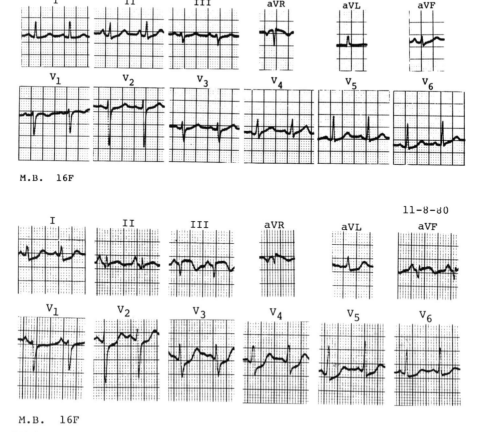

FIGURE 9–33. Acute inferior myocardial infarction in a 16-year-old girl with Kawasaki disease and coronary artery aneurysm. The aneurysm was demonstrated by coronary arteriogram before the development of myocardial infarction. The ECG on 5-12-80 (A) was obtained before and that on 11-8-80 (B) after the infarction occurred. Note the appearance of Q waves with ST-segment elevation and T-wave inversion in the inferior leads on the tracing of 11-8-80. (Courtesy of Dr. Samuel Kaplan.)

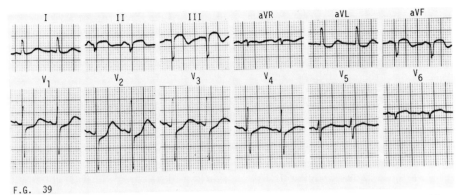

F.G. 39

FIGURE 9–34. Acute inferolateral myocardial infarction with normal coronary arteriogram. The patient was a 39-year-old woman who had a history of angina at rest and with exertion. She had the onset of an acute inferolateral myocardial infarction on the day before this ECG was recorded. The tracing shows a QS deflection in leads II, III, and aVF, with small R waves in leads V_5 and V_6. There is also ST-segment elevation with T-wave inversion in the inferior leads with reciprocal ST-segment depression in leads V_1 through V_4. Coronary arteriogram performed 6 days later was normal. The myocardial infarction was probably the result of coronary artery spasm.

of dissection of the aorta, when the coronary arteries are occluded by the dissecting hematoma.[131] The dissection also may be localized to the coronary artery.[51]

The ECG signs of myocardial infarction are frequently seen in patients who have undergone coronary artery bypass surgery. The reported incidence varies from 9 to 20 percent.[28,136,184] Iatrogenic myocardial infarction also may occur in connection with other types of cardiac surgery or therapeutic and diagnostic procedures such as pericardiocentesis, transthoracic left ventricular catheterization, and coronary arteriography. In 3079 patients who underwent percutaneous transluminal coronary angioplasty, myocardial infarction developed in 170 (5.5 percent).[64] The coro-

nary artery also may be lacerated by penetrating trauma. It is seldom injured by nonpenetrating trauma, however, which usually results in myocardial contusion.[208]

Myocardial infarction may be the result of coronary embolism.[278] This is seen in patients with bacterial endocarditis, mitral stenosis, cardiomyopathy with mural thrombus, prosthetic valves, myxoma of left atrium, and other rarer conditions.

In recent years, there has been a growing interest in the group of patients with myocardial infarction but angiographically normal coronary arteries (Figs. 9–34 and 9–35). Coronary spasm has been demonstrated in some of these patients and is believed to be one of the mechanisms responsible for myocardial infarc-

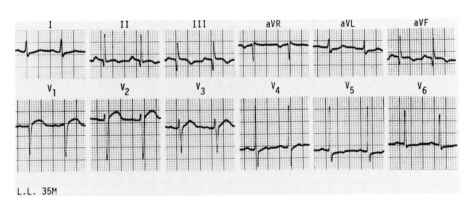

L.L. 35M

FIGURE 9–35. Inferior myocardial infarction with normal coronary arteries. The patient was a 35-year-old man with two episodes of myocardial infarction documented by serial ECG and cardiac enzyme changes. This tracing was recorded during the second episode and shows changes consistent with inferior myocardial infarction. There also are ST-segment and T-wave abnormalities in lead V_4 through V_6. Coronary arteriogram was performed shortly after each episode of myocardial infarction. It was normal on both occasions. The ventriculogram revealed hypokinesis of the inferoposterior wall of the left ventricle.

tion.[46,47,125,176,177,202,203] The observations made by Maseri and associates suggest that coronary artery spasm may lead to coronary thrombosis and myocardial infarction.[176,177] Another explanation proposed for the normal appearance of the coronary arteriogram in patients with myocardial infarction is acute coronary embolism with subsequent clot lysis, retraction, or recanalization.[8]

Case reports have accumulated since 1982 to indicate that angina pectoris and acute myocardial infarction may be associated with cocaine abuse.[10,58,139,210,234,251,288] The cardiac event may occur with intranasal administration, intravenous administration, or inhalation of the substance. The coronary arteries of the patients who suffer acute myocardial infarction are often normal. The prevailing theory for the genesis of cocaine-induced myocardial infarction is coronary spasm followed by thrombosis. Cocaine is known to be a sympathomimetic agent that causes tachycardia and blood pressure elevation. It produces systemic vasoconstriction. These pharmacologic effects increase the oxygen demand of the myocardium and may result in relative myocardial ischemia. Demonstration of cocaine-

induced focal constriction of the coronary arteries is still lacking, however. Figure 9–36 is an example of an acute anterolateral myocardial infarction related to cocaine use in a 27-year-old man.

The epicardial portion of the coronary arteries may be, in some instances, bridged by muscle bands. Such myocardial bridging has been noted in up to 7.5 percent of coronary arteriograms.[138] It involves exclusively the anterior descending artery. Although the narrowing of the vessel during ventricular systole seldom causes symptoms, angina, acute myocardial infarction, and sudden death have been reported.[85,87,183]

Young women taking oral contraceptives were reported to have an increased incidence of myocardial infarction.[170] The increased risk was not attributed to increased coronary atheroma, but the exact mechanism is not clear.[169]

Anomalous origin of the left coronary artery from the pulmonary artery is the most common cause of myocardial infarction that results from congenital abnormalities.[151,279] The ECG usually shows anterolateral myocardial infarction, often accompanied by signs of left

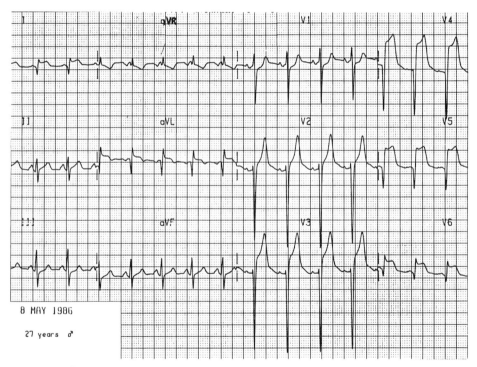

FIGURE 9–36. Acute anterolateral myocardial infarction related to cocaine. The patient was a 27-year-old man who developed severe chest pain several hours after the intranasal use of cocaine. The ECG shows abnormal Q waves with marked ST-segment elevations in leads I, aVL, and V₄ through V₆. ST-segment elevation is present also in lead V₃. The patient refused cardiac catheterization during that hospital admission. Coronary arteriogram peformed 6 months later revealed normal coronary arteries.

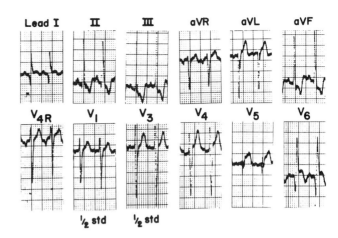

FIGURE 9–37. Autopsy-confirmed anomalous coronary artery arising from the pulmonary artery in a 4-month-old baby. Anterolateral myocardial infarction and left ventricular hypertrophy were present and are demonstrated in the ECG. (Courtesy of Dr. Samuel Kaplan.)

ventricular hypertrophy (Fig. 9–37). The latter probably results from compensatory hypertrophy of the unaffected portion of the left ventricle. Coronary arteriovenous fistula and coronary artery aneurysm with thrombosis are the other possible congenital causes of myocardial infarction.

Subendocardial infarction may be seen in patients with severe shock even in the presence of normal coronary arteries. It also has been described in carbon monoxide poisoning.[63]

DIFFERENTIAL DIAGNOSIS: PSEUDOINFARCTIONS

Although abnormal Q waves, especially in the presence of ST-segment displacement and T-wave changes, are the typical ECG findings in patients with Q-wave myocardial infarction, similar changes may be seen in patients without coronary artery disease. The various conditions that may present an ECG pseudoinfarction pattern are discussed in detail to emphasize the pitfalls of ECG interpretation when other clinical information is not taken into consideration.

Ventricular Hypertrophy

Left ventricular hypertrophy is one of the most common ECG abnormalities that may mimic myocardial infarction. Frequently there are QS deflections in the right precordial leads or poor progression of the R wave in the right and mid-precordial leads to suggest anterior myocardial infarction. The secondary repolarization abnormalities with ST-segment elevation in these leads may be mistaken as current of injury. An example is given in Figure 9–38. Although this pseudoinfarction pat-

tern may be seen in left ventricular hypertrophy of various origins, its presence in patients with aortic stenosis often creates a diagnostic problem, since angina pectoris is common in these patients in the absence of coronary artery disease. The pathogenesis of the abnormal initial QRS forces is not entirely clear. In many instances, there is patchy myocardial fibrosis.[14] Conduction disturbance may be responsible for the others. A rapid reversal of the abnormalities was observed in some patients with aortic valvular disease after aortic valve surgery.[15]

In analysis of patients with a QS or QR pattern in leads V_3 and V_4 without myocardial infarction, Surawicz and associates reported that the initial QRS vectors were usually directed downward.[260] Accordingly, initial R waves were almost invariably recorded in the leads taken below the standard level of leads V_3 and V_4. This was in contrast to most patients with myocardial infarction with a similar QRS pattern. The Q waves persisted in the lower leads.

In *right ventricular hypertrophy,* QR complexes with T-wave inversion may be seen in the right precordial leads. The abnormal Q waves in such cases seldom lead to the misinterpretation of myocardial infarction, since they usually are associated with a relatively severe degree of anatomic right ventricular hypertrophy. Other ECG changes suggestive of right heart involvement, such as abnormal right axis deviation in the frontal plane, tall R waves in the right precordial leads, deep S waves in the left precordial leads, and right atrial enlargement, often coexist. The genesis of the abnormal Q waves in the right precordial leads in patients with right ventricular hypertrophy is uncertain but it is probably related to abnormal septal depolarization.[90] The

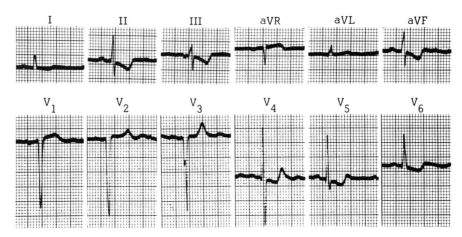

FIGURE 9–38. Left ventricular hypertrophy with pseudoinfarction pattern. The patient was a 48-year-old man with rheumatic heart disease, severe aortic stenosis, and moderate aortic insufficiency. In the tracing, deep S waves are present in leads V_1 through V_3, with ST-segment depression and T-wave inversion in the left precordial leads consistent with left ventricular hypertrophy. A small R wave is present in leads V_1 and V_2 but is absent in lead V_3. These changes suggest anterior myocardial infarction. Coronary arteriogram, however, was normal, and the coronary arteries also were found to be normal during surgery. (Reproduced from Chou TC: Pseudoinfarction. Cardiovasc Clin 5(3):199, 1973, by permission.)

normal left-to-right septal activation may be reversed, or the right septal force is greatly increased and becomes the dominant potential.

Abnormal QS deflections are seen in the precordial leads of a significant number of patients with chronic cor pulmonale. This is discussed in the following section.

Pulmonary Diseases

PULMONARY EMPHYSEMA AND CHRONIC COR PULMONALE

Leftward displacement of the transitional zone in the precordial leads is a common finding in patients with chronic obstructive lung disease and chronic cor pulmonale. The R waves in the right precordial and sometimes mid-precordial leads become small and may even disappear, thereby suggesting anterior myocardial infarction (Fig. 9–39).[161,186,217,260] This is especially true in cases of chronic cor pulmonale. Abnormal Q waves also may appear in the inferior leads to suggest inferior myocardial infarction.[161]

Abnormally small or absent R waves in the right and mid-precordial leads in patients with pulmonary emphysema have been explained mainly on the basis of the vertical displacement of the heart secondary to low-lying, flattened diaphragms and the intervention of hyperinflated lungs.[217] The position of

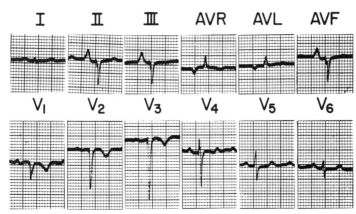

FIGURE 9–39. Pseudoinfarction pattern in a man with pulmonary emphysema and chronic cor pulmonale proved at autopsy. The ECG was recorded from a 65-year-old man. The limb leads show signs of right atrial enlargement, and the QRS axis is directed superiorly and slightly rightward. Abnormal Q waves are present in leads V_2 through V_4, with T-wave inversion in leads V_1 through V_3. At autopsy, severe pulmonary emphysema and right ventricular hypertrophy and dilatation were found. The heart weighed 465 g. The right ventricular weight was about three times that of the left ventricle. The coronary arteries revealed a slight degree of atherosclerosis. The myocardium demonstrated no evidence of infarction or fibrosis. (Reproduced from Chou TC: Pseudoinfarction. Cardiovasc Clin 5(3):199, 1973, by permission.)

the exploring electrode of the precordial leads becomes more superior in relation to the heart (Fig. 9–40A). If the initial QRS forces are directed inferiorly, they may either become perpendicular or be directed toward the negative side of the electrical axis of these leads, and a small R wave or a Q wave may, therefore, be recorded to suggest anterior

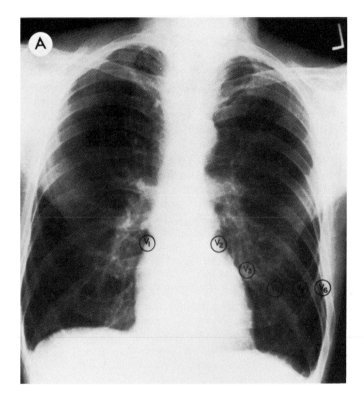

FIGURE 9–40. (A) The chest roentgenogram of a 58-year-old man with severe pulmonary emphysema showing the locations of the electrodes for the standard precordial leads V_1 through V_6 in relation to the heart. They are at a level close to the base of the heart.

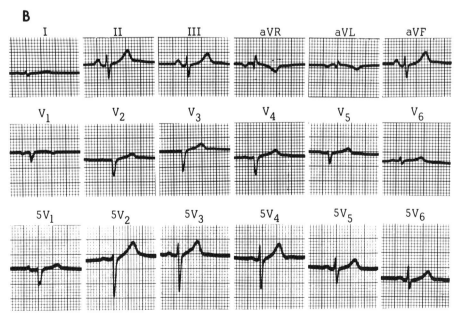

FIGURE 9–40 *Continued.* (B) The ECG of the same patient. It shows QS deflections in leads V_1 through V_4 to mimic anterior myocardial infarction. Additional precordial leads were recorded one intercostal space below the levels of the routine electrode locations. The QRS complexes are partially normalized. (Reproduced from Chou TC: Pseudoinfarction. Cardiovasc Clin 5(3):199, 1973, by permission.)

myocardial infarction. If the precordial leads are recorded one intercostal space lower ($5V_1$ through $5V_6$) the morphology of the precordial lead QRS complexes often is partially normalized (Fig. 9–40B). In patients who have right ventricular hypertrophy, these changes may be exaggerated and the abnormality of septal activation becomes an additional factor. Q waves are more likely to be recorded in the right precordial leads. In a series of 50 cases of chronic cor pulmonale, QS deflections in the right precordial leads were seen in about 36 percent.[291]

Although myocardial infarction may coexist in patients with pulmonary emphysema or chronic cor pulmonale, its detection is difficult, especially if serial ECGs and other clinical information are not available. In practice, when abnormal Q waves in the right and midprecordial leads are accompanied by P pulmonale, rightward displacement of the QRS and T axes, reduction of the size of the QRS complex in the limb leads and left precordial leads, large S waves in leads I, II, and III resulting in an $S_1S_2S_3$ pattern, or large S waves in leads V_5 and V_6 altering the R/S ratio of these leads, the abnormal Q waves are most likely the result of chronic obstructive lung disease rather than myocardial infarction.

SPONTANEOUS PNEUMOTHORAX

Both spontaneous and artificial pneumothorax may induce ECG changes in a significant number of patients.[8,62] In both left- and right-sided pneumothorax, the frontal plane QRS axis may be shifted to the right. The voltage of the QRS complex in lead I is reduced. T-wave inversion may occur in the limb leads or the precordial leads. The latter is especially common in left-sided pneumothorax. The inverted T waves often are symmetrical and peaked, with an upward convexity of the descending limb resembling ischemic T waves in coronary artery disease. Patients with left-sided pneumothorax often show a decrease or loss of the R wave in the precordial leads to mimic anterior myocardial infarction. The reduction of the voltage of the QRS complex may be generalized. P-wave changes also may be observed. The combined effect of displacement and rotation of the heart and interposition of air between the heart and chest wall has been suggested as the mechanism responsible for the ECG abnormalities. Figure 9–41 illustrates the appearance of ECG signs resembling acute myocardial infarction in a 26-year-old man with left-sided spontaneous pneumothorax (Fig. 9–42). The R wave in leads V_2 through V_4 returned after the left lung was reexpanded.

Pulmonary Embolism

It often is difficult to distinguish pulmonary embolism from acute myocardial infarction, both clinically and electrocardiographically. In acute pulmonary embolism, Q waves may

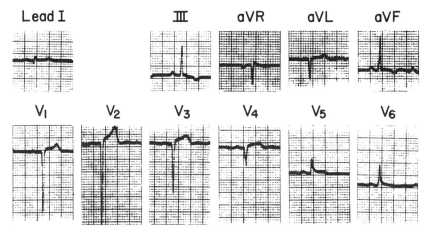

FIGURE 9–41. Left-sided spontaneous pneumothorax. The ECG was recorded from a 26-year-old man who complained of sudden onset of chest pain and dyspnea. It shows abnormal QS complexes with slight ST-segment elevation in leads V_1 through V_4. The T waves are inverted in leads III, aVF, and V_6. The changes in the precordial leads resemble those of acute anteroseptal myocardial infarction. His chest radiograph (see Fig. 9–42), however, showed massive left-sided pneumothorax with collapse of the lung. The heart and mediastinum were displaced to the right. Suction tube drainage was applied to the left pleural space. After the left lung was reexpanded, a repeat ECG showed the disappearance of the Q waves in leads V_2 through V_4. (Reproduced from Chou TC: Pseudoinfarction. Cardiovasc Clin 5(3):199, 1973, by permission.)

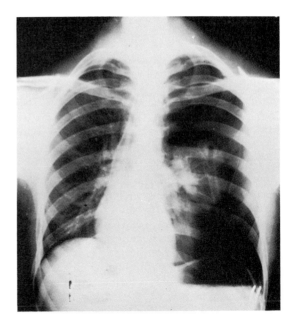

FIGURE 9–42. The chest roentgenogram of the patient with spontaneous pneumothorax whose ECG is shown in Figure 9–41. (Reproduced from Chou TC: Pseudoinfarction. Cardiovasc Clin 5(3):199, 1973, by permission.)

appear in lead III and sometimes in lead aVF accompanied by ST-segment and T-wave changes to suggest inferior myocardial infarction.[70,178,216] This is illustrated in Figure 9–43.

The abnormal Q waves in leads III and aVF in pulmonary embolism have been attributed to acute right ventricular dilatation with clockwise rotation of the heart along its longitudinal axis. The interventricular septum becomes so oriented that its right septal surface is directed superiorly. The initial left-to-right septal activation results in forces directed superiorly. Therefore, Q waves are recorded in leads III and aVF. In contrast to inferior myocardial infarction, Q waves seldom appear in lead II in acute pulmonary embolism.

Acute pulmonary embolism occasionally may simulate acute anterior myocardial infarction.[236] Figure 9–44 is a tracing recorded from a 60-year-old man. An ECG recorded 2 days earlier was normal. After an episode of severe dyspnea and retrosternal chest pain, the ECG revealed QS complexes in leads V_2 and V_3 and abnormal Q waves in leads V_4 and V_5, with slight ST-segment elevation and T-wave inversion in these leads. The diagnosis of acute anterior myocardial infarction was made. A pulmonary arteriogram, however, demonstrated multiple filling defects bilaterally. The R waves in the precordial leads reappeared a few days later. The patient died 10 days later. At autopsy, multiple and massive pulmonary emboli were found. The coronary arteries

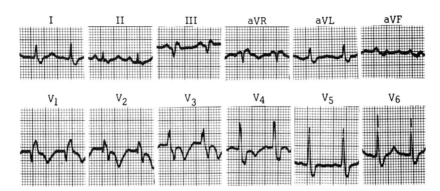

FIGURE 9–43. Pulmonary embolism. The ECG was obtained from a 61-year-old man with massive pulmonary embolism. The diagnosis was verified by autopsy. There was minimal coronary atherosclerosis, with no evidence of myocardial infarction. The ECG shows right bundle branch block with T-wave inversion in leads V_1 through V_5. A deep, wide Q wave is present in lead III, and a small QS complex appears in lead aVF. (Reproduced from Chou TC: Pseudoinfarction. Cardiovasc Clin 5(3):199, 1973, by permission.)

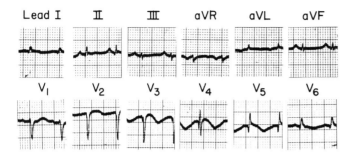

FIGURE 9–44. Massive pulmonary embolism simulating anterior myocardial infarction in a 60-year-old man. The diagnosis was confirmed by autopsy, which showed no evidence of myocardial infarction. (Reproduced from Romhilt D, Susilavorn B, Chou TC: Unusual electrocardiographic manifestation of pulmonary embolism. Am Heart J 80:237, 1970, by permission of CV Mosby.)

showed only mild atherosclerosis, and serial sections of the heart revealed no evidence of myocardial infarction. I have seen additional similar cases. The pathogenesis of these ECG changes is unclear. Acute right ventricular dilatation and strain with relative myocardial ischemia of the right ventricle are possible contributing factors.

Myocardial Diseases

PRIMARY MYOCARDIAL DISEASE

Abnormal Q waves that resemble myocardial infarction are particularly common in the obstructive type of cardiomyopathy.[26,91,173] In a series of 123 patients with idiopathic hypertrophic subaortic stenosis, Frank and Braumwald noted abnormal Q waves in 69 (56 percent).[91] A lower incidence was reported by other observers.[26,173] The pathologic Q waves are observed most commonly in leads V_4 through V_6 and lead I (Fig. 9–45) and generally have been attributed to ventricular septal hypertrophy. The normal left-to-right initial septal forces are markedly increased, resulting in an exaggeration of the septal Q waves.

Primary myocardial disease of the nonobstructive type also may cause an infarction pattern in the ECG even though this occurs less frequently than the obstructive variety[173,224,262] (Fig. 9–46). In most cases, the ECG findings are the result of localized area of myocardial destruction. In some instances, however, a gross fibrotic area cannot be found. Microscopic lesions were thought to be responsible for conduction disturbances that resulted in aberration of the initial portion of the QRS forces.[262]

SECONDARY MYOCARDIAL DISEASES

A pseudoinfarction pattern may be encountered in the ECGs of patients with various forms of myocarditis,[108] neuromuscular and neurologic disorders such as progressive muscular dystrophy,[214,250] Friedreich's ataxia,[127] scleroderma,[240,282] amyloidosis,[29] and primary and metastatic tumors of the heart.[97,124] In these patients, the abnormal Q waves are the result of replacement of the myocardium by fibrous or other electrically inert tissues. Figure 9–47 illustrates the ECG changes in a 20-year-old patient with progressive muscular dystrophy.

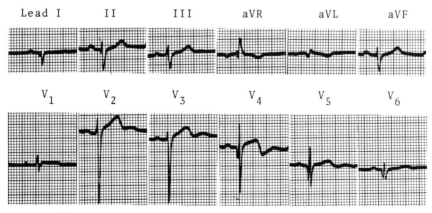

FIGURE 9–45. Idiopathic hypertrophic subaortic stenosis in a 23-year-old man. An intraventricular pressure gradient of 135 mm Hg was demonstrated during isoproterenol infusion. The ECG changes resemble those of anterolateral myocardial infarction. (Reproduced from Chou TC: Pseudoinfarction. Cardiovasc Clin 5(3):199, 1973, by permission.)

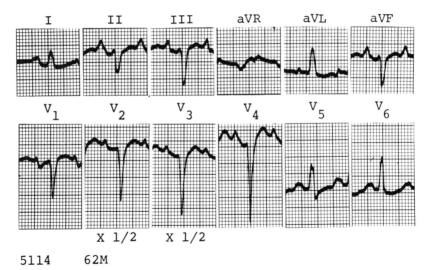

X 1/2   X 1/2

5114   62M

FIGURE 9–46. Idiopathic cardiomyopathy simulating myocardial infarction. The diagnosis of cardiomyopathy is supported by clinical and autopsy findings. The heart weighed 555 g, with biventricular hypertrophy. Only minimal coronary atherosclerosis was present. The myocardium showed microscopic evidence of scattered fibrosis but no gross sign of infarction. In the ECG, the P waves are consistent with biatrial enlargement. The QRS changes suggest left anterior hemiblock and left ventricular hypertrophy. The QS deflections in leads V_1 through V_3 mimic anteroseptal myocardial infarction. Some of the ST and T changes are probably due to digitalis effect.

Figure 9–48 demonstrates the findings in a 3-year-old child with myocardial fibroma.

Conduction Abnormalities

LEFT BUNDLE BRANCH BLOCK

Uncomplicated complete and incomplete left bundle branch block often presents small or no R waves in the right precordial leads.[187] QS deflections that extend from leads V_1 through V_4 or a reversal of the R-wave progression in these precordial leads also may occur in the absence of myocardial infarction. The secondary ST elevation in the right precordial leads in association with the QS deflection may falsely suggest the presence of an acute process. QS deflections also may be seen in leads II, III, and aVF to suggest inferior myocardial infarction.

LEFT ANTERIOR HEMIBLOCK

In left anterior hemiblock, the frontal plane QRS axis is displaced leftward to −30° or beyond. Lead I displays a qR pattern, and leads

FIGURE 9–47. Progressive muscular dystrophy in a 20-year-old man. Autopsy revealed patchy fibrosis throughout the myocardium. In the ECG, deep but narrow Q waves are present in leads V_5 and V_6 with a tall R wave in lead V_1, findings typical for this condition. (Reproduced from Chou TC: Pseudoinfarction. Cardiovasc Clin 5(3):199, 1973, by permission.)

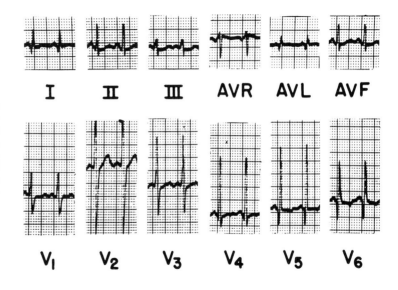

I   II   III   AVR   AVL   AVF

V_1 V_2 V_3 V_4 V_5 V_6

A

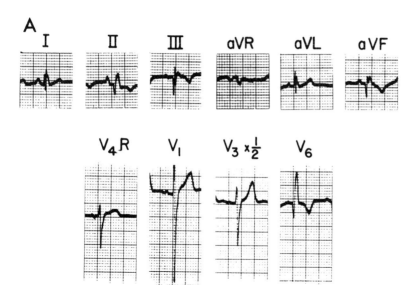

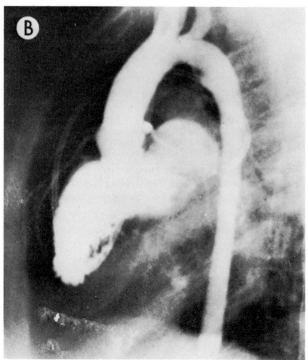

FIGURE 9–48. (A) Myocardial fibroma in a 3-year-old boy. The ECG changes mimic inferolateral myocardial infarction. (B) The left ventriculogram of the same child with myocardial fibroma demonstrating the filling defect in the inferoposterior aspect of the left ventricle. (Courtesy of Dr. Samuel Kaplan.)

C

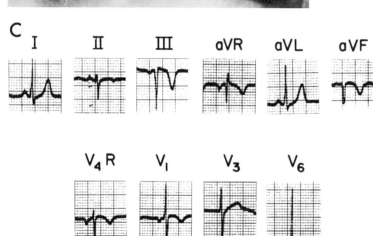

FIGURE 9–48 Continued. (C) The postoperative ECG of the same child taken 9 months after the removal of myocardial fibroma. (Courtesy of Dr. Samuel Kaplan. Reproduced from Chou TC: Pseudoinfarction. Cardiovasc Clin 5(3):199, 1973, by permission.)

II and III display an rS deflection. QRS changes also may occur in the precordial leads, which have previously received little attention. The transitional zone often is displaced to the left, with the appearance of deep S waves in the left precordial leads. Q waves may appear in the right and mid-precordial leads to mimic anterior myocardial infarction.[179,237] The abnormality of the initial QRS forces has been attributed to the delay of excitation of that portion of the ventricular septum that normally is supplied by the anterior division of the left bundle branch. The relative early activation of the part of the septum supplied by the posterior division results in a displacement of the initial vectors inferiorly. These vectors may now be oriented to the negative side of the lead axes of the right precordial leads, and Q waves are recorded. This explanation is supported by the demonstration of a change of the qRS deflection in leads V_1 and V_2 to RS deflection when these chest leads are placed one intercostal space lower.[179]

VENTRICULAR PREEXCITATION SYNDROME

In ventricular preexcitation syndrome, the early activation of an ectopic ventricular site through the accessory bundle alters markedly the direction of the initial QRS forces. If the initial vectors are directed superiorly, the delta wave is downward in the inferior leads and mimics the abnormal Q waves of inferior myocardial infarction. In my experience, this is the most common form of pseudoinfarction pattern in patients with ventricular preexcitation syndrome. It is observed in both types A and B of this anomaly. In type A ventricular preexcitation syndrome, the delta waves may be downward in leads I and aVL to resemble lateral wall myocardial infarction. The downward initial deflection in leads V_1 and V_2 in type B ventricular preexcitation syndrome may mislead to the interpretation of anterior myocardial infarction. Figure 9–49 gives an example of intermittent type B ventricular preexcitation syndrome in a 29-year-old man with atrial septal defect. The pseudoinfarction pattern appeared in the inferior leads when preexcitation occurred. This misinterpretation can usually be avoided when the short PR interval and the wide QRS complex with initial slurring are noted. Occasionally, however, in a variant form of the syndrome, the PR interval may be within normal limits, and the differential diagnosis may be more difficult.

Intracranial Hemorrhage

The association of ECG changes and diseases of the central nervous system has long been noted. This occurs most commonly in patients with intracranial bleeding, especially subarachnoid hemorrhage. The abnormalities

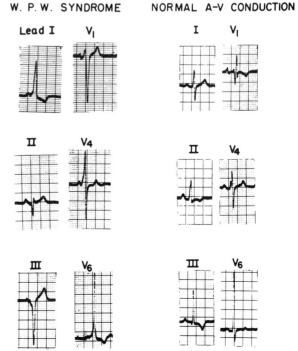

FIGURE 9–49. Ventricular preexcitation syndrome simulating inferior myocardial infarction. The ECG was recorded from a 29-year-old man with the secundum type of atrial septal defect and intermittent ventricular preexcitation syndrome. During the ventricular preexcitation syndrome, the delta vectors were directed superiorly, resulting in abnormal Q waves in the inferior leads.

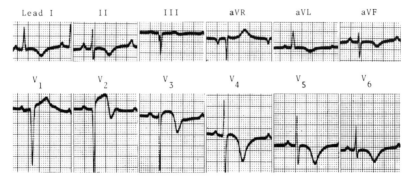

FIGURE 9–50. Subarachnoid hemorrhage in a 60-year-old woman. The ECG changes suggest acute anterior myocardial infarction. (Reproduced from Chou TC, Susilavorn B: Electrocardiographic changes in intracranial hemorrhage. J Electrocardiol 2:193, 1969, by permission.)

usually consist of ST-segment elevation or depression; large, wide, upright, or inverted T waves; a long QT interval; and prominent U waves.[33] Abnormal Q waves occasionally are observed.[49,68]

Figures 9–50 and 9–51 represent an example of pseudoinfarction that occurred in a 60-year-old woman who died of subarachnoid hemorrhage. The initial ECG was interpreted as acute anterior myocardial infarction. It was not until the second tracing was obtained 1 day later that the true nature of the responsible lesion was suspected.

Altered autonomic tone has been suggested as the most likely mechanism for the production of ECG changes in central nervous system diseases. It may affect the ECG as a result of functional alterations of ventricular recovery time or by the production of anatomic lesions or as a combination of both factors.[3] A few instances of subendocardial hemorrhage in patients with no evidence of significant coronary artery disease have been reported.[152] In a large pathologic series of patients who died of intracranial lesion, microscopic focal myocytolysis was found in 8 percent.[60]

Myocardial Contusion

In nonpenetrating injury to the heart, myocardial contusion is the most common lesion. Hemorrhage and necrosis of various degrees may occur. The ECG most commonly reveals some nonspecific ST and T-wave abnormalities.[209,274] When the conduction system is involved, AV block or intraventricular conduction defect may be observed. If the contusion, hemorrhage, and necrosis are extensive, the ECG may be indistinguishable from that seen in myocardial infarction. Figure 9–52 was re-

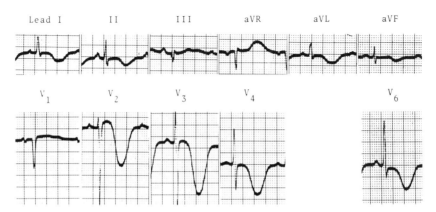

FIGURE 9–51. Tracing obtained from the patient in Figure 9–50 with subarachnoid hemorrhage 1 day later. It shows many of the findings frequently associated with central nervous system lesion. Careful autopsy examination revealed mild left ventricular hypertrophy and dilatation but no myocardial damage. (Reproduced from Chou TC, Susilavorn B: Electrocardiographic changes in intracranial hemorrhage. J Electrocardiol 2:193, 1969, by permission.)

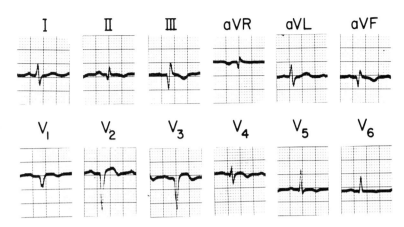

FIGURE 9–52. Myocardial contusion. The tracing was recorded from a 34-year-old man who sustained a nonpenetrating trauma to the chest. The ECG is suggestive of anteroseptal and inferior myocardial infarction. The coronary arteriogram was normal. (Reproduced from Chou TC: Pseudoinfarction. Cardiovasc Clin 5(3): 199, 1973, by permission.)

corded from a 34-year-old man who was involved in a motorcycle accident and sustained severe nonpenetrating trauma to his precordium. His ECG revealed changes suggestive of anterior and inferior myocardial infarction. His coronary arteriogram was normal.

Hyperkalemia

Levine and associates described the "dialyzable currents of injury" in potassium intoxication.[155] The ST-segment elevation occurred most commonly in the right precordial leads and resembled acute myocardial infarction or pericarditis. The changes subsided after hemodialysis. The ECG in Figure 9–53 was obtained from a patient with a serum potassium level of 9.6 mEq/L. The tracing revealed intraventricular conduction defect. The small R waves and marked ST-segment elevation in leads V_1 through V_4 were suggestive of acute anterior myocardial infarction. After the patient was treated with sodium bicarbonate and insulin, the record obtained 6 hours later (Fig. 9–54) showed a normal QRS duration, and the current of injury in the right and midprecordial leads was no longer present.

The ST-segment elevation in hyperkalemia probably is due to a marked derangement of the intracellular and extracellular potassium ratio.[99]

Mitral Valve Prolapse–Systolic Click Syndrome

In the mitral valve prolapse–systolic click syndrome the characteristic ECG abnormalities seen in some of the patients consist of ST-segment and T-wave changes in the inferior leads and occasionally in the left precordial leads to mimic myocardial ischemia. A few instances of abnormal Q waves consistent with myocardial infarction have been described in patients who had normal coronary arteriograms.[267] The abnormal Q waves may simulate either inferior or anterior myocardial infarction.

Acute Pericarditis

Although acute pericarditis is not associated with abnormal Q waves, it is mentioned here because it is frequently mistaken for acute myocardial infarction. ST-segment elevation is the common abnormal finding in the early

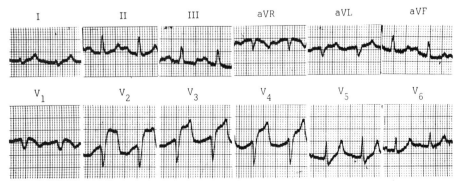

FIGURE 9–53. The ECG of a patient with hyperkalemia. The serum potassium was 9.6 mEq/L. (Reproduced from Chou TC: Pseudoinfarction. Cardiovasc Clin 5(3):199, 1973, by permission.)

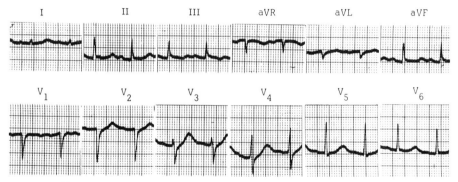

FIGURE 9-54. The ECG recorded from the patient in Figure 9-53 after the serum potassium level had returned to the normal range. (Reproduced from Chou TC: Pseudoinfarction. Cardiovasc Clin 5(3):199, 1973, by permission.)

stage of acute myocardial infarction. In acute pericarditis, however, the ST-segment elevation is diffuse and is usually present in all leads except lead aVR and sometimes leads V_1 and III. In myocardial infarction, the ST elevation is more localized and is accompanied by reciprocal ST depression in the opposite leads.

DIAGNOSIS OF MYOCARDIAL INFARCTION IN THE PRESENCE OF VENTRICULAR CONDUCTION ABNORMALITIES

Myocardial Infarction in the Presence of Right Bundle Branch Block

In uncomplicated right bundle branch block, the initial QRS forces are not altered. Because most myocardial infarctions result in abnormalities of the initial QRS vectors, the presence of right bundle branch block does not in-

terfere with the recognition of the infarcts (Fig. 9-55). The standard diagnostic criteria may still be applied. This also is true if right bundle branch block is accompanied by left anterior or left posterior hemiblock (Figs. 9-56 and 9-57). The only exception is in the case of true posterior myocardial infarction in which the major changes are not in the initial part of the QRS complex. Because right bundle branch block per se causes anterior and rightward displacement of the middle and late QRS forces, lead V_1 may display predominantly positive potential in the absence of posterior myocardial damage.

Horan and associates studied the reliability of Q waves of more than 0.03 second in duration in the diagnosis of myocardial infarction when right bundle branch block was present.[132] In 36 autopsied cases with myocardial infarction, abnormal Q waves were observed in 26, giving a sensitivity of 72 percent. In 40 cases without anatomic evidence of myocardial infarction, a false-positive ECG

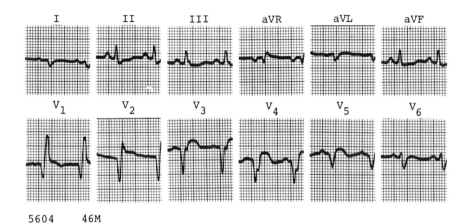

5604   46M

FIGURE 9-55. Acute extensive anterior myocardial infarction with right bundle branch block. The infarction was proved at autopsy.

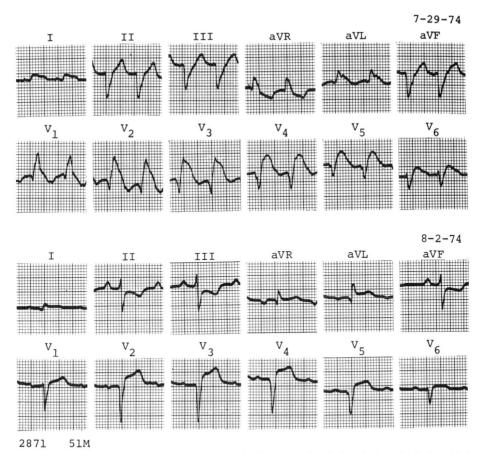

2871   51M

FIGURE 9-56. Acute extensive anterior myocardial infarction with right bundle branch block and left anterior hemiblock. The tracing on 7-29-74 was recorded on the third day after the onset of acute myocardial infarction. Both complete right bundle branch block and left anterior hemiblock are present in addition to signs of acute extensive anterior myocardial infarction. The tracing on 8-2-74 shows the disappearance of right bundle branch block. The patient died on 8-6-74. The left anterior descending and circumflex arteries were totally occluded. The presence of extensive anterior and septal myocardial infarction was confirmed. About 65 percent of the left ventricle was involved.

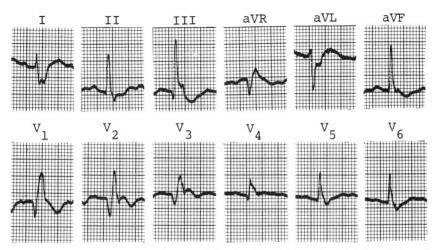

FIGURE 9-57. Acute anteroseptal myocardial infarction with complete right bundle branch block and left posterior hemiblock. The diagnosis of infarction is supported by typical clinical and laboratory findings. The diagnosis of left posterior hemiblock is based on the abnormal right axis of the first half of the QRS complex in the frontal plane.

diagnosis occurred in 25 percent. Most of these latter patients had right ventricular hypertrophy. The sensitivity of the ECG diagnosis of myocardial infarction in the presence of right bundle branch block is therefore comparable to that without right bundle branch block.[133]

Myocardial Infarction in the Presence of Left Bundle Branch Block

The diagnosis of myocardial infarction in the presence of left bundle branch block is difficult. The changes in the sequence of ventricular activation in left bundle branch block cause marked alterations of both the initial and late QRS forces. Many of the conventional criteria for the diagnosis of myocardial infarction are no longer applicable. As discussed, the leftward displacement of the initial QRS forces as a result of the right-to-left septal activation is accompanied by the appearance of Q waves or QS deflections in the right precordial leads. Therefore, the loss of R waves in the right and even mid-precordial leads can no longer be regarded as a sign of anterior myocardial infarction. In an autopsy series of cases of left bundle branch block reported by Horan and associates,[133] abnormal Q waves were found in leads V_1 through V_4 in 35 percent of the patients with infarction and in 40 percent of those without infarction.

The following criteria were suggested for the detection of myocardial infarction in the presence of left bundle branch block:

1. Q waves in leads I, V_5, or V_6.[120,252,254]
2. A reversal of R-wave progression in the right and mid-precordial leads.[120,206]
3. Early notching of the S waves to the right of the transitional zone (usually leads V_3 and V_4).[41]
4. Late wide notching of the S waves to the right of the transitional zone (usually V_3 and V_4).[36,120]
5. An rSR' pattern in leads I, V_5, and V_6.[41]
6. An RS complex in the left precordial leads.[17]
7. A W or QS deflection in leads II, III, and aVF.[77]
8. Primary ST and T-wave changes.[77,120,254]

The presence of Q waves in lead I, aVL, V_5, or V_6 generally is considered one of the most reliable signs of myocardial infarction in the presence of left bundle branch block. In left bundle branch block, the initial septal activation is from right to left. The leftward displacement of the corresponding QRS forces results in the absence of Q waves in leads I, V_5, and V_6, which is one of the diagnostic features of this conduction defect. When there is a massive infarction of the interventricular septum, the loss of the initial septal forces allows the potential generated from the free

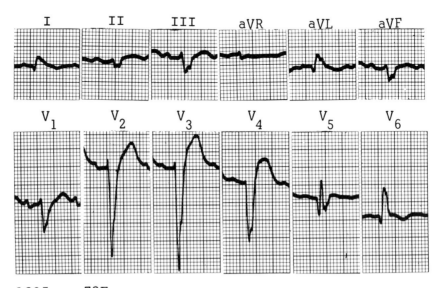

1395   72F

FIGURE 9–58. Complete left bundle branch block with myocardial infarction proved by autopsy. The ECG diagnosis of myocardial infarction is based on the Q waves in leads I, aVL, V_5, and V_6. An autopsy was performed 10 days later and showed severe generalized coronary atherosclerosis with total occlusion of left circumflex artery. There was an extensive recent lateral wall myocardial infarction in addition to a previous one. Left ventricular hypertrophy also was present.

wall of the right ventricle to be manifested. The early QRS vectors are displaced rightward and projected on the negative side of the lead axis of leads I, V_5, and V_6. As a result, Q waves are recorded. Although it was believed that any Q wave in these leads is a reliable sign of anteroseptal myocardial infarction,[151,253] this was not substantiated by Scott[247] in a study of 85 autopsied cases. Q waves were observed in these leads equally often in patients with or without myocardial infarction. He noted that if the duration of the Q waves was 0.04 second or longer, myocardial infarction was almost always present. In my experience, the septal location of the infarct is not always verified. Figure 9–58 illustrates an example of lateral myocardial infarction with Q waves in leads I, aVL, V_5, and V_6 in the presence of complete left bundle branch block.

In left bundle branch block, a reversal of the R-wave progression in the precordial leads may occur with massive infarction of the septum[206] (Fig, 9–59). The initial QRS forces from the free wall of the right ventricle become dominant and are directed anteriorly and rightward. Tall R waves may be recorded in the right precordial leads, but the R-wave amplitude decreases as the mid-precordial leads are taken. Although this criterion was met in many of the cases with proven anteroseptal myocardial infarction, it also gave a high incidence of false-positive diagnoses.[247]

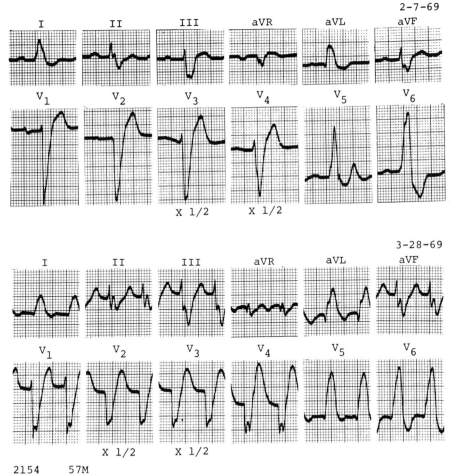

2154   57M

FIGURE 9–59. Left bundle branch block and myocardial infarction. The patient was a 57-year-old man with a history of hypertension and coronary artery disease. The tracing on 2-7-69 was recorded after he developed congestive heart failure and increasing frequency of angina pectoris. It shows first-degree AV block, complete left bundle branch block with a QRS duration of 0.18 second, and digitalis effect. On 3-28-69, he developed severe substernal chest pain and episodes of ventricular tachycardia. The ECG shows the loss of R waves in leads V_3 and V_4 and the development of a small Q wave in lead V_5. The patient died 5 days later. At autopsy, the heart weighed 1200 g, with marked biventricular hypertrophy. Severe coronary artery disease was present, with a massive acute anterior myocardial infarction. An old inferior myocardial infarction and fatty degeneration and infiltration of the interventricular septum also were observed.

Chapman and Pearce described early notching of the S wave or QS deflection in the precordial lead just to the right of the transitional zone (usually lead V_3 or V_4) in patients with autopsy-proven anteroseptal and apical myocardial infarction.[41] This notching begins about 0.03 second after the onset of the QRS complex, usually on the downstroke of the S wave or QS deflection, and is wide and deep. Earlier, Cabrera and Friedland suggested a similar sign in the same leads, the wide notching (greater than 0.05 second in duration) occurring at the terminal portion of the rS or QS complex.[36] When these signs were applied to autopsy cases, about one fourth of the cases with myocardial infarction were recognized, whereas a false-positive diagnosis was made in 8 percent of those without infarction by each of these criteria.[247] Scott also evaluated the criterion of rSR' pattern in leads I, V_5, and V_6 and found it to be nonspecific. An RS complex in the left precordial leads also was found to be an unreliable sign.[247]

The presence of Q waves in lead II, resulting in a W complex, was proposed by Dressler and associates[77] as an indication of inferior myocardial infarction in the presence of left bundle branch block. The degree of reliability of this criterion, especially in regard to the localization of the infarction, was questioned.[231,247] In an autopsy study by Horan and associates, all 8 cases with Q waves greater than 0.03 second in leads II, III, and aVF were accompanied by anatomic evidence of inferior myocardial infarction.[133] In a study of 256 patients with intermittent left bundle branch block, however, Abben and associates found that such Q waves in the inferior leads often disappear during normal ventricular conduction.

PRIMARY ST AND T-WAVE CHANGES

Because of the pronounced secondary ST and T-wave changes in left bundle branch block, additional primary repolarization abnormalities usually are not detectable. If they are observed, however, they are helpful and often serve as strong supporting evidence of acute myocardial infarction.[77,254] The directions of the ST and T vectors in uncomplicated left bundle branch block are discordant to the mean QRS vector. Therefore, ST-segment elevation and upright T waves are present in the leads with deep S waves, and the reverse occurs in leads with prominent R waves. If the ST segment is displaced toward the major area of the QRS complex, acute injury or myocar-

dial infarction may be suspected (Fig. 9–60). Negative T waves over the right precordial leads also are indicative of complicated left bundle branch block.[17] A disproportional elevation of the ST segment in leads V_1 and V_2 to more than 8 mm, or half of the height of the T wave (in the absence of digitalis), also is considered meaningful.[17] Both of these signs have been found to be specific, even though insensitive.

Myocardial Infarction in the Presence of Ventricular Preexcitation Syndrome

The preexcitation of an ectopic area of the ventricle through a bypass tract profoundly modifies the initial QRS forces. As discussed, a pseudoinfarction pattern may appear. On the other hand, the delta wave may mask the abnormal Q waves of true myocardial infarction. This problem is well illustrated in Figure 9–61. The signs of an old anterior and lateral myocardial infarction are obscured by the appearance of ventricular preexcitation, which in turn causes abnormal Q waves in the inferior leads to mimic myocardial infarction. Indeed, in most instances, the diagnosis of myocardial infarction cannot be made when ventricular preexcitation is present. Occasionally, however, acute infarction may be recognized because of additional primary ST-segment and T-wave changes. If there is marked ST-segment elevation in the leads with predominantly upright QRS complexes or ST-segment depression in those with essentially downward QRS deflections, myocardial injury may be suspected.[253,283] An example is given in Figure 9–62. In my experience, the polarity of the T wave in relation to the QRS complex is variable in uncomplicated cases of preexcitation syndrome. It is undependable for recognizing ischemic changes unless a previous record is available for comparison. The degree of preexcitation in the same individual may vary, resulting in a change in the secondary ST and T-wave abnormalities. Such a possibility should be considered before it is accepted as an indication of an acute event.[253,283]

DIAGNOSIS OF MYOCARDIAL INFARCTION IN PATIENTS WITH ARTIFICIAL VENTRICULAR PACEMAKERS

The diagnosis of myocardial infarction in patients with artificial ventricular pacemakers also is difficult because of the abnormal sequence of ventricular excitation. If the pace-

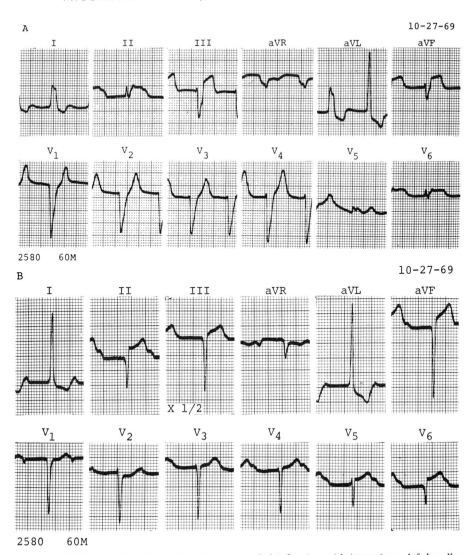

FIGURE 9–60. Acute inferior and anterior myocardial infarction with intermittent left bundle branch block. The patient was a 60-year-old man with hypertensive cardiovascular disease and acute myocardial infarction. (A) During complete left bundle branch block, the degree of the ST-segment elevation in leads II, aVF, and V_6 is disproportional to the amplitude of the QRS complex. In leads II and V_6, the ST segment is displaced toward the major deflection of the QRS. The presence of myocardial injury is, therefore, suspected. (B) During normal intraventricular conduction, the signs of acute inferior and anterior myocardial infarction become apparent. The tracing also is suggestive of left ventricular hypertrophy. First-degree AV block is seen in both tracings.

maker is of the demand type, effort should be given to find spontaneous QRS complexes. Otherwise, the diagnosis most likely depends on the presence of additional primary ST and T-wave changes, as in the case of left bundle branch block or ventricular preexcitation syndrome. In Figure 9–63, ST-segment elevation is present in leads I, V_5, and V_6, with T-wave inversion in leads V_5 and V_6 after the onset of acute myocardial infarction diagnosed clinically. No significant change of the QRS complexes can be detected, however.

VENTRICULAR ANEURYSM

Persistent ST-segment elevation in patients with myocardial infarction generally is considered the most helpful sign of ventricular aneurysm. The mechanism of such ST-segment displacement is not fully understood. The most attractive explanation proposed involves the generation of current of injury at the junction of the aneurysm with the surrounding myocardium. During ventricular systole, there is an outward bulging of the aneurysm as the

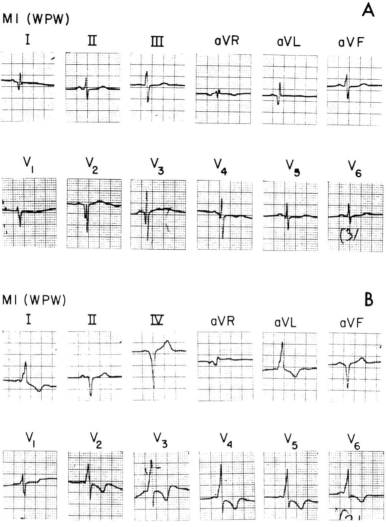

FIGURE 9–61. Effect of ventricular preexcitation syndrome on the diagnosis of myocardial infarction. The patient had intermittent ventricular preexcitation syndrome and a history of myocardial infarction. (A) During normal conduction, the ECG shows old anterior and high lateral myocardial infarctions and borderline abnormal left axis deviation. (B) When ventricular preexcitation syndrome appears, a pseudoinfarction pattern develops in the inferior leads, but the signs of anterior and high lateral myocardial infarctions are masked.

FIGURE 9–62. Wolff-Parkinson-White syndrome (ventricular preexcitation and paroxysmal tachycardia) with acute anterior myocardial infarction. The patient was a 47-year-old man who was known to have type A WPW syndrome. (A) The tracing of 1-10-73 is representative of his baseline ECG. (B) The tracing on 8-27-73 was recorded during an episode of acute myocardial infarction. There is a reduction of the amplitude of the QRS complex especially in the precordial leads. ST-segment elevation with T-wave inversion appears in leads V_2 through V_6. (C) During an episode of atrioventricular reentrant tachycardia with normal intraventricular conduction on 9-5-73, the typical signs of an extensive anterior myocardial infarction appear. The rhythm strip demonstrates the conversion of the paroxysmal tachycardia to normal sinus rhythm by carotid sinus massage with the reappearance of ventricular preexcitation.

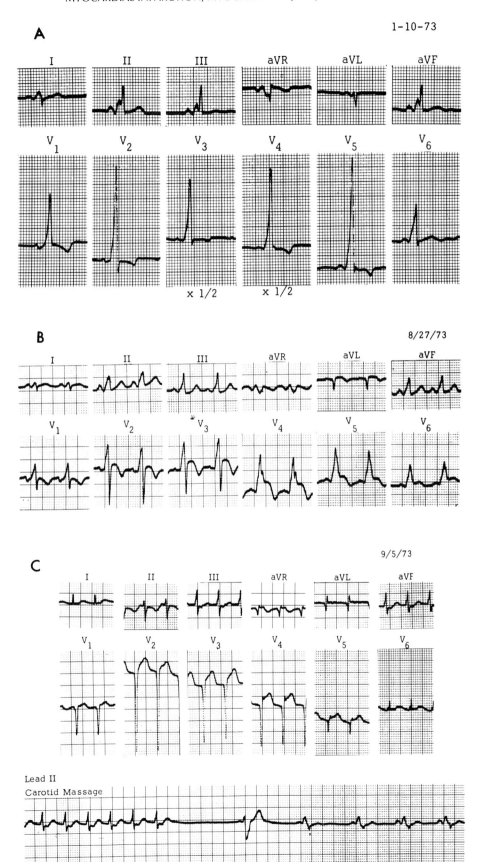

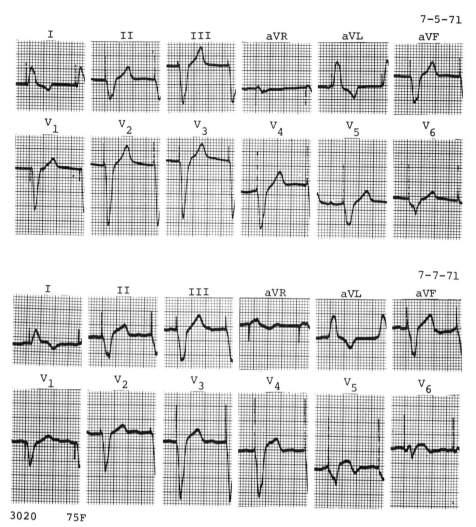

FIGURE 9–63. Acute myocardial infarction in a patient with artificial right ventricular pacemaker. The tracing on 7-7-71 was recorded after the patient developed clinical evidence of acute myocardial infarction. In comparison with the previous tracing on 7-5-71, there is ST-segment elevation in leads I, V5, and V6, with new inversion of the T waves in leads V5 and V6.

rest of the left ventricle moves toward the center of the ventricular cavity. This paradoxical movement produces an undue tension at the junction of these two portions of the ventricle, resulting in injury of the surviving myocardium next to the border of the aneurysm.

To discuss the reliability of the ECG in the diagnosis of ventricular aneurysm, it is necessary to give a precise definition of ventricular aneurysm because of the various criteria used in the literature. Pathologically, a ventricular aneurysm is defined as a protrusion of a localized portion of the external aspect of the ventricle, accompanied by a corresponding protrusion of the ventricular cavity.[78] In the cineventriculographic studies, most authors consider the presence of dyskinesis or local

systolic paradoxical expansile wall motion as evidence for aneurysm. Others also have included akinesis or local absence of wall motion as a sign of aneurysm.[78] My preference is to consider dyskinesis but not akinesis as the cineventriculographic evidence of ventricular aneurysm.

There is also the question of the definition of persistent ST-segment elevation. Most investigators regard ST-segment elevation that lasts for more than 1 month after the onset of acute myocardial infarction as the indication of persistent elevation.[78] In one study, however, it was noted that, when the ST-segment remained elevated for 2 weeks after the onset of acute myocardial infarction, the elevation seldom regressed.[182]

Electrocardiographic–Anatomic Correlation

Dubnow and associates reported the ECG findings in 64 cases of ventricular aneurysm found at autopsy.[78] Fifty patients had anterior aneurysm, 13 had posterior (inferior) aneurysm, and 1 had both anterior and posterior aneurysm. The ECG pattern of infarction was present in 54 of the 64 patients. Thirteen of the patients had intraventricular conduction defect, including 4 with left bundle branch block. Except in 3 patients, the ECG location of the infarction correlated well with the anatomic site of the aneurysm, but some patients had additional ECG signs of myocardial infarction in another area. Among the patients who had tracings taken more than 30 days after the onset of the myocardial infarction, 79 percent of those with anterior aneurysm had persistent ST-segment elevation and 50 percent of those with inferior infarction had this abnormality. Cokkinos and associates described the preoperative and postoperative ECG of 26 patients with left ventricular aneurysm who had undergone surgical resection.[57] In all the cases, the anatomic localization determined at the time of operation was correctly predicted by the ECG changes. There appeared to be a significant relation between the QRS duration and the age of the aneurysm, but its correlation with the size is equivocal. Twenty-one patients had abnormal Q waves. Those with wider distribution of the abnormal Q waves had larger aneurysms. Twenty-two patients had persistent ST-segment elevation. The size of the aneurysm cannot, however, be predicted by the degree of the ST-segment elevation. After aneurysmectomy, there usually was a decrease of the QRS duration, with an increase in the amplitude of the R waves. The number of leads with abnormal Q waves was reduced, and they disappeared completely from all leads in a few instances. The ST-segment elevation also tends to decrease, and it

was no longer present after surgery in about one-third of the cases. These anatomic correlation studies suggest that the ECG is a fairly sensitive tool in the detection of the ventricular aneurysm, especially the more common anteriorly located lesions. The available data, however, are inadequate to evaluate the specificity of the persistent ST-segment elevation as an indication of aneurysm anatomically.

Figures 9–64 through 9–67 give an example of the preoperative and postoperative findings in a 52-year-old man with a large ventricular aneurysm. He had an acute myocardial infarction 5 months before the illustrated preoperative tracing was made. Aneurysm resection was performed because of congestive heart failure and episodes of ventricular tachycardia. The preoperative and postoperative chest radiographs also are shown.

Electrocardiographic and Cineventriculographic Correlation

In 123 patients with coronary artery disease who had left ventriculograms, Miller and associates found 21 patients with localized dyskinesis.[181] Twenty of these patients had pathologic Q waves in the ECG suggestive of myocardial infarction. ST-segment elevation with T-wave inversion was present in 65 percent of the 21 patients. On the other hand, when the pattern of abnormal Q waves, ST elevation, and T-wave inversion was observed, dyskinesis was demonstrated in 68 percent of the patients. Others showed lesser degrees of asynergy (akinesis or hypokinesis). None of the patients had normal ventriculograms. Therefore, in patients with known coronary artery disease and signs of Q-wave myocardial infarction, both the sensitivity and the specificity of these ST and T-wave changes as an indication for ventricular dyskinesis were about two thirds. The incidence of dyskinesis in anterior myocardial infarction was higher when

FIGURE 9–64. Ventricular aneurysm. The patient was a 52-year-old man who had an acute extensive anterior myocardial infarction 5 months before the recording of this ECG. Note the persistent ST-segment elevation in the precordial leads and leads I and aVL. Left anterior hemiblock also is present. Chest roentgenogram taken at this time is illustrated in Figure 9–65.

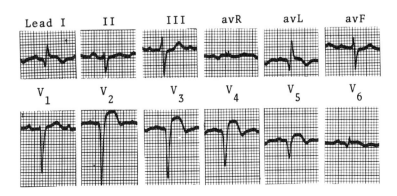

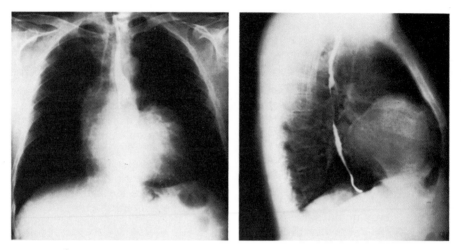

FIGURE 9–65. Ventricular aneurysm. The chest reontgenogram of the patient whose ECG is shown in Figure 9–64. A large ventricular aneurysm is demonstrated in both the posteroanterior and lateral views.

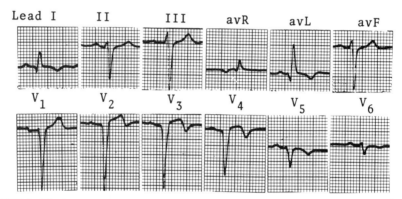

FIGURE 9–66. Electrocardiogram after ventricular aneurysmectomy. The tracing was recorded 5 months after the surgery from the same patient described in Figures 9–64 and 9–65. There is now less ST elevation. The Q waves in leads I and aVL are smaller, and small r waves are now seen in leads V_5 and V_6.

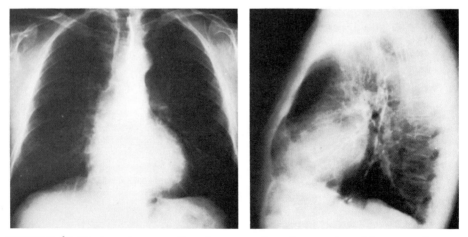

FIGURE 9–67. Chest roentgenogram from the same patient after resection of the ventricular aneurysm.

the number of the precordial leads with abnormal Q waves increased. Similar results in regard to the sensitivity of the persistent ST-segment elevation were obtained by Mills and associates in 65 patients with advanced anterior and apical asynergy.[182] Only 1 of 30 patients with coronary artery disease and normal ventriculogram had such ST abnormality, suggesting that the sign is highly specific for asynergy. These authors attributed the lower sensitivity of the ECG in the cine series from that of the anatomic studies to the more advanced stage of the disease in the anatomic cases. In some patients with dyskinesis, the ST segment became elevated after exercise.

Various arrhythmias may be seen in patients with ventricular aneurysm. The reported incidence varies between 12 to 41 percent.[72,86] Ventricular tachycardia is the most common associated arrhythmia.

ATRIAL INFARCTION

Atrial infarction is seldom recognized electrocardiographically, but it is reported to occur in from 1 to 17 percent of patients with myocardial infarction.[289] The low amplitude of the atrial depolarization forces and the masking of most of the atrial repolarization potential by the ventricular complex during sinus rhythm are chiefly responsible for the difficulty of the diagnosis. Because of the limited number of well-documented cases reported in the literature, no attempt is made here to describe the exact quantitative criteria. Only a general description of the ECG changes is given.

Displacement of the PQ interval, which represents a part of the atrial ST (STa) segment, is considered the most useful sign of atrial infarction. This may be best appreciated in patients with AV block. Elevation of the STa segment with reciprocal STa depression in the opposite leads suggests atrial injury. Depression of the STa segment alone is not a reliable sign unless the degree of the depression is marked.[162] Abnormal P waves having the shape of an M or a W or, being irregular or notched, are meaningful if they develop during an acute coronary episode.[289] Atrial infarction should be suspected in patients with ventricular myocardial infarction and any form of atrial arrhythmia.[162]

MYOCARDIAL INJURY

Acute ST-segment elevation *without* QRS changes is seen most commonly in the early phase of acute myocardial infarction. In most cases, evolutionary changes follow and abnormal Q waves develop. In non–Q-wave infarction, however, no appreciable change of the QRS complex occurs, but the clinical course and cardiac enzymes are indicative of acute myocardial necrosis.

ST-segment elevation with reciprocal ST depression may be seen transiently in patients with angina without infarction. The changes may occur during exertion or at rest. Angina at rest with ST-segment elevation is most likely due to coronary spasm. The subject of coronary spasm is discussed in more detail later in this chapter.

There are many other causes of ST-segment elevation that simulates myocardial injury. Most of the entities have been discussed in the section on pseudoinfarctions. The ST elevation may occur without abnormal Q waves. These include ventricular hypertrophy, conduction abnormalities, pulmonary embolism, spontaneous pneumothorax, intracranial hemorrhage, and hyperkalemia.

Among the noncoronary pathologic causes of ST-segment elevation, acute pericarditis is the most important. In acute pericarditis, the ST-segment elevation is diffuse and usually is present in all leads except lead aVR and sometimes leads V_1 and III. QRS changes are absent. In myocardial injury, the ST-segment elevation is more localized and accompanied by reciprocal ST depression in the opposite leads.

ST-segment elevation that mimics myocardial injury may occur in healthy individuals as a normal variant. It has been attributed to early repolarization. It is most commonly seen in the mid- and left precordial leads but also is seen in the limb leads (Fig. 9–68). The elevation in the precordial leads may be pronounced and may reach 4 or 5 mm in height. The ST segment has an upward concavity (whereas the ST segment in myocardial injury may have an upward convexity). It often is accompanied by a notched J point and a prominent T wave.[45,109,270] The elevation generally remains unchanged over a long period, but the degree of elevation may vary.

Marked ST-segment depression in patients with ischemic heart disease is often a manifestation of acute non–Q-wave infarction. In the absence of other laboratory information to suggest myocardial necrosis, it is difficult to decide whether the ST-segment depression represents myocardial injury or ischemia. Although on a theoretical basis, ST-segment depression in ischemic heart disease is indicative of myocardial injury, many cardiologists prefer the interpretation of subendocardial

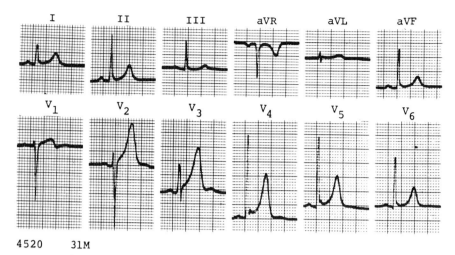

4520   31M

FIGURE 9–68. Prominent T waves in a healthy 31-year-old man. ST-segment elevation also is present in the precordial leads. They may be mistaken as signs of myocardial injury and ischemia or acute pericarditis.

ischemia, especially when the change is transient. Because the differences between the two entities are only in degrees and there is no anatomic distinction between the two, the choice of interpretation is arbitrary in most instances, especially when other clinical information is not available.

MYOCARDIAL ISCHEMIA

Ischemia of the myocardium may manifest in the ECG as one of the following changes:

1. Abnormally tall T waves
2. Symmetrically or deeply inverted T waves
3. Horizontal ST-segment depression with or without T-wave inversion
4. Nonspecific ST and T-wave changes
5. Normalization of abnormal T waves
6. Prolongation of the QT interval in addition to the above

Abnormally Tall T Waves

Tall and upright T waves may be seen in acute myocardial infarction at its earliest stage before changes of the QRS complex or ST segment occur (see Figs. 9–13 and 9–15). They are often refererd to as *hyperacute T waves*.[76,93,119,219] The T waves may be symmetrical or asymmetrical, peaked or blunted. ST-segment elevation may or may not coexist. Other ECG signs of acute myocardial infarction usually follow within a short time, however. Tall T waves also are seen in patients with angina but without acute myocardial in-

farction. They may be either transient or persistent. They usually are symmetrical and are seen most commonly in the precordial leads.[93,119,219,271] The QT interval usually is prolonged. Tall, symmetrical T waves may be recorded as a reciprocal change in myocardial infarction or ischemia that involves the opposite side of the heart. For example, inferior or inferoposterior myocardial infarction with deeply inverted T waves in leads II, III, and aVF may be accompanied by tall, symmetrical T waves in the precordial leads.

DIFFERENTIAL DIAGNOSIS

Prominent T waves may be seen in healthy individuals as a normal variant (Fig. 9–68). They are most commonly recorded in the midprecordial leads, often greater than 10 mm in height. ST-segment elevation often is present in the same leads.[270] Tall T waves also may be seen in patients with hyperkalemia. They are usually the earliest ECG sign of this electrolyte imbalance. Typically the T waves are tall, peaked (tented), narrow, and symmetrical. They are usually most prominent in the precordial leads. The QT interval is often normal or shortened in the absence of QRS prolongation, a finding that is often helpful in distinguishing the tall T waves of hyperkalemia from those due to myocardial ischemia.[259] Intracranial bleeding occasionally may be accompanied by tall T waves. The marked prolongation of the QT interval and the prominent U waves in this condition frequently make one suspect the correct cause. Other causes of prominent T waves include the secondary T-wave changes in left ventricular hypertrophy and left bundle branch block.

Symmetrically or Deeply Inverted T Waves

In the absence of QRS abnormalities, the presence of symmetrical or deep T-wave inversion often is considered as an indication of transmural myocardial ischemia. As discussed previously, this also is seen in non–Q-wave infarction. The routine interpretation of symmetrically or deeply inverted T waves as a sign of myocardial ischemia without considering other possibilities, however, is one of the most common errors in electrocardiography, often leading to undesirable consequences.

DIFFERENTIAL DIAGNOSIS

Normal Variant. T-wave inversion that simulates myocardial ischemia may occur in healthy individuals as a normal variant. The T waves in the right precordial leads, and some-

times also the mid-precordial leads, may be inverted in adults because of persistent juvenile pattern. This is more common in blacks, especially black women.[265] Benign T-wave inversion also is seen occasionally in healthy young adults in the left and mid-precordial leads in association with ST-segment elevation. This pattern is relatively more common in young black men and in trained athletes.[109,122,160,227] (Fig. 9–69).

Giant T-Wave Inversion Associated With Stokes-Adams Syncope. Massive T-wave inversion occasionally occurs after Stokes-Adams seizures in patients with complete heart block[137,141] (Fig. 9–70). Such T-wave changes may disappear after a few days or may persist for a few months. The pathophysiology of this repolarization abnormality is not clear.

Posttachycardia T-Wave Inversion. T-wave inversion is seen occasionally after an episode of supraventricular or ventricular tachycardia. The T waves may be symmetrical and appear ischemic. They are most commonly located in the left and mid-precordial leads and in the inferior limb leads. The QT

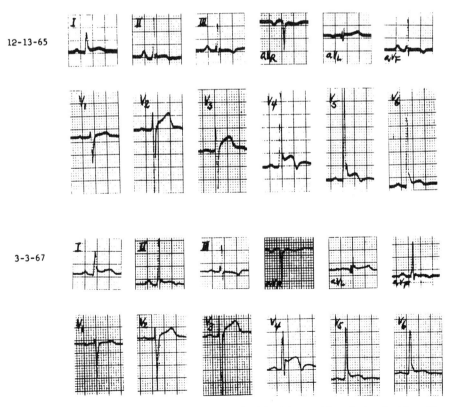

FIGURE 9–69. Benign ST and T-wave changes in a healthy 24-year-old professional athlete. The changes, especially in leads V_4 and V_5, mimic myocardial injury and ischemia and remained the same 15 months later.

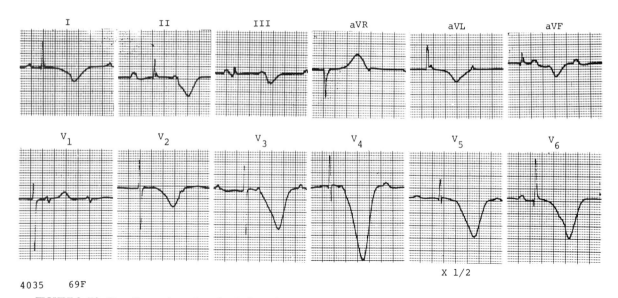

4035   69F

FIGURE 9–70. Giant T-wave inversion after Stokes-Adams seizures in a 69-year-old woman with complete AV block. The T waves gradually became upright later. Similar T-wave changes occurred again 5 years later after another episode of Stokes-Adams seizures. She died a few weeks later. Autopsy revealed 80 percent narrowing of the left anterior descending artery and 50 percent narrowing of the right coronary artery but no evidence of myocardial infarction.

interval is often prolonged, but ST-segment elevation is not seen. The changes usually persist for only a few hours but may last for days.[98,147,196,228,243] In my experience, they are more common in children than in adults.

Postpacemaker T-Wave Inversion. Striking T-wave inversion may appear in the non-paced beats after artificial ventricular pacing (Fig. 9–71). The characteristics of the T waves are similar to those seen after paroxysmal tachycardia. They are usually broad and associated with QT prolongation and most often are located in the left precordial and inferior leads. They may persist for a variable duration, which appears to be related to the duration of and power used in the artificial pacing.[42,43,116]

Other Conditions. Many of the pathologic entities discussed in the sections on pseudoinfarction and myocardial injury may present T-wave changes simulating ischemia without being accompanied by abnormal Q waves or ST elevation. These conditions are listed below without further discussion:

Intracranial disease, especially bleeding
Mitral valve prolapse–systolic click syndrome
Pericarditis
Myocardial diseases, either primary or secondary
Pulmonary embolism
Spontaneous pneumothorax
Myocardial contusion
Ventricular hypertrophy
Ventricular conduction defects

Horizontal ST-Segment Depression With or Without T-Wave Inversion

Horizontal depression or downward sloping of the ST segment is one of the more typical signs of subendocardial ischemia or injury. As mentioned, it may be seen in patients with non–Q-wave infarction. The question of whether it represents injury or ischemia also has been discussed. In the absence of myocardial necrosis, it is often observed in patients with spontaneous or induced angina pectoris (Fig. 9–72). It should be distinguished from the junctional type of ST-segment depression, which often is found in normal individuals. The T waves that follow the depressed ST segment may be either upright or inverted. These changes are found most often in the left and mid-precordial leads, as well as in leads II, III, and aVF. They may last for a few minutes but often persist for hours, days, or weeks. The duration is likely to be longer in patients with unstable angina. Because left and right ventricular hypertrophy or strain also may be associated with ST-segment depression and T-wave inversion, these conditions should be included in the differential diagnosis. When these abnormalities are present in leads with a predominantly downward QRS deflection, they are more likely to be caused by suben-

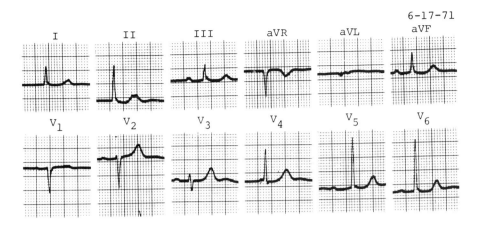

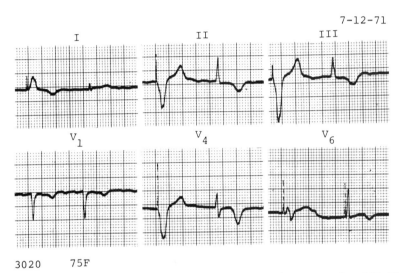

FIGURE 9–71. Postpacemaker T-wave inversion. The tracing on 6-17-71 reveals variable PR interval as a result of complete AV block. The QRS and T complexes are within normal limts. A right ventricular artificial pacemaker was implanted on 7-9-71. Three days later (7-12-71), the patient developed atrial fibrillation. The spontaneous ventricular complexes show T-wave inversion in the inferior and precordial leads. The second QRS complex in lead V_6 on 7-12-71 is the result of normal ventricular depolarization, but it is preceded by a pacemaker spike.

docardial ischemia. Isolated ST-segment depression without T-wave inversion is also more suggestive of the diagnosis of ischemia. If the ST and T changes are acute, the presence of ischemia is favored, but acute cor pulmonale still cannot be excluded. Digitalis also may induce similar ST and T changes, but the QT interval usually is shortened.

Nonspecific ST and T-Wave Changes

Many patients with coronary artery disease have ST-segment and T-wave changes that are considered nonspecific. The ST segment may be slightly depressed. The T wave may be low, flat, or slightly inverted. Because such ST and T-wave changes may be associated with nu-

merous physiological and pathologic conditions, any definitive interpretation of the ECG without correlation with the clinical data and serial tracings is hazardous and unjustified.

Normalization of Abnormal T Waves

In patients with coronary artery disease and inverted T waves, a reversal of the T waves to normal upright position occasionally occurs during an ischemic episode.[198] The ST segment, if depressed before the anginal episode, may become isoelectric. The normalization probably results from the opposing and cancelling effect of the acute event. An example of this phenomenon is given in Figure 9–73, recorded when the patient was experi-

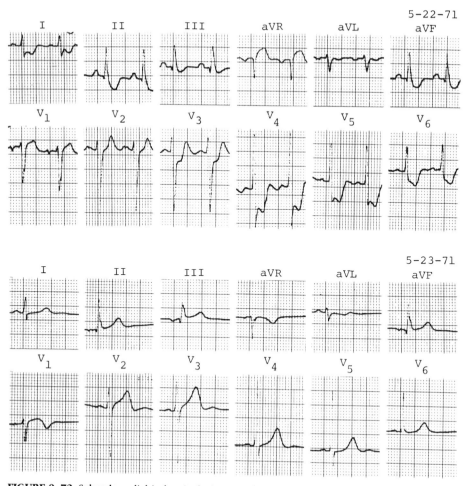

FIGURE 9–72. Subendocardial ischemia during angina pain. The tracing on 5-22-71 was recorded during an episode of angina. There is marked ST-segment depression in leads I, II, III, aVF, and V₃ through V₆. The tracing returned to normal (except for an ectopic atrial pacemaker) on the next day.

encing angina pectoris. In some cases, reciprocal ST-segment depression is noted in the leads opposite to the area of ischemia, where the ST elevation is masked. This finding may lead to the erroneous conclusion that a different coronary artery is involved.[198]

Prolongation of the QT Interval

In addition to the above mentioned ST and T-wave changes, myocardial ischemia may cause marked prolongation of the QT interval (Fig. 9–74). Indeed, it is the most common cause of QT prolongation, a subject that is discussed in detail in Chapter 25. Prolonged QT interval is a useful sign in the differential diagnosis of T-wave abnormalities. Other than what has already been mentioned in this section, its presence speaks against T-wave changes as a normal variant. T-wave inversion due to peri-

carditis is not associated with QT prolongation unless myocarditis exists.

CORONARY ARTERY SPASM

Increasing evidence indicates that angina pectoris and myocardial infarction may be caused by coronary artery spasm.[46,47,125,176,177,202,203] Such spasm may involve vessels with or without organic obstructive lesions. Maseri and associates and other investigators have demonstrated by angiography the vasospastic origin of the ischemic episodes in patients who had angina at rest. During the anginal episodes, the ECG may reveal ST-segment elevation, ST-segment depression (Fig. 9–75), an increase in T-wave amplitude, or pseudonormalization of inverted T waves. Such ECG changes also may be seen in the same patients during asymptomatic periods. Among the various pre-

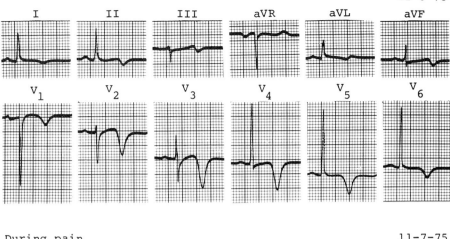

During pain   11-7-75

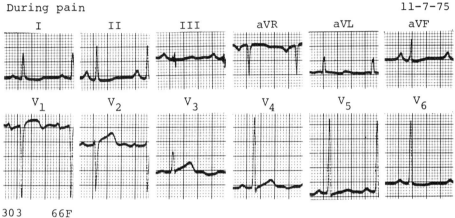

303   66F

FIGURE 9–73. Normalization of the T waves during angina. The patient was a 66-year-old woman with unstable angina. The tracing on 11-6-75 represents her baseline ECG. There is diffuse T-wave inversion that is most marked in the precordial leads. During an episode of angina on 11-7-75, the T waves in leads V_2 through V_5 become upright. Those in the other leads also are less abnormal. After the pain subsided, the T-wave changes, as shown on 11-6-75, returned. The patient also has hypertension, and the ECGs show left ventricular hypertrophy.

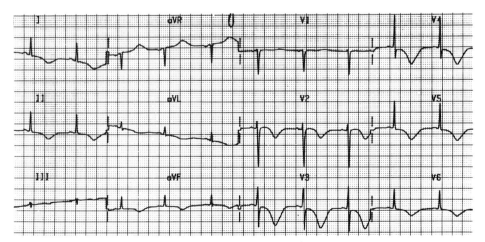

FIGURE 9–74. Diffuse T-wave inversion and prolongation of the QT interval due to myocardial ischemia. The patient is a 56-year-old woman with a history of non–Q-wave myocardial infarction and severe three-vessel coronary artery disease demonstrated by arteriogram 3 years earlier. The tracing was recorded during a hospital stay due to unstable angina. There are deeply inverted T waves in most of the leads, with marked prolongation of the QT interval. The QT interval measures 0.51 second with a QTc interval of 0.54 second. The ECGS taken 2 days before and 3 days after the tracing was made showed only nonspecific ST and T-wave changes, with an almost normal QT interval.

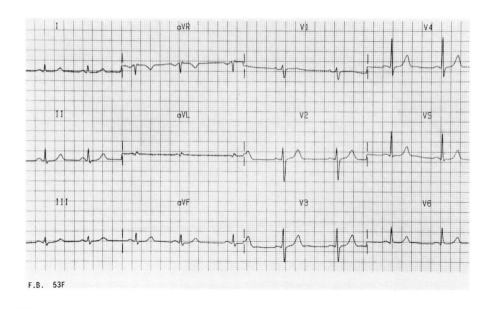

F.B. 53F

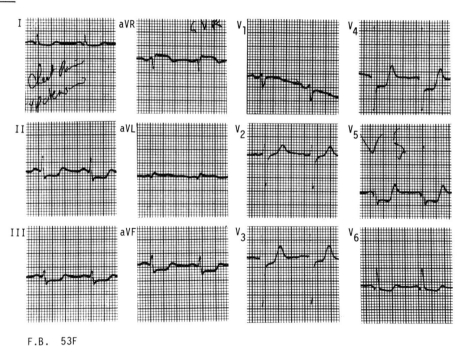

F.B. 53F

FIGURE 9–75. Coronary spasm causing ST-segment depression. The patient is a 53-year-old woman with recurrent episodes of chest pain followed by near syncope. (A) Normal tracing recorded when she was symptom free. (B) Tracing obtained during an episode of chest pain associated with severe hypotension showing ST-segment depression in all of the leads except leads aVR and V_1. The ST segment became isoelectric a few minutes later when the chest pain subsided. Coronary arteriogram performed the next day was normal. The ST-segment changes most likely were due to myocardial ischemia secondary to coronary spasm.

sentations of vasospastic angina, variant angina is the most widely recognized.

VARIANT ANGINA PECTORIS

In Prinzmetal's original description, which was based on 23 cases, this variant form of an-gina is characterized clinically by the development of chest pain when the patient is at rest or relatively inactive.[159,223] Exertion or emotional upset usually does not precipitate pain. The pain is frequently more severe and of longer duration than it is in the classical type of angina. The pain is recurrent, often occurring in a cyclic and regular pattern and, in some cases, at about the same time each day. In the ECG, transient ST-segment elevation with reciprocal depression is observed during chest pain. This is in contrast to the classical type of angina in which only ST-segment depression is observed. The leads that show the ST-segment elevation usually correspond to the distribution of a major coronary artery. In patients with abnormal baseline ECGs with T-wave inversion or ST-segment depression, the changes during pain may appear to "improve" the ECG. The area of ST-segment elevation often is the site of future myocardial infarction. During the episode of angina the R

waves in these leads may become taller. Arrhythmias, most often ventricular in origin, occur in about half of the cases during pain. AV conduction defect also may be observed.[222,223]

Many additional cases of this variant form of angina have been reported in recent years. Its incidence among patients with angina pectoris is estimated to be between 2 and 3 percent.[166] Although many variations of this syndrome have been described, it generally is agreed that its major features consist of recurrent angina at rest associated with transient ST-segment elevation in the ECG. Figures 9–76 through 9–79 illustrate this as well as other

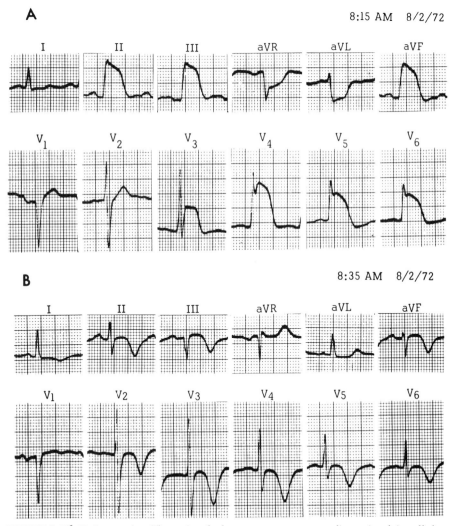

FIGURE 9–76. Variant angina. The patient had severe coronary artery disease involving all three major vessels, especially the anterior descending branch, as demonstrated by coronary arteriogram. (A) Tracing recorded during angina at rest. (B) Tracing recorded 20 minutes later, after the pain had subsided. The latter tracing is representative of the patient's baseline ECG. During angina (A), marked ST-segment elevation is present in leads II, III, aVF, and V$_3$ through V$_6$, with reciprocal ST-segment depression in leads aVR and aVL. There is also an increase of the amplitude of the R wave in leads II, III, and aVF, with the disappearance of the S waves in leads showing marked ST-segment elevation. The resulting complexes resemble the monophasic transmembrane potential. Many similar episodes were observed.

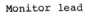

Monitor lead

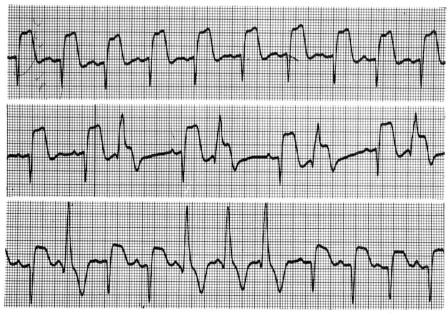

1887   60F

FIGURE 9–77. Variant angina. The rhythm strip was recorded from the same patient whose 12-lead ECGS are illustrated in Figure 9–76. This tracing was recorded during another episode of angina at rest. It demonstrates the marked ST-segment elevation, which gradually decreased. There are premature ventricular beats from two foci, with a short run of bigeminal rhythm in the middle strip. In the bottom strip, there is a short episode of accelerated idioventricular rhythm.

additional ECG findings seen in patients with variant angina. The ST elevation may be pronounced and merge with the R wave, resulting in a wide R-ST and T complex resembling a monophasic action potential (see Fig. 9–76). The increase in the R-wave amplitude may be accompanied by a decrease or disappearance of the S wave[166] (see Fig. 9–76). In some patients, when the ECG is monitored continuously during the attacks, the ST-segment elevation is noted to increase to a maximum level over a few minutes, remain constant for a few minutes, and then recede. Transient ST-segment elevation also has been recorded without symptoms in some patients who experienced angina on other occasions with identical ECG changes. Transient decrease of the amplitude of or loss of R waves during the episode also has been reported.[180]

The frequency of associated cardiac arrhythmias described by Prinzmetal[222,223] also is supported by the more recent reports.[146,221] Arrhythmias are more likely to develop when the ST-segment elevation during the ischemic episode is more pronounced (e.g., 4 mm or greater).[146] Premature ventricular beats, classical ventricular tachycardia, accelerated idioventricular rhythm, and ventricular fibrilla-

tion have been observed and are illustrated in Figures 9–77 and 9–78. The second most common type of arrhythmia is AV conduction defect, varying between first degree and complete AV block (Fig. 9–79). The AV block occurs mainly in patients with the ST-segment elevation that involves the inferior leads. The escape rhythm may be either junctional or idioventricular in origin. Supraventricular tachycardia and bundle branch block also have been observed during the ischemic episode.

Although Prinzmetal and associates[222,223] reported ST-segment depression in some of the patients during exercise, later studies revealed that the response to exercise was variable. The ST-segment may be depressed or elevated or remain unchanged during exercise.[166,261]

The findings of the coronary arteriogram in patients with variant angina are also variable. Although it was originally believed that a high-grade obstruction is present in at least one of the major coronary vessels, a significant number of patients showed normal arteriograms.[46,130] A considerable amount of information is available to indicate that spasm of a major coronary artery with transient complete

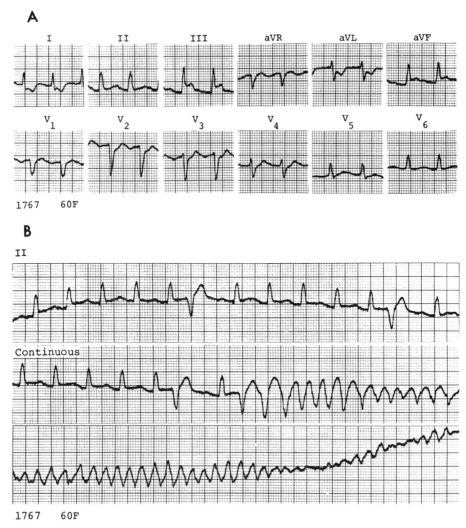

FIGURE 9-78. Variant angina. The patient was a 60-year-old woman with recurrent angina at rest. (A) Tracing recorded during one of the episodes, revealing ST-segment elevation in leads II, III, and aVF, with reciprocal ST-segment depression in leads I, aVL, V₂, and V₃. Tracing B was recorded a few minutes later and shows the appearance of premature ventricular beats and the development of ventricular tachycardia and fibrillation.

occlusion of that vessel is responsible for the syndrome in these patients. Such a mechanism may be responsible in patients with normal coronary artery, as well as in those with diseased vessels. In a review of 65 patients with variant angina in whom coronary arteriogram was performed, Arnett and Roberts found that the coronary arteries were severely narrowed in 43 (66 percent) and normal in 22 (34 percent).[9] Coronary spasm was demonstrated in 14 (22 percent) of the 65 patients, including patients both with and without narrowing of the vessels.[9]

Finally, it should be emphasized that the diagnosis of variant angina should not be made without the demonstration of the recurrent

and transient nature of the ST-segment elevation and the absence of enzyme changes to suggest myocardial infarction. ST-segment elevation may be the only ECG sign of acute myocardial infarction at its early stage.

Ergonovine Provocative Test for Coronary Artery Spasm

In patients with symptoms suggestive of coronary spasm the chest pain and ST-segment displacement may be provoked by the intravenous administration of ergonovine maleate (Fig. 9-80). The test has been found highly sensitive and specific for the detection of symptomatic coronary spasm in patients with

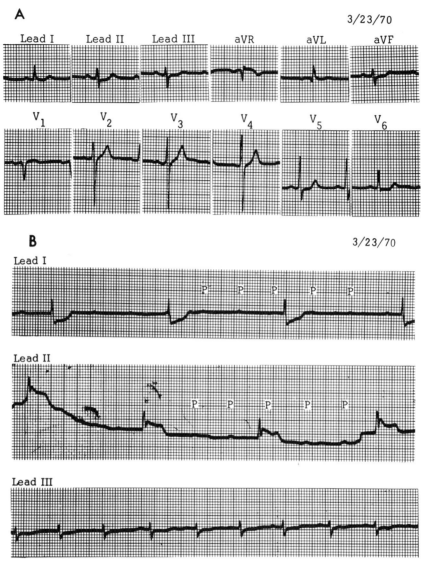

FIGURE 9–79. Variant angina with AV block. The patient has recurrent angina at rest. Tracing A is representative of his baseline ECG. It shows left axis deviation. Minimal ST-segment depression is present in the inferior leads and left precordial leads. Leads I and II of tracing B were recorded while the patient had chest pain. Lead III was recorded 10 minutes later, when the pain had subsided. ST-segment elevation is present in lead II during the pain, with reciprocal ST depression in lead I. Complete AV block is present during this time. Sinus rhythm with normal AV conduction is present in lead III during the asymptomatic period.

normal coronary arteriograms.[69,128,129,273] In a review by Heupler and associates, the ergonovine test was positive in 110 (98 percent) of 112 patients with Prinzmetal's variant angina and normal arteriograms.[129] Among the 15 patients with noncardiac chest pain or valvular heart disease studied by them, the test was negative in all.[129] It also was negative in 63 of 66 patients with angina-like chest pain and in all 6 patients with myocardial infarction but without history of variant angina.

The performance of ergonovine provocative test is not without risk. Serious arrhythmias may develop. Occasional death and myocardial infarction due to refractory induced coronary spasm have been reported.[34] It is a general consensus that the test should not be performed outside of the catheterization laboratory or in patients with severe fixed coronary artery lesions.

SILENT MYOCARDIAL ISCHEMIA

Evidence has accumulated to indicate that myocardial ischemia may occur in the absence of symptoms. Silent myocardial ischemia is

3/27/70

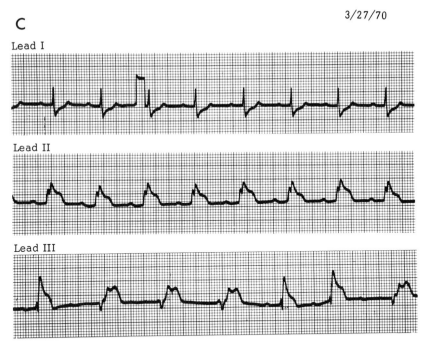

FIGURE 9–79 *Continued.* Tracing C demonstrates the changes during another similar episode. The ST-segment changes are again demonstrated. In lead III, there is transient complete AV block with ventricular escape rhythm, as indicated by the second, third, fourth, and last QRS complexes. (B reproduced from Fowler NO: Angina pectoris: Clinical diagnosis. Circulation 46:1079, 1972. By permission of the American Heart Association.)

observed in patients with asymptomatic coronary artery disease,[55,82] in postinfarction patients,[56] and in patients with angina during the painless period.[47a,73,175,268] Silent ischemia usually is demonstrated electrocardiographically by the appearance of ST-segment depression or, less commonly, ST-segment elevation during exercise tests or ambulatory or bedside monitoring. Hemodynamic measurements and radionuclide myocardial perfusion and ventriculographic studies in some patients have substantiated the relation between such asymptomatic ST-segment changes and myocardial ischemia.[47a,54,73] Transient coronary occlusion during percutaneous transluminal coronary angioplasty (PTCA) may be associated with both painless and painful ischemic episodes.[53] The specificity of the ST-segment depression as an indication for silent myocardial ischemia depends on the type of patients studied, however. The likelihood of a false-positive diagnosis is higher among subjects with a low probability of coronary artery disease. This is particularly true in asymptomatic individuals who are undergoing ambulatory ECG monitoring.

Erikssen and associates performed exercise testing in 2014 male office workers, 40 to 59 years of age.[82] Fifty patients (2.5 percent) had abnormal exercise test results and significant

coronary artery disease proved by coronary angiography but were asymptomatic. Thirty-six other patients also had abnormal exercise test results and no symptoms but had normal coronary arteriograms. Cohn and associates studied the ambulatory ECGs of 10 patients without symptoms and with angiographically proved coronary artery disease and abnormal exercise test results for myocardial ischemia.[55] Silent myocardial ischemia, as indicated by ST-segment depression of 1 mm or more for at least 1 minute, was found in all 10 patients, with a frequency that varied from 1 to 17 episodes per patient per 48 hours.

In a review of literature, Rozanski and Berman found that, among patients known to have coronary artery disease, about one third of the episodes of ST-segment depression observed during exercise testing occur silently.[239] Ambulatory ECG monitoring in patients with histories of angina and abnormal exercise test results revealed that about 75 percent of the ischemic episodes (ST-segment depression) are silent.[239] ST-segment elevation instead of depression may be seen but occurs less often.[268] The frequency of myocardial ischemia, silent or symptomatic, follows a typical circadian rhythm, with the highest frequency of episodes that occur in the morning hours.[226,233] The heart rate at the onset of the

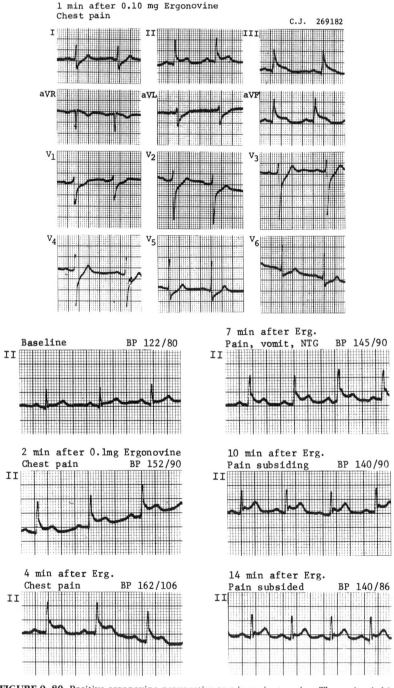

FIGURE 9–80. Positive ergonovine provocative test in variant angina. The patient's history is suggestive of variant angina. The coronary arteriogram revealed a 40 percent stenotic lesion of the left anterior descending artery. (A) Tracing recorded 1 minute after the administration of 0.1 mg of ergonovine intravenously when the patient developed chest pain similar to what he had previously without provocation. It shows ST-segment elevation in leads II, III, and aVF, with ST-segment depression in leads I, aVL, and V_1 through V_6. (B) Tracing of lead II recorded at various intervals after ergonovine was administered. The chest pain subsided, and the ST segment returned nearly to the baseline level 7 minutes after sublingual nitroglycerin administration and 14 minutes after ergonovine administration.

episodes during ambulatory monitoring is significantly lower than that during treadmill exercise tests.[55] The severity of the coronary artery disease does not appear to be a factor in determining the frequency of pain or painless episodes.[226] In the Coronary Artery Surgery Study (CASS), 53 (3.6 percent) of 1477 patients who had left main coronary artery disease had no symptoms.[263] No significant difference was noted in the severity of the left main coronary artery stenosis, the extent of overall coronary artery disease, and the left ventricular function between these patients and those who had symptoms.

Information about the prognosis of patients with asymptomatic coronary artery disease and silent myocardial ischemia is limited. In the 50 patients without symptoms followed for more than 8 years by Erikssen and colleagues, angina developed in 16 patients and myocardial infarction occurred in 7, 2 of them being silent cases.[82] The prognosis of patients with chronic, stable symptomatic coronary artery disease and exercise-induced silent ischemia over several years is similar to the prognosis of those in whom the ischemia is associated with angina.[84,275] Transient myocardial ischemia documented during submaximal exercise testing after myocardial infarction identifies patients at high risk of future cardiac events and death, whether or not the ischemia is accompanied by angina.[80, 101,264] In patients with unstable angina, the documentation of silent myocardial ischemia by continuous ECG monitoring, however, has been shown to provide important prognostic information.[114,115,197] The probability of acute myocardial infarction and death in the following months or years is higher in patients with silent ischemic ST-segment changes.[114,115] This is particularly true if the duration of the silent ischemia is more than 1 hour per each 24-hour monitoring period.[114,197]

REFERENCES

1. Abben R, Denes P, Rosen KM: Evaluation of criteria for diagnosis of myocardial infarction: Study of 256 patients with intermittent left bundle branch block. Chest 75:575, 1979
2. Abbott JA, Scheinman MM: Nondiagnostic electrocardiogram in patients with acute myocardial infarction: Clinical and anatomic correlations. Am J Med 55:608, 1973
3. Abildskov JA: Electrocardiographic wave form and the nervous system (Editorial). Circulation 41:371, 1970
4. Andersen HR, Falk E, Nielsen D: Right ventricular infarction: Frequency, size and topography in coronary heart disease. A prospective study comprising 107 consecutive autopsies from a coronary care unit. J Am Coll Cardiol 10:1223, 1987
5. Anderson JL, Marshall HW, Bray BE, et al: A randomized trial of intracoronary streptokinase in the treatment of acute myocardial infarction. N Engl J Med 308:1312, 1983
6. Anderssen N, Skaeggestad O: The electrocardiogram in patients with previous myocardial infarction. Acta Med Scand 176:123, 1964
7. Antaloczy Z, Barcsak J, Magyaar E: Correlation of electrocardiologic and pathologic findings in 100 cases of Q wave and non–Q wave myocardial infarction. J Electrocardiol 21:331, 1988
8. Armen RN, Frank TV: Electrocardiographic patterns in pneumothorax. Dis Chest 15:709, 1949
9. Arnett EN, Roberts WC: Acute myocardial infarction and angiographically normal coronary arteries. Circulation 53:395, 1976
10. Ascher EK, Stauffer JE, Gaasch WH: Coronary artery spasm, cardiac arrest, transient electrocardiographic waves and stunned myocardium in cocaine-associated acute myocardial infarction. Am J Cardiol 61:939, 1988
11. Bairey CN, Shah PK, Lew AS, Hulse S: Electrocardiographic differentiation of occlusion of the left circumflex versus the right coronary artery as a cause of inferior acute myocardial infarction. Am J Cardiol 60:456, 1987
12. Bar FW, Brugada P, Dassen WR, et al: Prognostic value of Q waves, R/S ratio, loss of R wave voltage, ST-T segment abnormalities, electrical axis, low voltage and notching: Correlation of electrocardiogram and left ventriculogram. Am J Coll Cardiol 4:17, 1984
13. Barker JM: The Unipolar Electrocardiogram: A Clinical Interpretation. New York, Appleton-Century-Crofts, 1952
14. Beamer V, Amidi M. Scheuer J: Vectorcardiographic findings simulating myocardial infarction in aortic valve disease. J Electrocardiol 3:71, 1970
15. Bell H, Pugh D, Dunn M: Vectorcardiographic evolution of left ventricular hypertrophy. Br Heart J 30:70, 1968
16. Benchimol A, Harris CL, Desser KB, et al: Resting electrocardiogram in major coronary artery disease. JAMA 224:1489, 1973
17. Besoain-Santander M, Gomez-Ebensperguer G: Electrocardiographic diagnosis of myocardial infarction in cases of complete left bundle branch block. Am Heart J 60:886, 1960
18. Blanke H, Cohen M, Schlueter GU, et al: Electrocardiographic and coronary arteriographic correlations during acute myocardial infarction. Am J Cardiol 54:249, 1984
19. Blanke H, Scherff F, Karsch KR, et al: Electrocardiographic changes after streptokinase-induced recanalization in patients with acute left anterior descending artery obstruction. Circulation 68:406, 1983
20. Boden WE, Gibson RS, Schechtman KB, et al: ST segment shifts are poor predictors of subsequent Q wave evolution in acute myocardial infarction: A natural history of early non–Q wave infarction. Circulation 79:537, 1989
21. Bodenheimer MM, Banka VS, Helfant RH: Q waves and ventricular asynergy: Predictive value and hemodynamic significance of anatomic localization. Am J Cardiol 35:615, 1975
22. Bonfiglio TA, Botti RE, Hagstrom JWC: Coronary arteritis, occlusion and myocardial infarction due to lupus erythematosus. Am Heart J 83:153, 1972

23. Bor I: Myocardial infarction and ischaemic heart disease in infants and children: Analysis of 29 cases and review of the literature. Arch Dis Child 44:268, 1969

24. Bough EW, Korr KS: Prevalence and severity of circumflex coronary artery disease in electrocardiographic posterior myocardial infarction. J Am Coll Cardiol 7:990, 1986

25. Braat S, Brugada P, DeZwaan C, et al: Value of electrocardiogram in diagnosing right ventricular involvement in patients with an acute inferior wall myocardial infarction. Br Heart J 49:368, 1983

26. Braudo M, Wigle ED, Keith JD: A distinctive electrocardiogram in muscular subaortic stenosis due to ventricular septal hypertrophy. Am J Cardiol 14:599, 1964

27. Bren GB, Wasserman AG, Ross AM: Electrocardiographic infarct evolution is accelerated by successful thrombolysis: A report from the NHIBI. Thrombolysis in Myocardial Infarction (TIMI) trial. J Am Coll Cardiol 9:63A, 1987

28. Brewer DL, Bilbro RH, Bartel AG: Myocardial infarction as a complication of coronary bypass surgery. Circulation 47:58, 1973

29. Buja LM, Khoi NB, Roberts WC: Clinically significant cardiac amyloidosis. Am J Cardiol 26:394, 1970

30. Buja LM, Willerson JT: Clinicopathologic correlates of acute ischemic heart disease syndromes. Am J Cardiol 47:343, 1981

31. Bulkley BH, Roberts WC: The heart in systemic lupus erythematosus and changes induced in it by corticosteroid therapy: A study of 36 necropsy patients. Am J Med 58:243, 1975

32. Burch GE, Horan LG, Ziskind J, et al: A correlative study of postmortem electrocardiographic and spatial vectorcardiographic data in myocardial infarction. Circulation 18:325, 1958

33. Burch GE, Meyers R, Abildskov JA: A new electrocardiographic pattern observed in cerebrovascular accidents. Circulation 9:719, 1954

34. Buxton A, Goldberg S, Hirshfeld JW, et al: Refractory ergonovine induced coronary vasospasm: Importance of intracoronary nitroglycerin. Am J Cardiol 46:329, 1980

35. Cabin HS, Clubb KS, Wackers F, Zaret B: Right ventricular myocardial infarction with anterior wall left ventricular infarction: An autopsy study. Am Heart J 113:16, 1987

36. Cabrera E, Friedland C: La onda de activacion ventricular en el bloqueo de rama izquierda con infarto (un nuevo signo electrocardiografico). Arch Inst Cardiol Mex 23:441, 1953

37. Camara EJN, Chandra N, Ouyang P, et al: Reciprocal ST change in acute myocardial infarction: Assessment by electrocardiography and echocardiogram. J Am Coll Cardiol 2:251, 1983

38. Candell-Riera J, Figueras J, Valle V, et al: Right ventricular infarction: Relationships between ST segment elevation in V_{4R} and hemodynamic, scintigraphic and echocardiographic findings in patients with acute inferior myocardial infarction. Am Heart J 101:281, 1981

39. Cardenas M, Diaz del Tio A, Gonzalez-Hermosillo JA, et al: El infarto agudo del myocardio del ventriculo derecho. Arch Inst Cardiol Mex 50:295, 1980

40. Cercek B, Lew AS, Laramee P, et al: Time course and characteristics of ventricular arrhythmias after reperfusion in acute myocardial infarction. Am J Cardiol 60:214, 1987

41. Chapman MG, Pearce ML: Electrocardiographic diagnosis of myocardial infarction in the presence of left bundle-branch block. Circulation 16:558, 1957

42. Chatterjee K, Harris A, Davies G, et al: Electrocardiographic changes subsequent to artificial ventricular depolarization. Br Heart J 31:770, 1969

43. Chatterjee K, Harris AM, Davies JG, et al: T-wave changes after artificial pacing. Lancet 1:759, 1969

44. Cheitlin MD, Carter PB: Takayasu's disease. Arch Intern Med 116:283, 1965

45. Chelton LG, Burchell HB: Unusual RT segment deviations in the electrocardiogram of normal persons. Am J Med Sci 230:54, 1955

46. Cheng TO, Bashour T, Kelser GA, et al: Variant angina of Prinzmetal with normal coronary arteriograms: A variant of the variant. Circulation 47:476, 1973

47. Cheng TO, Bashour T, Singh BK, et al: Myocardial infarction in the absence of coronary arteriosclerosis: Result of spasm? Am J Cardiol 30:680, 1972

47a. Chierchia S, Lazzari M, Freedman B, et al: Impairment of myocardial perfusion and function during painless myocardial ischemia. J Am Coll Cardiol 1:924, 1983

48. Chou TC, Fowler NO, Gabel M, et al: Electrocardiographic and hemodynamic changes in experimental right ventricular infarction. Circulation 67:1258, 1983

49. Chou TC, Susilavorn B: Electrocardiographic–pathological conference: Electrocardiographic changes in intracranial hemorrhage. J Electrocardiol 2:193, 1969

50. Chou TC, van der Bel-Kahn J, Allen J, et al: Electrocardiographic diagnosis of right ventricular infarction. Am J Med 70:1175, 1981

51. Claudon DG, Claudon DB, Edwards JE: Primary dissection aneurysm of coronary artery. Circulation 45:259, 1972

52. Cohn JN: Right ventricular infarction revisited. Am J Cardiol 43:666, 1979

53. Cohn PF: Silent myocardial ischemia: Present status. Mod Conc Cardiovasc Dis 56:1, 1987

54. Cohn PF, Brown EJ Jr, Wynne J, et al: Global and regional left ventricular ejection fraction abnormalities during exercise in patients with silent myocardial ischemia. J Am Coll Cardiol 1:931, 1983

55. Cohn PF, Lawson WE: Characteristics of silent myocardial ischemia during out-of-hospital activities in asymptomatic angiographically documented coronary artery disease. Am J Cardiol 59:746, 1987

56. Cohn PF, Sodums MT, Lawson WE, et al: Frequent episodes of silent myocardial ischemia after apparently uncomplicated myocardial infarction. J Am Coll Cardiol 8:982, 1986

57. Cokkinos DV, Hallman GL, Cooley DA, et al: Left ventricular aneurysm: Analysis of electrocardiographic features and postresection changes. Am Heart J 82:149, 1971

58. Coleman DL, Ross TF, Naughton JL: Myocardial ischemia and infarction related to recreational cocaine use. West J Med 136:444, 1982

59. Coll S, Betriu Am, De Flores T, et al: Significance of Q-wave regression after transmural acute myocardial infarction. Am J Cardiol 61:739, 1988

60. Connor RCR: Heart damage associated with intracranial lesions. Br Med J 3:29, 1968

61. Cook RW, Edward JE, Pruitt RD: Electrocardiographic changes in acute subendocardial infarction: I. Large subendocardial and large nontransmural infarcts. Circulation 18:603, 1958

62. Copeland RB, Omenn GS: Electrocardiogram changes suggestive of coronary artery disease in pneumothorax: Their reversibility with upright posture. Arch Intern Med 125:151, 1970

63. Cosby RS, Bergeron M: Electrocardiographic changes in carbon monoxide poisoning. Am J Cardiol 11:93, 1963

64. Cowley MJ, Dorros G, Kelsey SF, et al: Acute coronary events associated with percutaneous transluminal coronary angioplasty. Am J Cardiol 53:12, 1984

65. Cox CJB: Return to normal of the electrocardiogram after myocardial infarction. Lancet 1:1194, 1967

66. Croft CH, Nicod P, Corbett JR, et al: Detection of acute right ventricular infarction by right precordial electrocardiography. Am J Cardiol 50:421, 1982

67. Croft CH, Woodward W, Nicod P, et al: Clinical implications of anterior S-T segment depression in patients with acute inferior myocardial infarction. Am J Cardiol 50:428, 1982

68. Cropp GJ, Manning GW: Electrocardiographic changes simulating myocardial ischemia and infarction associated with spontaneous intracranial hemorrhage. Circulation 22:25, 1960

69. Curry RC, Pepine CJ, Sabom MB, et al: Effects of ergonovine in patients with and without coronary artery disease. Circulation 56:803, 1977

70. Cutforth RH, Oram S: The electrocardiogram in pulmonary embolism. Br Heart J 20:41, 1958

71. Davies MJ, Woolf N, Robertson WB: Pathology of acute myocardial infarction with particular reference to occlusive coronary thrombi. Br Heart J 38:659, 1976

72. Davis RW, Ebert PA: Ventricular aneurysm: A clinical-pathologic correlation. Am J Cardiol 29:1, 1972

73. Deanfield JE, Shea M, Ribiero P, et al: Transient ST-segment depression as a marker of myocardial ischemia during daily life. Am J Cardiol 54:1195, 1984

74. DeWood MA, Spores J, Notske R, et al: Prevalence of total coronary occlusion during the early hours of transmural myocardial infarction. N Engl J Med 303:897, 1980

75. DeWood MA, Stifter WF, Simpson CS, et al: Coronary arteriographic findings soon after non–Q wave myocardial infarction. N Engl J Med 315:417, 1986

76. Dressler W, Roesler H: High T waves in the earliest stage of infarction. Am Heart J 34:627, 1947

77. Dressler W, Roesler H, Schwager A: The electrocardiographic signs of myocardial infarction in the presence of bundle branch block: I. Myocardial infarction with left bundle branch block. Am Heart J 39:217, 1950

78. Dubnow MH, Burchell HB, Titus JL: Post-infarction ventricular aneurysm. A clinicomorphologic and electrocardiographic study of 80 cases. Am Heart J 70:753, 1965

79. Dunn WJ, Edwards JE, Pruitt RD: The electrocardiogram in infarction of the lateral wall of the left ventricle: A clinicopathologic study. Circulation 14:540, 1956

80. Epstein SE, Palmeri ST, Patterson RE: Evaluation of patients after acute myocardial infarction: Indications for cardiac catheterization and surgical intervention. N Engl J Med 307:1487, 1982

81. Erhardt LR, Sjogren A, Wahlberg I: Single right-sided precordial lead in the diagnosis of right ventricular involvement in inferior myocardial infarction. Am Heart J 91:571, 1976

82. Erikssen J, Thaulow E: Follow-up of patients with asymptomatic myocardial ischemia. In Rutishauser

W, Roskamm H (eds): Silent myocardial ischemia. Berlin, Springer-Verlag, 1984, p 154

83. Essen RV, Merx W, Effert S: Spontaneous course of ST-segment elevation in acute anterior myocardial infarction. Circulation 59:105, 1979

84. Falcone C, deServi S, Poma E, et al: Clinical significance of exercise-induced silent myocardial ischemia in patients with coronary artery disease. J Am Coll Cardiol 9:295, 1987

85. Faruqui AM, Maloy WC, Felner JM, et al: Symptomatic myocardial bridging of coronary artery. Am J Cardiol 41:1305, 1978

86. Favaloro RG, Effler DB, Groves LK, et al: Ventricular aneurysm: Clinical experience. Ann Thorac Surg 6:227, 1968

87. Feldman AM, Baughman KL: Myocardial infarction associated with a myocardial bridge. Am Heart J 111:784, 1986

88. Flatley FJ, Atwell ME, McEvoy RK: Pseudoxanthoma elasticum with gastric hemorrhage. Arch Intern Med 112:106, 1963

89. Forman MB, Goodin J, Phelan B, et al: Electrocardiographic changes associated with isolated right ventricular infarction. J Am Coll Cardiol 4:640, 1984

90. Fowler NO, Westcott RN, Scott RC: The Q wave in precordial electrocardiograms overlying the hypertrophied right ventricle intracavity leads. Circulation 5:441, 1952

91. Frank S, Braunwald E: Idiopathic hypertrophic subaortic stenosis. Circulation 37:759, 1968

92. Freifeld AG, Schuster EH, Bulkley BH: Nontransmural versus transmural myocardial infarction. Am J Med 75:423, 1983

93. Freundlich J: The diagnostic significance of tall upright T-waves in the chest leads. Am Heart J 52:749, 1956

94. Fuchs RM, Achuff SC, Grunwald L, et al: Electrocardiographic localizations of coronary artery narrowings: Studies during myocardial ischemia and infarction in patients with one-vessel disease. Circulation 66:1168, 1982

95. Ganz W, Geft I, Shah PK, et al: Intravenous streptokinase in evolving acute myocardial infarction. Am J Cardiol 53:1209, 1984

96. Geft IL, Shah PK, Rodriguez L, et al: ST elevations in leads V_1 to V_5 may be caused by right coronary artery occlusion and acute right ventricular infarction. Am J Cardiol 53:991, 1984

97. Geha AS, Weidman WH, Soule EH, et al: Intramural ventricular cardiac fibroma: Successful removal in two cases and review of the literature. Circulation 36:427, 1967

98. Geiger AJ: Electrocardiogram simulating those of coronary thrombosis after cessation of paroxysmal tachycardia. Am Heart J 26:555, 1943

99. Gelzayd EA, Holzman D: Electrocardiographic changes of hyperkalemia simulating acute myocardial infarction: Report of a case. Dis Chest 51:211, 1967

100. Georas CS, Dahlquist E, Cutts FB: Subendocardial infarction: Correlation of clinical, electrocardiographic, and pathologic data in 17 cases. Arch Intern Med 111:146, 1963

101. Gibson RS, Beller GA, Gheorghiade M, et al: The prevalence and clinical significance of residual myocardial ischemia 2 weeks after uncomplicated non–Q wave infarction: A prospective natural history study. Circulation 73:1186, 1986

102. Gibson RS, Crampton RS, Watson DD, et al: Precordial ST-segment depression during acute inferior

myocardial infarction: Clinical, scintigraphic and angiographic correlations. Circulation 66:732, 1982

103. Gibson RS, Watson DD, Craddock GB, et al: Prediction of cardiac events after uncomplicated myocardial infarction: A prospective study comparing pre-discharge exercise thallium-201 scintigraphy and coronary angiography. Circulation 68:321, 1983

104. Goldberg HL, Borer JS, Jacobstein JG, et al: Anterior S-T segment depression in acute inferior myocardial infarction: Indicator of posterolateral infarction. Am J Cardiol 48:1009, 1981

105. Goldberg RJ, Gore JM, Alpert JS, Dalen JE: Non–Q wave myocardial infarction: Recent changes in occurrence and prognosis. A community-wide perspective. Am Heart J 113:273, 1987

106. Goldberg S, Greenspon AJ, Urban PL, et al: Reperfusion arrhythmia: A marker of restoration of antegrade flow during intracoronary thrombolysis for acute myocardial infarction. Am Heart J 105:26, 1983

107. Goldberger E: Unipolar Lead Electrocardiography and Vectorcardiography, 3rd ed. Philadelphia, Lea & Febiger, 1953

108. Goldman AM: Acute myocarditis simulating myocardial infarction. Dis Chest 41:61, 1962

109. Goldman MJ: RS-T segment elevation in the mid- and left precordial leads as a normal variant. Am Heart J 46:817, 1953

110. Goldman MJ: Normal variants in the electrocardiogram leading to cardiac invalidism. Am Heart J 59:71, 1960

111. Gorgels APM, Vos MA, Letsch IS, et al: Usefulness of the accelerated idioventricular rhythm as a marker for myocardial necrosis and reperfusion during thrombolytic therapy in acute myocardial infarction. Am J Cardiol 61:231, 1988

112. Gorlin R, Klein MD, Sullivan JM: Prospective correlative study of ventricular aneurysm: Mechanistic concept and clinical recognition. Am J Med 42:512, 1967

113. Gottlieb RS, Duca PR, Kasparian H, et al: Correlation of abnormal Q waves, coronary pathology and ventricular contractility. Am Heart J 90:451, 1975

114. Gottlieb SO, Weisfeldt ML, Ouyang P, et al: Silent ischemia as a marker for early unfavorable outcomes in patients with unstable angina. N Engl J Med 314:1214, 1986

115. Gottlieb SO, Weisfeldt ML, Ouyang P, et al: Silent ischemia predicts infarction and death during 2 year follow-up of unstable angina. J Am Coll Cardiol 10:756, 1987

116. Gould L, Venkataraman K, Goswami MK, et al: Pacemaker-induced electrocardiographic changes simulating myocardial infarction. Chest 63:829, 1973

117. Gunnar RM, Pietras RJ, Blackaller J, et al: Correlation of vectorcardiographic criteria for myocardial infarction with autopsy findings. Circulation 35:158, 1967

118. Halsinger DR, Osmundson PJ, Edwards JE: The heart in periarteritis nodosa. Circulation 25:610, 1962

119. Handjani AM: Significance of positive tall and peaked electrocardiographic T waves in early diagnosis of ischemic heart disease. Chest 62:24, 1972

120. Hands ME, Cook EF, Stone PH, et al: Electrocardiographic diagnosis of myocardial infarction in the presence of complete left bundle branch block. Am Heart J 116:23, 1988

121. Hands ME, Lloyd BL, Robinson JS, et al: Prognostic significance of electrocardiographic site of infarc-

tion after correction for enzymatic size of infarction. Circulation 73:885, 1986

122. Hanne-Paparo N, Wendkos MH, Brunner D: T wave abnormalities in the electrocardiograms of top-ranking athletes without demonstrable organic heart disease. Am Heart J 81:743, 1971

123. Haraphongse M, Tanomsup S, Jugdutt BI: Inferior ST segment depression during acute anterior myocardial infarction: Clinical and angiographic correlations. J Am Coll Cardiol 4:467, 1984

124. Harris TR, Copeland GD, Brody DA: Progressive injury current with metastatic tumor of the heart: Case report and review of the literature. Am Heart J 69:392, 1965

125. Hart NJ, Silverman ME, King SB: Variant angina caused by coronary artery spasm. Am J Med 56:269, 1974

126. Heggtveit HA: Syphilitic aortitis: A clinicopathologic autopsy study of 100 cases, 1950 to 1960. Circulation 29:346, 1964

127. Hejtmancik MR, Bradfield JY, Miller GV: Myocarditis and Friedreich's ataxia. Am Heart J 38:757, 1948

128. Heupler FA: Provocative testing for coronary arterial spasm: Risk, method and rationale. Am J Cardiol 46:335, 1980

129. Heupler FA, Proudfit WL, Razavi M, et al: Ergonovine maleate provocative test for coronary arterial spasm. Am J Cardiol 41:631, 1978

130. Higgins CB, Wexler L, Silverman JF, Schroeder JS: Clinical and arteriographic features of Prinzmetal's variant angina: Documentation of etiologic factors. Am J Cardiol 37:831, 1976

131. Hirst AE, Johns VJ, Kime SW: Dissecting aneurysm of the aorta: A review of 505 cases. Medicine 37:217, 1958

132. Horan LG, Flowers NC, Johnson JC: Significance of the diagnostic Q wave of myocardial infarction. Circulation 43:428, 1971

133. Horan LG, Flowers NC, Tolleson WJ, et al: The significance of diagnostic Q waves in the presence of bundle branch block. Chest 58:214, 1970

134. Huey BL, Beller GA, Kaiser DL, Gibson RS: A comprehensive analysis of myocardial infarction due to left circumflex artery occlusion: Comparison with infarction due to right coronary artery and left anterior descending artery occlusion. J Am Coll Cardiol 12:1156, 1988

135. Huey BL, Gheorghiade M, Crampton RS, et al: Acute non–Q wave myocardial infarction associated with early ST segment elevation: Evidence for spontaneous coronary reperfusion and implications for thrombolytic trials. J Am Coll Cardiol 9:18, 1987

136. Hultgren H, Miyagawa M, Buck W, et al: Ischemic myocardial injury during coronary artery surgery. Am Heart J 82:624, 1971

137. Ippolito TL, Blier JS, Fox TT: Massive T-wave inversion. Am Heart J 48:88, 1954

138. Irvin RG: The angiographic prevalence of myocardial bridging in man. Chest 81:198, 1982

139. Isner JM, Estes M, Thompson PD, et al: Acute cardiac events temporally related to cocaine use. N Engl J Med 315:1438, 1986

140. Isner JM, Roberts WC: Right ventricular infarction complicating left ventricular infarction secondary to coronary heart disease. Am J Cardiol 42:885, 1978

141. Jacobson D, Schrire V: Giant T wave inversion associated with Stokes-Adams syncope. S Afr Med J 40:641, 1966

142. James TN: The coronary circulation and conduction

system in acute myocardial infarction. Prog Cardiovasc Dis 10:410, 1968

143. Kalbfleisch JM, Shadaksharappa KS, Conrad LL, et al: Disappearance of the Q-deflection following myocardial infarction. Am Heart J 76:193, 1968

144. Kaplan BM, Berkson DM: Serial electrocardiograms after myocardial infarction. Ann Intern Med 60:430, 1964

145. Karten I: Arteritis, myocardial infarction and rheumatoid arthritis. JAMA 210:1717, 1969

146. Kerin NZ, Rubenfire M, Naini M, et al: Arrhythmias in variant angina pectoris: Relationship of arrhythmias to ST segment elevation and R-wave changes. Circulation 60:1343, 1979

147. Kernohan RJ: Post-paroxysmal tachycardia syndrome. Br Heart J 31:803, 1969

148. Kircher BJ, Topol EJ, O'Neill WW, Pitt B: Prediction of infarct coronary artery recanalization after intravenous thrombolytic therapy. Am J Cardiol 59:513, 1987

149. Kitamura S, Kawashima Y, Kawachi K, et al: Left ventricular function in patients with coronary arteritis due to acute febrile mucocutaneous lymph node syndrome or related diseases. Am J Cardiol 40:156, 1977

150. Klein LW, Helfant RH: The Q-wave and non-Q wave myocardial infarction: Differences and similarities. Prog Cardiovasc Dis 29:205, 1986

151. Koops B, Kerber RE, Wexler L, et al: Congenital coronary artery anomalies. JAMA 226:1425, 1973

152. Koskelo P, Punsar S, Sipila W: Subendocardial hemorrhage and ECG changes in intracranial bleeding. Br Med J 1:1479, 1964

153. Krone RJ, Friedman E, Thanavaro S, et al: Long-term prognosis after first Q-wave (transmural) or non-Q-wave (nontransmural) myocardial infarction: Analysis of 593 patients. Am J Cardiol 52:234, 1983

154. Levine HD, Philips E: An appraisal of the newer electrocardiography: Correlations in one hundred and fifty consecutive autopsied cases. N Engl J Med 245:833, 1951

155. Levine HD, Wanzer SH, Merrill JP: Dialyzable currents of injury in potassium intoxication resembling acute myocardial infarction or pericarditis. Circulation 13:29, 1956

156. Lew AS, Hod H, Cercek B, et al: Inferior ST segment changes during acute anterior myocardial infarction: A marker of the presence or absence of concomitant inferior wall ischemia. J Am Coll Cardiol 10:519, 1987

157. Lew AS, Isner JM: Right ventricular infarction. Cardiovasc Clin 17:203, 1987

158. Lew AS, Maddahi J, Shah PK, et al: Factors that determine the direction and magnitude of precordial ST-segment deviations during inferior wall acute myocardial infarction. Am J Cardiol 55:883, 1985

159. Lew AS, Weiss AT, Shah PK, et al: Precordial ST segment depression during acute inferior myocardial infarction: Early thallium-201 scintigraphic evidence of adjacent posterolateral or inferoseptal involvement. J Am Coll Cardiol 5:203, 1985

160. Lichtman J, O'Rourke RA, Klein A, et al: Electrocardiogram of the athlete: Alterations simulating those of organic heart disease. Arch Intern Med 132:763, 1973

161. Littman D: The electrocardiographic findings in pulmonary emphysema. Am J Cardiol 5:339, 1960

162. Liu CK, Greenspan G, Piccirillo RT: Atrial infarction of the heart. Circulation 23:331, 1961

163. Lopez-Sendon J, Coma-Canella I, Alcasena S, et al:

Electrocardiographic findings in acute right ventricular infarction: Sensitivity and specificity of electrocardiographic alterations in right precordial leads V_{4R}, V_{3R}, V_1, V_2 and V_3. J Am Coll Cardiol 6:1273, 1985

164. Lorell B, Leinbach RC, Pohost GM, et al: Right ventricular infarction: Clinical diagnosis and differentiation from cardiac tamponade and pericardial constriction. Am J Cardiol 43:465, 1979

165. Lown B, Vassaux C, Hood WB, et al: Unresolved problems in coronary care. Am J Cardiol 20:494, 1967

166. MacAlpin RN, Kattus AA, Alvaro AB: Angina pectoris at rest with preservation of exercise capacity: Prinzmetal's variant angina. Circulation 47:946, 1973

167. Mahony C, Hindman MC, Aronin N, et al: Prognostic differences in subgroups of patients with electrocardiographic evidence of subendocardial or transmural myocardial infarctions. Am J Med 69:183, 1980

168. Maisel AS, Ahnve S, Gilpin E, et al: Prognosis after extension of myocardial infarct: The role of Q wave or non-Q wave infarction. Circulation 71:211, 1985

169. Mann JI, Inman WHW: Oral contraceptives and death from myocardial infarction. Br Med J 2:245, 1975

170. Mann JI, Vessey MP, Thorogood M, et al: Myocardial infarction in young women with special reference to oral contraceptive practice. Br Med J 2:241, 1975

171. Marmor AI, Geltman EM, Schectman K, et al: Recurrent myocardial infarction: Clinical predictors and prognostic implications. Circulation 66:415, 1982

172. Marmor A, Sobel BE, Roberts R: Factors presaging early recurrent myocardial infarction ("extension"). Am J Cardiol 48:603, 1981

173. Marriott HJL: Electrocardiographic abnormalities, conduction disorders and arrhythmias in primary myocardial disease. Prog Cardiovasc Dis 7:99, 1964

174. Martinez-Rios MA, Bruto Da Costa BC, Cecena-Seldner FA, et al: Normal electrocardiogram in the presence of severe coronary artery disease. Am J Cardiol 25:320, 1970

175. Maseri A: Role of coronary artery spasm in symptomatic and silent myocardial ischemia. J Am Coll Cardiol 9:249, 1987

176. Maseri A, L'Abbata A, Baroldi G, et al: Coronary vasospasm as a possible cause of myocardial infarction. N Engl J Med 299:1271, 1978

177. Maseri A, L'Abbate A, Chierchia S, et al: Significance of spasm in the pathogenesis of ischemic heart disease. Am J Cardiol 44:788, 1979

178. McGinn S, White PD: Acute cor pulmonale resulting from pulmonary embolism. JAMA 104:1473, 1935

179. McHenry PL, Phillips JF, Fisch C, et al: Right precordial qrS pattern due to left anterior hemiblock. Am Heart J 81:498, 1971

180. Meller J, Conde CA, Donoso E, et al: Transient Q waves in Prinzmetal's angina. Am J Cardiol 35:691, 1975

181. Miller RR, Amsterdam EA, Bogren HG, et al: Electrocardiographic and cineangiographic correlations in assessment of the location, nature and extent of abnormal left ventricular segmental contraction in coronary artery disease. Circulation 49:447, 1974

182. Mills RM, Young E, Gorlin R, et al: Natural history of S-T segment elevation after acute myocardial infarction. Am J Cardiol 35:609, 1975

183. Morales AR, Romanelli R, Boucek RJ: The mural left

anterior descending coronary artery, strenuous exercise and sudden death. Circulation 62:230, 1980

184. Morris GC, Reul GJ, Howell JF, et al: Follow-up results of distal coronary artery bypass for ischemic heart disease. Am J Cardiol 29:180, 1972

185. Mukharji J, Murray S, Lewis SE, et al: Is anterior ST depression with acute transmural inferior infarction due to posterior infarction? A vectorcardiographic and scintigraphic study. J Am Coll Cardiol 4:28, 1984

186. Murata K, Hashiba K, Ikeda M, et al: QS- and QR-pattern in leads V_3 and V_4: Electrocardiographic and pathologic correlation of 41 cases, including 25 cases without myocardial infarction. Jpn Circ J 27:359, 1963

187. Myers GB: QRS-T patterns in multiple precordial leads that may be mistaken for myocardial infarction: III. Bundle branch block. Circulation 11:60, 1960

188. Myers GB, Klein HA, Stofer BE: I. Correlation of electrocardiographic and pathologic findings in anteroseptal infarction. Am Heart J 36:535, 1948

189. Myers GB. Klein HA, Hiratzka T: II. Correlation of electrocardiographic and pathologic findings in large anterolateral infarcts. Am Heart J 36:838, 1948

190. Myers GB, Klein HA, Hiratzka T: III. Correlation of electrocardiographic and pathologic findings in anteroposterior infarction. Am Heart J 37:205, 1949

191. Myers GB, Klein HA, Hiratzka T: IV. Correlation of electrocardiographic and pathologic findings in infarction of the interventricular septum and right ventricle. Am Heart J 37:720, 1949

192. Myers GB, Klein HA, Hiratzka T: V. Correlation of electrocardiographic and pathologic findings in posterior infarction. Am Heart J 38:547, 1949

193. Myers, GB, Klein HA, Hiratzka T: VI. Correlation of electrocardiographic and pathologic findings in posterolateral infarction. Am Heart J 38:837, 1948

194. Myers GB, Klein HA, Stofer BE: VII. Correlation of electrocardiographic and pathologic findings in lateral infarction. Am Heart J 37:374, 1949

195. Myers GB, Sears CH, Hiratzka T: Correlation of electrocardiographic and pathologic findings in ringlike subendocardial infarction of the left ventricle. Am J Med Sci 222:417, 1951

196. Myerson RM: Transient inversion of T waves after paroxysmal tachycardia. JAMA 148:193, 1952

197. Nademanee K, Intarachot V, Josephson MA, et al: Prognostic significance of silent myocardial ischemia in patients with unstable angina. J Am Coll Cardiol 10:1, 1987

198. Nobel RJ, Rothbaum DA, Knoebel SB, et al: Normalization of abnormal T waves in ischemia. Arch Intern Med 136:391, 1976

199. Norell MS, Lyons JP, Gardener JE, et al: Significance of "reciprocal" ST segment depression: Left ventriculographic observations during left anterior descending coronary angioplasty. J Am Coll Cardiol 13:1270, 1989

200. Ogawa H, Hiramori K, Haze K, et al: Classification of non–Q-wave myocardial infarction according to electrocardiographic changes. Br Heart J 54:473, 1985

201. Ogawa H, Hiramori K, Haze K, et al: Comparison of clinical features of non–Q wave and Q wave myocardial infarction. Am Heart J 111:513, 1986

202. Oliva PB, Breckinridge JC: Arteriographic evidence of coronary arterial spasm in acute myocardial infarction. Circulation 56:366, 1977

203. Oliva PB, Potts DE, Pluss RG: Coronary arterial spasm in Prinzmetal angina: Documentation by coronary arteriography. N Engl J Med 288:745, 1973

204. Oppenheimer BS, Rothschild MA: The value of the electrocardiogram in the diagnosis and prognosis of myocardial disease. Trans Assoc Am Physicians 39:247, 1924

205. Palmeri ST, Harrison DG, Cobb FR, et al: A QRS scoring system for assessing left ventricular function after myocardial infarction. N Engl J Med 306:4, 1982

206. Pantridge JF: Observations on the electrocardiogram and ventricular gradient in complete left bundle branch block. Circulation 3:589, 1951

207. Pardee HEB: Heart disease and abnormal electrocardiograms, with special reference to coronary T wave. Am J Med Sci 169:270, 1925

208. Parkinson J, Bedford DE: Successive changes in the electrocardiogram after cardiac infarction (coronary thrombosis). Heart 14:195, 1927

209. Parmley LF, Manion WC, Mattingly TW: Nonpenetrating traumatic injury of the heart. Circulation 18:371, 1958

210. Pasternack PF, Colvin SB, Baumann FG: Cocaine-induced angina pectoris and acute myocardial infarction in patients younger than 40 years. Am J Cardiol 55:847, 1985

211. Paton BC: The accuracy of diagnosis of myocardial infarction: A clinicopathologic study. Am J Med 23:761, 1957

212. Pearce ML, Chapman MG: The evaluation of Q aVF by the initial sagittal QRS vectors in 70 autopsied cases. Am Heart J 53:782, 1957

213. Perloff JK: The recognition of strictly posterior myocardial infarction by conventional scalar electrocardiography. Circulation 30:706, 1964

214. Perloff JK, Roberts WC, DeLeon AC, et al: The distinctive electrocardiogram of Duchenne's progressive muscular dystrophy. Am J Med 42:179, 1967

215. Phibbs B: "Transmural" versus "subendocardial" myocardial infarction: An electrocardiographic myth. J Am Coll Cardiol 1:561, 1983

216. Phillips E, Levine HD: A critical evaluation of extremity and precordial electrocardiography in acute cor pulmonale. Am Heart J 39:205, 1950

217. Phillips JH, Burch GE: Problems in the diagnosis of cor pulmonale. Am Heart J 66:818, 1963

218. Pierard LA, Sprynger M, Gilis F, Carlier J: Significance of precordial ST-segment depression in inferior acute myocardial infarction as determined by echocardiography. Am J Cardiol 57:82, 1986.

219. Pinto IJ, Nanda NC, Biswas AK, et al: Tall upright T waves in the precordial leads. Circulation 36:708, 1967

220. Pipberger HV, Lopez EA: "Silent" subendocardial infarcts: Fact or fiction? Am Heart J 100:597, 1980

221. Previtali M, Klersy C, Salerno JA, et al: Ventricular tachyarrhythmias in Prinzmetal's variant angina: Clinical significance and relation to the degree and time course of S-T segment elevation. Am J Cardiol 52:19, 1983

222. Prinzmetal M, Ekmekei A, Kennamer R, et al: Variant form of angina pectoris: Previously undelineated syndrome. JAMA 174:102, 1960

223. Prinzmetal M, Kennamer R, Merliss R, et al: Angina pectoris. I. A variant form of angina pectoris: Preliminary report. Am J Med 27:375, 1959

224. Pruitt RD, Curd GW, Leachman R: Simulation of electrocardiogram of apicolateral myocardial in-

farction by myocardial destructive lesions of obscure etiology (myocardiopathy). Circulation 25:506, 1962

225. Przybojewski JZ: Polyarteritis nodosa in the adult: Report of a case with repeated myocardial infarction and a review of cardiac involvement. S Afr Med J 60:512, 1981

226. Quyyumi A, Wright CM, Mockus LJ, Fox KM: How important is a history of chest pain in determining the degree of ischaemia in patients with angina pectoris? Br Heart J 54:22, 1985

227. Rafilzadeh M, Luria MH, Lochaya E, et al: Physiologic studies in a healthy adolescent with inverted precordial T waves. Dis Chest 52:101, 1967

228. Rakov HI: Prolonged benign T-wave inversion following paroxysmal ventricular tachycardia. NY J Med 64:2100, 1964

229. Ratliff NB, Hackel DB: Combined right and left ventricular infarction: Pathogenesis and clinicopathologic correlation. Am J Cardiol 45:217, 1980

230. Raunio H, Rossanen V, Romppanen, et al: Changes in the QRS complex and ST segment in transmural and subendocardial myocardial infarction: A clinicopathologic study. Am Heart J 98:176, 1979

231. Rhoads DV, Edwards JE, Pruitt RD: The electrocardiogram in the presence of myocardial infarction and intraventricular block of the left bundle-branch block type. Am Heart J 62:735, 1961

232. Richardson SG, Morton P, Murtagh JG, et al: Relation of coronary arterial patency and left ventricular function to electrocardiographic changes after streptokinase treatment during acute myocardial infarction. Am J Cardiol 61:961, 1988

233. Rocco MB, Barry J, Campbell S, et al: Circadian variation of transient myocardial ischemia in patients with coronary artery disease. Circulation 75:395, 1987

234. Rod JL, Zucker RP: Acute myocardial infarction shortly after cocaine inhalation. Am J Cardiol 59:161, 1987

235. Rodrigues B, Dewhurst NG, Smart LM, et al: Diagnosis and prognosis of right ventricular infarction. Br Heart J 56:19, 1986

236. Romhilt D, Susilavorn B, Chou TC: Unusual electrocardiographic manifestation of pulmonary embolism. Am Heart J 80:237, 1970

237. Rosenbaum MB. Elizari MV, Lazzari JO: The Hemiblocks. Oldsmar, Fla, Tampa Tracings, 1970.

238. Rosenberg BA, Malach M: Acute myocardial infarction in a city hospital: Follow-up study of 131 survivors. Am J Cardiol 8:799, 1961

239. Rozanski A, Berman DS: Silent myocardial ischemia: I. Pathophysiology, frequency of occurrence, and approaches toward detection. Am Heart J 114:615, 1987

240. Sackner MA, Heinz ER, Steinberg AJ: The heart in scleroderma. Am J Cardiol 17:542, 1966

241. Salcedo JR, Baird MG, Chambers RJ, et al: Significance of reciprocal S-T segment depression in anterior precordial leads in acute inferior myocardial infarction: Concomitant left anterior descending coronary artery disease? Am J Cardiol 48:1003, 1981

242. Sanerkin NG: Extracardiac anastomisis in coronary ostial occlusion. Br Heart J 30:440, 1968

243. Sargin O, Demirkol C: Deeply inverted T-waves after supraventricular paroxysmal tachycardia. Dis Chest 48:321, 1965

244. Savage RM, Wagner GS, Ideker RE, et al: Correlation of postmortem anatomic findings with electrocardiographic changes in patients with myocardial infarction. Circulation 55:279, 1977

245. Schiebler GL, Loring AE, Brogdon BG, et al: Cardiovascular manifestation of Hurler's syndrome. Circulation 26:782, 1962

246. Schimke RN, McKusick VA, Huang T, et al: Homocystinuria: Studies of 20 families with 38 affected members. JAMA 193:711, 1965

247. Scott RC: Left bundle branch block: A clinical assessment. Part II. Am Heart J 70:691, 1965

248. Shah PK, Pichler M, Berman DS, et al: Noninvasive identification of a high-risk subset of patients with acute inferior myocardial infarction. Am J Cardiol 46:915, 1980

249. Sheldon W, Favaloro R, Sones F, et al: Reconstructive coronary artery surgery: Venous autograft technic. JAMA 213:78, 1970

250. Slucka C: The electrocardiogram in Duchenne progressive muscular dystrophy. Circulation 38:933, 1968

251. Smith HWB, Liberman HA, Brody SL, et al: Acute myocardial infarction temporally related to cocaine use. Ann Intern Med 107:13, 1987

252. Sodeman WA, Johnston FD, Wilson FN: The Q_1 deflection of the electrocardiogram in bundle branch block and axis deviation. Am Heart J 28:271, 1944

253. Sodi-Pallares D, Cisneros F, Medrano GA, et al: Electrocardiographic diagnosis of myocardial infarction in the presence of bundle branch block (right and left), ventricular premature beats and Wolff-Parkinson-White syndrome. Prog Cardiovasc Dis 6:107, 1963

254. Sodi-Pallares D, Rodriguez MI: Morphology of the unipolar leads recorded at the septal surfaces: Its application to the diagnosis of left bundle branch block complicated by myocardial infarction. Am Heart J 43:27, 1952

255. Spodick DH: Q-wave infarction versus S-T infarction. Am J Cardiol 51:913, 1983

256. Stimmel B, Katz AM, Donoso E: Q-wave development in acute subendocardial infarction. Arch Intern Med 131:676, 1973

257. Stone PH, Raabe DS, Jaffe AS, et al: Prognostic significance of location and type of myocardial infarction: Independent adverse outcome associated with anterior location. J Am Coll Cardiol 11:453, 1988

258. Sullivan W, Vlodaver Z, Tuna N, et al: Correlation of electrocardiographic and pathologic findings in healed myocardial infarction. Am J Cardiol 42:724, 1978

259. Surawicz B: Relationship between electrocardiogram and electrolytes. Am Heart J 73:814, 1967

260. Surawicz B, VanHorne RG, Urbach JR, et al: QS- and QR-pattern in leads V_3 and V_4 in absence of myocardial infarction: Electrocardiographic and vectorcardiographic study. Circulation 12:391, 1955

261. Sweet RL, Sheffield LT: Myocardial infarction after exercise-induced electrocardiographic changes in a patient with variant angina pectoris. Am J Cardiol 33:813, 1974

262. Tabel ME, Fisch C: Abnormal Q waves simulating myocardial infarction in diffuse myocardial diseases. Am Heart J 68:534, 1964

263. Taylor HA, Deumite NJ, Chaitman BR, et al: Asymptomatic left main coronary artery disease in Coronary Artery Surgery Study (CASS) registry. Circulation 79:1171, 1989

264. Theroux P, Waters DD, Halphen D, et al: Prognostic value of exercise testing soon after myocardial infarction. N Engl J Med 301:341, 1979

265. Thomas J, Harris E, Lassiter G: Observations on the T wave and S-T segment changes in the precordial electrocardiograms of 320 negro adults. Am J Cardiol 5:468, 1960

266. Timmis GC: Electrocardiographic effects of reperfusion. Cardiol Clinics 5:427, 1987

267. Tuqan SK, Mau RD, Schwartz MJ: Anterior myocardial infarction patterns in the mitral valve prolapse–systolic click syndrome. Am J Med 58:719, 1975

268. vonArnim T, Hofling B, Schreiber M: Characteristics of episodes of ST elevation or ST depression during ambulatory monitoring in patients subsequently undergoing coronary angiography. Br Heart J 54:484, 1985

269. Wartman WB, Hellerstein HK: The incidence of heart disease in 2,000 consecutive autopsies. Ann Intern Med 28:41, 1948

270. Wasserberger RH, Alt WJ: The normal RS-T segment elevation variant. Am J Cardiol 8:184, 1961

271. Wasserberger RH, Corliss RJ: Prominent precordial T waves as an expression of coronary insufficiency. Am J Cardiol 16:195, 1965

272. Wasserman AG, Bren GB, Ross AB, et al: Prognostic implications of diagnostic Q waves after myocardial infarction. Circulation 65:1451, 1982

273. Waters DD, Szlachcic J, Bonan R, et al: Comparative sensitivity of exercise, cold pressor and ergonovine testing in provoking attacks of variant angina in patients with active disease. Circulation 67:310, 1983

274. Watson JH, Bartholomae WM: Cardiac injury due to nonpenetrating chest trauma. Ann Intern Med 52:871, 1960

275. Weiner DA, Ryan TJ, McCabe CH, et al: Significance of silent myocardial ischemia during exercise testing in patients with coronary artery disease. Am J Cardiol 59:725, 1987

276. Weinshel AM, Isner JM, Salem EN, et al: The coronary anatomy of right ventricular myocardial infarction: Relationship between the site of right coronary occlusion and origin of the right ventricular free wall branches. Circulation 68:III-351, 1983

277. Weiss, MM, Weiss MM Jr: The electrocardiogram in myocardial infarction. Arch Intern Med 101:1126, 1958

278. Wenger NK, Bauer S: Coronary embolism: Review of the literature and presentation of fifteen cases. Am J Med 25:549, 1958

279. Wesselhoeft H, Fawcett JS, Johnson AL: Anomalous origin of the left coronary artery from the pulmonary trunk: Its clinical spectrum, pathology and pathophysiology, based on a review of 140 cases with seven further cases. Circulation 38:403, 1968

280. Williams RA, Cohn PF, Vokonas PS, et al: Electrocardiographic, arteriographic and ventriculographic correlations in transmural myocardial infarction. Am J Cardiol 31:595, 1973

281. Willich SN, Stone PH, Muller JE, et al: High-risk subgroups of patients with non-Q wave myocardial infarction based on direction and severity of ST segment deviation. Am Heart J 114:1110, 1987

282. Windesheim JH, Parkin TW: Electrocardiograms of ninety patients with acrosclerosis and progressive diffuse sclerosis (scleroderma). Circulation 17:874, 1959

283. Wolff L, Richman JL: The diagnosis of myocardial infarction in patients with anomalous atrioventricular excitation (Wolff-Parkinson-White syndrome). Am Heart J 45:545, 1953

284. Woods JD, Laurie W, Smith WG: The reliability of the electrocardiogram in myocardial infarction. Lancet 2:265, 1963

285. Yanagihara R, Todd JK: Acute febrile mucocutaneous lymph node syndrome. Am J Dis Child 134:603, 1980

286. Young E, Cohn PF, Gorlin R, et al: Vectorcardiographic diagnosis and electrocardiographic correlation in left ventricular asynergy due to coronary artery disease: I. Severe asynergy of the anterior and apical segments. Circulation 51:467, 1975

287. Yu PN, Stewart JM: Subendocardial myocardial infarction with special reference to the electrocardiographic changes. Am Heart J 39:862, 1950

288. Zimmerman FH, Gustafson GM, Kemp HG: Recurrent myocardial infarction associated with cocaine abuse in a young man with normal coronary arteries: Evidence for coronary artery spasm culminating in thrombosis. J Am Coll Cardiol 9:964, 1987

289. Zimmerman HA, Bersano E, Dicosky C: The Auricular Electrocardiogram. Springfield, Ill, Charles C Thomas, 1968

290. Zmyslinski RW, Akiyama T, Biddle TL, et al: Natural course of the S-T segment and QRS complex in patients with acute anterior myocardial infarction. Am J Cardiol 43:29, 1979

291. Zuckerman, R, Cabrera CA, Fishleder BL, et al: Electrocardiogram in chronic cor pulmonale. Am Heart J 35:421, 1948

Stress Test

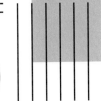

10

The electrocardiographic (ECG) stress test is widely used for the detection of myocardial ischemia, especially in patients with coronary artery disease (CAD). During exercise, the increase of oxygen requirements is associated with increased cardiac output and myocardial oxygen consumption. In patients with significant CAD the increased demand may exceed the reserve capacity of the coronary blood flow. Relative myocardial ischemia may occur in other types of heart disease if the increased myocardial oxygen consumption during exercise cannot be met even though the coronary arteries are normal. If myocardial ischemia occurs, it may be associated with ECG changes that are not apparent while the patient is at rest. Modern exercise testing is not limited to ECG observation only. Hemodynamic response to the exercise also is an important part of the information to be gained. In addition, the stress test is useful in the assessment of the severity of the CAD, prognosis, and functional capacity of the patient after the presence of ischemic heart disease is known. It also is used for the evaluation of the efficacy of antianginal therapy and revascularization procedures. Indeed, it probably is used more often for these purposes than for the diagnosis of CAD. The stress test also is performed for the exposure of cardiac arrhythmia.

The evaluation of the clinical usefulness and limitations of the stress test for ischemic heart disease is complicated by the fact that there is no uniformity among medical institutions in regard to the type of stress given, the exercise protocol, the recording techniques, and the ECG criteria used.

The following conditions generally are considered contraindications for the test:

1. Recent onset of chest pain or a change in the pattern of pain to suggest unstable angina.

2. Acute myocardial infarction within a week after its onset.

3. The presence of congestive heart failure, excessive hypertension, or severe aortic stenosis in the adults.

4. Uncontrolled ventricular arrhythmias.

5. Known critical stenosis of left main or proximal coronary artery.

A more detailed discussion of the indications and contraindications for exercise testing is included in the guidelines prepared by the task force from the American College of Cardiology and American Heart Association.[119] Conditions that may affect the accuracy of the test are discussed later in the chapter.

TYPES OF STRESS TESTS

The most commonly performed ECG stress test is the graded exercise test using either the treadmill or bicycle ergometer. It often is carried out in conjunction with the administration of radionuclides (e.g., thallium, technetium) to evaluate myocardial perfusion and ventricular function. In this text, the discussion is confined to the ECG changes.

Some years ago, the two-step exercise test, described by Master, was a commonly used ECG stress test.[98] It involves walking up and down two standardized steps within a certain period of time for a number of trips as determined by the age, weight, and sex of the patient. When the exercise is completed, the ECG is recorded in the supine position immediately and several times afterwards. The test is no longer used because the stress usually is inadequate and the patient is not monitored during exercise.

Graded Exercise Test

In the graded exercise test (GXT), the patient begins with a low level of work load that he or she is able to perform without difficulty. The work load is then increased in small increments during continuous ECG monitoring until the target heart rate is reached or symptoms or signs of myocardial ischemia develop.

The GXT is terminated also if the patient is unable to continue because of dyspnea, fatigue, or leg pain. A decrease of the blood pressure or the appearance of frequent premature ventricular contractions or other significant arrhythmias also calls for the discontinuation of the exercise. Examination of the ECG changes during the exercise is important, because 5 to 11 percent of the patients with abnormal responses may not display such findings after the cessation of the exercise.[96,97]

The protocol used in the GXT varies among different medical centers. In addition to variations in the equipment used, the work load may be maximal or submaximal for the individual. In our institution, the treadmill is used, and the procedure follows essentially that suggested by Sheffield and co-workers.[123] The test is done at least 2 hours after a meal. The baseline ECGs include tracings taken in the supine position at rest and during hyperventilation, in the sitting position, and while standing with and without hyperventilation. The exercise consists of five stages at 3-minute intervals as outlined by Bruce and Hornsten.[19] It begins with the subject walking at a speed of 1.7 miles per hour (mph) at 10 percent grade (stage 1). Stages 2 through 5 involve a stepwise increase from a speed of 2.5 to 3.4, 4.2, and 5.0 mph, with a grade of 12, 14, 16, and 18 percent, respectively. The target point is 85 percent of the predicted maximal heart rate for the subject's age (Table 10–1). The ECG is monitored continuously with an oscilloscope during the exercise, and short strips of leads V_4, V_5, and V_6 are recorded simultaneously every minute at a paper speed of 50 mm/sec. The blood pressure is taken every 3 minutes during the exercise. At the end of the exercise, leads V_4, V_5, and V_6 and a complete 12-lead ECG are recorded immediately in the sitting position. Leads V_4, V_5, and V_6 are repeated every minute after the exercise for at least 6 minutes or until the tracing returns to the resting pattern. An additional 12-lead ECG is recorded at 4 minutes after exercise and is repeated if necessary. The blood pressure reading is taken at 2, 4, and 6 minutes after exercise.

RECORDING TECHNIQUES

The results of exercise testing are affected by the recording technique. The conventional 12-lead ECG, the XYZ leads of the Frank lead system, and several bipolar lead systems are in use. The conventional 12-lead ECG is the most widely chosen one for the GXT. The relative sensitivity of the various leads was tested by Blackburn and associates.[8,9] When the conventional 12 leads were recorded nearly simultaneously, almost all the ST-segment changes were demonstrated in leads II, aVF, and V_3 through V_6; 89 percent of that information is contained in lead V_5 and 94 percent in leads V_3 through V_6.[9] Braat and associates found that the addition of lead V_4R improved the diagnostic accuracy in patients with proximal stenosis of the right coronary artery.[14] The Frank XYZ leads were found to be less sensitive than the 12-lead ECG.[8] In 90 percent of the cases, the ST changes could be found in the X (horizontal) lead, whereas changes limited to the Y (vertical) lead were found in only 10 percent of the patients.[8] The bipolar lead systems are claimed to have sensitivity equal to that of the 12-lead ECG. The exploring electrode generally is placed at V_5, and the reference electrode is placed over the manubrium sterni or right lateral subclavicular area.

CRITERIA FOR A POSITIVE EXERCISE TEST

1. Horizontal or downsloping ST-segment depression of 1 mm or more with a duration of 0.08 second or more (Fig. 10–1). The PR segment is the reference point with which the ST segment is compared. The degree of ST-segment depression considered as an abnormal test result varies between 0.5 and 2.0 mm or more. The criterion of 1 mm or more depression is the most generally accepted. Slowly

TABLE 10–1. Predicted Maximal Heart Rate for Various Age Groups

	Age (yr)							
	30	*35*	*40*	*45*	*50*	*55*	*60*	*65*
Men	193	191	189	187	184	182	180	178
Women	190	185	181	177	172	168	163	159

Ischemic S-T segment
depression

Junctional S-T segment
depression

horizontal   downsloping

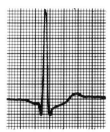

FIGURE 10-1. Examples of ischemic and junctional types of ST-segment depression.

upsloping ST-segment depression also is considered by some authorities to be an abnormal response.[90,112] The definition of slow upsloping varies. One commonly used criterion is ST-segment depression of 1 mm or more 0.08 second after the J junction.

2. ST-segment elevation of 1 mm or more.

3. U-wave inversion.[54,90] Gerson and associates found that, in patients with chest pain, exercise-induced U-wave inversion had a sensitivity of 21 percent and a specificity of 99 percent for the diagnosis of significant CAD.[54] It was particularly suggestive of severe stenosis of the proximal left anterior descending or left main coronary artery. In some cases, the U-wave inversion occurred in the absence of abnormal ST-segment response.

4. The ST-segment/heart rate (ST/HR) slope. The degree of ST-segment displacement in relation to the increase in heart rate with exercise has been found by some investigators to be a more accurate indicator of the presence or absence and severity of CAD.[36,37,43,106] In the analysis, the ST-segment shift 0.08 seconds after the J point is measured and averaged for 5 to 10 beats at each heart rate increments of 10 beats/min or every 3 minutes. The changes in the ST segment in relation to the heart rate are plotted using the ST measurements for the ordinate and heart rate for the abscissa. The line best fitting the relation is determined by means of linear regression analysis. The steepest slope obtained from the leads chosen for the analysis is used. A slope of greater than 130 or 220×10^{-4} mm/beat/min is considered an abnormal response, depending on the investigators.[36,43] The overall diagnostic accuracy of the ST/HR slope in angiographically proved cases of CAD was found to be significantly superior to that of the conventional ST criterion. Okin and colleagues found that an ST/HR slope of 600×10^{-4} mm/beat/min or greater identified three-vessel coronary disease with a sensitivity of 93 percent compared with 66 percent with the conventional criterion.[106] Further studies are needed to confirm these rather encouraging results.

5. Increase in R-wave amplitude. Bonoris and co-workers reported an increase in the R-wave amplitude immediately after exercise in patients with severe multivessel coronary artery narrowing and ventricular dysfunction.[11] It was postulated that the increased R-wave amplitude was due to ventricular dilatation secondary to poor ventricular function. The results of later studies varied, some supporting and others not supporting the original observation.[3,5,6,45,69,146]

6. Decrease in the Q-wave amplitude in lead V_5. Regression of the Q-wave amplitude in lead V_5 during exercise was found by Nohara and associates to correlate well with interventricular septal perfusion defect and left anterior descending artery stenosis.[104] Progression or no change of Q wave or the appearance of a new Q wave in lead V_5 was associated with normal septal perfusion. Morales-Ballejo and colleagues, using a modified lead V_5, reported similar findings a few years earlier.[101] The changes in Q-wave amplitude are not widely used in the routine stress test.

Other changes that once were considered to be abnormal responses are no longer used in the diagnosis of CAD. They include (1) marked junctional type of ST depression of 1.5 mm or greater[15,99]; (2) QX/QT ratio of greater than 0.5[61,84] (the QX interval is measured from the beginning of the Q wave to the point X where ST segment returns to the iso-electric line); (3) development of serious arrhythmia, such as multifocal premature ventricular contractions, ventricular tachycardia, atrioventricular block, atrial tachycardia, or atrial fibrillation[99]; and (4) T-wave inversion with the amplitude of the T wave greater than 1.5 mm.[99]

The significance of exercise-induced bundle branch block is a controversial subject. Some investigators found that it occurred primarily in association with CAD, especially in the case of exercise-induced right bundle branch block.[149,158] Others reported normal coronary arteries in most of these patients, especially if the bundle branch block developed at a rate of 125 beats/min or greater.[145] The different results probably are related to the populations studied.

DIAGNOSTIC ACCURACY OF THE EXERCISE TEST IN CORONARY ARTERY DISEASE: SENSITIVITY AND SPECIFICITY

Arteriographic Correlation. Although coronary arteriogram may underestimate the severity of the lesions and is unable to exclude coronary spasm, it remains the standard against which the diagnostic value of the various noninvasive tests for CAD is measured.

ST-Segment Depression

The reliability of exercise-induced ST-segment depression in the diagnosis of CAD is affected by the following factors:

1. Presence or absence of chest pain
2. Sex
3. Degree of ST-segment depression
4. Time of onset and duration of the positive response
5. Severity of the CAD

One of the most important factors that affects the reliability of the stress test is the population examined.[111] According to the Bayes theorem, a low incidence of the disease is associated with a high incidence of false-positive responses to the test, and a high incidence of the disease is accompanied by a high occurrence of false-negative responses. The results listed in Table 10-2 were obtained from symptomatic patients. With the criterion of 1 mm or more ST-segment depression, the sensitivity of the test varied between 57 and 82 percent. The specificity for the presence of significant CAD ranged from 57 to 95 percent (i.e., a false-positive diagnosis was made in 5 to 43 percent). In one of the largest series consisting of 1472 patients reported by McNeer and associates the sensitivity was 57 percent and the specificity was 90 percent.[95] The results from the different series had no apparent relation to the arteriographic criteria used or the target point chosen. Figures 10-2 through 10-4 represent cases with true-positive, false-negative, and false-positive responses proved by angiography or autopsy.

The specificity of the test is much lower in subjects without symptoms (see Fig. 10-4). Froelicher and associates studied 76 air crewmen without symptoms but with a positive re-

TABLE 10–2. Correlation of Graded Exercise Test with Findings of Coronary Arteriography in Patients with Symptoms

Study	No. of Patients	Exercise, Target Point	Cine Criteria for CAD (% luminal narrowing)	ECG Criteria for Positive Test (mm ST Displacement)	Sensitivity (%)	Specificity (%)
McHenry et al[93]	166	Treadmill, 90% predicted max HR	≥ 75	≥ 1.0	82	95
Martin and McConahay[96]	100	Treadmill, max effort	≥ 50	≥ 0.5	84	57
				≥ 0.75	68	72
				≥ 1.0	62	89
Bartel et al[4]	465	Treadmill, 85% predicted max HR	≥ 70	≥ 1.0	65	92
Goldschlager et al[58]	410	Treadmill, 85% predicted max HR	≥ 50	≥ 1.0	64	93
McNeer et al[95]	1472	Treadmill, 85% predicted max HR	≥ 75 > 50 LM	≥ 1.0	57	90
Weiner et al[154]	2045	Treadmill, 85% predicted max HR	≥ 70 (diameter) > 50 LM	≥ 1.0	80 (M) 76 (F)	74 (M) 65 (F)

CAD = coronary artery disease; max HR = maximal heart rate; LM = left main coronary artery; M = male; F = female.

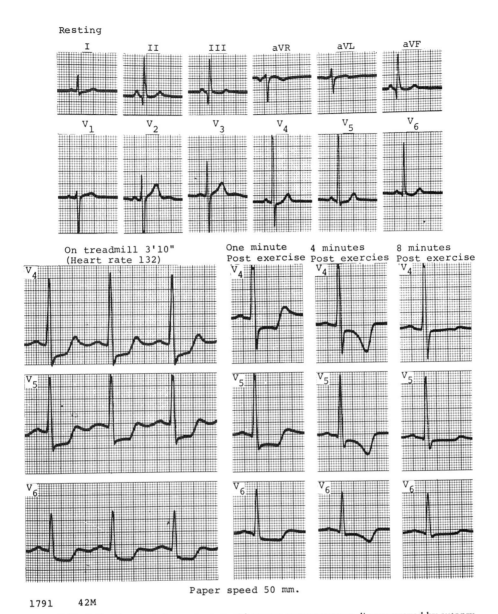

Resting

I   II   III   aVR   aVL   aVF

V_1 V_2 V_3 V_4 V_5 V_6

On treadmill 3'10"   One minute   4 minutes   8 minutes
(Heart rate 132)   Post exercise Post exercies Post exercise

V_4 V_4 V_4 V_4

V_5 V_5 V_5 V_5

V_6 V_6 V_6 V_6

Paper speed 50 mm.

1791   42M

FIGURE 10–2. Positive graded exercise test with severe coronary artery disease proved by autopsy. The patient was a 42-year-old man with a history of moderate hypertension and recent onset of angina. In the resting ECG, relatively deep Q waves are present in leads II, III, and aVF to suggest possible previous inferior myocardial infarction. The QRS voltage in the precordial leads is consistent with left ventricular hypertrophy. Three minutes after the beginning of the exercise on a treadmill, marked ST-segment depression developed even though the patient did not experience chest pain. The exercise was discontinued. The serial changes of the ST segment and T waves are shown. The ECG returned to the resting pattern 10 minutes after exercise. Coronary arteriogram performed 6 weeks later revealed 70 to 90 percent luminal narrowing of the left main coronary artery and the three major branches at various locations. The patient died 5 days later. The lesions in the coronary arteries were verified at autopsy. Inferior myocardial infarction, both earlier and recent, was found to involve about 25 percent of the left ventricular myocardium. A moderate degree of left ventricular hypertrophy also was demonstrated.

sponse (1 mm ST-segment depression) to maximal treadmill exercise testing.[49] Eighteen men had normal resting ECGs, whereas the other 58 had ST and T-wave abnormalities on their resting ECGs after at least one normal tracing. Only 43 percent of the men had angiographically demonstrated significant CAD with 50 percent or more luminal narrowing.[49] In the subjects without symptoms studied by Borer and co-workers, only 37 percent of those with abnormal test results had significant disease.[13]

Resting

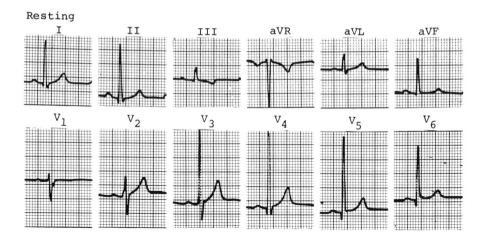

On treadmill 11.5 minutes (Heart rate 160)

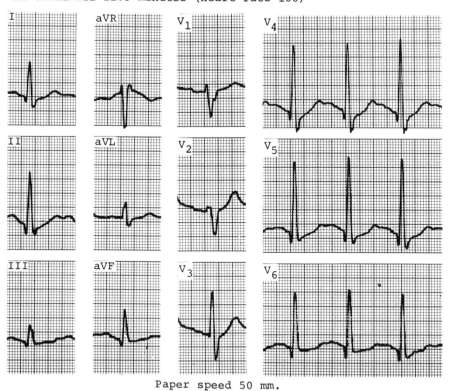

Paper speed 50 mm.

FIGURE 10–3. False-negative exercise test. The patient is a 49-year-old man with a history of chest pain. Coronary arteriogram revealed 80 percent occlusion of the right coronary artery, 80 percent of the left anterior descending artery, and 50 percent narrowing of the left circumflex artery. The resting ECG is within normal limits. The exercise ECG shows only junctional type ST-segment depression when the target rate was reached. (Courtesy of Dr. Evelyn McCall.)

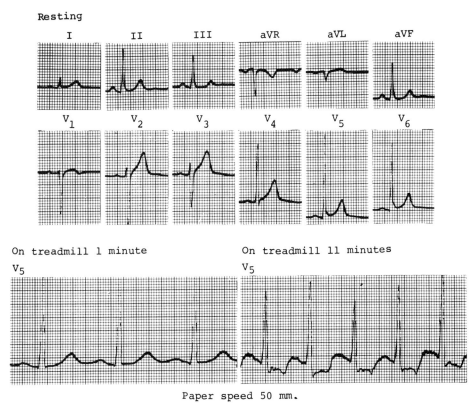

Resting

I   II   III   aVR   aVL   aVF

V₁   V₂   V₃   V₄   V₅   V₆

On treadmill 1 minute
V₅

On treadmill 11 minutes
V₅

Paper speed 50 mm.

FIGURE 10–4. False-positive graded exercise test. The patient is a healthy 49-year-old mountain climber who has no symptoms. His physical examination, chest roentgenogram, and other laboratory findings are all within normal limits. Although the resting ECG suggests the possibility of left ventricular hypertrophy because of the tall R wave in lead V₅, no other evidence supports this diagnosis. The exercise ECG shows marked horizontal ST-segment depression after 7 minutes of treadmill exercise. A coronary arteriogram was done and was normal. (Courtesy of Dr. Evelyn McCall.)

The differences in exercise response between men and women were evaluated by Sketch and colleagues.[126] The study included 195 men and 56 women with chest pain who were evaluated by multistage submaximal stress testing and selective coronary arteriogram. Among patients with abnormal exercise test results, significant CAD was found in 89 percent of the men but in only 33 percent of the women. Among patients with normal exercise test results, 37 percent of the men and 12 percent of the women had significant CAD. Therefore, the authors concluded that a positive exercise test was of little value in predicting significant CAD in women, whereas a negative test was useful in excluding it. Their results were confirmed by later observations.[144,154] Among the 2045 patients included in the coronary artery surgery study (CASS), Weiner and associates found that women were 4.5 times more likely to have a false-positive response than men.[154] This difference prevailed whether the resting ST segments and T waves were abnormal or not.[154]

The magnitude of the ST-segment depression affects the reliability of the test significantly. There is a decrease in the sensitivity but an increase in the specificity as the degree of ST-segment depression required for a positive response is more pronounced.[23,96,97] For example, in the Cohn series (based on Master two-step test), the sensitivity of the test decreased from 84 to 34 percent when the criterion of the ST-segment depression was changed from ≥ 0.5 to ≥ 2.0 mm, and the specificity was increased from 73 to 100 percent.[23] Although marked ST-segment depression generally is associated with the presence of multivessel disease, many exceptions do occur. An example is given in Figure 10–4.

The configuration, time of onset, and duration of depressed ST segment during and after treadmill exercise were evaluated by Goldschlager and associates.[58] False-positive response was rare with depressed, downsloping ST segments. Two- or three-vessel disease or main left CAD was present in about 90 percent of patients who had depressed, down-

Control

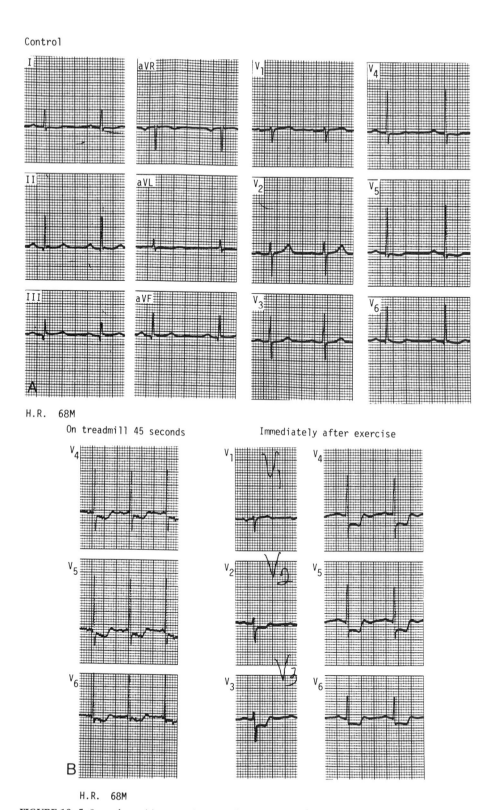

H.R. 68M

On treadmill 45 seconds   Immediately after exercise

H.R. 68M

FIGURE 10–5. Strongly positive exercise test. The patient is a 68-year-old man with a history of myo-cardial infarction 10 years ago followed by exertional angina since then. (A) The resting ECG shows nonspecific ST-segment and T-wave changes. (B) Forty-five seconds after the beginning of exercise on the treadmill, the patient had chest pain and downsloping ST-segment depression appeared in leads V_4 through V_6. The exercise was discontinued immediately, but the ST-segment depression continued to increase.

12 minutes after exercise   22 minutes after exercise   30 minutes after exercise

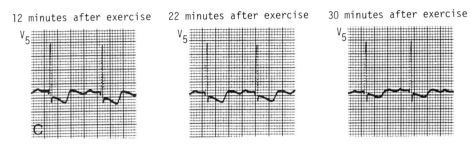

H.R.   68M

FIGURE 10–5. *Continued.* (C) The ST-segment depression persisted and was present, although improved, 30 minutes after exercise. Coronary arteriogram revealed an 80 percent occlusive lesion of the left main artery and complete occlusion of the proximal left anterior descending and right coronary arteries. The first marginal branch of the left circumflex artery also had marked stenosis.

sloping ST segments or ischemic changes appearing in the first 3 minutes of exercise or persisting for more than 8 minutes after exercise. In the 1472 patients studied by McNeer and co-workers, more than 97 percent of those who had a positive response at Bruce stage I or II had significant CAD.[95] Such a relation between early onset of a positive response and extensive CAD also was found by other investigators.[25] Figure 10–5 gives a remarkable example of a patient with early and prolonged positive response. Karnegis and co-workers found that a positive response occurring during the recovery phase after exercise had the same significance as that during exercise.[74]

When the extent of the CAD is taken into consideration, the sensitivity of the exercise test is enhanced when the number of vessels involved is increased. McHenry and associates found that 61 percent of the patients with single-vessel disease had abnormal ST-segment response as compared to 93 percent of those with two- or three-vessel disease.[93] Others reported a sensitivity of 40, 66, and 76 percent for one-, two-, and three-vessel disease, respectively.[4] When only one vessel is involved, the stress test was found by some to be more sensitive to disease of the left anterior descending artery than to disease of one of the two other vessels.[93] This observation, however, was not shared by other investigators.[4,73] The site of the ST-segment depression does not appear to be helpful in the localization of the CAD.[34,46,73]

The development of typical angina during the test added significantly to its diagnostic accuracy. Its presence alone is almost as predictive as ischemic ST-segment displacement.[151] Failure of the blood pressure to rise or the development of hypotension during exercise testing usually indicates the presence of severe CAD.[118,151] Ischemic ventricular dysfunc-

tion is probably the underlying cause for the abnormal blood pressure response.

Because of the prognostic and therapeutic implications of left main or severe three-vessel CAD, much attention has been given to changes during exercise testing that may identify their presence. These changes include the following:[10,25,58,95,102,118,120,150,161]

1. ST-segment depression of 2 mm or more
2. Downsloping ST-segment depression
3. Early positive response (Bruce stage 1 or 2)
4. Persistence of ST depression more than 6 minutes into recovery
5. ST-segment depression in 5 or more leads
6. Exertional hypotension

When several of these changes are observed, the presence of significant left main or severe three-vessel CAD is likely (see Figs. 10–5 and 10–6). Separation of left main from severe three-vessel disease by these criteria is difficult, however.[153]

In summary, the GXT for the detection of significant CAD is more useful in males than in females. False-positive results are more common in subjects who exhibit no symptoms. When more ST-segment depression is required for the interpretation of a positive response, the test becomes less sensitive but more specific. It is more likely to be positive in multivessel disease, which usually is present if the ST-segment depression is 2 mm or more. The distribution of the ST-segment depression is of no value in localizing the arterial lesion.

ST-Segment Elevation

Although horizontal or downsloping ST-segment depression is the typical abnormal response in stress testing, some patients exhibit

Resting   BP 112/90

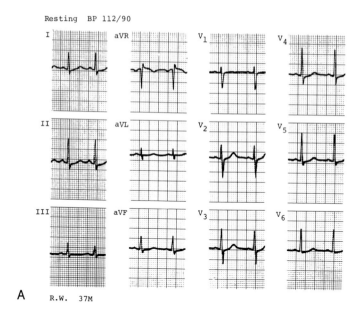

A   R.W.   37M

3 min. exercise   Chest pain   BP 60/40

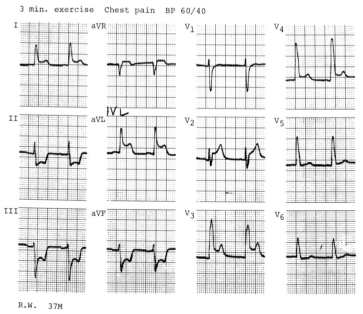

B   R.W.   37M

FIGURE 10–6. Severe left main coronary artery disease. The patient is a 37-year-old man with a history of chest pain. (A) In the resting ECG, there is a slight junctional segment depression in some of the leads. His blood pressure before the exercise was 112/90. Three minutes after treadmill exercise was begun, he had chest pain and hypotension, with a blood pressure of 60/40. The exercise was discontinued immediately. (B) The 12-lead ECG reveals ST-segment elevation in leads I, aVL, and V_2 through V_4, with ST-segment depression in leads II, III, and aVF. Coronary arteriogram revealed 90 percent occlusion of left main artery.

ST-segment elevation (Figs. 10–6 and 10–7). Generally, ST-segment elevation implies a more severe degree of myocardial ischemia than does ST-segment depression. The reported incidence of exercise-induced ST-segment elevation is related to the population ex- amined and the degree of elevation required for a positive response. In 1275 healthy men studied by Bruce and associates, 0.5 percent were found to display ST-segment elevation of 1.0 mm or more.[18] Using the criterion of ST-segment elevation of 1 mm or more, most

Control

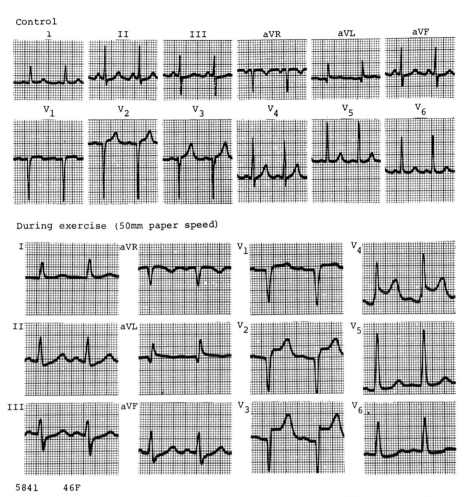

During exercise (50mm paper speed)

5841   46F

FIGURE 10–7. Positive graded exercise test with ST-segment elevation. The patient is a 46-year-old woman with a typical history of angina pectoris. The resting ECG shows poor progression of the R wave in the right precordial leads, suggesting possible old anterior myocardial infarction. The exercise ECG reveals marked ST-segment elevation in leads V_1 through V_4 2 minutes after the beginning of exercise on a treadmill when the patient had chest pain. Coronary arteriogram revealed, however, only a 30 percent narrowing in the anterior descending branch of the left coronary artery. The left ventricular cineangiogram was normal. Exercise-induced coronary spasm may be the cause of the ST-segment elevation.[107] (Courtesy of Dr. Donald Romhilt.)

studies of patients with symptoms showed an incidence of 3.0 to 6.5 percent.[21,33,44,131,148] The incidence is higher when ST-segment elevation of 0.5 mm or more is considered a positive response.[65,88]

Exercise-induced ST-segment elevation is seen most commonly in patients who have had previous myocardial infarctions.[134,148] Most series reported an incidence of 14 to 27 percent.[82,108,128,142,152] Patients with anterior myocardial infarction are more likely to have exercise-induced ST-segment elevation than are those with inferior myocardial infarction.[22,30] The ST-segment elevation almost always occurs in the leads with Q waves.[33,68] It also is associated with left ventricular wall motion abnormality, either dyskinetic or aki-

netic, in the corresponding site in over 90 percent of cases.[22,33,148] This segmental left ventricular wall motion abnormality is believed to be the underlying mechanism for the ST-segment elevation.

In postinfarction patients, exercise-induced ST-segment elevation may or may not be associated with reciprocal ST-segment depression. It has been suggested that the ST-segment depression in such instances is more likely caused by myocardial ischemia associated with multivessel disease.[152]

Ten to 30 percent of patients with variant angina also may have ST-segment elevation with exercise.[22] The leads that show ST-segment elevation are usually the same leads that record elevation during angina at rest. The ST elevation is most likely due to coronary spasm. Specchia and associates performed coronary arteriograms in 7 patients at the time of exercise-induced ST-segment elevation. Coronary spasm of a major coronary vessel was found in all.[130] Yasue and colleagues also reported similar findings in the large artery supplying the area of the myocardium corresponding to the site of the ST-segment elevation.[159] Most patients with variant angina and exercise-induced ST-segment elevation, however, also have significant fixed lesions.[31]

In the absence of previous myocardial infarction or variant angina, exercise-induced ST-segment elevation is uncommon. The reported incidence among patients with symptoms ranged from 0.2 to 1.7 percent.[22] Severe stenosis of a coronary artery is usually found (Fig. 10–6). The correlation between the site of the ST-segment elevation and the artery involved is generally good if the changes are in the anterior and lateral leads but not in the inferior leads.[35,88] The mechanism of the ST elevation in these cases is still uncertain.

CONDITIONS OFTEN ASSOCIATED WITH FALSE-POSITIVE OR FALSE-NEGATIVE EXERCISE TEST FOR CORONARY ARTERY DISEASE

Causes of False-Positive Response

The positive response in many of the following conditions does reflect myocardial ischemia. The response is referred to as *false*-positive only in terms of CAD.

1. Rheumatic heart disease with severe valvular dysfunction[67]
2. Aortic insufficiency from other cause[100]
3. Congenital aortic or pulmonary stenosis[100]
4. Pulmonary hypertension, either primary or secondary[100]
5. Constrictive pericarditis[100]
6. Severe anemia
7. Left ventricular hypertrophy[64]
8. Systemic hypertension[84,115]
9. Digitalis,[76,105,126] quinidine, procainamide
10. Hypokalemia[53,129]
11. Postprandial changes[113]
12. Hyperventilation[70,83]
13. Postural changes[81]
14. Vasoregulatory abnormalities[47,50,75]
15. Mitral valve prolapse syndrome[40,51]
16. Pectus excavatum[75]
17. Intraventricular conduction defect including bundle branch block and Wolff-Parkinson-White (WPW) syndrome[42,52,136]

In patients with severe valvular heart disease, either congenital or acquired, the associated reduction of cardiac output may interfere with adequate coronary perfusion and result in myocardial ischemia during exercise. The ischemic response in the ECG stress testing may indeed indicate relative coronary insufficiency. It is considered a false-positive result only in the sense that there is no intrinsic CAD. A similar mechanism is probably also responsible for the abnormal response in patients with pulmonary hypertension, constrictive pericarditis, or anemia. Figure 10–8 gives an example of a "false"-positive exercise test in a patient with congenital aortic stenosis. Relative coronary insufficiency is probably also the responsible mechanism in patients with left ventricular hypertrophy because of the increased muscle mass and increased oxygen demand. In 16 patients with ECG evidence of left ventricular hypertrophy and normal coronary arteriograms who were subjected to a submaximal treadmill exercise test, 6 (38 percent) were found to have positive test results.[64] Two of the patients did not have valvular heart diease. Lepeschkin and Surawicz found that subjects without symptoms and with systemic hypertension may have false-positive ECG exercise response even if left ventricular hypertrophy is not detectable.[84] Such a finding also was observed by later investigators.[115]

Digitalis is known to cause a false-positive exercise test in patients with various types of heart disease and in normal subjects.[76,105,127] In 16 young healthy subjects with normal two-step Master test results before the administration of digoxin, 8 (50 percent) had postexercise ischemic ST-segment depression of at least 1 mm after they received digitalis.[76] In another study of 98 healthy men, 25 percent had digoxin-induced positive submaximal graded exercise test results.[127] A direct relation was seen between increasing age and higher incidence of the digoxin-induced positive response. The results of the study suggested that the drug should be withdrawn for 12 days to remove its effect.[127] Administration of potassium salts lessened or abolished the changes that occurred during exercise.[76] It was proposed that loss of potassium from the myocardium may be the responsible mechanism. This explanation is supported by the finding that hypokalemia is often associated

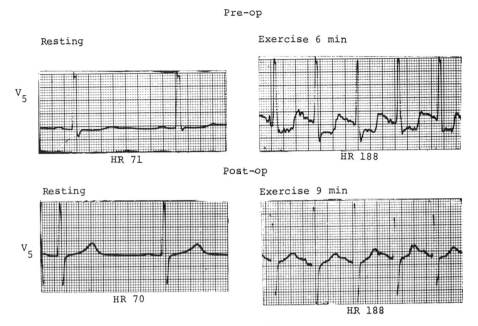

Paper speed 50mm.

FIGURE 10–8. False-positive exercise in aortic stenosis. The patient is an 11-year-old boy with severe congenital aortic stenosis. A systolic pressure gradient of 110 mm Hg across the aortic valve was demonstrated during cardiac catheterization. In the ECG, ischemic ST-segment depression is present during exercise before surgery but is not after aortic valvectomy. (Courtesy of Dr. Frederick James.)

with abnormal exercise response.[53] In one study, 8 of 12 patients with low serum potassium level showed ST-segment depression and T-wave changes after exercise, and these changes were abolished after potassium repletion. Therefore, in patients who are taking diuretics, the results of the ECG stress test should be interpreted with caution. Patients receiving quinidine or procainamide also may exhibit false-positive exercise response, the cause of which is uncertain.

Food intake may induce ST-segment and T-wave changes in the resting ECG. A "meal test" was once suggested as a form of ECG stress test.[125] Abnormal exercise response also may develop after glucose ingestion in subjects who otherwise had normal exercise ECGs.[113] It is a generally adopted practice to perform exercise testing at least 2 hours after a meal to avoid this source of variability.

Hyperventilation is known to produce ST-segment and T-wave changes that mimic those of myocardial ischemia. False-positive ECG response to exercise secondary to hyperventilation has been demonstrated in patients with normal coronary arteriogram.[70,83,89] In 46 patients with normal coronary vessels, Lary and Goldschlager observed ischemic types of ST-segment changes by hyperventilation in 7 (15 percent) of the patients.[83] In contrast, only 6 (3 percent) of 192 patients with angiographically proven CAD had such changes during hyperventilation. The mechanism for the false-positive response during hyperventilation is still unclear.

ST-segment and T-wave changes that simulate myocardial ischemia may occur with standing. This is especially common when bipolar leads are used. In a study of 200 normal subjects between the ages of 15 and 30 years, 32 (16 percent) showed such a postural change.[81] A high incidence of false-positive response on standing or with hyperventilation in healthy subjects with labile ST and T-wave changes also was reported by McHenry and associates.[94]

Several reports described a syndrome seen in young and middle-aged women consisting of angina pectoris and abnormal exercise ECG but normal coronary arteriogram.[77,78,86] The cause of the syndrome is unclear. Exercise-induced coronary spasm may be a possibility.[130] The course of the syndrome is generally benign, and the chest pain is often transient.[78]

Freisinger and associates described 40 patients, including both males and females, who had abnormal exercise test results but no other evidence of ischemic heart disease.[47] An unusual increase in heart rate on standing, ST-T wave changes on standing, ischemic ECG changes without chest discomfort, which occurred early during exercise but disappeared as exercise proceeded, were noted in these patients. Propranolol tended to abolish these changes. The authors believed this syndrome was probably due to vasoregulatory abnormalities (vasoregulatory asthenia). Similar cases were reported by others.[75]

Patients with the mitral valve prolapse syndrome and normal coronary arteriograms may have false-positive exercise responses.[39,40] This phenomenon is clinically important because chest pain is a frequent symptom in these patients. Engel and associates found that patients with vasoregulatory abnormalities often had mitral valve prolapse.[44] Mitral valve prolapse also is found to be common in patients with hyperventilation-induced ST changes.[51]

A false-positive exercise test as a result of marked pectus excavatum also has been reported in patients with normal coronary arteries.[75] The explanation for such a relation was not given.

The secondary ST-segment and T-wave changes in patients with intraventricular conduction defect such as bundle branch block and WPW syndrome interfere with proper interpretation of the exercise response. Both false-positive and false-negative responses may be seen in patients with bundle branch block.[42,107] Studies in a limited number of patients, however, suggested that the exercise test may be useful even if bundle branch block is present.[26,85,114] Further investigation in a larger number of patients is needed. False-positive diagnosis is particularly common in patients with the WPW syndrome. Gazes reported abnormal two-step Master exercise test results in 20 of 23 such patients who had no other evidence of heart disease.[52] An example is given in Figure 10–9. Strasberg and co-workers observed a false-positive response in all of the 18 patients whose preexcitation pattern persisted during treadmill exercise.[136]

Causes of False-Negative Response

Other than the inherent limitations of the exercise test in the detection of CAD, certain drugs are known to impair its sensitivity. Propranolol and other beta-adrenergic blocking agents reduce the heart rate and maximum systolic arterial blood pressure during exer-

cise and therefore decrease the left ventricular work and myocardial oxygen requirements. In 11 patients studied by Gianelli and associates, the maximum ST-segment depression was reduced from an average of 2.3 mm to 1 mm.[56] In some patients, the ST-segment depression induced by exercise became minimum or was completely prevented. The increase in exercise tolerance with nitrates in patients with angina pectoris is well known. The changes in exercise ECG also may be modified for the duration of the action of the drug.[60] Quinidine and phenothiazines also have been reported to cause false-negative response.[137]

EXERCISE TESTING IN PATIENTS WITH ABNORMAL RESTING ELECTROCARDIOGRAMS

A number of reports suggest that exercise testing may be of value even when the resting ECG is abnormal.[24,72,87] Linhart and Turnoff studied 121 patients with abnormal resting ECGs and compared the results of their maximal exercise test and coronary arteriograms with those of 57 patients who had normal resting tracings.[87] Most of the patients with abnormal resting ECGs showed nonspecific ST-segment and T-wave changes. In these patients, there was only a slight reduction of the reliability of the stress test. The sensitivity and specificity of the test were 76 and 79 percent as compared with 85 and 100 percent in patients with normal control ECGs. Kansal and associates reported on 37 patients with chest pain and ST-segment depression at rest but without obvious nonischemic causes of ST depression.[72] When correlated with coronary arteriograms, additional ischemic ST depression of 1 mm or more with submaximal grade exercise had a diagnostic sensitivity of 92 percent and a specificity of 75 percent.

ST-segment elevation may be seen in the resting ECGs of healthy subjects because of early repolarization. Although it is not an abnormal finding, the usual criteria for the interpretation of the exercise test are probably still applicable. In a study involving a relatively small number of subjects, the ST segment returned to the isoelectric baseline in patients with normal coronary arteriograms, whereas those with significant CAD had horizontal ST-segment depression.[2]

Intraventricular conduction defects, including bundle branch block, generally are considered one of the conditions that will interfere with proper interpretation of the results

Resting

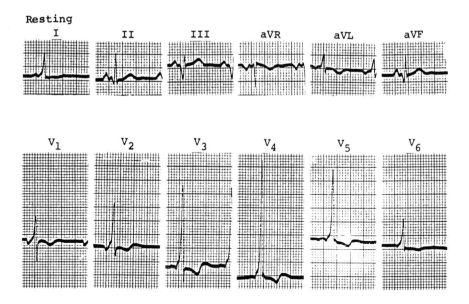

Immediately after exercise

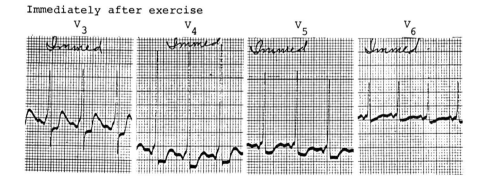

2 minutes after exercise

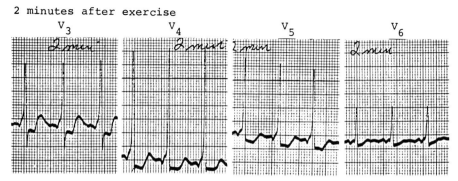

FIGURE 10–9. False-positive exercise test in Wolf-Parkinson-White syndrome. The patient is a 19-year-old man who has atypical chest pain. The resting ECG shows type A WPW pattern. The ECG recorded immediately and 2 minutes after a double Master two-step test reveals marked horizontal and downsloping ST-segment depression in leads V_3 through V_5.

of the exercise test.[52] Although earlier reports suggested that exercise-induced ST-segment depression in patients with left bundle branch block was more likely to be associated with advanced CAD,[85] the results of a later study were unable to support such a conclusion.[107] Tanaka and associates studied 30 patients with right bundle branch block.[138] Eighteen of the patients had significant CAD. They found that the exercise test had a sensitivity rate of 69 percent and a specificity rate of 45 percent in detecting CAD. The specificity of the treadmill test was greater if the ST-segment depression was recorded in leads V_4 through V_6. ST-segment depression limited to leads V_1 through V_3 often represented a false-positive response.

PROGNOSTIC VALUE OF EXERCISE TESTING

The available data indicate that the results of exercise testing have significant prognostic implications. Abnormal exercise response is associated with an increased risk of future cardiac events and mortality in both those with and those without symptoms. In addition to abnormal ST-segment changes, marked limitation in the ability to exercise is also an important sign of unfavorable prognosis.

Froelicher and associates reported on a group of 1390 air crewmen *without symptoms* who were screened for patent CAD by maximal treadmill testing.[48] They were followed for an average of 6.3 years. Angina, acute myocardial infarction, or sudden death was used as the end point for CAD. The maximal treadmill test had a sensitivity of 61 percent and a specificity of 92 percent in predicting future coronary events. Bruce and colleagues performed exercise tests in 2365 clinically healthy men and followed them for an average of 5.6 years.[16] Eleven percent of the subjects had exercise-induced ischemic ST-segment depression. The incidence of coronary events during the follow-up period in these individuals was 4.7 percent, compared with an incidence of 1.4 percent among those with normal ST-segment changes. Inability to exercise more than 6 minutes and inability to increase the heart rate to 90 percent of age-predicted normal values also were significant indicators of increased risk of coronary events. Giagnoni and associates prospectively studied 135 normotensive subjects without symptoms but with exercise-induced ischemic ST-segment depression of 1 mm or more and compared them with 379 control individuals with normal stress test results.[55] In a follow-up period of 6 years, coronary events occurred 5.5

times more often in the subjects with abnormal exercise responses. A group of 916 apparently healthy men between the age of 27 and 55 years (mean age, 37 years) were exercised and followed by McHenry and associates for an average of 12.7 years.[92] During the initial examination, 23 subjects had abnormal ST-segment responses; 9 (39 percent) of these subjects had coronary events during the follow-up period. An additional 38 subjects had conversion to an abnormal ST-segment response during serial testing; 12 (32 percent) of them had coronary events. The incidence of coronary events among the 833 subjects with normal ST-segment response to exercise was 5.3 percent (44 patients).

In a prospective study by Doyle and Kinch, 2003 *unselected* men underwent repeated treadmill exercise testings and were followed for up to 13 years.[32] Twenty-eight men had abnormal exercise test results when entered in the study; 17 (61 percent) of them had other evidence of ischemic heart disease during the follow-up period. Seventy-five men had normal responses initially but had an abnormal response during the follow-up period. Thirty-four (45 percent) of them subsequently showed clinical manifestations of CAD or experienced sudden death. Ellestad and Wan reported the results of maximal treadmill stress testing in 2700 subjects, including those with and without symptoms.[38] ST-segment depression of 1.5 mm, 0.08 second from the J point, or ST-segment elevation of 1 mm or more was used as the criterion of an abnormal test result. An abnormal response predicted an incidence of some new coronary event at a rate of 9.5 percent a year, as compared with 1.7 percent in those patients with normal test results. Early onset of ischemia occurring during the exercise was associated with a higher incidence of coronary events. The magnitude of the ST-segment depression, however, had no demonstrable relation to the incidence of coronary events. In the Multiple Risk Factor Intervention Trial (MRFIT), 6205 men between the age of 35 to 57 years underwent exercise testing and routine medical care.[110] An abnormal ST-segment depression was observed in 734 (12 percent) of the men. There was a nearly fourfold increase in 7-year coronary mortality among men with abnormal ST-segment responses to exercise compared with those with normal responses.

Degenais and associates studied 220 patients with *chest pain* and strongly abnormal (≥ 2 mm horizontal or downsloping ST-segment depression) exercise test results.[28] They found that the 5-year survival rate decreased with decreased exercise duration. In the 107 patients who had coronary arteriograms and 103 of those who had significant disease, the overall survival rate was 74 percent. All patients who achieved Bruce stage 4 survived. The survival rate was 86 percent when the patients terminated their exercise during stage 3, 73 percent during stage 2, and only 52 percent during stage 1. Weiner and associates analyzed the clinical and exercise data in 4083 medically treated patients with symptomatic CAD.[155] Among the exercise variables, the ST-segment response and the final exercise stage achieved were the most important predictors of survival. The probability of survival at 5 years was 72 percent for those patients who had 1 mm or greater ST-segment depression and who were able to achieve a level of exercise equivalent to only Bruce stage 1 or lower. It was 95 percent for those patients with less than 1 mm of ST-segment depression who were able to exercise to stage 3 or higher. Left ventricular function and number of diseased coronary vessels were the overall most important predictors of survival.

More recently, it has been shown that the survival rate in patients with silent ischemia during exercise is similar to that of patients with angina during exercise.[12,156] Patients with ST-segment elevation on exercise have poorer ventricular function and prognosis than those with ST-segment depression on exercise.[16]

Exercise Testing After Myocardial Infarction

PATIENTS WITH OLD MYOCARDIAL INFARCTION

The GXT in patients with myocardial infarction that occurred 2 or more months previously has been found useful in predicting the extent of CAD, the presence or absence of left ventricular aneurysm, and left ventricular dysfunction. Weiner and co-workers exercised 154 patients with a single previous myocardial infarction and correlated the ST-segment changes with angiography.[152] They concluded that ST-segment depression with or without ST-segment elevation in other leads suggests multivessel disease. ST-segment elevation alone or normal exercise test results suggest single-vessel disease, and ST-segment elevation with or without ST-segment depression in other leads predicts left ventricular aneurysm. The relation between ST-segment depression and multivessel CAD also was observed by others.[108,117] Patients with previous myocardial infarction and exercise-induced ST-segment el-

evation also were found to have lower left ventricular ejection fractions.[108] Stone and co-workers performed submaximal treadmill exercise 6 months after myocardial infarction in 473 patients and followed them for 12 months.[135] The mortality was significantly greater in patients who exhibited any of the following: inability to perform the exercise test because of cardiac limitations, the development of ST-segment elevation of 1 mm or greater during the exercise test, an inadequate blood pressure response during exercise, the development of any ventricular premature depolarizations during exercise or the recovery period, and inability to exercise beyond stage 1 of the modified Bruce protocol. The estimated risk or mortality ranged from 1 percent if none of these features was present to 17 percent if three or four were present.

PATIENTS WITH RECENT MYOCARDIAL INFARCTION

Limited exercise testing soon after an uncomplicated myocardial infarction has gained increasing clinical application in recent years. It is useful in evaluating the patient's prognosis and in guiding therapy.[29,133,139,140,157] The test usually is performed 2 or 3 weeks after myocardial infarction, before the patient is discharged from the hospital. In some institutions, it has been done as early as 1 week or less after infarction.[133,140] The level of exercise on the treadmill is limited by the heart rate, which is generally 120 or 130 beats/min, or 70 percent of predicted maximum heart rate for age. Some clinicians prefer to use a time limit during use of a modified Bruce protocol.[157] The exercise is terminated sooner if symptoms, unfavorable hemodynamic findings, or ventricular tachyarrhythmias develop. In patients with uncomplicated myocardial infarction who are free of angina and congestive heart failure, the risk of the limited exercise testing is low, but recurrent acute myocardial infarction or ventricular fibrillation has been reported.[109,157]

Exercise-induced angina, ST-segment displacement, hypotension, repetitive ventricular arrhythmias, and poor exercise tolerance have been predictive of higher risk for future cardiac events such as unstable angina, recurrent myocardial infarction, and cardiac death.[29,79,121,133,140,147,157] Krone and colleagues performed a low-level exercise test early after acute myocardial infarction, mostly before hospital discharge, in 667 patients and followed them for 1 year.[80] They found that patients who were unable to increase their blood pressure to 110 mm Hg or higher or to complete 9 minutes of exercise (equivalent to Bruce stage 1), or who developed ventricular arrhythmias had a 1-year mortality of 13 percent as compared with 1 percent among those who were able to do so and without ventricular arrhythmias. Senaratne and associates found the predictive value of low-level predischarge exercise test to be similar to that of symptom-related testing performed 6 weeks after infarction.[122] It also has been found that the development of ST-segment depression, especially in association with angina, and abnormal blood pressure response to exercise are highly predictive of the presence of multivessel disease.[62] This relation is observed both in patients with Q-wave and in those with non–Q-wave infarction.[124] A poor blood pressure response during the limited exercise also is suggestive of reduced left ventricular function.[132] Exercise-induced ST-segment elevation usually is associated with greater impairment of left ventricular function due to more extensive damage rather than extent of the CAD.[63]

EXERCISE TESTING FOR THE EXPOSURE OF VENTRICULAR ARRHYTHMIAS

Premature ventricular beats may be induced by exercise. In the 196 middle-aged men without overt heart disease studied by Blackburn and associates, 3 percent had premature ventricular beats at rest, but the percentage increased to 30 at the top workload.[7] Jelinek and Lown performed 1000 GXTs on 625 subjects with and without heart disease. Compared with the control resting period, the incidence of premature ventricular beats more than doubled with exercise.[71] The incidence of repetitive premature ventricular beats increased almost by eightfold. More arrhythmias were seen on recovery than during exercise. They were more easily evoked in patients with CAD than in normal subjects. Although 24-hour ambulatory ECG has been shown to be more effective in the exposure of ventricular arrhythmias, a significant number of patients developed the arrhythmias with exercise testing alone.[27,116]

The incidence and significance of exercise-induced ventricular arrhythmias depends in a large extent on the population examined. In populations without symptoms, premature ventricular beats occur in 19 to 50 percent of the subjects,[48,91] 2 to 6 percent of them having the complex form of ventricular arrhythmias. The incidence appears to increase with age[41] and with increased workload.[7] The prognostic implications of exercise-induced ventricular arrhythmias in subjects without symptoms are unclear. In the 1390 men who had no symptoms studied by Froelicher and associates and

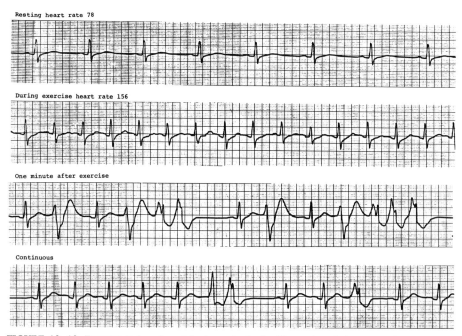

FIGURE 10–10. Exercise-induced ventricular arrhythmia. The patient is known to have coronary artery disease. No arrhythmia is seen in the resting ECG before or during the treadmill exercise test. Repetitive ventricular ectopic beats are present in the tracing 1 minute after the exercise was terminated.

followed for 6 years, the development of ventricular arrhythmias alone during exercise was found to have no predictive value for CAD.[48]

In patients with CAD, the reported incidence of exercise-induced ventricular arrhythmias ranges from 38 to 65 percent (Fig. 10–10).[59,71,91] Most studies suggest that the survival rate of patients with CAD, including those with recent myocardial infarction, is decreased if they have exercise-induced com-

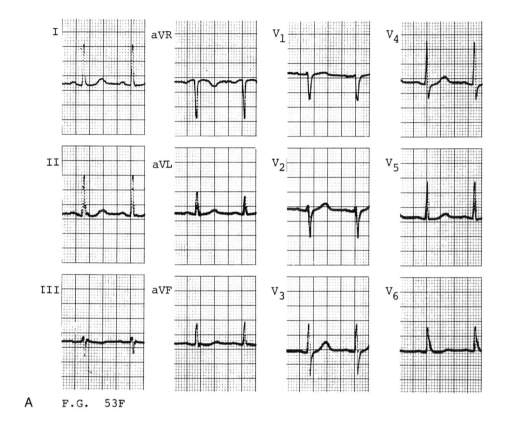

A   F.G.   53F

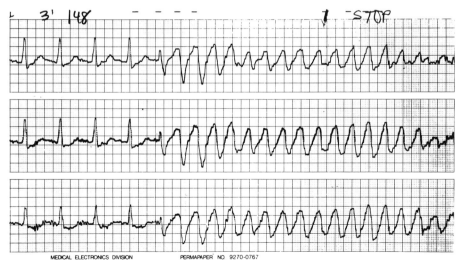

B   F.G.   53F

FIGURE 10–11. Ventricular fibrillation developed during exercise. The patient is a 53-year-old woman with a history of hypertension, diabetes, and chest pain. (A) The resting ECG shows minor nonspecific ST and T-wave abnormalities. Three minutes after the beginning of the treadmill exercise, she had a sensation of tightness in her chest. (B) The ECG revealed the appearance of ventricular tachycardia followed by ventricular fibrillation. She underwent successful defibrillation.

plex ventricular arrhythmias.[20,68,80,147] Some reports dispute such an association, however.[103,117] Significant multivessel disease is likely to be present in patients with angina and exercise-induced ventricular arrhythmias.[59,66,91] This is especially true if ST-segment changes consistent with myocardial ischemia also are present. The importance of the ischemic ST-segment changes in association with the ventricular arrhythmias is exemplified by the study of Udall and Ellestad.[143] They followed 1327 patients with known or suspected heart disease who had ventricular ectopic beats during the control, exercise, or recovery phase of treadmill exercise test for five years. The annual incidence of new coronary events (myocardial infarction, angina, cardiac deaths) was 6.4 percent in 758 patients with ventricular ectopic beats alone, 9.5 percent in 609 patients with ischemic ST-segment changes alone, and 11.4 percent in 569 patients with both premature ventricular beats and ST-segment changes.

Cardiac diseases other than CAD that also may have increased incidence of ventricular arrhythmias related to exercise include mitral valve prolapse, cardiomyopathy (congestive and hypertrophic), aortic stenosis, and long QT syndromes. The prognostic significance of exercise-induced arrhythmias in these conditions is unknown.[57]

SAFETY OF THE EXERCISE TEST

Rochmis and Blackburn reported a survey of the safety experience of 170,000 exercise stress tests performed in 73 medical centers.[114] Sixteen documented deaths were attributed to the exercise, a mortality of 1 in 10,000 tests. Nonfatal complications that required hospitalization within 1 week of the test occurred at the rate of about 3 per 10,000 tests. In a report of 1377 symptom-limited exercise tests performed in 263 patients with histories of ventricular tachycardia or fibrillation, serious but nonfatal arrhythmia complications occurred during 2.3 percent of the tests, involving 9.1 percent of the patients.[160] The incidence of such complications in 8221 maximal exercise tests involving 3444 patients without histories of sustained ventricular arrhythmias performed in the same institution was 0.05 percent. Although exercise test generally is safe, the occasional patients that develop serious complications (Fig. 10–11) remind us that this noninvasive test should not be performed indiscriminately.

REFERENCES

1. Abarquez RF Jr, Kintanar QL, Valdez EV, et al: Evaluation of some criteria for the dynamic and post-exercise electrocardiogram in diagnosing coronary insufficiency. Am J Cardiol 13:310, 1964
2. Alimurung BN, Gilbert CA, Felner JM, et al: The influence of early repolarization variant on the exercise electrocardiogram: A correlation with coronary arteriograms. Am Heart J 99:739, 1980
3. Baron DW, Ilsley C, Sheiban I, et al: R wave amplitude during exercise: Relation to left ventricular function and coronary artery disease. Br Heart J 44:512, 1980
4. Bartel AG, Behar VS, Peter RH, et al: Graded exercise stress tests in angiographically documented coronary artery disease. Circulation 49:348, 1974
5. Battler A, Froelicher V, Slutsky R, et al: Relationship of QRS amplitude changes during exercise to left ventricular function and volumes and the diagnosis of coronary artery disease. Circulation 60:1004, 1979
6. Berman JL, Wynne J, Cohn PF: Multiple-lead QRS changes with exercise testing: Diagnostic value and hemodynamic implications. Circulation 61:53, 1980
7. Blackburn H, Taylor HL, Hamrell B, et al: Premature ventricular complexes induced by stress testing. Am J Cardiol 31:441, 1973
8. Blackburn H, Taylor HL, Okamoto N, et al: The exercise electrocardiogram: A systematic comparison of chest lead configurations employed for monitoring during exercise, In Karvonen M, Barry A (eds): Physical Activity and the Heart. Springfield, IL, Charles C Thomas, 1966
9. Blackburn H, Katigbak R: What electrocardiographic leads to take after exercise? Am Heart J 67:184, 1964
10. Blumenthal DS, Weiss JL, Mellits ED, et al: The predictive value of a strongly positive stress test in patients with minimal symptoms. Am J Med 70:1005, 1981
11. Bonoris PE, Greenberg PS, Christison GW, et al: Evaluation of R wave amplitude changes versus ST-segment depression in stress testing. Circulation 57:904, 1978
12. Bonow RO, Bacharach ST, Green MV, et al: Prognostic implications of symptomatic versus asymptomatic (silent) myocardial ischemia induced by exercise in mildly symptomatic and in asymptomatic patients with angiographically documented coronary artery disease. Am J Cardiol 60:778, 1987
13. Borer JS, Brensike JF, Redwood DR, et al: Limitations of the electrocardiographic response to exercise in predicting coronary artery disease. N Engl J Med 293:367, 1975
14. Braat SH, Kingma JH, Brugada P, Wellens HJJ: Value of lead V_{4R} in exercise testing to predict proximal stenosis of the right coronary artery. J Am Coll Cardiol 5:1308, 1985
15. Brody AJ: Master two-step exercise test in clinically unselected patients. JAMA 171:1195, 1959
16. Bruce RA, DeRouen TA, Hossack KF: Value of maximal exercise tests in risk assessment of primary coronary artery disease events in healthy men: Five years' experience of the Seattle Heart Watch Study. Am J Cardiol 46:371, 1980
17. Bruce RA, Fisher LD, Pettinger M, et al: ST segment elevation with exercise: A marker for poor ventricular function and poor prognosis. Coronary Artery

Surgery Study (CASS) confirmation of Seattle Heart Watch results. Circulation 77:897, 1988

18. Bruce RA, Gey CO, Cooper MN, et al: Seattle Heart Watch: Initial clinical, circulatory and electrocardiographic responses to maximal exercise. Am J Cardiol 33:459, 1974

19. Bruce RA, Hornsten TR: Exercise stress testing in evaluation of patients with ischemic heart disease. Prog Cardiovasc Dis 11:371, 1969

20. Califf RM, McKinnis RA, McNeer JF, et al: Prognostic value of ventricular arrhythmias associated with treadmill exercise testing in patients studied with cardiac catheterization for suspected ischemic heart disease. J Am Coll Cardiol 2:1060, 1983

21. Chahine RA, Raizner AE, Ishimori T: The clinical significance of exercise-induced ST-segment elevation. Circulation 54:209, 1976

22. Chaitman BR, Waters DD, Theroux P, et al: S-T segment elevation and coronary spasm in response to exercise. Am J Cardiol 47:1350, 1981

23. Cohn PF, Vokonas PS, Herman MV, et al: Postexercise electrocardiogram in patients with abnormal resting electrocardiograms. Circulation 43:648, 1971

24. Cohn PF, Vokonas PS, Most AS, et al: Diagnostic accuracy of two-step postexercise ECG. JAMA 220:501, 1972

25. Colby J, Hakki AH, Iskandrian AS, et al: Hemodynamic, angiographic and scintigraphic correlates of positive exercise electrocardiograms: Emphasis on strongly positive exercise electrocardiograms. J Am Coll Cardiol 2:21, 1983

26. Cooksey JD, Parker BM, Bahl OP: The diagnostic contribution of exercise testing in left bundle branch block. Am Heart J 88:482, 1974

27. Crawford M, O'Rourke RA, Ramakrishna N, et al: Comparative effectiveness of exercise testing and continuous monitoring for detecting arrhythmias in patients with previous myocardial infarction. Circulation 50:301, 1974

28. Dagenais GR, Rouleau JR, Christen A, et al: Survival of patients with a strongly positive exercise electrocardiogram. Circulation 65:452, 1982

29. Davidson DM, DeBusk RF: Prognostic value of a single exercise test 3 weeks after uncomplicated myocardial infarction. Circulation 61:236, 1980

30. de Feyter PJ, Majid PA, van Eenige MJ, et al: Clinical significance of exercise-induced ST-segment elevation. Br Heart J 46:84, 1981

31. de Servi S, Falcone C, Gavazzi A, et al: The exercise test in variant angina: Results in 114 patients. Circulation 64:684, 1981

32. Doyle JT, Kinch SH: The prognosis of an abnormal electrocardiographic stress test. Circulation 41:545, 1970

33. Dunn RF, Bailey IK, Uren R, et al: Exercise-induced ST-segment elevation: Correlation of thallium-201 myocardial perfusion scanning and coronary arteriography. Circulation 61:989, 1980

34. Dunn RF, Freedman B, Bailey IK, et al: Localization of coronary artery disease with exercise electrocardiography: Correlation with thallium-201 myocardial perfusion scanning. Am J Cardiol 48:839, 1981

35. Dunn RF, Freedman B, Kelly DT, et al: Exercise-induced ST-segment elevation in leads V_1 or aVL: A predictor of anterior myocardial ischemia and left anterior descending coronary artery disease. Circulation 63:1357, 1981

36. Elamin MS, Boyle R, Kardash MM, et al: Accurate detection of coronary heart disease by new exercise test. Br Heart J 48:311, 1982

37. Elamin MS, Mary DASG, Smith DR, Linden RJ: Prediction of severity of coronary artery disease using slope of submaximal ST segment/heart rate relationship. Cardiovasc Res 14:681, 1980

38. Ellestad MH, Wan MKC: Predictive implications of stress testing: Follow-up of 2700 subjects after maximum treadmill stress testing. Circulation 51:363, 1975

39. Engel PJ, Alpert BL, Hickman JR Jr: The nature and prevalence of the abnormal exercise electrocardiogram in mitral valve prolapse. Am Heart J 98:716, 1979

40. Engel PJ, Alpert BL, Triebwasser JH, et al: Exercise testing in mitral valve prolapse. Am J Cardiol 41:430, 1978

41. Faris JV, McHenry PL, Jordan JW, et al: Prevalence and reproducibility of exercise-induced ventricular arrhythmias during maximal exercise testing in normal men. Am J Cardiol 37:617, 1976

42. Feil H, Brofman BL: The effect of exercise on the electrocardiogram of bundle branch block. Am Heart J 45:665, 1953

43. Finkelhor RS, Newhouse KE, Vrobel TR, et al: The ST segment/heart rate slope as a predictor of coronary artery disease: Comparison with quantitative thallium imaging and conventional ST segment criteria. Am Heart J 112:296, 1986

44. Fortuin NJ, Friesinger GC: Exercise-induced S-T segment elevation. Am J Med 49:459, 1970

45. Fox K, England D, Jonathan A, et al: Inability of exercise-induced R wave changes to predict coronary artery disease. Am J Cardiol 49:674, 1982

46. Fox RM, Hakki AH, Iskandrian AS: Relation between electrocardiographic and scintigraphic location of myocardial ischemia during exercise in one-vessel coronary artery disease. Am J Cardiol 53:1529, 1984

47. Friesinger GC, Biern RO, Likar I, et al: Exercise electrocardiography and vasoregulatory abnormalities. Am J Cardiol 30:733, 1972

48. Froelicher VF, Thomas MM, Pillow C, et al: Epidemiologic study of asymptomatic men screened by maximal treadmill testing for latent coronary artery disease. Am J Cardiol 34:770, 1974

49. Froelicher VF, Yanowitz FG, Thompson AJ, et al: The correlation of coronary angiography and the electrocardiographic response to maximal treadmill testing in 76 asymptomatic men. Circulation 48:597, 1973

50. Furberg C: Adrenergic beta-blockade and electrocardiographic ST-T changes. Acta Med Scand 181:21, 1967

51. Gardin JM, Isner JM, Ronan JA, et al: Pseudoischemic "false positive" S-T segment changes induced by hyperventilation in patients with mitral valve prolapse. Am J Cardiol 45:952, 1980

52. Gazes PC: False-positive exercise test in the presence of the Wolff-Parkinson-White syndrome. Am Heart J 78:13, 1969

53. Georgopoulos AJ, Proudfit WL, Page IH: Effect of exercise on electrocardiograms of patients with low serum potassium. Circulation 23:567, 1961

54. Gerson MC, Phillips JF, Morris SN, et al: Exercise-induced U-wave inversion as a marker of stenosis of the left anterior descending coronary artery. Circulation 60:1014, 1979

55. Giagnoni E, Secchi MB, Wu SC, et al: Prognostic value of exercise EKG testing in asymptomatic normotensive subjects: A prospective matched study. N Engl J Med 309:1085, 1983

56. Gianelli RD, Treister BL, Harrison DC: The effect of

propranolol on exercise induced ischemic S-T depression. Am J Cardiol 24:161, 1969

57. Goldschlager N, Cohn K, Goldschlager A: Exercise-related ventricular arrhythmias. Mod Concepts Cardiovasc Dis 48:67, 1979

58. Goldschlager N, Selzer A, Cohn K: Treadmill stress tests as indicators of presence and severity of coronary artery disease. Ann Intern Med 85:277, 1976

59. Goldschlager N, Cake D, Cohn K: Exercise-induced ventricular arrhythmias in patients with coronary artery disease: Their relationship to angiographic findings. Am J Cardiol 31:434, 1973

60. Goldstein RE, Rosing DR, Redwood DR, et al: Clinical and circulatory effects of isosorbide dinitrate: Comparison with nitroglycerin. Circulation 43:629, 1971

61. Greenberg PS, Friscia DA, Ellestad MH: Predictive accuracy of Q-X/Q-T ratio, Q-Tc interval, S-T depression and R wave amplitude during stress testing. Am J Cardiol 44:18, 1979

62. Griffith L, Varnauskas E, Wall J, et al: Correlation of coronary arteriography after acute myocardial infarction with predischarge limited exercise test response. Am J Cardiol 61:201, 1988

63. Haines DE, Beller GA, Watson DD, et al: Exercise-induced ST segment elevation 2 weeks after uncomplicated myocardial infarction: Contributing factors and prognostic significance. Am J Coll Cardiol 9:996, 1987

64. Harris CN, Aronow WS, Parker DP, et al: Treadmill stress test in left ventricular hypertrophy. Chest 63:353, 1973

65. Hegge FN, Tuna N, Burchell HB: Coronary arteriographic findings in patients with axis shifts or S-T segment elevations on exercise-stress testing. Am Heart J 86:603, 1973

66. Helfant RH, Pine R, Kabde V, et al: Exercise-related ventricular premature complexes in coronary heart disease: Correlations with ischemia and angiographic severity. Ann Intern Med 80:589, 1974

67. Hellerstein HK, Prozan GB, Leibow IM, et al: The two-step exercise test as a test of cardiac function in chronic rheumatic heart disease and in arteriosclerotic heart disease with old myocardial infarction. Am J Cardiol 7:234, 1961

68. Henry RL, Kennedy GT, Crawford MH: Prognostic value of exercise-induced ventricular ectopic activity for mortality after acute myocardial infarction. Am J Cardiol 59:1251, 1987

69. Hopkirk JA, Uhl GS, Hickman JR, Fischer J: Limitation of exercise-induced R wave amplitude changes in detecting coronary artery disease in asymptomatic men. J Am Coll Cardiol 3:821, 1984

70. Jacobs WF, Battle WE, Ronan JA: False-positive ST-T wave changes secondary to hyperventilation and exercise. Ann Intern Med 81:479, 1974

71. Jelinek MV, Lown B: Exercise stress testing for exposure of cardiac arrhythmia. Prog Cardiovasc Dis 16:497, 1974

72. Kansal S, Roitman D, Sheffield LT: Stress testing and ST-segment depression at rest. Circulation 54:636, 1976

73. Kaplan MA, Harris CM, Aronow WS, et al: Inability of the submaximal treadmill stress test to predict the location of coronary disease. Circulation 47:250, 1973

74. Karnegis JN, Matts J, Tuna N, et al: Comparison of exercise-positive with recovery-positive treadmill graded exercise tests. Am J Cardiol 60:544, 1987

75. Katts AA: Exercise electrocardiography: Recognition of the ischemic response, false positive and negative patterns. Am J Cardiol 33:721, 1974

76. Kawai C, Hultgren HN: The effect of digitalis upon the exercise electrocardiogram. Am Heart J 68:409, 1964

77. Kemp HG, Elliott WC, Gorlin R: The anginal syndrome with normal coronary arteriography. Trans Assoc Am Physician 80:59, 1967

78. Kimbiris D, Waxler E, Dreifus LS: Fate of women with chest pain resembling angina pectoris and normal coronary arteriography (Abstract). Circulation 42(Suppl III):73, 1970

79. Koppes GM, Kruyer W, Beckmann CH, et al: Response to exercise early after uncomplicated acute myocardial infarction in patients receiving no medication: Long-term follow-up. Am J Cardiol 46:764, 1980

80. Krone RJ, Gillespie JA, Weld FM, et al: Low-level exercise testing after myocardial infarction: Usefulness in enhancing clinical risk stratification. Circulation 71:80, 1985

81. Lachman AB, Semler HJ, Gustafson RH: Postural S-T-T changes in the radioelectrocardiogram simulating myocardial ischemia. Circulation 31:557, 1965

82. Lahiri A, Balasubramanian V, Millar-Craig MW, et al: Exercise-induced ST segment elevation: Electrocardiographic, angiographic, and scintigraphic evaluation. Br Heart J 43:582, 1980

83. Lary D, Goldschlager N: Electrocardiographic changes during hyperventilation resembling myocardial ischemia in patients with normal coronary arteriograms. Am Heart J 87:383, 1974

84. Lepeschkin E, Surawicz B: Characteristics of true positive and false positive results of electrocardiographic Master two-step exercise test. N Engl J Med 258:511, 1958

85. Lewis CM, Dagenais GR, Friesinger CG, et al: Coronary arteriographic appearance in patients with left bundle branch block. Circulation 41:299, 1970

86. Likoff W, Segal BL, Kasparian H: Paradox of normal selective coronary arteriograms in patients considered to have unmistakable coronary heart disease. N Engl J Med 276:1063, 1967

87. Linhart JW, Turnoff HB: Maximum treadmill exercise test in patients with abnormal control electrocardiograms. Circulation 49:667, 1974

88. Longhurst JC, Kraus WL: Exercise-induced ST elevation in patients without myocardial infarction. Circulation 60:616, 1979

89. McHenry PL, Cogan OJ, Elliott WC, et al: False positive ECG response to exercise secondary to hyperventilation: Cineangiographic correlation. Am Heart J 79:683, 1970

90. McHenry PL, Fisch C: Clinical applications of the treadmill exercise test. Mod Concepts Cardiovasc Dis 46:21, 1977

91. McHenry PL, Morris SN, Kavalier M, et al: Comparative study of exercise-induced ventricular arrhythmias in normal subjects and patients with documented coronary artery disease. Am J Cardiol 37:609, 1976

92. McHenry PL, O'Donnell J, Morris SN, Jordan JJ: The abnormal exercise electrocardiogram in apparently healthy men: A predictor of angina pectoris as an initial coronary event during long-term follow-up. Circulation 70:547, 1984

93. McHenry PL, Phillips JF, Knoebel SB: Correlation of computer-quantitated treadmill exercise electrocardiogram with arteriographic location of coronary artery disease. Am J Cardiol 30:747, 1972

94. McHenry PL, Richmond HW, Weisenberger BL, et al: Evaluation of abnormal exercise electrocardiogram in apparently healthy subjects: Labile repolar-

ization (ST-T) abnormalities as a cause of false-positive responses. Am J Cardiol 47:1152, 1981

95. McNeer JF, Margolis JR, Lee KL, et al: The role of the exercise test in the evaluation of patients for ischemic heart disease. Circulation 57:64, 1978

96. Martin CM, McConahay DR: Maximal treadmill exercise electrocardiography: Correlations with coronary arteriography and cardiac hemodynamics. Circulation 46:956, 1972

97. Mason RE, Likar I, Biern RO, et al: Multiple-lead exercise electrocardiography: Experience in 107 normal subjects and 67 patients with angina pectoris, and comparison with coronary cinearteriography in 84 patients. Circulation 36:517, 1967

98. Master AM: The two-step test of myocardial function. Am Heart J 10:495, 1935

99. Master AM: The Master two-step test. Am Heart J 75:809, 1968

100. Mattingly TW: The postexercise electrocardiogram: Its value in the diagnosis and prognosis of coronary arterial disease. Am J Cardiol 9:395, 1962

101. Morales-Ballejo H, Greenberg PS, Ellestad MH, Bible M: Septal Q wave in exercise testing: Angiographic correlation. Am J Cardiol 48:247, 1981

102. Morris SN, Phillips JF, Jordan JW, et al: Incidence and significance of decreases in systolic blood pressure during graded treadmill exercise testing. Am J Cardiol 41:221, 1978

103. Nair CK, Aronow WS, Sketch MH, et al: Diagnostic and prognostic significance of exercise-induced premature ventricular complexes in men and women: A four year follow-up. J Am Coll Cardiol 5:1201, 1985

104. Nohara R, Kambara H, Suzuki Y, et al: Septal Q wave in exercise testing: Evaluation by single-photon emission computed tomography. Am J Cardiol 55:905, 1985

105. Nordstrom-Ohrberg G: Effect of digitalis glycosides on electrocardiogram and exercise test in healthy subjects. Acta Med Scand 176(Suppl 420):1, 1964

106. Okin PM, Kligfield P, Ameisen O, et al: Identification of anatomically extensive coronary artery disease by the exercise ECG ST segment/heart rate slope. Am Heart J 115:1002, 1988

107. Orzan F, Garcia E, Mathur VS, et al: Is the treadmill exercise test useful for evaluating coronary artery disease in patients with complete left bundle branch block? Am J Cardiol 42:36, 1978

108. Paine RD, Dye LE, Roitman DI, et al: Relation of graded exercise test findings after myocardial infarction to extent of coronary artery disease and left ventricular dysfunction. Am J Cardiol 42:716, 1978

109. Pederson A, Grande P, Saunamaki K, et al: Exercise testing after myocardial infarction (Letter). N Engl J Med 302:174, 1980

110. Rautaharju PM, Prineas RJ, Eifler WJ, et al: Prognostic value of exercise electrocardiogram in men at high risk of future coronary heart disease: Multiple risk factor intervention trial experience. J Am Coll Cardiol 8:1, 1986

111. Redwood DR, Borer JS, Epstein SE: Whither the ST segment during exercise? Circulation 54:703, 1976

112. Rijneke AD, Ascoop CA, Talmon JL: Clinical significance of upsloping ST segments in exercise electrocardiography. Circulation 61:671, 1980

113. Riley CP, Oberman A, Sheffield LT: Electrocardiographic effects of glucose ingestion. Arch Intern Med 130:703, 1972

114. Rochmis P, Blackburn H: Exercise tests: A survey of procedures, safety and litigation experience in approximately 170,000 tests. JAMA 217:1061, 1971

115. Roitman D, Jones WB, Sheffield LT: Comparison of submaximal exercise ECG test with coronary cineangiocardiogram. Ann Intern Med 72:641, 1970

116. Ryan M, Lown B, Horn H: Comparison of ventricular ectopic activity during 24-hour monitoring and exercise testing in patients with coronary heart disease. N Engl J Med 292:224, 1975

117. Sami M, Chaitman B, Fisher L, et al: Significance of exercise-induced ventricular arrhythmia in stable coronary artery disease: a Coronary Artery Surgery Study project. Am J Cardiol 54:1182, 1984

118. Sanmarco ME, Pontius S, Selvester RH: Abnormal blood pressure response and marked ischemic ST-segment depression as predictors of severe coronary artery disease. Circulation 61:572, 1980

119. Schlant RC, Blomqvist CG, Brandenburg RO, et al: Guidelines for exercise testing: A report of the American College of Cardiology/American Heart Association Task Force on Assessment of Cardiovascular Procedures. J Am Coll Cardiol 8:725, 1986

120. Schneider RM, Seaworth JF, Dohrmann ML, et al: Anatomic and prognostic implications of an early positive treadmill exercise test. Am J Cardiol 50:682, 1982

121. Schwartz KM, Turner JD, Sheffield LT, et al: Limited exercise testing soon after myocardial infarction. Ann Intern Med 94:727, 1981

122. Senaratne MPJ, Hsu L, Rossall RE, Kappagoda T: Exercise testing after myocardial infarction: Relative values of the low level predischarge and postdischarge exercise test. J Am Coll Cardiol 12:1416, 1988

123. Sheffield LT, Holt JH, Reeves TJ: Exercise graded by heart rate in electrocardiographic testing for angina pectoris. Circulation 32:622, 1965

124. Sia STB, MacDonald PS, Horowitz JD, et al: Usefulness of early exercise testing after non–Q-wave myocardial infarction in predicting prognosis. Am J Cardiol 57:738, 1986

125. Simonson E: Electrocardiographic stress tolerance tests. Prog Cardiovasc Dis 13:269, 1970

126. Sketch MH, Mohiuddin SM, Lynch JD, et al: Significant sex differences in the correlation of electrocardiographic exercise testing and coronary arteriograms. Am J Cardiol 36:169, 1975

127. Sketch MH, Mooss AN, Butler ML, et al: Digoxin-induced positive exercise tests: Their clinical and prognostic significance. Am J Cardiol 48:655, 1981

128. Smith JW, Dennis CA, Gassmann A, et al: Exercise testing three weeks after myocardial infarction. Chest 75:12, 1979

129. Soloff LA, Fewell JW: Abnormal electrocardiographic responses in exercise in subjects with hypokalemia. Am J Med Sci 242:724, 1961

130. Specchia G, de Servi S, Falcone C, et al: Significance of exercise-induced ST-segment elevation in patients without myocardial infarction. Circulation 63:46, 1981

131. Sriwattanakomen S, Ticzon AR, Zubritzky SA, et al: S-T segment elevation during exercise: Electrocardiographic and arteriographic correlation in 38 patients. Am J Cardiol 45:762, 1980

132. Starling MR, Crawford MH, Richards KL, et al: Predictive value of early postmyocardial infarction modified treadmill exercise testing in multivessel coronary artery disease detection. Am Heart J 102:169, 1981

133. Starling MR, Crawford MH, Henry RL, et al: Prognostic value of electrocardiographic exercise testing and noninvasive assessment of left ventricular ejection fraction soon after acute myocardial infarction. Am J Cardiol 57:532, 1986

134. Stiles GL, Rosati RA, Wallace AG: Clinical relevance of exercise-induced S-T segment elevation. Am J Cardiol 46:931, 1980

135. Stone PH, Turi ZG, Muller JE, et al: Prognostic significance of the treadmill exercise test performance 6 months after myocardial infarction. J Am Coll Cardiol 8:1007, 1986

136. Strasberg B, Ashley WW, Wyndham CRC, et al: Treadmill exercise testing in the Wolff-Parkinson-White syndrome. Am J Cardiol 45:742, 1980

137. Surawicz B, Saito S: Exercise testing for detection of myocardial ischemia in patients with abnormal electrocardiograms at rest. Am J Cardiol 41:943, 1978

138. Tanaka T, Friedman MJ, Okada RD, et al: Diagnostic value of exercise-induced ST segment depression in patients with right bundle branch block. Am J Cardiol 41:670, 1978

139. Theroux P, Marpole DG, Bourassa MG: Exercise stress testing in the post-myocardial infarction patient. Am J Cardiol 52:664, 1983

140. Theroux P, Water DD, Halphen C, et al: Prognostic value of exercise testing soon after myocardial infarction. N Engl J Med 301:341, 1979

141. Topol EJ, Juni JE, O'Neill WW, et al: Exercise testing three days after onset of acute myocardial infarction. Am J Cardiol 60:958, 1987

142. Tubau JF, Chaitman BR, Bourassa MG, et al: Detection of multivessel coronary disease after myocardial infarction using exercise stress testing and multiple ECG lead systems. Circulation 61:44, 1980

143. Udall JA, Ellestad MH: Predictive implications of ventricular premature contractions associated with treadmill stress testing. Circulation 56:985, 1977

144. Val PG, Chaitman BR, Waters DD, et al: Diagnostic accuracy of exercise ECG lead systems in clinical subsets of women. Circulation 65:1465, 1982

145. Vasey C, O'Donnell J, Morris S, McHenry P: Exercise-induced left bundle branch block and its relation to coronary artery disease. Am J Cardiol 56:892, 1985

146. Wagner S, Cohn S, Selzer A: Unreliability of exercise-induced R wave changes as indexes of coronary artery disease. Am J Cardiol 44:1241, 1979

147. Waters DD, Bosch X, Bouchard A, et al: Comparison of clinical variables and variables derived from a limited predischarge exercise test as predictors of early and late mortality after myocardial infarction. J Am Coll Cardiol 5:1, 1985

148. Waters DD, Chaitman BR, Bourassa MG, et al: Clin-

ical and angiographic correlates of exercise-induced ST-segment elevation: Increased detection with multiple ECG leads. Circulation 61:286, 1980

149. Wayne V, Bishop R, Cook L, Spodick D: Exercise-induced bundle branch block. Am J Cardiol 52:283, 1983

150. Weiner DA: Exercise testing for the diagnosis and severity of coronary disease. J Cardiac Rehab 1:438, 1981

151. Weiner DA, McCabe CH, Cutler SS, et al: Decrease in systolic blood pressure during exercise testing: Reproducibility, response to coronary bypass surgery and prognostic significance. Am J Cardiol 49:1627, 1982

152. Weiner DA, McCabe CH, Klein MD, et al: ST segment changes postinfarction: Predictive value for multivessel coronary disease and left ventricular aneurysm. Circulation 58:887, 1978

153. Weiner DA, McCabe CH, Ryan TJ: Identification of patients with left main and three vessel coronary disease with clinical and exercise test variables. Am J Cardiol 46:21, 1980

154. Weiner DA, Ryan TJ, McCabe CH, et al: Correlations among history of angina: ST-segment response and prevalence of coronary artery disease in the Coronary Artery Surgery Study (CASS). N Engl J Med 301:230, 1979

155. Weiner Da, Ryan TJ, McCabe CH, et al: Prognostic importance of a clinical profile and exercise test in medically treated patients with coronary artery disease. J Am Coll Cardiol 3:772, 1984

156. Weiner DA, Ryan TJ, McCabe CH, et al: Significance of silent myocardial ischemia during exercise testing in patients with coronary artery disease. Am J Cardiol 59:725, 1987

157. Weld FM, Chu KL, Bigger JT, et al: Risk stratification with low-level exercise testing 2 weeks after acute myocardial infarction. Circulation 64:306, 1981

158. Williams MA, Esterbrooks DJ, Nair CK, et al: Clinical significance of exercise-induced bundle branch block. Am J Cardiol 61:346, 1988

159. Yasue H, Omote S, Takizawa A, et al: Circadian variation of exercise capacity in patients with Prinzmetal's variant angina: Role of exercise-induced coronary arterial spasm. Circulation 59:938, 1979

160. Young DZ, Lampert S, Graboys TB, et al: Safety of maximal exercise testing in patients at high risk for ventricular arrhythmia. Circulation 70:184, 1984

161. Young SG, Froelicher VF: Exercise testing: An update. Mod Concepts Cardiovas Dis 52:25, 1983

Pericarditis

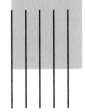

11

In acute pericarditis, the most characteristic electrocardiographic (ECG) finding is the diffuse ST-segment displacement (Fig. 11–1). This finding generally is attributed to the associated subepicardial myocarditis.[3] The inflammatory process induces a zone of injury in the superficial layer of the myocardium. According to the blocking of depolarization theory,* the injured zone is only partially depolarized and becomes electrically more positive than the rest of the myocardium at the end of depolarization. Abnormal ST vectors appear that are directed away from the ventricular cavity and toward the epicardium. The sum of these forces, or the mean ST vector, is oriented toward the cardiac apex (i.e., leftward, inferiorly, and anteriorly). The direction is therefore similar to that of the normal ST vector as well as to that of the mean QRS vector. Leads that face the epicardial surface record ST-segment elevation, and those that face the endocardium or the ventricular cavity record ST-segment depression. ST-segment elevation is present in most of the conventional leads except lead aVR, in which it is depressed. Lead V_1 may show ST-segment depression, since it faces the surface of the right atrium. If the QRS axis is horizontal, ST-segment depression occasionally may be seen in lead III; if the axis is vertical, it may be seen in lead aVL.

If the subepicardial injury is less severe or is subsiding, diffuse T-wave inversion rather than ST-segment displacement is observed (Fig. 11–2). The T-wave changes are probably due to a delay in the recovery of the injured subepicardial myocardium. The ventricular repolarization now proceeds from the endocardium toward the epicardium, which is the reverse of the normal process. The resultant T vector is directed to the right, posteriorly, and superiorly. T-wave inversion is therefore observed in leads that normally display upright T waves.

When pericardial fluid accumulates, its short-circuiting effect may reduce the amplitude of the QRS complex. In some instances, the voltage is decreased because of the insulating effect of fibrin deposit.[44] The genesis of electrical alternans in pericardial effusion is discussed later in this chapter.

In chronic constrictive pericarditis, subepicardial fibrosis is probably responsible for the persistence of T-wave abnormalities. The QRS voltage may be markedly reduced because of myocardial atrophy.[10] The compression scar involving the atrial musculature may cause abnormal P waves and atrial fibrillation.

ELECTROCARDIOGRAPHIC CHANGES IN ACUTE PERICARDITIS WITH OR WITHOUT PERICARDIAL EFFUSION

1. P wave, PR-segment changes, and atrial arrhythmias
2. Low voltage of the QRS complex
3. Electrical alternans
4. Diffuse ST-segment elevation and T-wave inversion.

P Wave, PR-Segment Changes, and Atrial Arrhythmias

The P wave usually is not affected in acute pericarditis. Its amplitude remains normal even when pericardial effusion is present. This is explained by the absence of effusion over the posterior surface of the atria, which is only partly covered by the pericardium.[44]

Spodick[39–41] and others[7] described PR-segment (STa) shift in patients with acute pericarditis. It was reported in as many as 82 percent of the patients and occurred mainly in the early stage of the disease while the ST segment was elevated or returning to the baseline but before the T waves became inverted. The

---

*For the sake of simplicity, other theories are not discussed here. They were described in an article by Fowler.[13]

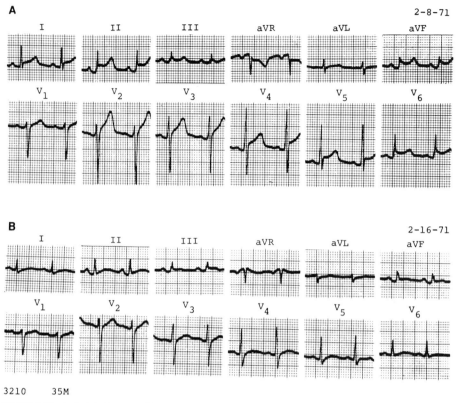

3210   35M

FIGURE 11–1. Serial changes of acute idiopathic pericarditis in a 36-year-old man. (A) Diffuse ST-segment elevation involving all the leads except aVR and aVL. In lead aVR, the ST-segment is depressed. The QRS complex is normal. (B) The ST segment is almost isoelectric, and the T waves are flattened or notched. (C) (*See facing page*) The T waves are definitely inverted in tracing recorded 1 week later but are limited to leads II, III, aVF, V5, and V6. (D) Tracing shows partial return of the T waves to normal pattern 7 weeks after the onset of the illness.

PR segment was depressed in all leads except lead aVR and occasionally lead V_1. In lead aVR, it was always elevated. These changes are attributed to subepicardial atrial injury. Because the atria are located posteriorly, to the right, and superior to the ventricles, the electrical forces generated from the epicardial injury are therefore oriented in this direction. Their orientation, in fact, is the same as the normal atrial ST and T vector, but the magnitude is increased. It was proposed that any PR-segment depression of more than 0.8 mm or elevation of more than 0.5 mm may be considered consistent with atrial injury.[7]

Figure 11–3 is the ECG of a 19-year-old man with idiopathic pericarditis. The PR-segment displacement is seen best in leads II, aVR, aVF, and V_4 through V_6. In my experience, a definite PR-segment displacement is not common. In many cases, it is difficult to establish the level of isoelectric line because of tachycardia and ST-segment elevation.

As a rule, cardiac arrhythmias are not common in *acute* pericarditis. When they occur, they usually are supraventricular in origin. Bellet and McMillan described atrial arrhythmias in 6 of their 57 cases of acute pericarditis of various causes.[3] In a prospective study of 100 consecutive cases, Spodick found arrhythmias, all atrial, in 7 patients.[38] All 7 patients had associated underlying heart disease, and 5 of the 7 had atrial fibrillation. Junctional tachycardia and atrial flutter were seen in the other 2 patients. In my experience, atrial flutter is encountered almost as often as atrial fibrillation. James' pathologic studies in patients who had pericarditis and atrial arrhythmias showed that the sinus node was involved in all.[22]

Low Voltage of the QRS Complex

In acute pericarditis without significant pericardial effusion, the QRS complex usually is

2-23-71

C

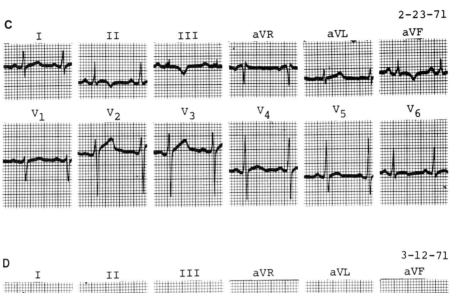

3-12-71

D

3210   35M

FIGURE 11–1. *Continued*

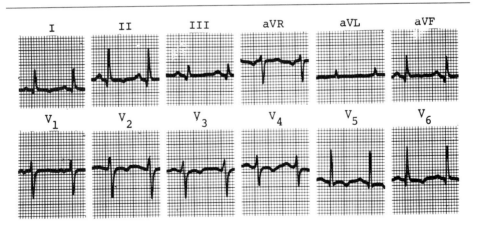

5378   29F

FIGURE 11–2. Diffuse T-wave inversion in acute idiopathic pericarditis. The tracing was recorded from a 29-year-old woman 4 days after the onset of substernal chest pain accompanied by a pericardial friction rub. ST-segment elevation is not present in this tracing or those recorded later.

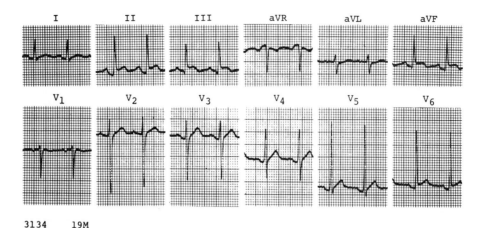

3134   19M

FIGURE 11–3. PR-segment depression in acute pericarditis. The patient is a 19-year-old man with acute idiopathic pericarditis. The PR-segment depression is seen best in leads II, aVF, and V₃ through V₆. It is elevated in lead aVR. ST-segment elevation is seen best in the inferior and left precordial leads.

normal. A reduction of the amplitude of the complex may occur when pericardial fluid accumulates. The relation between the amount of fluid and the decrease in voltage, however, is not consistent.[19] In most instances, there is a return to normal amplitude after pericardiocentesis (see Fig. 11–11). If this fails to occur, the low voltage probably is the result of the insulating effect of fibrin deposit.[32]

Low voltage of the QRS complex may be seen in pathologic states other than pericardial effusion due to pericarditis. It may occur in pericardial effusion caused by congestive heart failure and myxedema; in the latter, the low voltage may partly be the result of myocardial involvement. Low QRS voltage is a common finding in chronic constrictive pericarditis. It also is seen in various types of diffuse myocardial disease such as amyloidosis, scleroderma, or cardiac neoplasm. Diffuse myocardial damage as a result of coronary artery disease may reduce the QRS amplitude. Extracardiac causes of low voltage include pleural effusion and chronic obstructive lung disease.

Electrical Alternans

Alternation of the amplitude of the P, QRS, or T waves may be seen in patients with large pericardial effusion. This, however, is neither a common nor a specific finding for pericardial effusion. When it occurs, it is most often associated with malignancy. It usually involves only the QRS complex. If there is total alternans with the involvement of the P, QRS,

and T waves, the finding is almost diagnostic of cardiac tamponade. More detailed discussion of this phenomenon is given at the end of this chapter.

Diffuse ST-Segment Elevation and T-Wave Inversion

Diffuse ST-segment elevation is the most characteristic finding in acute pericarditis. When this is followed by typical serial changes, the ECG is highly suggestive of the diagnosis (see Fig. 11–1). Spodick described four stages of evolutionary ST and T-wave changes.[39] In stage 1, there is ST-segment elevation in almost all leads that face the epicardial surface of the ventricles, with ST-segment depression in those leads oriented toward the ventricular cavity (e.g., lead aVR). In stage 2, the ST junction returns to the baseline and the T-wave amplitude begins to decrease. During this stage, the ECG may appear normal. In stage 3, the T waves are inverted. Stage 4 represents ECG resolution with a return to the normal pattern. One or more stages of the ECG changes may be absent, depending on the time of the recording in relation to the disease process, the frequency of observation, and the severity of the disease. The typical ST changes were reported in 90 percent or more of the patients with acute pericarditis.[40,44] The true sensitivity of the ECG in the diagnosis of this disease is difficult to estimate, however, since many milder cases probably are not recognized clinically.

Although the ST-segment and T-wave

changes in pericarditis are typically widespread, they are not always present in all leads. In the precordial leads, ST-segment elevation is seen most commonly in V_5 and V_6 and is present in decreasing frequency from V_4 to V_1. In the limb leads, it occurs most often in leads I and II and less often in leads aVF, III, and aVL. If the ST segment in lead aVR is displaced, it is always depressed. ST-segment depression appears in decreasing order in leads aVR, V_1, III, and aVL. The T-wave changes have similar distribution, but exceptions do occur. In Figure 11–1C, the T-wave inversion is limited to the inferolateral leads only. In some instances, only a biphasic T wave is observed.

The incidence of typical ST and T-wave changes also depends on the cause of pericarditis. In idiopathic pericarditis, the characteristic ST-segment elevation occurred in about 64 percent of the 325 cases reviewed by Soffer,[37] and normal ECGs were recorded in only 6 percent. The classic changes are present in most patients with purulent pericarditis (Fig. 11–4). Benzing and associates described the typical findings in 7 of 8 such patients.[4] In 35 patients with tuberculous pericarditis reported by Rooney and co-workers, only 9 percent showed ST elevation typical of pericarditis, but 84 percent had T-wave inversion compatible with the diagnosis.[35] The ST changes also are rarely seen in patients with chronic effusive pericarditis resulting from other causes.[2] In 33 patients with uremic pericarditis reported on by Bailey and associates, only 1 had the typical changes.[1] Pericarditis complicating acute myocardial infarction is difficult to diagnose by the ECG. This may be because the pericarditis is usually limited to the area of infarction and the ECG changes are difficult to distinguish from those due to the acute infarction. When transient ST segment is

present in all the epicardial leads but is associated with QRS changes of a localized infarction, or if reciprocal ST-segment depression is absent in acute myocardial infarction, the presence of complicating pericarditis should be considered. In postmyocardial infarction syndrome, the diagnosis is less difficult if the ST and T changes recur after the acute changes of the infarct have subsided[11,25] In Dressler's series, half of the 44 cases had ECG changes compatible with pericarditis.[11] The ECG is less helpful than expected in postpericardiotomy syndrome.[12,27] In postpericardiotomy syndrome after traumatic hemopericardium, however, the typical changes may be seen in two-thirds of the patients.[45] ECG changes of pericarditis frequently are seen during the early postoperative period after cardiac surgery but they are transient, lasting only for a few days. In pericarditis due to radiation therapy, the symptoms and signs of pericarditis are commonly delayed for a few months to several years, but generally less than a year, after the treatment.[43] The ECG shows either ST and T-wave changes of acute pericarditis or the findings associated with pericardial effusion (see Fig. 11–12). In rheumatic, rheumatoid, or neoplastic pericarditis, the ECG changes are observed only occasionally.[14,44]

The duration of the ECG changes in pericarditis also depends on its cause and the extent of the associated myocardial damage. Persistent ECG abnormalities occur most often in purulent, tuberculous, and neoplastic pericarditis. In idiopathic pericarditis, the ST-segment changes usually return to normal within a week but may last longer. The T-wave inversion may persist for weeks or months. In a review of 234 patients who had follow-up examinations reported in the literature, 13 patients had persistent changes lasting more than 3 months. The T-wave inversion often

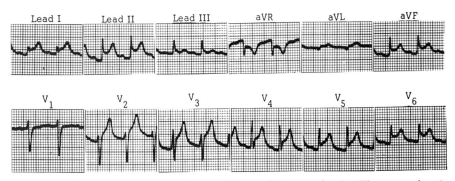

FIGURE 11–4. Pneumococcal pericarditis in a 20-year-old woman showing ST-segment elevation in all leads except lead aVR, in which it is depressed, and lead V_1, in which it is isoelectric.

showed variations in depth and contour from day to day despite absence of other evidence of active disease.[28]

DIFFERENTIAL DIAGNOSIS

Myocardial Infarction

The ST-segment and T-wave changes of acute pericarditis often are mistaken as signs of acute myocardial infarction. Although the absence of abnormal Q waves is in favor of pericarditis, this also may occur in patients with myocardial infarction, especially in its early stage. The following signs are useful in separating these two conditions[20]:

1. Reciprocal ST-segment displacements are typically seen in patients with myocardial infarction. They are not seen in acute pericarditis except in the leads that face the ventricular cavity, such as lead aVR and occasionally leads V_1, III, and aVL.

2. Marked ST-segment elevation of more than 4 or 5 mm is unusual in acute pericarditis.

3. A fusion of the ST segment and T wave into a single monophasic curve is seldom seen in patients with pericarditis.

4. In acute pericarditis the elevated ST segment usually has an upward concavity. The T wave remains upright until the ST segment returns to the isoelectric line. In myocardial infarction, the T wave often begins to invert while the ST segment is still elevated, resulting in an upward convexity of the ST segment.

5. The T-wave inversion in pericarditis is more diffuse but less deep than in myocardial infarction. An incompletely inverted T wave, such as a diphasic or notched T wave, often is seen in pericarditis.

6. A definite prolongation of the QT interval is more in favor of myocardial infarction than pericarditis,[44] unless myocarditis coexists with pericarditis.

Normal Variant

Diffuse ST-segment elevation often is seen in healthy young individuals because of early repolarization (Fig. 11–5). The distribution of the ST-segment changes is similar to that in acute pericarditis, being most marked in the precordial leads. However, the elevation remains stable and essentially unchanged on serial observations. It usually is associated with tall T waves in the same leads. The terminal part of the QRS complex often is slurred or notched.

Myocarditis

Diffuse T-wave inversion is one of the most common ECG findings in myocarditis. ST-segment displacement, usually depression, may occur occasionally. In many cases, both myocarditis and pericarditis coexist. The presence of ventricular arrhythmias or atrioventricular

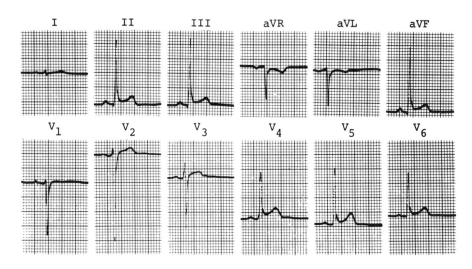

4486   20M

FIGURE 11–5. Diffuse ST-segment elevation as a normal variant. The patient is a healthy 20-year-old man. Repeated ECGs showed no change. Notching of the terminal part of the QRS complex is visible.

or intraventricular conduction defect is suggestive of the diagnosis of myocarditis.

Pulmonary Embolism, Pneumothorax, Cerebrovascular Accident, Hyperkalemia

Pulmonary embolism, pneumothorax, cerebrovascular accident, and hyperkalemia all may cause ST-segment elevation to mimic acute pericarditis or myocardial infarction. They were discussed in Chapter 9 in association with the pseudoinfarction pattern. Similar findings have been described in patients with pneumomediastinum.[30] I have seen a case of pneumopericardium that exhibited findings identical to those of acute pericarditis. Figure 11–6 demonstrates a rather unusual case of diffuse ST elevation as a result of intracranial bleeding.

Subepicardial Hemorrhage

Subepicardial hemorrhage, an uncommon cause of diffuse ST and T-wave changes simulating pericarditis, is illustrated in Figure 11–7. The subepicardial hemorrhage was the result of a dissecting aneurysm.

ELECTROCARDIOGRAPHIC FINDINGS IN CHRONIC CONSTRICTIVE PERICARDITIS

The ECG abnormalities in constrictive pericarditis are nonspecific. One or more of the following changes usually are present, however. If the ECG is normal, the diagnosis of constrictive pericarditis should be reconsidered.

1. Atrial arrhythmias
2. Abnormal P waves

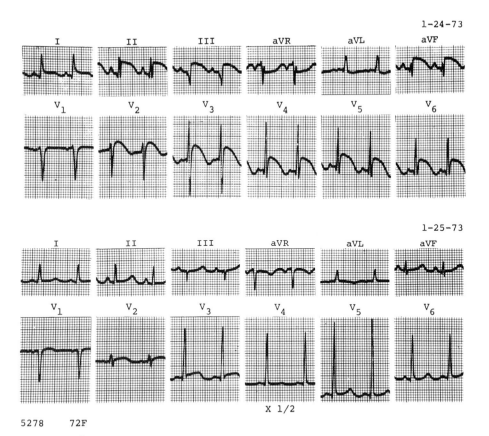

FIGURE 11–6. Diffuse ST-segment elevation as a result of a cerebrovascular accident. The patient was a 72-year-old woman who became comatose on 1-23-73. The tracing on 1-24-73 shows diffuse ST-segment elevation. The QT interval is prolonged, however, and the T waves in leads V_2 through V_6 are inverted while the ST segment is elevated. These findings are atypical for acute pericarditis. The ST-segment elevation has subsided almost completely on the tracing taken on the next day. She died 5 days later. Autopsy revealed bilateral cerebral, cerebellar, and pontine hemorrhage. Examination of the heart showed 50 to 70 percent narrowing of the three major coronary vessels. No evidence was found of pericarditis or myocardial infarction, however.

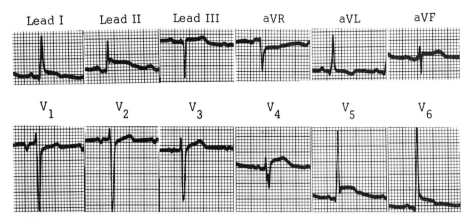

FIGURE 11-7. Subepicardial hemorrhage. The patient was a 61-year-old man who had a dissecting aneurysm. At autopsy, it was found that the dissection had extended subepicardially. The ECG shows abnormal P waves consistent with left atrial enlargement and left ventricular hypertrophy. There is diffuse ST-segment elevation with T-wave inversion in some of the leads.

3. Low voltage of the QRS complex
4. Abnormal right axis deviation
5. T-wave abnormalities

Atrial Arrhythmias

In contrast to the situation in acute pericarditis, atrial arrhythmias are common in constrictive pericarditis. Atrial fibrillation was reported in 23 to 36 percent of the cases, whereas atrial flutter was reported in 6 to 10 percent.[6,9,47] Paroxysmal atrial tachycardia is seldom seen.

Abnormal P Waves

In patients with sinus rhythm, the P waves often are notched or abnormally wide. They are abnormal in about two thirds of the cases

and may assume the pattern of P mitrale (Fig. 11-8). Both the atrial arrhythmias and the abnormal P waves have been attributed to atrial involvement by the compressing scar.

Low Voltage of the QRS Complex
(Fig. 11-9)

In the reported series, abnormally low amplitude of the QRS complex was seen in 55 to 90 percent of the cases.[9,17,33] In a pathologic study of 11 cases by Dines and associates, myocardial atrophy was found uniformly throughout the myocardium.[10]

Right Axis Deviation

Right axis deviation or right ventricular hypertrophy pattern occasionally is seen in pa-

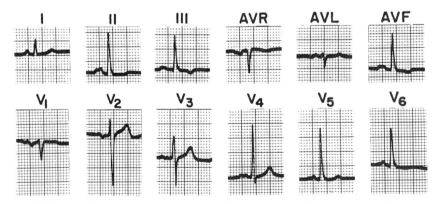

FIGURE 11-8. Abnormal P waves in constrictive pericarditis. The patient is a 58-year-old man who has a severely calcified pericardium. The P mitrale type of P waves are seen best in leads II and aVF and in some of the precordial leads. Abnormal T waves are present in the inferior and left precordial leads.

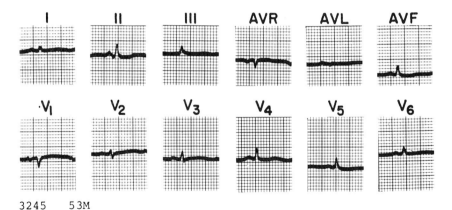

3245 53M

FIGURE 11–9. Constrictive pericarditis proved by surgery. The ECG shows low voltage of the QRS complex in all of the leads. Diffuse ST-segment and T-wave abnormalities are also present.

tients with constrictive pericarditis.[8] In some patients, this can be explained by the presence of severe fibrotic annular subpulmonary constriction resulting in anatomic right ventricular hypertrophy. An example of this is given in Figure 11–10. More often, however, the pathophysiology of the right axis deviation is unclear. It was postulated that cardiac rotation and distortion may be responsible.[8]

T-Wave Abnormalities

Flattening or inversion of the T waves is the most common finding in constrictive pericarditis (see Fig. 11–9). In the larger reported series, they were present in 90 to 100 percent of the cases.[6,9,17,47]

ELECTRICAL ALTERNANS

Electrical alternans refers to a regular alternation in the configuration or magnitude of the ECG complexes that arise from the same pacemaker and is independent of periodic extracardiac phenomena. The alternation may involve the P, QRS, or T wave, or all three. When all three waves are involved, the condition is called *total electrical alternans*. In the diagnosis of electrical alternans, one should be certain that the RR interval is unchanged. In most, the alternation is 2:1, but changes occasionally occur on every third beat.

Electrical alternans is uncommon. It has been estimated to occur in about 1 to 6 of 10,000 ECGs.[42] Among the reported cases, al-

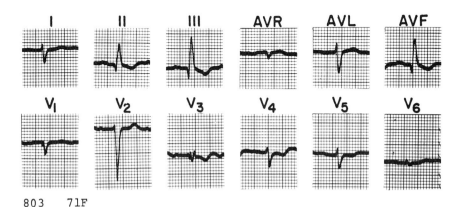

803 71F

FIGURE 11–10. Constrictive pericarditis with abnormal right axis deviation. The patient was a 71-year-old woman with autopsy-proven constrictive pericarditis. The pericardium was calcified. There was compression of the outflow tract of the right ventricle. Right ventricular hypertrophy was demonstrated. A grade III ejection systolic murmur was heard along the left sternal border during life. In the ECG, the P waves are notched in the inferior leads. There is right axis deviation. The R waves are small in all the precordial leads. The S waves in leads V_4 and V_5 are relatively deep. The right axis deviation and R/S ratio in V_5 are consistent with right ventricular hypertrophy. Diffuse ST and T-wave abnormalities are present, some of which may be related to digitalis.

ternation of the QRS complex with or without T-wave changes (i.e., ventricular electrical alternans) is the most common (Figs. 11–11 through 11–13). Isolated T-wave alternans is rare. ST-segment alternans has been described in patients with Prinzmetal's angina and during percutaneous transluminal coronary angioplasty.[23] I have encountered several cases of U-wave alternans, one of which is illustrated in Figure 11–14. A case of electrical alternans of U waves associated with multiple electrolyte deficits was reported.[36] I recently saw a case of U-wave alternans in a patient with acquired immunodeficiency syndrome treated with pentamidine.[6]

Clinical Correlation

Although electrical alternans is best known for its association with pericardial effusion, the latter is responsible in only about one third of the cases that display electrical alternans. When there is total electrical alternation with simultaneous involvement of the atrial and

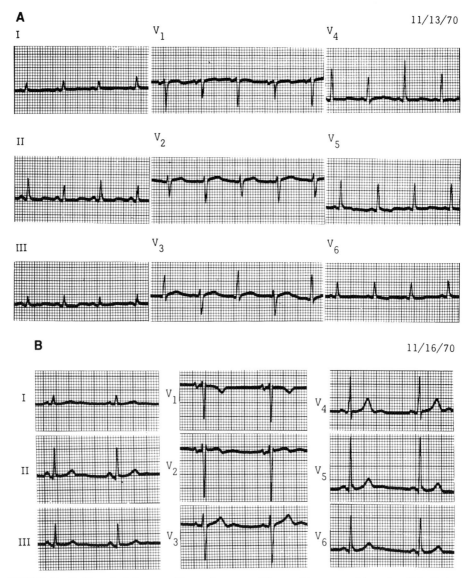

FIGURE 11–11. Electrical alternans. The patient was a 50-year-old woman with pericardial effusion and cardiac tamponade as a result of neoplasm. The tracing made on 11-13-70 (*A*) demonstrates the alternation of the QRS complex during cardiac tamponade. The electrical alternans is no longer present in the tracing of 11-16-70 (*B*) after the tamponade was relieved. The voltage of the QRS complex is increased, and the T waves are more normal in appearance. (Reproduced from Fowler NO: The electrocardiogram in pericarditis. Cardiovasc Clin 5:256, 1973, by permission of the author and FA Davis.)

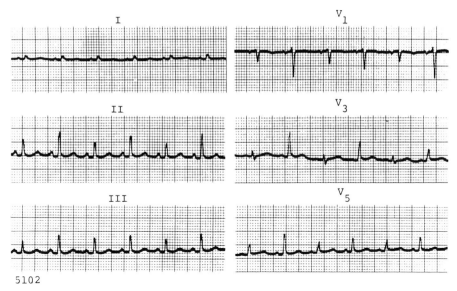

FIGURE 11–12. Electrical alternans involving the QRS complex in a 26-year-old man with pericardial effusion secondary to radiation for reticulum cell sarcoma.

ventricular components, however, pericardial effusion with tamponade almost invariably is present.[26] Conversely, total electrical alternans was found in only 4 of 56 patients with cardiac tamponade reported on by Guberman and associates.[16] An additional 7 of their patients had alternans of the QRS complex only. Six of the 11 patients with either total alternans or only QRS alternans had malignant pericardial effusion (see Fig. 11–11).

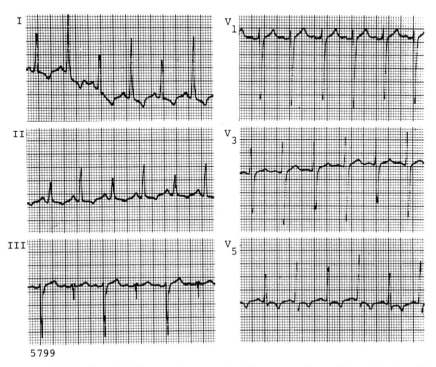

FIGURE 11–13. Electrical alternans in postpericardiotomy syndrome. The patient is a 30-year-old man who developed pericarditis and pericardial effusion 3 weeks after aortic valve surgery. In the ECG, in addition to the alternation of the QRS complex, T-wave alternans can be seen in lead III.

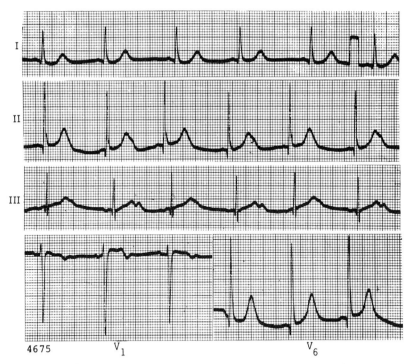

4675 V₁ V₆

FIGURE 11–14. U-wave alternans. The patient is a 38-year-old woman with hypertension and coronary artery disease. The tracing was recorded while she was in congestive heart failure. There is alternation of the U wave as well as the QRS complex and T wave. The patient was not receiving digitalis at the time.

In patients with pericardial effusion but without cardiac tamponade, electrical alternans is observed even less frequently. Therefore, this phenomenon is of limited value in the recognition of pericardial effusion.

Hypertension and coronary artery disease is the next largest entity that is associated with electrical alternans. This phenomenon is illustrated in Figure 11–15 in a patient with hypertensive cardiovascular disease and angina

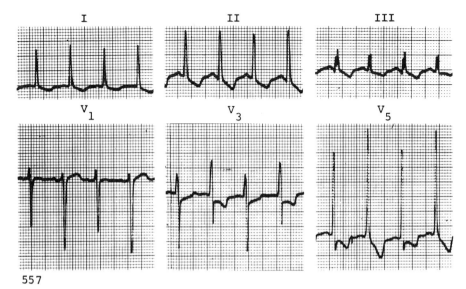

557

FIGURE 11–15. Electrical alternans in a patient with coronary artery and hypertensive cardiovascular disease. No evidence of pericardial effusion was found. The alternans involves both the QRS complex and T wave.

pectoris and in Figure 11–16 in a patient with coronary artery disease and left bundle branch block. The alternation involves both the QRS and T waves. The condition also has been observed in other types of organic heart disease, including rheumatic heart disease and cor pulmonale.

Although most cases of electrical alternans are seen in patients with sinus rhythm, many are encountered in patients with ectopic tachycardias. The tachycardia may be supraventricular or ventricular and, in the former, may have narrow or wide QRS complexes.[24] In cases of narrow QRS tachycardia, electrical alternans occurs most frequently in patients with the Wolff-Parkinson-White syndrome. An example of supraventricular tachycardia with electrical alternans is given in Figure 11–17. Figure 11–18 is an example of nonparoxysmal ventricular tachycardia with QRS and T-wave alternans.

Mechanism of Electrical Alternans

In cases associated with pericardial effusion, electrical alternans is most likely to result from an anatomic alternation of the cardiac position. With pericardial effusion, the restraining interference of the lungs on the heart is decreased. Echocardiographic and angiocardiographic studies have given considerable support to this explanation.[34,46]

In the absence of pericardial effusion, the probable mechanism is an alternation in the pattern of depolarization. The refractory phase in some portion of the heart may be prolonged, so that after activation a subsequent normal impulse finds that region of the myocardium still refractory. Consequently, the response of every alternate beat is different from the previous beat.[18] In narrow QRS tachycardia, the appearance of QRS alternans often is rate-related.[29] The alternans usually is seen when the cycle length is short and is independent of the mechanism of the tachycardia.[29]

CONGENITAL DEFECT OF THE PERICARDIUM

Congenital defect or absence of the pericardium is uncommon. The left side of the pericardium is usually affected.[31] The ECG findings may mimic those of right ventricular hypertrophy or anterior myocardial infarction (Fig. 11–19). An erroneous clinical diagnosis of pulmonary hypertension, pulmonic stenosis, or left-to-right shunt often is made because of the prominent pulmonary artery segment seen on the chest radiograph.[14]

In a review of the ECG findings of 41 cases of uncomplicated complete defect of the left pericardium, Inoue and associates found right axis deviation in 56 percent, incomplete right bundle branch block in 47 percent, clockwise rotation in 47 percent, and tall and peaked P waves in the right pericardial leads in 26 percent of the cases.[21] These changes are attrib-

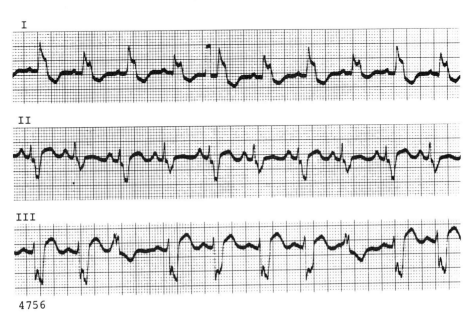

4756

FIGURE 11–16. Electrical alternans involving the QRS complex and T wave in a patient with coronary artery disease and left bundle branch block. (Two premature ventricular beats are seen in lead III.)

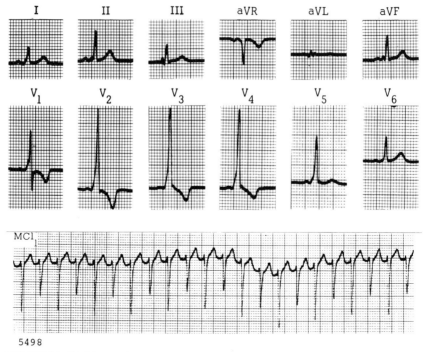

FIGURE 11–17. Electrical alternans during supraventricular tachycardia. The patient is a 23-year-old woman with type A Wolff-Parkinson-White syndrome without other evidence of organic heart disease. Alternation of the QRS complex is seen during the tachycardia.

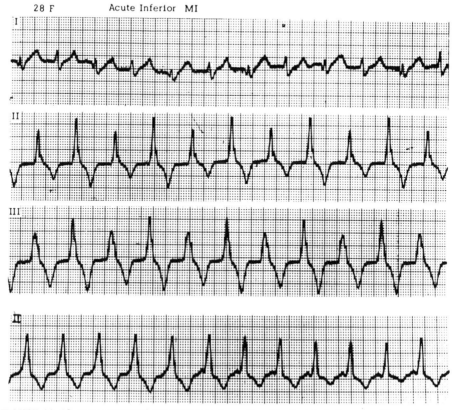

FIGURE 11–18. Nonparoxysmal ventricular tachycardia with electrical alternans. The patient is a 27-year-old woman with acute inferior myocardial infarction. The bottom strip supports the diagnosis of nonparoxysmal ventricular tachycardia by demonstrating the presence of AV dissociation and fusion beats (last 6 or 7 beats). The top three strips (leads I, II and III) show QRS and T-wave alternans.

29 JAN 1989

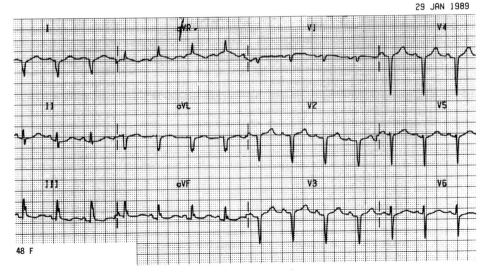

FIGURE 11–19. Congenital defect of the left pericardium. The patient is a 48-year-old woman who is known to have had the defect since the age of 20 years. The diagnosis was confirmed by the appearance of air in the pericardial space after intrapleural injection. Clinical examination and right heart catheterization revealed no evidence of other cardiac abnormality. The patient was previously reported by Fowler.[14]

uted to marked clockwise rotation of the heart along its longitudinal axis.

REFERENCES

1. Bailey GL, Hampers CL, Hager EB, et al: Uremic pericarditis: Clinical features and management. Circulation 38:582, 1968
2. Bedford ED: Chronic effusive pericarditis. Br Heart J 26:499, 1964
3. Bellet S, McMillan TM: Electrocardiographic patterns in acute pericarditis: Evolution, causes and diagnostic significance of patterns in limb and chest leads. A study of 57 cases. Arch Intern Med 61:381, 1938
4. Benzing G, Kaplan S: Purulent pericarditis. Am J Dis Child 106:289, 1963
5. Chamblis JR, Jaruszewski EJ, Brofman BL, et al: Chronic cardiac compression. Circulation 4:816, 1951
6. Bibler MR, Chou TC, Toltzis RJ, Wade PA: Recurrent ventricular tachycardia due to pentamidine-induced cardiotoxicity. Chest 94:1303, 1988
7. Charles MA, Bensinger TA, Glasser SP: Atrial injury current in pericarditis. Arch Intern Med 131:657, 1973
8. Chesler E, Mitha AS, Matisonn RE: The ECG of constrictive pericarditis: Pattern resembling right ventricular hypertrophy. Am Heart J 91:420, 1976
9. Dalton JC, Pearson RJ, White PD: Constrictive pericarditis: A review and long-term follow-up of 78 cases. Ann Intern Med 45:445, 1956
10. Dines DE, Edwards JE, Burchell HB: Myocardial atrophy in constrictive pericarditis. Proc Staff Meet Mayo Clin 33:93, 1958
11. Dressler W: The post-myocardial infarction syndrome. Arch Intern Med 103:28, 1959
12. Engle MA, Ito T: The postpericardiotomy syndrome. Am J Cardiol 7:73, 1961
13. Fowler NO: The electrocardiogram in pericarditis. Cardiovasc Clin 5:256, 1973
14. Fowler NO: Congenital defect of the pericardium: Its resemblance to pulmonary artery enlargement. Circulation 26:114, 1962
15. Franco AE, Levine HD, Hall AP: Rheumatoid pericarditis: Report of 17 cases diagnosed clinically. Ann Intern Med 77:837, 1972
16. Guberman BA, Fowler NO, Engel PJ, et al: Cardiac tamponade in medical patients. Circulation 64:633, 1981
17. Gimlette TMD: Constrictive pericarditis. Br Heart J 21:9, 1959
18. Hamburger WW, Katz LN, Saphir L: Electrical alternans: Clinical study with report of 2 necropsies. JAMA 106:902, 1936
19. Harvey AN, Whitehill MR: Tuberculous pericarditis. Medicine 16:45, 1937
20. Hull E: The electrocardiogram in pericarditis. Am J Cardiol 7:21, 1961
21. Inoue H, Fujii J, Mashima S, Murao S: Pseudo right atrial overloading pattern in complete defect of the left pericardium. J Electrocardiol 14:413, 1981
22. James TN: Pericarditis and the sinus node. Arch Intern Med 110:305, 1962
23. Joyal M, Feldman RL, Pepine CJ, et al: ST-segment alternans during percutaneous transluminal coronary angioplasty. Am J Cardiol 54:915, 1984
24. Kremers MS, Miller JM, Josephson ME: Electrical alternans in wide complex tachycardia. Am J Cardiol 56:305, 1985
25. Likoff W: Pericarditis complicating myocardial infarction. Am J Cardiol 7:69, 1961
26. Littman D, Spodick DH: Total electrical alternation in pericardial disease. Circulation 17:912, 1958
27. McGuinness JB, Taussig HB: The postpericardiotomy syndrome: Its relationship to ambulation in the presence of "benign" pericardial and pleural reaction. Circulation 26:500, 1962
28. McGuire J, Helm RA, Iglauer A, et al: Nonspecific pericarditis and myocardial infarction. Circulation 14:874, 1956
29. Morady F, DiCarlo LA, Baerman JM, et al: Determi-

nants of QRS alternans during narrow QRS tachycardia. J Am Coll Cardiol 9:489, 1987

30. Munsell WP: Pneumomediastinum: A report of 28 cases and reviews of the literature. JAMA 202:129, 1967

31. Nasser WK, Helmen C, Tavel ME, et al: Congenital absence of the left pericardium: Clinical, electrocardiographic, radiographic, hemodynamics, and angiographic findings in six cases. Circulation 41:469, 1970

32. Nizet PM, Marriott HJL: Electrocardiogram and pericardial effusion. JAMA 198:169, 1966

33. Portal RW, Besterman EMM, Chambers RJ, et al: Prognosis after operation for constrictive pericarditis. Br Med J 1:563, 1966

34. Price EC, Dennis EW: Electrical alternans: Its mechanism demonstrated. Circulation 39-III:165, 1969

35. Rooney JJ, Crocco JA, Lyons HA: Tuberculous pericarditis. Ann Intern Med 72:73, 1970

36. Shimoni Z, Flatau E, Schiller D, et al: Electrical alternans of giant U waves with multiple electrolyte deficits. Am J Cardiol 54:920, 1984

37. Soffer A: Electrocardiographic abnormalities in acute, convalescent and recurrent stages of idiopathic pericarditis. Am Heart J 60:729, 1960

38. Spodick DH: Arrhythmias during acute pericarditis: A prospective study of 100 consecutive cases. JAMA 235:39, 1976

39. Spodick DH: The electrocardiogram in acute pericarditis: Distributions of morphologic and axial changes in stages. Am J Cardiol 33:470, 1974

40. Spodick DH: Diagnostic electrocardiographic sequences in acute pericarditis: Significance of PR segment and PR vector changes. Circulation 48:575, 1973

41. Spodick DH: Differential diagnosis of acute pericarditis. Prog Cardiovasc Dis 14:192, 1971

42. Stewart JR, Fajardo LF: Radiation-induced heart disease: An update. Prog Cardiovasc Dis 27:173, 1984

43. Spodick DH: Electric alternation of the heart: Its relation to the kinetics and physiology of the heart during cardiac tamponade. Am J Cardiol 10:155, 1962

44. Surawicz B, Lasseter KC: Electrocardiogram in pericarditis. Am J Cardiol 26:471, 1970

45. Tabatznik B, Isaacs JP: Postpericardiotomy syndrome following traumatic hemopericardium. Am J Cardiol 7:83, 1961

46. Usher BW, Popp RL: Electrical alternans: Mechanism in pericardial effusion. Am Heart J 83:459, 1972

47. Wood P: Chronic constrictive pericarditis. Am J Cardiol 7:48, 1961

Myocardial Diseases

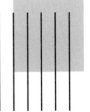

12

Myocardial diseases, or cardiomyopathies, may be divided according to their cause or physiological effect. Under the physiological or functional classification, they are divided into the dilated (or congestive), hypertrophic, and restrictive types. Based on the cause, they may be classified as follows:

1. Idiopathic cardiomyopathy
   a. Dilated (or congestive)
   b. Hypertrophic—obstructive and non-obstructive
2. Secondary cardiomyopathy
   a. Neuromuscular disease, such as Friedreich's ataxia, progressive muscular dystrophy, myotonic dystrophy, and Kearns-Sayre syndrome
   b. Connective tissue disease, such as scleroderma, disseminated lupus erythematosus, polyarteritis nodosa, polymyositis, and rheumatoid heart disease
   c. Neoplastic heart disease, primary or metastatic
   d. Metabolic disease, such as hemochromatosis, and myxedema
   e. Granulomatous cardiomyopathy, such as sarcoidosis
   f. Amyloidosis
   g. Myocarditis, such as rheumatic, viral, parasitic, and that associated with acquired immunodeficiency syndrome (AIDS)

Because the myocardial diseases generally involve a diffuse process, various cardiac chambers and conduction systems may be affected. The electrocardiographic (ECG) abnormalities are therefore expected to be diverse. Abnormality of the atrial activation or excitation potential may be accompanied by abnormal P waves, atrial arrhythmias, or signs of atrial enlargement. Abnormality of ventricular activation or excitation potential may result in ventricular arrhythmias, signs of ventricular hypertrophy, intraventricular conduction defect, or bundle branch block. Abnormal Q waves or reduction of the QRS voltage may appear because of replacement of the myocardial tissue by electrically inert tissue, altered sequence of activation, or abnormal forces generated from asymmetrical hypertrophy. Various degrees of atrioventricular (AV) block may occur if the AV conduction system is involved.

As a rule, the ECG findings in cardiomyopathy are not diagnostic. They are helpful only when interpreted in conjunction with other clinical data. Indeed, under proper clinical setting the information may be most valuable, and sometimes the ECG is the only clinical evidence of cardiac involvement.

IDIOPATHIC DILATED (CONGESTIVE) CARDIOMYOPATHY

P Waves

In patients with sinus rhythm, abnormal P waves were reported to be present in 14 to 32 percent of those with dilated cardiomyopathy.[34,67] In a small series of 40 cases that I analyzed, abnormal P waves were present in 15 cases. Signs of left atrial enlargement with wide, notched P waves in the limb leads or large negative component of the P waves in lead V_1 were the most common findings. Many of the cases showed large biphasic P waves in lead V_1 to suggest biatrial enlargement (Fig. 12–1). They are often conspicuous in appearance. Their frequent presence in patients with cardiomyopathy was emphasized by Hamby and Raia.[47] Changes consistent with right atrial enlargement alone are uncommon.

QRS Complex

Left ventricular hypertrophy is the most common abnormal finding in dilated cardiomyopathy (see Fig. 12–1). It occurs in about one third or more of the reported series.[34,47,67] Because anatomic left ventricular hypertrophy is almost always present at autopsy, the inci-

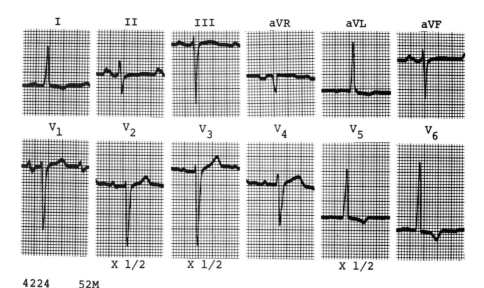

4224   52M

FIGURE 12–1. Idiopathic dilated cardiomyopathy. The patient was a 52-year-old man, and the diagnosis of dilated cardiomyopathy was supported by autopsy findings. The heart was markedly enlarged and weighed 650 g. There was severe dilatation of both atria and ventricles as well as biventricular hypertrophy with multiple areas of severe myocardial fibrosis. The coronary arteries were normal. In the ECG, the P-wave changes are consistent with biatrial enlargement. There is a large diphasic P wave in lead V_1. Abnormal left axis deviation is present. The QRS voltage and ST-T changes are consistent with left ventricular hypertrophy.

dence of this ECG finding is actually lower than expected. This is probably due to the frequent occurrence of bundle branch block in this disease. Diffuse myocardial fibrosis may account for the reduction of the QRS voltage in some cases. Anatomic right ventricular hypertrophy, which is commonly seen at autopsy, may cancel out some of the leftward forces. ECG signs of combined ventricular hypertrophy are relatively uncommon, however, and those of isolated right ventricular hypertrophy are rare. Some patients have low voltage of the QRS complex in the limb leads. Rarely, the amplitude is also low in the precordial leads[47,67] (Fig. 12–2).

Intraventricular conduction defect is common in these patients. This is particularly true of left bundle branch block (Fig. 12–3). The review of literature by Flowers and Horan described an incidence of about 9 percent in a

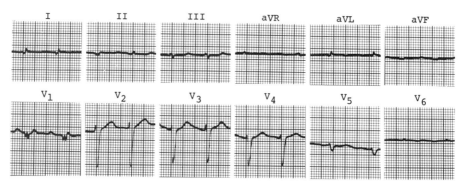

231W HH 61M

FIGURE 12–2. Dilated cardiomyopathy proved by autopsy. The patient was a 61-year-old man with recurrent biventricular congestive heart failure. At autopsy, the heart weighed 800 g, with four-chamber dilatation and hypertrophy. There was severe diffuse myocardial and interstitial fibrosis but no evidence of recent or old myocardial infarction. Coronary artery disease was present, but the stenotic lesions were not severe. The ECG shows first-degree AV block. The P waves are small and difficult to recognize except in lead V_1. The QRS voltage is low in all leads except leads V_2 through V_4.

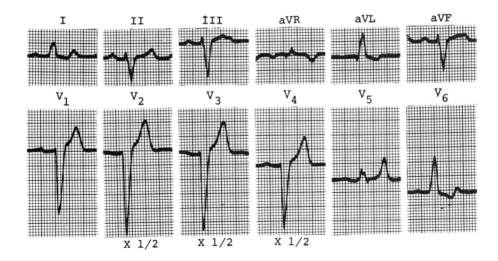

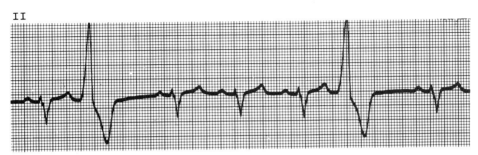

FIGURE 12–3. Idiopathic dilated cardiomyopathy in a 34-year-old man. The diagnosis is based on clinical data. The ECG shows first-degree AV block and complete left bundle branch block. The patient also has frequent premature ventricular contractions.

collected series of more than 1000 patients.[34] Some authors, however, reported a higher incidence of 15 to 20 percent, which is also my experience.[47,67] The difference may be related to the patient population and the severity of the disease. In an autopsy series of 36 cases reported by Stapleton and associates, it was present in 44 percent.[97] It is probably reasonable to say that the relative incidence of left bundle branch block in idiopathic dilated cardiomyopathy is higher than that in ischemic heart disease. In a patient with cardiomegaly of unknown cause, the presence of left bundle branch block further supports the diagnosis of primary myocardial disease. Abnormal left axis deviation consistent with left anterior hemiblock also is common, occurring in as many as 42 percent in some series.[47] On the other hand, right bundle branch block is seen in less than 4 percent of the patients.[30,34] In some cases, there is a prolongation of the QRS duration, but the morphology of the QRS complex is not typical of either left or right bundle branch block.

Abnormal Q waves that simulate myocardial infarction are often seen in patients with dilated cardiomyopathy, even though the incidence is lower than that in the hypertrophic variety. Myocardial fibrosis is responsible for the pseudoinfarction pattern in most cases. In some hearts, no gross fibrotic lesion can be found, and conduction disturbances may be the responsible mechanism.[67,82,98] Abnormal Q waves are most often present in the right and mid-precordial leads. Figures 12–4 and 12–5 are examples of autopsy-proven cases of dilated cardiomyopathy that mimic anterior and inferior myocardial infarction.

ST Segment and T Waves

Most of the ST-segment and T-wave changes in dilated cardiomyopathy are secondary to left ventricular hypertrophy or conduction defect. In some patients, however, they are the only ECG abnormalities identifiable and are seen most often in the left precordial leads.

Arrhythmias and AV Block

Rhythm disturbances are often a prominent feature of the disease. Atrial fibrillation and

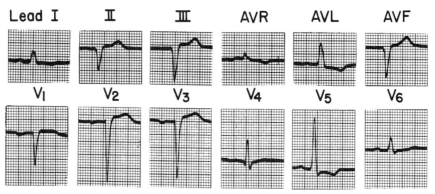

FIGURE 12–4. Idiopathic dilated cardiomyopathy with changes suggestive of myocardial infarction. The patient was a 75-year-old man with autopsy findings consistent with dilated cardiomyopathy. The heart weighed 505 g. There was a moderate degree of left ventricular hypertrophy. The coronary arteries showed a mild degree of atherosclerosis. No evidence of myocardial infarction was found on gross examination, but widespread, filled-out areas of fibrosis were revealed on microscopic examination. The ECG shows first-degree AV block. The QRS changes are suggestive of anterior and inferior myocardial infarction.

frequent premature ventricular beats are particularly prevalent. Huang and associates obtained 24-hour ambulatory (Holter) ECGs from 35 patients with idiopathic dilated cardiomyopathy.[57] Premature ventricular beats were found in all of the patients, 83 percent having frequent (more than 30 per hour) and 77 percent having complex premature ventricular beats. Twenty-one (60 percent) of the 35 patients had nonsustained (defined as less than 1 minute in duration) ventricular tachycardia. Frequent premature atrial beats, supraventricular tachycardia, atrial flutter, and junctional rhythm have all been reported.[30,34]

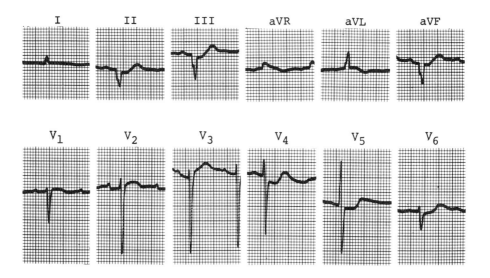

5529   56F

FIGURE 12–5. Idiopathic dilated cardiomyopathy with pseudoinfarction pattern. The patient was a 56-year-old woman with pathologic findings consistent with dilated cardiomyopathy. The heart weighed 540 g, with biventricular hypertrophy. The myocardium revealed diffuse multiple small areas of myocardial fibrosis. A larger area of fibrosis was present in the inferior wall of the left ventricle extending to the apex. The coronary arteries were patent, with only minimal atherosclerosis in the left anterior descending artery. In the ECG, a QS deflection is present in leads II, III, and aVF to suggest inferior myocardial infarction. The QRS changes also are suggestive of coexisting left anterior hemiblock. The small R wave in lead V_6 probably is related to the apical fibrosis. ST and T-wave abnormalities also are present, some of which are probably due to digitalis.

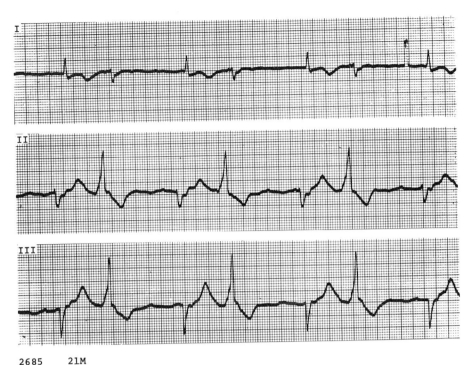

I

II

III

2685   21M

FIGURE 12-6. Arrhythmias in dilated cardiomyopathy. The patient was a 20-year-old man, and the diagnosis of cardiomyopathy was confirmed at autopsy. In the ECG, there is sinus tachycardia with complete AV block. The frequent premature ventricular beats result in a bigeminal rhythm.

Ventricular tachycardia and fibrillation may be responsible for sudden death in some of the patients.

First-degree AV block occurs in about 6 to 30 percent of the patients[47] (see Fig. 12-4). The incidence is even higher in the autopsy series.[97] Complete AV block is rare. Such a case is illustrated in Figure 12-6 during the terminal stage of this disease.

HYPERTROPHIC CARDIOMYOPATHY, OBSTRUCTIVE AND NONOBSTRUCTIVE

Idiopathic hypertrophic subaortic stenosis and *asymmetrical septal hypertrophy* were the terms most commonly used previously to describe this disease entity characterized by myocardial hypertrophy of unknown cause. Because many of the patients do not have obstruction of the left ventricular outflow, it is generally agreed that the term *hypertrophic cardiomyopathy*, divided into the *obstructive* and *nonobstructive* types, is more descriptive and inclusive.

Most patients with hypertrophic cardiomyopathy have abnormal ECGs. In the 134 cases reported by Savage and associates, only 7 percent had normal tracings,[89] and they were more common in patients without symptoms and who had nonobstructive and localized lesions.[66,89] None of the abnormal findings, however, are diagnostic of the disease. Although some of the changes occur more frequently in the obstructive than in the nonobstructive type, the ECG is not helpful in separating the two types.

P Waves

Signs of left atrial enlargement are seen frequently. The decrease in left ventricular compliance in this disease increases the resistance to left atrial systole leading to its hypertrophy. If mitral insufficiency coexists, the atrial chamber is further enlarged. Although changes suggestive of right atrial enlargement have been reported, I believe that they most likely represent the so-called pseudo P-pulmonale seen occasionally in patients with left atrial enlargement (see Chapter 2).

QRS Complex

Most patients have a normal QRS axis. Left axis deviation is seen in about 10 to 30 percent,[36,89] whereas right axis deviation is uncommon.

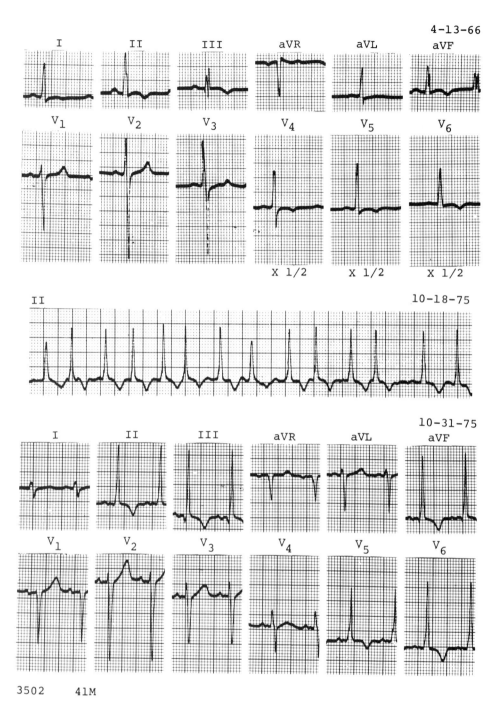

3502   41M

FIGURE 12–7. Hypertrophic obstructive cardiomyopathy. The diagnosis of muscular subaortic stenosis was made in 1959 when the patient was 25 years old and was based on hemodynamic and surgical findings. There was a systolic gradient of 85 mm Hg between the main body and outflow tract of the left ventricle. No corrective surgery was performed at that time. The tracing of 4-13-66 is essentially unchanged from that recorded in 1959. It shows left ventricular hypertrophy. The patient had episodes of atrial fibrillation in 1975, which is illustrated in the rhythm strip. There also is a rightward shift of the QRS axis in the tracing of 1975. The cause of the right axis deviation is unclear. There is no clinical evidence of right ventricular hypertrophy. Left posterior hemiblock may be responsible for the axis shift.

Electrocardiographic evidence of left ventricular hypertrophy is present in about one half to two thirds of patients[20,46,52,58,66,89] (Fig. 12–7). Anatomically, hypertrophy of the free wall of the left ventricle may develop as a result of outflow tract obstruction[13] or represent primary involvement of the free wall myocardium.

The reports on the relation of the ECG findings of left ventricular hypertrophy with the echocardiographic changes are conflicting. It was found that the ECG signs of left ventricular hypertrophy were related to the thickness of the interventricular septum, the posterior wall of the left ventricle, or the extensiveness of the hypertrophy.[58,66,89] Others were unable to substantiate the relationship.[46] When there is ECG evidence of progressive hypertrophy, however, the prognosis is usually poor.[70]

Hollister and Goodwin reported a high incidence (48 percent) of combined ventricular hypertrophy in their 28 patients.[55] Such experience is not shared by others. The difference in the ECG criteria used for the diagnosis is probably responsible for this discrepancy.

One of the distinctive ECG abnormalities in hypertrophic cardiomyopathy is the presence of abnormal Q waves often mimicking that of myocardial infarction (Figs. 12–8 and 12–9). Although Frank and Braunwald[36] described such a finding in over 50 percent of their original series of patients with idiopathic hypertrophic subaortic stenosis, its overall incidence in hypertrophic cardiomyopathy is considerably lower and is about 20 to 32 per-

cent.[4,30,34,60,66,89] In young patients, such a pseudoinfarction pattern often leads to the suspicion and recognition of this disease. The abnormal Q waves are seen most commonly in the anterolateral leads (leads I, aVL, V$_4$ through V$_6$) but also may be observed in the inferior and anterior leads. They are generally believed to be the result of septal hypertrophy. The initial QRS forces that represent the left-to-right septal activation become abnormally prominent. They are directed rightward, anteriorly, and superiorly as in the normal subjects but are abnormal in amplitude and duration. The exaggeration of the septal Q waves in leads I, aVL, V$_5$, V$_6$, and sometimes in the inferior leads accounts for the frequent appearance of the pseudoinfarction pattern. This explanation is supported by the finding that, after surgical resection of the hypertrophied septum, the abnormal Q waves may become smaller or disappear.[105] In 184 cases of hypertrophic cardiomyopathy studied by Savage and associates, however, the presence of abnormal Q waves did not significantly correlate with increased septal thickness or septum-to-free wall ratio seen on the echocardiogram.[89] VanDam and associates studied 10 patients with epicardial and intramural electrograms during surgery.[100] They suggested that the abnormal Q waves may be related to an array of abnormal initial depolarization fronts in the inner layers of the left ventricular wall. The findings from electrophysiological studies in 6 patients by Cosio and associates suggest that the Q waves are septal in origin

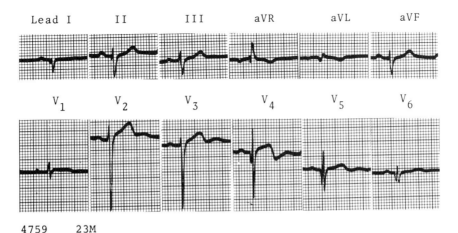

4759   23M

FIGURE 12–8. Idiopathic hypertrophic obstructive cardiomyopathy with pseudoinfarction pattern. The tracing was recorded from a 23-year-old man with an intraventricular pressure gradient of 135 mm Hg developed during Isoprel infusion. In the ECG, abnormal Q waves are present in leads I and V$_4$ through V$_6$. The R/S ratio in lead V$_1$ is greater than 1. (This tracing is the same as that in Fig. 9–45.)

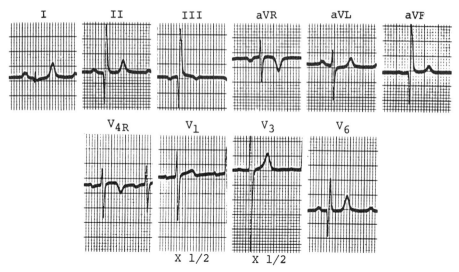

1982   12M

FIGURE 12-9. Idiopathic hypertrophic cardiomyopathy, nonobstructive, in a 12-year-old boy. The diagnosis was based on clinical and angiographic findings. No intraventricular pressure gradient was demonstrable during cardiac catheterization. The ECG shows left ventricular hypertrophy. Abnormal Q waves are present in leads II, III, aVF, and V6. (Courtesy of Dr. Samuel Kaplan.)

and that the myopathic septal muscle has electrophysiological properties different from those of the remainder of the myocardium.[24]

Abnormal Q waves are seen in both the obstructive and nonobstructive types of hypertrophic cardiomyopathy. In the obstructive variety, they have no apparent relation to the severity of the outflow tract obstruction. During the course of the disease, the abnormal Q waves may develop or disappear and increase or decrease in amplitude.[36] Because the forces generated from the interventricular septum and the free wall of the left ventricle are diametrically opposed, their relative degree of hypertrophy at various stages of the disease may account for the changes in the amplitude of the Q waves. In the later stages of the disease, the hypertrophied septal myocardial fibers may be replaced by fibrous tissue that is associated with a decrease in the initial septal forces or Q waves in the anterolateral leads.[104]

In patients with obstructive hypertrophic cardiomyopathy, tall R waves with inverted T waves in lead V_1 are occasionally seen to simulate right ventricular hypertrophy.[13] They also are attributed to marked septal hypertrophy. Most of the patients also have abnormal Q waves in the left precordial leads, but occasionally the tall R waves are observed in their absence.

Patients with hypertrophic cardiomyopathy have a lower incidence of intraventricular conduction defect than do those with dilated cardiomyopathy. In my experience, right bundle branch block is particularly uncommon. The typical Wolff-Parkinson-White syndrome was described in 4 of the 123 patients with obstructive cardiomyopathy reported by Frank and Braunwald.[36] These authors also noted 11 patients with atypical forms of the syndrome in which one of the triad of the syndrome (short PR, delta wave, prolonged QRS duration) was absent.

ST-Segment and T-Wave Changes

ST-segment and T-wave abnormalities are the most common findings in this disease.[31,89] They are usually secondary to left ventricular hypertrophy or conduction defects. In the absence of QRS changes, these findings are most often nonspecific in nature. Yamaguchi and associates described 30 patients with hypertrophic nonobstructive cardiomyopathy and giant negative T waves in the precordial leads. The ventriculograms and echocardiograms revealed marked concentric apical hypertrophy.[107] Similar findings were reported by others.[59]

Arrhythmias and AV Block

Recognition of rhythm disturbances is of particular importance in patients with hypertrophic cardiomyopathy. The most common mode of demise in these patients is sudden death. In the 254 patients with hypertrophic cardiomyopathy followed by McKenna and associates for 1 to 23 years (mean 6 years), 58 died, 32 of them suddenly.[69] Similar high incidence of sudden death also was reported by other institutions.

Twenty-four– to 48-hour ambulatory ECG monitoring reveals supraventricular tachyarrhythmias in 15 to 46 percent of patients with hypertrophic cardiomyopathy.[17,68,90] Atrial fibrillation occurs in 7 to 16 percent[35,40,68,90] (see Fig. 12–7). It usually appears late in the course of the disease and does not seem to be related to the severity of the left ventricular outflow obstruction. Its onset is often accompanied by significant clinical deterioration. Complex ventricular premature beats are observed in 33 to 48 percent of the patients and ventricular tachycardia in 15 to 26 percent.[17,68,90] Maron and associates found that patients with nonsustained ventricular tachycardia had about an eightfold greater risk of sudden death than patients without such ventricular arrhythmias.[65] In a recently reported case, ventricular tachycardia followed by ventricular fibrillation was documented by ambulatory ECG as the mechanism of sudden death.[73]

Sinoatrial nodal disease is uncommon in patients with hypertrophic cardiomyopathy and so is high-degree AV block.[17,68,96]

RESTRICTIVE CARDIOMYOPATHY

In restrictive cardiomyopathy, there is a decrease in ventricular diastolic compliance. It may be the result of a variety of pathologic processes that involve the myocardium or endocardium such as amyloidosis, hemochromatosis, and fibrosis from various causes. The ECG findings are nonspecific. They are discussed under the disease entities that may be associated with such hemodynamic changes.

SECONDARY CARDIOMYOPATHY

No attempt is made in this text to describe in detail the ECG findings in the various disease entities included in the secondary cardiomyopathies. Only the more common or distinctive changes are discussed.

Neuromuscular Disease

FRIEDREICH'S ATAXIA

The association of cardiac lesions and Friedreich's ataxia is well known and has been at-

tributed to a common genetic origin. Pathologically diffuse interstitial fibrosis and degeneration of myocardial fibers were observed in all autopsied cases. Some hearts showed intimal thickening of the small coronary vessels.[53] Hypertrophy of one or both ventricles is a frequent finding, with the hypertrophy sometimes being eccentric.

The ECG findings are abnormal in 75 to 92 percent of the cases.[21,48,99] ST-segment and T-wave changes are the most common abnormalities, being present in about 60 to 75 percent of the patients.[21,48] Right axis deviation occurs more often than left axis deviation. Left and right ventricular hypertrophy patterns are seen in 10 to 16 percent of the larger series.[21,48] Tall and broad R waves may be seen in the right precordial leads in the absence of echocardiographic evidence of right ventricular hypertrophy or asymmetrical septal hypertrophy.[21] Abnormal Q waves, mostly in the inferolateral leads, were reported in 14 to 20 percent of the cases[21,37] and are probably related to myocardial fibrosis. Various atrial arrhythmias and ventricular extrasystoles are observed. AV conduction delay is uncommon, but short PR interval was observed in 24 percent of the patients in one series.[21] Figure 12–10 is an example that illustrates some of the abnormalities seen in a patient with Friedreich's ataxia.

PROGRESSIVE MUSCULAR DYSTROPHY

An abnormal ECG is frequently seen in the Duchenne or pseudohypertrophic type of muscular dystrophy. In the larger series, it occurs in about 68 to 95 percent of patients.[94] The most common findings are tall R waves in lead V_1 with or without deep but narrow Q waves in the left precordial and sometimes the limb leads (see Fig. 9–47). An RSr' pattern or polyphasic R waves in lead V_1 suggestive of right ventricular conduction defect also are seen. The PR interval is often abnormally short. Although sinus tachycardia usually is the only arrhythmia encountered, premature atrial and ventricular contractions, atrial flutter, and paroxysmal ventricular tachycardia were reported.[78] Abnormal ECG findings are more likely to be seen in older patients and in those with longstanding and disabling skeletal muscle disease; they are present in all fatal cases.[39] The presence of abnormal Q waves is considered evidence of late changes.

The rather distinctive ECG changes of tall R waves in V_1 and deep Q waves in leads V_5 and

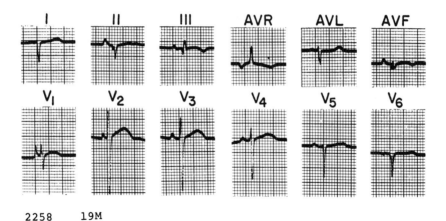

2258   19M

FIGURE 12–10. Friedreich's ataxia. The patient was 19 years old. The ECG shows abnormal P waves, especially in lead V_1, to suggest right atrial enlargement. There is abnormal right axis deviation. The amplitude of the R waves is decreased in leads V_3 through V_5, and a QS deflection is present in leads I, II and V_6. The T waves are inverted in leads III and aVF. (Courtesy of Dr. Samuel Kaplan.)

V_6 were attributed by Perloff and associates[78] to selective myocardial scarring of the postero-basal portion of the left ventricle, which allowed the anterior forces (R in V_1) to become more prominent. The abnormal deep Q waves in the left precordial leads reflected lateral extension of this scarring. My autopsy case, illustrated in Figure 9–47, appears to support this view, which was, however, questioned by Slucka.[94]

Various rhythm and conduction disturbances are seen in Duchenne's muscular dystrophy. These include sinus pauses, atrial, ectopic beats and rhythm, junctional rhythm, atrial flutter, ventricular premature beats, intraatrial conduction defect, Mobitz type I second-degree AV block, short PR interval, left hemiblocks, and right bundle branch block.[78,88,102]

Abnormal ECG changes are uncommon in the facio-scapulohumeral type of progressive muscular dystrophy.

MYOTONIA DYSTROPHY (STEINERT'S DISEASE)

Although myocardial fibrosis is often seen in patients with myotonia dystrophy, the most prominent cardiac abnormality in this familial muscular disease involves the conduction tissue, especially the His-Purkinje system.[71,72,79] Fibrosis, fatty infiltration, and atrophy of the sinus node, AV node, bundle of His, and bundle branches are observed in most cases at autopsy.[72]

The ECG is abnormal in 45 to 85 percent of patients with the disease.[22,26,71,74,75,79] The com-

mon findings are low P waves, prolonged PR interval, abnormal left axis deviation, intraventricular conduction defect, bundle branch block, abnormal Q waves, and ST-segment and T-wave abnormalities (Fig. 12–11). Various arrhythmias, particularly atrial fibrillation and atrial flutter, also are seen. Ventricular tachycardia and sudden death may occasionally occur.[45] In 65 patients reported on by Olofsson and colleagues, first-degree AV block and left anterior hemiblock were encountered most commonly in patients with mild and moderate neuromuscular symptoms and functional limitations. Atrial fibrillation and flutter, abnormal Q waves, and repolarization abnormalities were more common in patients with severe disease.[74]

KEARNS-SAYRE SYNDROME

Kearns-Sayre syndrome is uncommon. It is a mitochondrial myopathy characterized clinically by progressive external ophthalmoplegia, pigmentary retinopathy, and cardiac conduction defect. In one large series of 66 patients reported on by Petty and associates,[80] the ECGs showed abnormal findings in 11 (17 percent). The abnormalities include first- and second-degree AV block, right bundle branch block, left anterior hemiblock, nonspecific intraventricular conduction defect, and ST-segment and T-wave changes. Impairment of cardiac function due to cardiomyopathy is uncommon but has been reported.[19,38] Figure 12–12 illustrates the presence of bifascicular block in a 20-year-old man with this syndrome.

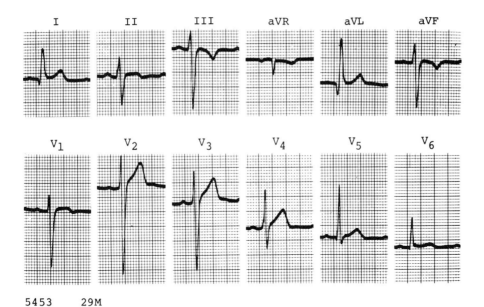

5453   29M

FIGURE 12–11. Myotonia dystrophy in a 29-year-old man. The diagnosis is based on clinical data and a strong family history. The tracing shows abnormal left axis deviation, consistent with left anterior hemiblock. The T waves are abnormal in the inferior leads.

Connective Tissue Disease

SCLERODERMA HEART DISEASE

The heart may be involved directly or indirectly in scleroderma. The myocardium may be the site of widespread fibrous degneration. Right ventricular hypertrophy sometimes occurs because of pulmonary hypertension sec-

ondary to pulmonary vascular abnormalities or pulmonary fibrosis. Left ventricular hypertrophy is observed in patients with systemic hypertension as a result of renal involvement. The pericardium is often involved, with possible development of large pericardial effusion.

The reported incidence of abnormal ECGs in patients with scleroderma ranges from 9 to

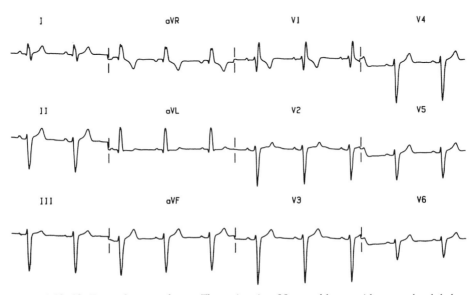

FIGURE 12–12. Kearns-Sayre syndrome. The patient is a 22-year-old man with external ophthalmoplegia, pigmentary retinopathy, and complete right bundle branch block with left anterior hemiblock as illustrated in the ECG.

85 percent.[87,106] The highest incidence was seen in the series reported by Sackner and associates.[87] In 60 patients with clinical or pathologic evidence of cardiac involvement, the ECGs showed signs of right ventricular hypertrophy in 16 (27 percent) cases. Signs of left ventricular hypertrophy were observed in 9 (15 percent). Some patients had changes suggestive of combined ventricular hypertrophy, low voltage of the QRS complexes, or abnormal Q waves simulating myocardial infarction. Other abnormalities included signs of pericarditis, abnormal P waves with P pulmonale pattern, notched P waves in the limb leads, bundle branch block, first- or second-degree AV block, atrial arrhythmias, and ventricular extrasystoles. Low voltage of the QRS complex (up to 20 percent) was more common in other series.[30] This finding and the pseudoinfarction pattern are attributable to myocardial fibrosis. Atrial fibrosis was present in many cases with notching of the P waves.[30]

SYSTEMIC LUPUS ERYTHEMATOSUS

Electrocardiographic findings are reported to be abnormal in 34 to 62 percent of patients with systemic lupus erythematosus.[28] In autopsied cases, the incidence of abnormal ECGs was even higher.[61] The most common changes involve the T waves, but they are nonspecific in nature. In many instances, the T-wave changes are the results of pericarditis, and their correlation with anatomic evidence of myocarditis is poor.[61] Low voltage of the QRS complex in the limb leads was seen in 23 (17 percent) of 137 patients studied by Hejtmancik and associates.[51] Pericardial effusion may be responsible for some of the cases. Other signs of myocardial involvement, such as AV and intraventricular conduction defects, are seen only occasionally. Myocardial infarction may occur as a result of lupus vasculitis of the larger coronary branches.[28] Findings suggestive of left ventricular hypertrophy were observed in a few patients who had hypertension.[93] Both supraventricular and ventricular tachyarrhythmias are infrequent. A notable phenomenon is the high incidence (20 percent) of congenital complete AV block in infants born to mothers who have systemic lupus erythematosus.[3]

POLYARTERITIS NODOSA

In polyarteritis nodosa, evidence of coronary arteritis is present in 50 to 62 percent of autopsied cases.[56,92] Aneurysm of the coronary arteries is seen occasionally. Myocardial infarcts of various sizes may be observed, but gross infarcts were identified in only a small number of cases in more recent series.[92] Pericarditis, diffuse or focal interstitial myocarditis, and ventricular hypertrophy are other pathologic findings; most of the hypertrophy is probably caused by associated systemic hypertension.

Electrocardiographic findings were abnormal in 85 percent of Holsinger's 41 autopsy cases.[56] The most common abnormality was T-wave changes, most of which were nonspecific. Some were probably due to pericarditis, myocardial ischemia, or ventricular hypertrophy. Three of the patients had ECG changes of acute myocardial infarction. Low QRS voltage, left axis deviation, supraventricular tachycardia such as atrial fibrillation, and atrial flutter also were seen in some patients.

POLYMYOSITIS

Cardiac involvement is recognized with increasing frequency in patients with polymyositis.[25,43,50,63,64,76,91] The prominent pathologic changes consist of fibrosis of the conduction system (including AV node, His bundle, and both bundle branches), the sinoatrial node, and the atrial and ventricular myocardium. Pericarditis also has been described. The ECG may reveal atrial and ventricular arrhythmias, AV block, bundle branch block, hemiblocks, abnormal Q waves, and ST-segment and T-wave abnormalities.[25,43,50,63,64,76,91]

RHEUMATOID HEART DISEASE

Fibrinoid granulomas were reported in all parts of the heart, including the myocardium, in some patients with rheumatoid arthritis. ST-segment and T-wave abnormalities may be seen in patients with myocarditis, but they are more often related to pericarditis.[12]

Myocardial Tumors

In both primary and secondary (metastatic) tumors of the heart, the ECG manifestations depend in a large measure on the location and extent of the space-occupying lesion. Tumor involvement of the atrium may cause abnormal P waves and atrial arrhythmias, especially atrial fibrillation and atrial flutter. AV block or bundle branch block occasionally occurs because of the invasion of the AV junction or interventricular septum (Fig. 12–13). The QRS voltage is decreased when there is extensive

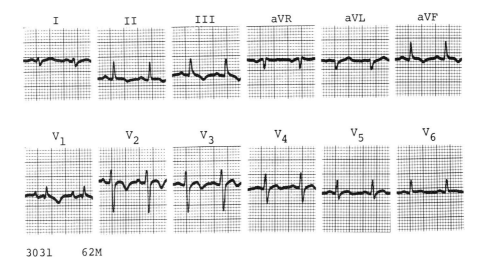

3031   62M

FIGURE 12–13. Metastatic tumor of the heart. The patient was a 62-year-old man with carcinoma of the lung and widespread metastasis. The metastatic lesions involved both ventricles but particularly the right ventricle, apex, and posterior wall of the left ventricle. The coronary arteries were normal. There was no sign of either left or right ventricular hypertrophy. In the ECG, there is a borderline right axis deviation. An rSR′ pattern is present in lead V_1, but the duration of the QRS complex is within normal limits. T-wave inversion is present in the inferior and right precordial leads. In the absence of anatomic evidence of right ventricular hypertrophy, the right axis deviation and rSR′ pattern in lead V_1 probably represent right ventricular conduction defect.

destruction of the myocardium.[9] In many cases, however, this is the result of pericardial effusion secondary to pericardial involvement. Infarction pattern may be observed with both primary and metastatic tumors of the heart. Progressive and prolonged ST-segment elevation is occasionally seen in patients who have metastatic tumors.[49] By far the most common abnormalities in secondary cardiac tu-

mors are nonspecific ST-segment and T-wave changes[8,10,18] (see Figs. 12–13 and 12–14).

Metabolic Disease

HEMOCHROMATOSIS

Myocardial degeneration and fibrosis occur in hemochromatosis when the deposition of he-

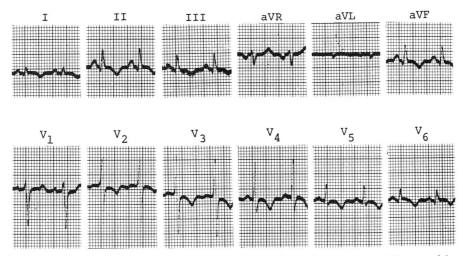

FIGURE 12–14. Malignant lymphoma with extensive and diffuse lymphomatous infiltration of the pericardium and myocardium. The patient was a 37-year-old man, and the diagnosis was confirmed at autopsy. About 80 percent of the myocardium was replaced by the tumor tissue. In the ECG, the amplitude of the R waves in the left precordial leads is reduced. Diffuse symmetrical T-wave inversion involves most of the leads.

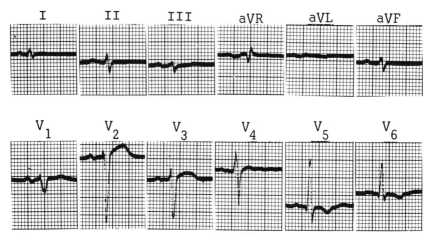

FIGURE 12–15. Autopsy-proven hemochromatosis with extensive involvement of the myocardium. The heart weighed more than 500 g. There was minimal atherosclerosis of the coronary arteries. The ECG shows low voltage of the QRS complex in the limb leads. The frontal plane QRS axis is indeterminate. T-wave abnormalities are present in the limb leads and leads V_4 through V_6.

mosiderin is extensive. The ECG may reveal low voltage of the QRS complexes and flat or inverted T waves[101] (Fig. 12–15). Supraventricular arrhythmias are common[29] and appear to correlate with the extent of iron deposits in the atrial myocardium.[15] Ventricular tachycardia, AV block, and intraventricular conduction defect, particularly right bundle branch block, are seen.[29]

MYXEDEMA HEART

Electrocardiographic changes are often part of the prominent manifestations of hypothyroid heart disease. The degree of the changes, however, may not be in proportion to that in the other tissues.[108] The typical findings include low voltage of all the complexes and flattening or inversion of the T waves (Fig. 12–16).

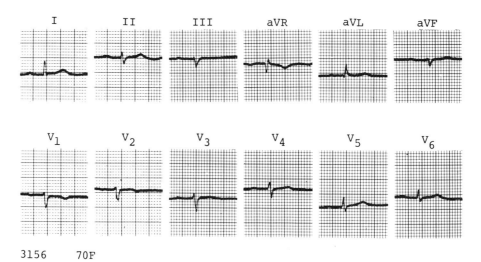

3156   70F

FIGURE 12–16. Myxedema heart disease. The patient is a 70-year-old woman with a 15-year history of myxedema. She had a recurrence of the symptoms and signs of myxedema after she stopped taking her medication for 1 year. She has no symptoms of coronary artery disease. The heart is not enlarged on radiographic examination. The ECG shows first-degree AV block. There is low voltage of the P waves and the QRS complexes with abnormal left axis deviation. The T waves are inverted in leads V_1 through V_3.

Low voltage of the QRS complex was observed in 35 percent of 92 cases reported by Douglas and Samuel.[27] It was most noticeable in leads I and II. T-wave changes and low P waves are even more common. Occasionally, the PR interval may be prolonged. All of these abnormalities usually improve with thyroid therapy within 3 weeks. Changes may even be noticed within 24 to 48 hours.[108]

In many cases, some of the ECG abnormalities are probably due to pericardial effusion, but they are also seen in its absence. Interstitial myocardial edema is believed to be the most likely explanation for the changes. Many of the patients also have coronary artery disease, which may account for some of the ECG abnormalities.

Granulomatous Cardiomyopathy

MYOCARDIAL SARCOIDOSIS

The outstanding ECG abnormalities resulting from sarcoid involvement of the myocardium are conduction disturbances and arrhythmias (Fig. 12–17). Indeed, conduction disturbance is the most common clinical manifestation in the reported autopsy series of myocardial sarcoidosis.[5,44] In 47 cases summarized from the literature, complete AV block occurred in 22 and incomplete AV block in 12.[44] Intraventricular conduction defect, mostly right bundle branch block, was observed in 15.[44] This high incidence of conduction disorder can be explained by the frequent involvement of the interventricular septum and conduction pathways, which were demonstrable in over 40 percent of the autopsied hearts with sarcoidosis.[5,44,81] Ectopic impulse formation is the second most common clinical manifestation. Both ventricular and supraventricular arrhythmias are seen, with the former being slightly more prevalent. Several different types of arrhythmias may be observed in the same patient. This is illustrated in Figure 12–17.

The granulomatous infiltration of the myocardium occasionally may be accompanied by ECG pattern of Q-wave infarction because of the loss of electrical forces from the involved area.[41] Nonspecific T-wave changes are often present, but they are of no diagnostic help. Unrelated to direct myocardial involvement are signs of right ventricular hypertrophy, which may be seen in patients with cor pulmonale resulting from extensive pulmonary sarcoidosis.

Amyloid Heart Disease

The frequency of ECG changes in cardiac amyloidosis depends a great deal on the amount of amyloid deposits in the heart. When the deposits are extensive and cardiac dysfunction is clinically evident, the ECG is almost always abnormal.

In a review of 339 cases reported in the literature, Buja and colleagues found low voltage of the complexes in 50 percent, left axis deviation in 59 percent, and conduction or rhythm disturbance in 58 percent of the patients.[14] Sixty-four percent of the patients had a pseudoinfarction pattern, most displaying small or absent R waves in leads V_1 through V_3. Although none of these ECG changes are specific, cardiac amyloidosis should be considered when a combination of these findings is present in an elderly patient in intractable congestive heart failure without a history of heart disease[32] (Fig. 12–18). Amyloid deposition in the intramural coronary arteries and conduction system, in addition to that in the myocardium, is responsible for these abnormal findings. Occasionally occlusion of the intramural coronary artery by amyloid is responsible for the appearance of ECG and pathologic evidence of recent myocardial infarction.[14]

Myocarditis

ACUTE RHEUMATIC FEVER AND RHEUMATIC MYOCARDITIS

Prolongation of the PR interval is the most frequent and outstanding ECG abnormality in patients with acute rheumatic fever. Its incidence varies considerably (from 25 to 95 percent) in different reported series.[86] Second-degree AV block of the Wenckebach type also may occur, but complete AV block is uncommon[23] (see Fig. 12–19). The presence of AV conduction defect, however, does not necessarily mean rheumatic involvement of the AV junction, as it may occur in the absence of carditis. Clarke and Keith analyzed the AV conduction time in 508 patients with acute rheumatic fever and found no significant difference in the PR interval between patients with and without carditis.[23] The prolongation also is not significantly related to the severity of carditis nor to subsequent evidence of cardiac damage.[33] Although increased vagal tone is thought to be responsible for the AV conduction defect, the exact mechanism is still unknown.

A

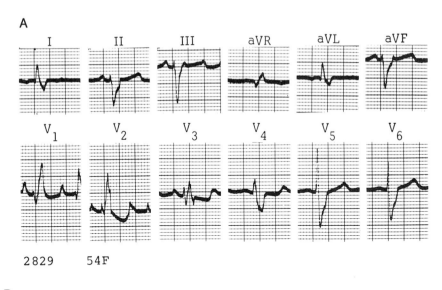

2829   54F

B

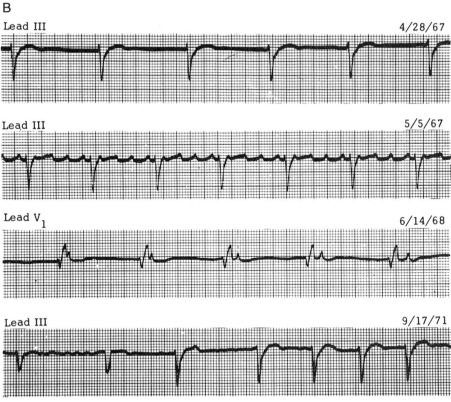

2829   54F

FIGURE 12–17. Myocardial sarcoidosis. The patient was a 54-year-old woman who was known to have had sarcoidosis for 15 years. She died suddenly, and no autopsy was performed. The diagnosis of myocardial sarcoidosis was based on clinical data. (A) Abnormal P waves suggestive of right atrial enlargement. Left anterior hemiblock and complete right bundle branch block also are present. (B) Tracing illustrating some of the arrhythmias that the patient had. They include AV junctional rhythm (4-28-67), atrial flutter (5-5-67), AV dissociation (6-14-68), and atrial fibrillation (9-17-71).

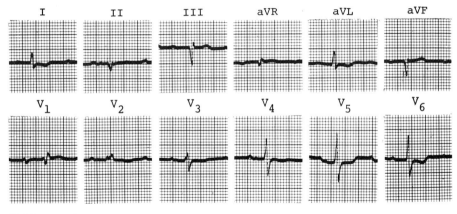

3900   68M

FIGURE 12–18. Cardiac amyloidosis. The patient was a 68-year-old man with primary systemic amyloidosis. There was extensive cardiac involvement, and the patient had severe congestive heart failure. The heart weighed 500 g with marked dilatation of the atria and severe dilatation and hypertrophy of both ventricles. The coronary arteries were normal. In the ECG, there is a first-degree AV block. The P waves are abnormally notched. There is an abnormal left axis deviation, and the QRS changes in the inferior leads suggest the possibility of inferior myocardial damage. An rSr' pattern is present in lead V_1 with notched R wave in lead V_2. It is uncertain whether these changes are due to right ventricular hypertrophy or to incomplete right bundle branch block. Diffuse ST and T-wave abnormalities also are present.

Almost equally common findings are ST-segment and T-wave changes, which were observed in 61 percent of one series.[11] Some of these are related to pericardial involvement, especially when the ST-segment is elevated. The QT interval also may be prolonged.

Various other arrhythmias have been observed. One of the more distinctive rhythm disturbances is AV junctional rhythm with or without AV dissociation.[6,23] In one series, this occurred in 9.4 percent of patients.[23] Left or right bundle branch block also is seen but is uncommon (see Figs. 7–3 and 12–19).

VIRAL MYOCARDITIS

An abnormal ECG that consists mostly of ST-segment and T-wave changes and occasionally AV block is not uncommon in many of the viral illnesses. Such a finding is present on about 5 percent of patients with mumps[7] and in 5 to 10 percent of those with infectious mononucleosis.[54,102] From 17 to 44 percent of patients with viral hepatitis are noted to have ECG abnormalities. Although both myocarditis and pericarditis were found in some of the autopsied cases, the ECG abnormalities are not necessarily always accompanied by inflammatory lesions in the heart. Figure 12–20 gives an example of a case of acute myocarditis, presumably of viral origin.

Coxsackievirus infection is known to be associated with ECG changes, including occasional cases with abnormal Q waves suggestive of myocardial infarction.[95] Such an example is given in Figure 12–21. Pseudoinfarction pattern also is observed in acute myocarditis that results from other causes.[42]

ACQUIRED IMMUNODEFICIENCY SYNDROME

Cardiac involvements in patients with AIDS include fibrinous pericarditis, pericardial effusion with or without cardiac tamponade, myocarditis, dilated cardiomyopathy, metastatic Kaposi's sarcoma, and nonbacterial thrombotic endocarditis.[1,2,16] In a series of 71 consecutive autopsied patients reported by Anderson and colleagues, myocarditis was the most common pathologic finding and was found in 52 percent of the cases.[2] Biventricular dilatation was present in 7 of these patients. Although opportunistic pathogens were found in the myocardium in some hearts, the cause of myocarditis was not identified in most of the patients.[2]

Electrocardiographic findings are abnormal in 33 to 58 percent of patients with AIDS, and ST-segment and T-wave changes are the most common findings.[62,83] Bundle branch block, infarction pattern, and low QRS voltage are sometimes present. Ventricular tachycardia may occasionally occur.[62,84] Figure 12–22 illustrates some of the changes in a patient with AIDS and dilated cardiomyopathy.

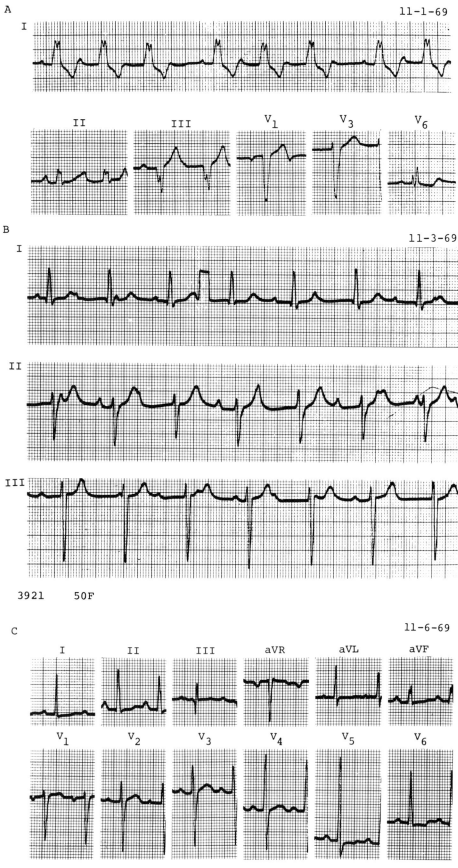

A   11-1-69

I

II   III   V₁   V₃   V₆

B   11-3-69

I

II

III

3921   50F

C   11-6-69

I   II   III   aVR   aVL   aVF

V₁   V₂   V₃   V₄   V₅   V₆

3921   50F

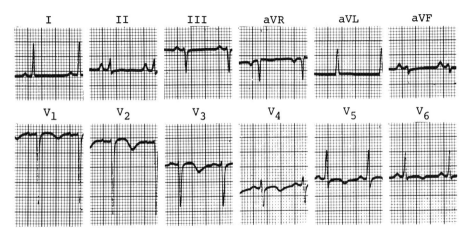

1906   37F

FIGURE 12–20. Actue myocarditis. The patient is a 37-year-old woman with a history of flu-like symptoms followed by the development of cardiomegaly, S_3 and S_4 gallops, and congestive heart failure. The ECG shows diffuse T-wave abnormalities with symmetrical T-wave inversion in the precordial leads. There is poor progression of the R wave in the precordial leads. It cannot be determined if anterior myocardial damage is present.

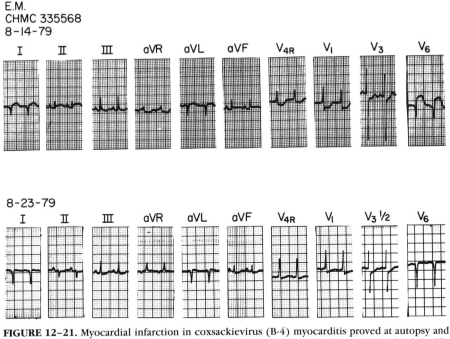

FIGURE 12–21. Myocardial infarction in coxsackievirus (B-4) myocarditis proved at autopsy and postmortem myocardial culture. In the ECG of 4-14-78, QR deflections are present in leads I, aVL, and V_6, with ST-segment elevation in these leads as well as leads II and aVF. Reciprocal ST-segment depression is present in leads V_{4R}, V_1, and V_3. The tracing is consistent with acute anterolateral myocardial infarction and inferior wall injury. The follow-up tracing on 8-23-79 shows the resolution of most of the ST-segment changes. (Courtesy of Dr. David Schwartz.)

←—————————————————————

FIGURE 12–19. Acute rheumatic fever with carditis. The patient was a 50-year-old woman with rheumatic heart disease, aortic insufficiency, and a recurrence of acute rheumatic fever with carditis. (A) Tracing illustrating the development of second-degree AV block with Wenckebach phenomenon and complete left bundle branch block. (B) Two days later, the patient had complete AV block and idioventricular rhythm. She was treated with steroids. (C) Tracing showing the return to 1:1 AV conduction with borderline first-degree AV block. Intraventricular conduction is now normal. The morphology of the ventricular complexes is consistent with left ventricular hypertrophy.

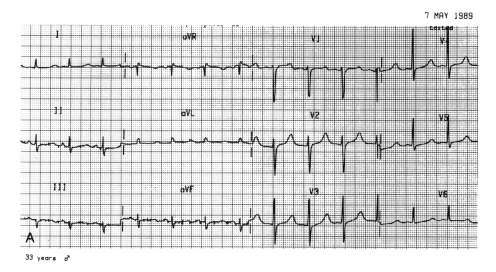

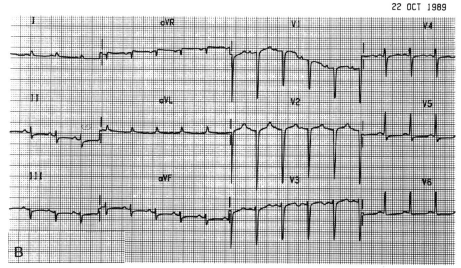

FIGURE 12–22. Dilated cardiomyopathy associated with acquired immunodeficiency syndrome. The patient was a 33-year-old man with AIDS. The diagnosis of dilated cardiomyopathy with congestive heart failure was made in June 1989. Radionuclide ventriculogram at the time revealed biventricular dilatation with hypokinesis. The right ventricular ejection fraction was 7 percent, and the left, 12 percent. (A) Tracing recorded on 5-7-89, before any evidence of cardiac involvement was recognized clinically, showing borderline abnormal left axis deviation. The QT interval is prolonged and is due to hypocalcemia secondary to his renal disease. (B) Tracing obtained on 10-22-89, 4 months after the diagnosis of cardiomyopathy was made, when the patient was again in congestive heart failure. There is low QRS voltage in the limb leads, left anterior hemiblock, and marked reduction of the R-wave amplitude in leads V_1 through V_4 suggestive of anteroseptal myocardial damage. Nonspecific ST and T-wave changes also are present.

CHAGAS' DISEASE

Involvement of the myocardium is almost a constant feature of Chagas' disease, a South American *Trypanosoma* disease. In its chronic form, many different forms of arrhythmias and conduction defects are observed. The ECGs are abnormal in nearly 90 percent of the cases.[85] The most characteristic finding is right bundle branch block (occurring in 57 percent) with or without left anterior hemiblock. Other more common changes are T-wave abnormalities and multifocal premature ventricular contractions.

REFERENCES

1. Acierno LJ: Cardiac complications in acquired immunodeficiency syndrome (AIDS): A review. J Am Coll Cardiol 13:1144, 1989

2. Anderson DW, Virmani R, Reilly JM, et al: Prevalent myocarditis at necropsy in the acquired immunodeficiency syndrome. Am Coll Cardiol 11:792, 1988

3. Ansari A, Larson PH, Bates HD: Cardiovascular manifestations of systemic lupus erythematosus: Current perspective. Prog Cardiovasc Dis 27:421, 1985

4. Bahl OP, Walsh TJ, Massie E: Electrocardiography and vectorcardiography in idiopathic hypertrophic subaortic stenosis. Am J Med Sci 259:262, 1970

5. Bashour FA, McConnell T, Skinner W, et al: Myocardial sarcoidosis. Dis Chest 53:413, 1968

6. Bates RC: Acute rheumatic fever: A study of 132 cases in young adults. Ann Intern Med 48:1017, 1958

7. Bengtsson E, Orndahl G: Complications of mumps with special reference to the incidence of myocarditis. Acta Med Scand 149:381, 1954

8. Berge T, Sievers J: Myocardial metastases: A pathological and electrocardiographic study. Br Heart J 30:383, 1968

9. Biran S, Hochman A, Levij IS, et al: Clinical diagnosis of secondary tumors of the heart and pericardium. Dis Chest 55:202, 1969

10. Bisel HF, Wroblewski F, La Due JS: Incidence and clinical manifestation of cardiac metastases. JAMA 153:712, 1953

11. Blackman NS, Hamilton CI: Serial electrocardiographic changes in young adults with acute rheumatic fever: Reports of 62 cases. Ann Intern Med 29:416, 1948

12. Bonfiglio T, Atwater TC: Heart disease in patients with seropositive rheumatoid arthritis. Arch Intern Med 124:714, 1969

13. Braudo M, Wigle ED, Keith JD: A distinctive electrocardiogram in muscular subaortic stenosis due to ventricular septal hypertrophy. Am J Cardiol 14:599, 1964

14. Buja LM, Khoi NB, Roberts WC: Clinically significant cardiac amyloidosis: Clinicopathologic findings in 15 patients. Am J Cardiol 26:394, 1970

15. Buja LM, Roberts WC: Iron in the heart: Etiology and clinical significance. Am J Med 51:209, 1971

16. Cammarosano C, Lewis W: Cardiac lesions in acquired immune deficiency syndrome (AIDS). J Am Coll Cardiol 5:703, 1985

17. Canedo MI, Frank MJ, Abdulla AM: Rhythm disturbances in hypertrophic cardiomyopathy: Prevalence, relation to symptoms and management. Am J Cardiol 45:848, 1980

18. Cates CU, Virmani R, Vaughn WK, et al: Electrocardiographic markers of cardiac metastasis. Am Heart J 112:1297, 1986

19. Channer KS, Channer JL, Campbell MJ, Rees JR: Cardiomyopathy in the Kearns-Sayre syndrome. Br Heart J 59:486, 1988

20. Chen CH, Nobuyoshi M, Kawai C: ECG pattern of left ventricular hypertrophy in nonobstructive hypertrophic cardiomyopathy: The significance of the mid-precordial changes. Am Heart J 97:687, 1979

21. Child JS, Perloff JK, Bach PM, et al: Cardiac involvement in Friedreich's ataxia: A clinical study of 75 patients. J Am Coll Cardiol 7:1370, 1986

22. Church SC: The heart in myotonia atrophica. Arch Intern Med 119:176, 1967

23. Clarke M, Keith JD: Atrioventricular conduction in acute rheumatic fever. Br Heart J 34:472, 1972

24. Cosio FG, Moro C, Alonso M, et al: The Q waves of hypertrophic cardiomyopathy: An electrophysiologic study. N Engl J Med 302:96, 1980

25. Denbow CE, Lie JT, Tancredi RG, et al: Cardiac involvement in polymyositis: A clinicopathologic study of 20 autopsied patients. Arthritis Rheum 22:1088, 1979

26. DeWind LT, Jones RJ: Cardiovascular observations in dystrophia myotonica. JAMA 144:299, 1950

27. Douglas AH, Samuel P: Analysis of electrocardiographic patterns in hypothyroid heart disease. NY J Med 60:2227, 1960

28. DuBois EL: Lupus Erythematosus, ed 2. Los Angeles, University of Southern California Press, 1974

29. Engle MA, Erlandson M, Smith CH: Late cardiac complications of chronic, severe, refractory anemia with hemochromatosis. Circulation 30:698, 1964

30. Escudero J, McDevitt E: The electrocardiogram in scleroderma: Analaysis of 60 cases and review of the literature. Am Heart J 56:846, 1958

31. Estes EH, Whalen RE, Roberts SR, et al: The electrocardiographic and vectorcardiographic findings in idiopathic hypertrophic subaortic stenosis. Am Heart J 65:155, 1963

32. Farrokh A, Walsh TJ, Massie E: Amyloid heart disease. Am J Cardiol 13:750, 1964

33. Feinstein AR, Wood HF, Spagnuolo M, et al: Rheumatic fever in children and adolescents: A long-term epidemiologic study of subsequent prophylaxis, streptococcal infections, and clinical sequelae. VII. Cardiac changes and sequelae. Ann Intern Med 60(Suppl 5):87, 1964

34. Flowers NV, Horan LG: Electrocardiographic and vectorcardiographic features of myocardial disease. In Fowler NO (ed): Myocardial Diseases. New York, Grune & Stratton, 1973

35. Fowler, NO: Cardiac Diagnosis and Treatment, ed 2. New York, Harper & Row, 1976

36. Frank S, Braunwald E: Idiopathic hypertrophic subaortic stenosis: Clinical analysis of 126 patients with emphasis on the natural history. Circulation 37:759, 1968

37. Gach JV, Andriange M, Franck G: Hypertrophic obstructive cardiomyopathy and Friedreich's ataxia: Report of a case and review of literature. Am J Cardiol 27:436, 1971

38. Gallastegui J, Hariman RJ, Handler B, et al: Cardiac involvement in the Kearns-Sayre syndrome. Am J Cardiol 60:385, 1987

39. Gilroy J, Cahalan JL, Berman K, et al: Cardiac and pulmonary complications in Duchenne's progressive muscular dystrophy. Circulation 27:484, 1963

40. Glancy DL, O'Brien KP, Gold HK, et al: Atrial fibrillation in patients with idiopathic hypertrophic subaortic stenosis. Br Heart J 32:652, 1970

41. Gold JA, Cantor PJ: Sarcoid heart disease: A case with an unusual electrocardiogram. Arch Intern Med 104:101, 1959

42. Goldman AM: Acute myocarditis simulating myocardial infarction. Dis Chest 41:61, 1962

43. Gottdiener JS, Sherber HS, Hawley RJ, et al: Cardiac manifestations in polymyositis. Am J Cardiol 41:1141, 1978

44. Gozo EG, Cosnow I, Cohen HC, et al: Heart in sarcoidosis. Chest 60:379, 1971

45. Grigg LE, Chan W, Mond HG, et al: Ventricular tachycardia and sudden death in myotonic dystrophy: Clinical, electrophysiologic and pathologic features. J Am Coll Cardiol 6:254, 1985

46. Halpern SW, Mandel WJ, Allen HN, et al: Disparity between echocardiographic and electrocardiographic findings in asymmetric septal hypertrophy (Abstract). Clin Res 25:89A, 1977

47. Hamby RI, Raia F: Electrocardiographic aspects of

primary myocardial disease in 60 patients. Am Heart J 76:316, 1968

48. Harding AE, Hewer RL: The heart disease of Friedreich's ataxia: A clinical and electrocardiographic study of 115 patients, with an analysis of serial electrocardiographic changes in 30 cases. Q J Med 208:489, 1983

49. Harris TR, Copeland GD, Brody DA: Progressive injury current with metastatic tumor of the heart. Am Heart J 69:392, 1965

50. Haupt HM, Hutchins GM: The heart and cardiac conduction system in polymyositis-dermatomyositis: A clinicopathologic study of 16 autopsied patients. Am J Cardiol 50:998, 1982

51. Hejtmancik MR, Wright JC, Quint R, et al: The cardiovascular manifestations of systemic lupus erythematosus. Am Heart J 68:119, 1964

52. Henderson MA, Ruddy TD, Rakowski H, et al: Left ventricular hypertrophy by ECG in hypertrophic cardiomyopathy (Abstract). J Am Coll Cardiol 1:693, 1983

53. Hewer RS: The heart in Friedreich's ataxia. Br Heart J 31:5, 1969

54. Hoagland RJ: Cardiac involvement in infectious mononucleosis. Am J Med Sci 232:252, 1956

55. Hollister RM, Goodwin JF: The electrocardiogram in cardiomyopathy. Br Heart J 25:357, 1963

56. Holsinger DR, Osmundson PJ, Edward JE: The heart in periarteritis nodosa. Circulation 25:610, 1962

57. Huang SK, Messer JV, Denes P: Significance of ventricular tachycardia in idiopathic dilated cardiomyopathy: Observations in 35 patients. Am J Cardiol 51:507, 1983

58. Joye J, DeMaria AN, Neumann A, et al: Electrocardiographic abnormalities in hypertrophic cardiomyopathy: Relation to cardiac hypertrophy and intraventricular obstruction (Abstract). Circulation 54:(Suppl II):II-209, 1976

59. Keren G, Belhassen B, Sherez B, et al: Apical hypertrophic cardiomyopathy: Evaluation by noninvasive and invasive techniques in 23 patients. Circulation 71:45, 1985

60. Klein MD, Mathur V, Levine HD, et al: Electromechanical correlations in hypertrophic subaortic stenosis. Circulation 38:635, 1968

61. Kong TQ, Kellum RE, Haserick JR: Clinical diagnosis of cardiac involvement in systemic lupus erythematosus: A correlation of clinical and autopsy findings in thirty patients. Circulation 26:7, 1962

62. Levy WS, Simon GL, Rios JC, Ross AM: Prevalence of cardiac abnormalities in human immunodeficiency virus infection. Am J Cardiol 63:86, 1989

63. Lightfoot PR, Bharati S, Lev M: Chronic dermatomyositis with intermittent trifascicular block. Chest 71:413, 1977

64. Lynch PG: Cardiac involvement in chronic polymyositis. Br Heart J 33:416, 1971

65. Maron BJ, Savage DD, Wolfson JK, et al: Prognostic significance of 24 hour ambulatory electrocardiographic monitoring in patients with hypertrophic cardiomyopathy: A prospective study. Am J Cardiol 48:252, 1981

66. Maron BJ, Wolfson JK, Ciro E, et al: Relation of electrocardiographic abnormalities and pattern of left ventricular hypertrophy identified by 2-dimensional echocardiography in patients with hypertrophic cardiomyopathy. Am J Cardiol 51:189, 1983

67. Marriott HJ: Electrocardiographic abnormalities, conduction disorders and arrhythmias in primary myocardial disease. Prog Cardiovasc Dis 7:99, 1964

68. McKenna WJ, Chetty S, Oakley CM, et al: Arrhyth-

mia in hypertropic cardiomyopathy: Exercise and 48 hour ambulatory electrocardiographic assessment with and without beta adrenergic blocking therapy. Am J Cardiol 45:1, 1980

69. McKenna WJ, Deanfield J, Faruqui A, et al: Prognosis in hypertrophic cardiomyopathy: Role of age and clinical, electrocardiographic and hemodynamic features. Am J Cardiol 47:532, 1981

70. McKenna WJ, Borggrefe M, England D, et al: The natural history of left ventricular hypertrophy in hypertrophic cardiomyopathy: An electrocardiographic study. Circulation 66:1233, 1982

71. Moorman JR, Coleman RE, Packer DL, et al: Cardiac involvement in myotonic muscular dystrophy. Medicine 64:371, 1985

72. Nguyen HH, Wolfe JT, Holmes DR, Edwards WD: Pathology of the cardiac conduction system in myotonic dystrophy: A study of 12 cases. J Am Coll Cardiol 11:662, 1988

73. Nicod P, Rolikar R, Peterson KL: Hypertrophic cardiomyopathy and sudden death. N Engl J Med 318:1255, 1988

74. Olofsson B, Forsberg H, Andersson S, et al: Electrocardiographic findings in myotonic dystrophy. Br Heart J 59:47, 1988

75. Payne CA, Greenfield JC: Electrocardiographic abnormalities associated with myotonic dystrophy. Am Heart J 65:436, 1963

76. Pearson CM, Bohan A: The spectrum of polymyositis and dermatomyositis. Med Clin North Am 61:439, 1977

77. Perloff JK: Cardiac rhythm and conduction in Duchenne's muscular dystrophy: A prospective study of 20 patients. J Am Coll Cardiol 3:1263 1984

78. Perloff JK, Roberts WC, DeLeon AC, et al: The distinctive electrocardiogram of Duschenne's progressive muscular dystrophy: An electrocardiographic–pathologic correlative study. Am J Med 42:179, 1967

79. Perloff JK, Stevenson WG, Roberts NK, et al: Cardiac involvement in myotonic muscular dystrophy (Steinert's disease): A prospective study of 25 patients. Am J Cardiol 54:1074, 1984

80. Petty RKH, Harding EA, Morgan-Hughes JA: The clinical features of mitochondrial myopathy. Brain 109:915, 1986

81. Porter GH: Sarcoid heart disease. N Engl J Med 263:1350, 1960

82. Pruitt RD, Curd GW, Leachman R: Simulation of electrocardiogram of apicolateral myocardial infarction by myocardial destructive lesions of obscure etiology (myocardiopathy). Circulation 25:506, 1962

83. Raffanti SP, Chiaramida AJ, Sen P, et al: Assessment of cardiac function in patients with the acquired immunodeficiency syndrome. Chest 93:592, 1988

84. Reilly JM, Cunnion RE, Anderson DW, et al: Frequency of myocarditis, left ventricular dysfunction and ventricular tachycardia in the acquired immune deficiency syndrome. Am J Cardiol 62:789, 1988

85. Rosenbaum MB: Chagasic myocardiopathy. Prog Cardiovasc Dis 7:199, 1964

86. Rothschild MA, Sachs B, Libman E: The disturbances of the cardiac mechanism in subacute bacterial endocarditis and rheumatic fever. Am Heart J 2:356, 1927

87. Sackner MA, Heinz ER, Steinberg AJ: The heart in scleroderma. Am J Cardiol 17:542, 1966

88. Sanyal SK, Johnson WW: Cardiac conduction abnormalities in children with Duchenne's progressive muscular dystrophy: Electrocardiographic features

and morphologic correlates. Circulation 66:853, 1982

89. Savage DD, Seides SF, Clark CE: Electrocardiographic findings in patients with obstructive and nonobstructive hypertrophic cardiomyopathy. Circulation 58:402, 1978

90. Savage DD, Seides SF, Maron BJ: Prevalence of arrhythmias during 24-hour electrocardiographic monitoring and exercise testing in patients with obstructive and nonobstructive hypertrophy cardiomyopathy. Circulation 59:866, 1979

91. Schaumburg HH, Nielsen SL, Yurchak PM: Heart block in polymyositis. N Engl J Med 284:480, 1971

92. Schrader ML, Hochman JS, Bulkley BH: The heart in polyarteritis nodosa: A clinicopathologic study. Am Heart J 109:1353, 1985

93. Shearn MA, Pirofsky B: Disseminated lupus erythematosus. Arch Intern Med 90:590, 1952

94. Slucka C: The electrocardiogram in Duchenne progressive muscular dystrophy. Circulation 38:933, 1968

95. Smith WG: Coxsackie B myopericarditis in adults. Am Heart J 80:34, 1970

96. Spilkin S, Mitha AS, Matisonn RE, et al: Complete heart block in a case of idiopathic hypertrophic subaortic stenosis. Circulation 55:418, 1977

97. Stapleton JF, Segal JP, Harvey WP: The electrocardiogram of myocardiopathy. Prog Cardiovasc Dis 13:217, 1970

98. Tavel ME, Fisch C: Abnormal Q waves simulating myocardial infarction in diffuse myocardial disease. Am Heart J 68:534, 1964

99. Thoren C: Cardiomyopathy in Friedreich's ataxia: With studies of cardiovascular and respiratory function. Acta Paediatr (Stockh) 53(Suppl 153):1, 1964

100. VanDam RTh, Roos JP, Durrer D: Electrical activation of ventricles and interventricular septum in hypertrophic obstructive cardiomyopathy. Br Heart J 34:100, 1972

101. Vigorita VJ, Hutchins GM: Cardiac conduction system in hemochromatosis: Clinical and pathologic features of six patients. Am J Cardiol 44:418, 1979

102. Welsh JD, Lynn TN, Haase GR: Cardiac findings in 73 patients with muscular dystrophy. Arch Intern Med 112:199, 1963

103. Weschsler HF, Rosenblum AH, Sills CT: Infectious mononucleosis: Report of an epidemic in an army post. Part II. Ann Intern Med 25:236, 1946

104. Wigle ED: Muscular subaortic stenosis: The clinical syndrome with additional evidence of ventricular septal hypertrophy. Int Ciba Symposium: Cardiomyopathies. London, J&A Churchill, 1965

105. Wigle ED, Baron RH: The electrocardiogram in muscular subaortic stenosis: Effect of a left septal incision and right bundle branch block. Circulation 34:585, 1966

106. Windesheim JH, Parkin TW: Electrocardiograms of ninety patients with acrosclerosis and progressive diffuse sclerosis (scleroderma). Circulation 17:874, 1958

107. Yamaguchi H, Ishimura T, Nishiyama S, et al: Hypertrophic nonobstructive cardiomyopathy with giant negative T waves (apical hypertrophy): Ventriculographic and echocardiographic features in 30 patients. Am J Cardiol 44:401, 1979

108. Zondek H: The electrocardiogram in myxedema. Br Heart J 26:227, 1964

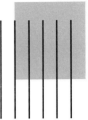

Chronic Obstructive Pulmonary Disease, Pneumothorax, Pulmonary Embolism $\quad$ **13**

CHRONIC OBSTRUCTIVE PULMONARY DISEASE

In chronic obstructive pulmonary disease (COPD), hyperinflation of the lungs is accompanied by a low position of the diaphragm. The heart becomes more vertical, and there is a clockwise rotation of the heart along its longitudinal axis. In the electrocardiogram (ECG), there is a rightward shift of the P and QRS axes in the frontal plane and posterior displacement of the QRS forces in the horizontal plane. The P waves become smaller in lead I and more prominent in the inferior leads. The amplitude of the QRS complexes in the limb leads are often small, since the major QRS forces are directed posteriorly and perpendicular to the frontal plane resulting in small projections in this plane. This also is true in the left precordial leads, because the posterior QRS vectors are more or less perpendicular to the lead axis of V_5 and V_6. The reduction of the voltage is further accentuated by the insulatory effect of the hyperinflated lungs, since the lung is a poor electrical conductor. The posterior displacement of the QRS forces also accounts for the leftward shift of the transitional zone. The relatively high position of the precordial electrodes in relation to the downward displaced heart contributes further to the increased negativity of the QRS complexes in these leads.

Electrocardiographic Criteria of Chronic Obstructive Pulmonary Disease

Chronic obstructive pulmonary disease may be suspected if one or more of the P-wave changes plus one or more of the QRS changes listed below are present.

1. P waves ≥2.5 mm in leads II, III, or aVF[16,20,24,30]
2. P-wave axis ≥80° (or >70°) in the frontal plane[11,16,20]

3. Lead I sign with an isoelectric P wave, QRS amplitude less than 1.5 mm, and T-wave amplitude less than 0.5 mm[11,20]
4. QRS axis ≥90° in the frontal plane
5. QRS amplitude in all the limb leads ≤5 mm[11,20,30]
6. QRS amplitude ≤5 mm in lead V_5 or V_6, or R wave ≤7 mm in lead V_5, or R wave ≤5 mm in lead V_6[11,20,30]
7. R/S ratio ≤1 in lead V_5 or V_6[3,11,20,34]
8. $S_1 S_2 S_3$ syndrome with R/S ratio less than 1 in leads I, II, and III, or S wave in these leads that exceeds the upper limits of normal for the various age groups as defined by Simonson[21]·

OTHER ELECTROCARDIOGRAPHIC CHANGES

1. Prominent negative P waves in lead V_1 (see Fig. 2–4)
2. Pseudoinfarction pattern (see Figs. 9–39 and 9–40)

Figures 13–1 through 13–3 were recorded from patients with COPD and various levels of pulmonary arterial pressure.

Correlation with Clinical and Other Laboratory Findings

Although most patients with severe COPD have some ECG abnormalities, normal ECGs are observed in about 21 to 27 percent of the patients.[24,30] Because a mild or even moderate degree of cor pulmonale is often difficult to detect clinically in a patient with COPD, the findings described in the various reports may not be due to the lung pathology alone.

*Age (yr)	S_1 (mm)	S_2 (mm)	S_3 (mm)
20–29	4	5	6
30–39	4	4	8
40–59	3	4	8

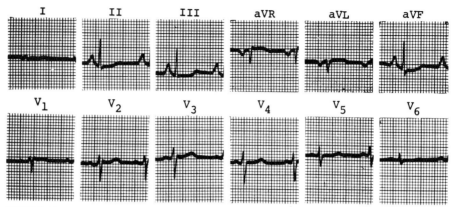

FIGURE 13–1. Chronic obstructive pulmonary disease without pulmonary hypertension. The patient is a 56-year-old man with moderately severe airway obstruction. Right heart catheterization revealed a pulmonary arterial pressure of 28/12 mm Hg. In the ECG there is a P pulmonale with a frontal plane P-wave axis of nearly +90°. Lead I sign is present. The R waves in V_5 and V_6 are small, and the R/S ratio in V_5 is less than 1. The ST-segment depression in leads II, III, and aVF may be the result of prominent Ta waves. The patient was not receiving any cardiac drugs at the time.

P-WAVE CHANGES

Spodick and associates analyzed 301 patients with various degrees of pulmonary emphysema.[24] Seventy-seven percent of the patients had P axes between +70° and +90°. The verticalization of the P axis was clearly related to an increasing degree of airway obstruction. The P pulmonale pattern, with tall and peaked P waves of greater than 2.5 mm in the inferior leads, was present in 14 percent. It was seen mostly in patients with moderately severe or severe disease (see Figs. 13–1 and 13–2). Peaked P waves with normal amplitude (Gothic P waves) were observed in 54 per-

cent of the cases, but their presence had no relation to the degree of functional impairment (see Fig. 13–3).

Calatayud and associates studied 173 patients with pulmonary emphysema.[5] P-wave axes in the frontal plane to the right of +70° were found in 56 percent of the cases. However, the axis was rarely greater than +90°. In 46 percent of the patients, the maximum P-wave amplitude in the limb leads was greater than 2.5 mm. The frequency of these abnormal findings increased as the functional impairment became more severe. They also believed that rightward shift of the P axis is the most helpful P-wave change for estimating the

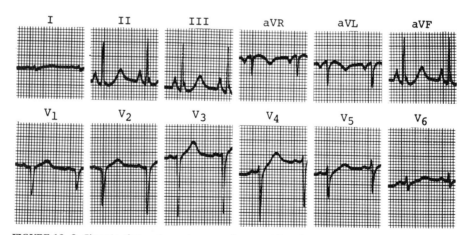

FIGURE 13–2. Chronic obstructive pulmonary disease with pulmonary hypertension. The patient is a 58-year-old man with a pulmonary arterial pressure of 42/25 mm Hg at rest. The ECG shows P pulmonale with a vertical P axis. The QRS complexes in lead I are small, and the frontal plane QRS axis is +90°. There is poor progression of the R wave in the precordial leads, with an R/S ratio in leads V_5 and V_6 of less than 1. The amplitude of the QRS complexes in V_6 also is small.

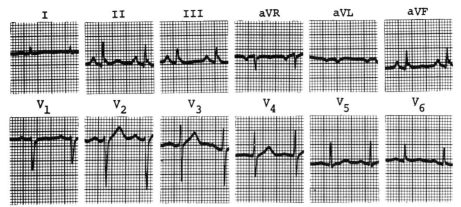

FIGURE 13–3. Chronic obstructive pulmonary disease. The patient is a 42-year-old man with severe COPD. Right heart catheterization revealed a resting pulmonary arterial pressure of 30/15 mm Hg, but the pressure rose to 50/24 mm Hg with moderate exercise. The ECG shows a P-wave axis of about +80°. The P waves in the inferior leads are peaked but not tall (Gothic). The R waves in V_6 have a borderline voltage. Otherwise, the tracing is unremarkable.

severity of the lung disease. Other investigators found a lower incidence (29 to 35 percent) of rightward deviation of the P axis.[6,14] The relation between the axis shift and the ventilatory capacity of the patient was not established in another study.[4]

The tall P waves in the inferior leads are often associated with a depression of the PR segment because of the prominent atrial T waves. For the same reason, the ST segment also is often depressed (see Fig. 13–1).

Occasionally, prominent negative P waves are present in lead V_1 or leads V_1 and V_2 to suggest left atrial enlargement (see Fig. 2–4). They may be seen in patients without evidence of left heart disease. This pseudo–left atrial enlargement pattern probably is due to the relatively high position of the electrodes in relation to the heart. The inferior direction of the P vector results in a projection on the negative side of the lead V_1 axis.

QRS CHANGES

Frontal plane QRS axes of +60° or greater or indeterminate axes occur in about 60 percent of the patients.[14,24] An axis of greater than +90° is, however, less common and was observed in only 8 percent in one series.[14] The degree of right axis deviation is significantly related to the degree of airway obstruction.[24] About one fourth of the patients have an $S_1S_2S_3$ pattern, which has no apparent relation to the severity of the disease.[24]

Abnormal left axis deviation is occasionally seen in patients with severe pulmonary emphysema.[2] It is attributed by some investigators to coexisting left ventricular disease. Others proposed that the left axis deviation is the result of an "axis illusion" phenomenon.[16,22,23] Because the QRS forces are essentially perpendicular to the frontal plane in many patients with COPD, a slight upward shift of the forces results in their projection in the left superior quadrant of the frontal plane instead of the left inferior quadrant. In my experience, there is often actually a marked right axis deviation, the mean QRS vector being directed toward the right superior quadrant (Fig. 13–4). The rather deep S waves in leads II and III give the erroneous impression of abnormal left axis deviation. In patients with pulmonary emphysema, however, the S_2 is greater than the S_3. In true left axis deviation, S_3 is greater than S_2.

Only limited data are available about the incidence of low QRS voltage in the limb leads and left precordial leads. In the 200 patients with COPD analyzed by Kilcoyne and colleagues, the QRS voltage was less than 5 mm in all the limb leads in 10 percent of the cases.[14] A leftward displacement of the transitional zone, with an R/S ratio in leads V_5 and V_6 of less than 1, was present in 12.5 percent. In my experience, the incidence of this latter finding is higher.

After studying 150 adults with moderately severe or severe pulmonary emphysema, Wasserburger and associates proposed an ECG pattern that they called "the electrocardiographic pentalogy of pulmonary emphysema."[30] It consists of (1) exaggerated P waves in leads II, III, and aVF; (2) a prominent Ta wave in leads II, III, and aVF; (3) ver-

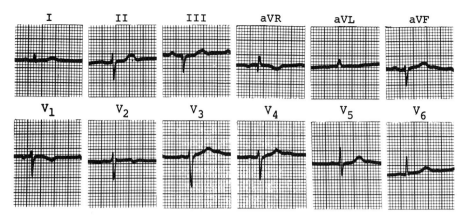

FIGURE 13–4. Chronic obstructive pulmonary disease with deep S_2 and S_3 mimicking abnormal left axis deviation. The patient is a 52-year-old man with severe COPD. The pulmonary arterial pressure was 30/14 mm Hg at rest and 58/30 mm Hg during mild exercise. There is no clinical evidence of left ventricular disease. The deep S waves in the inferior leads may lead to the misinterpretation of abnormal left axis deviation. S_2 is greater than S_3, however, suggesting the major QRS forces are directed superiorly and rightward. There also is poor progression of the R wave in the right and mid-precordial leads.

tical cardiac position; (4) clockwise rotation along the longitudinal cardiac axis; and (5) a tendency to low voltage, particularly in the left precordial leads. They found such a pattern in 34 percent of their patients, all of whom had severe emphysema based on pulmonary function tests.

SPECIFICITY OF THE CRITERIA

In a prospective study, Kamper and associates from my institution tested the reliability of the various criteria listed previously.[13] Patients who met one or more of the criteria were evaluated for the presence or absence of COPD by clinical examination, pulmonary function tests, and arterial gas studies. As expected, because none of the individual criteria is specific for COPD, only 46 percent of the patients were found to have airway obstruction (i.e., 54 percent false-positive diagnosis). When at least two criteria were met, however, especially when they included both P-wave and QRS changes, the specificity of the criteria was much improved. For example, in the 23 patients with P-wave axes greater than +80° and QRS axes greater than +90°, or low voltage of the QRS complexes in lead V_5 or V_6, or an R/S ratio of less than 1 in V_5 or V_6, all were found to have significant COPD. Five of 6 patients with the P pulmonale pattern and right axis deviation of the QRS complex had evidence of airway obstruction. Furthermore, when more of the criteria were met, there was an increase in the severity of the COPD.

Differential Diagnosis

Other disease entities that may be associated with one or more of the various abnormal findings seen in patients with pulmonary emphysema have been discussed in the previous chapters. Only a brief summary is given here. The P pulmonale pattern also is observed in patients with chronic cor pulmonale without pulmonary emphysema. It occurs in patients with congenital heart disease, such as pulmonary stenosis, tetralogy of Fallot, and Eisenmenger's syndrome. In such cases, however, the P axis is usually less vertical than that of patients with COPD or cor pulmonale. Transient P pulmonale pattern may be seen in patients with acute pulmonary embolism; with bronchial asthma, especially during the acute episode; or even with arterial oxygen desaturation alone. Tall and peaked P waves may also be seen in healthy subjects with asthenic body build or during standing. The P wave increases in amplitude during tachycardia or exercise or during expiratory effort against pressure. A significant number of patients with left ventricular disease present a pseudo P pulmonale pattern[7] (see Chapter 2). This is especially true in patients with hypertensive heart disease, but the pattern also is encountered in those with coronary artery disease.

A vertical QRS axis is a normal finding in children and young adults. Pathologic states other than COPD that are associated with a vertical axis include right ventricular hypertrophy, left posterior hemiblock, and lateral wall myocardial infarction. The $S_1S_2S_3$ pattern may be a normal variant, but it also is seen in patients with right ventricular hypertrophy that results from other causes.

Low voltage of the QRS complex also is observed in patients with pericardial disease with effusion or constriction. Various types of diffuse myocardial disease, such as amyloidosis and scleroderma may be accompanied by a reduction of the amplitude of the QRS complex. In myxedema, the reduction of the voltage is the result of either pericardial effusion or myocardial involvement or both. In patients with coronary artery disease, small QRS complexes may be the result of diffuse muscle damage.

Of special clinical importance is the poor progression of the R wave in the precordial leads in many patients with chronic obstructive lung disease (see Figs. 13–2 and 13–5). In some cases, the rS complexes are replaced by QS complexes in the right and mid-precordial leads to simulate anterior wall myocardial wall infarction (see Figs. 9–39 and 9–40). This finding is explained by the relatively high position of the precordial electrodes in relation to the heart. They are often at the level of the base of the heart (see Fig. 9–40) and therefore record negative ventricular potential. The abnormal complexes can be partially normalized by recording the leads at lower intercostal spaces. A pseudoinfarction pattern also may be seen in the inferior leads. Its genesis is unclear.

Arrhythmia in Chronic Obstructive Pulmonary Disease

Persistent or chronic arrhythmias other than sinus tachycardia are uncommon in patients with COPD. Transient arrhythmias, however, are not uncommon when the patients have intercurrent respiratory infections, respiratory failure, or pulmonary embolism. Most of the patients already have chronic cor pulmonale. The arrhythmias are mostly supraventricular in origin. They include paroxysmal atrial tachycardia, multifocal atrial tachycardia, atrial fibrillation, and occasionally atrial flutter. In 1482 hospitalized patients with severe COPD, Thomas and Valabhji reported arrhythmias in 7 percent of the cases.[29] Most of the patients also had ECG evidence of right ventricular hypertrophy. They believed that the underlying mechanism for the appearance of arrhythmias is an increase in the degree of pulmonary hypertension because of the superimposed respiratory complications.

Diagnosis of Right Ventricular Hypertrophy in Patients with Chronic Obstructive Pulmonary Disease

The diagnosis of chronic cor pulmonale may be made when the ECG meets one or more of the usual signs of right ventricular hypertrophy. In the autopsied cases with chronic cor pulmonale, ECG evidence of right ventricular hypertrophy is present in about 60 to 70 percent. It is present in only slightly more than one fourth of the cases diagnosed clinically, however. The accuracy of the diagnosis is further compromised by the fact that some of the ECG signs may be seen in patients with COPD but without cor pulmonale. These include the P pulmonale pattern, the $S_1S_2S_3$ pattern, and the leftward shift of the transitional zone with a reversal of the R/S ratio in the left precordial leads. When, however, the signs of right atrial

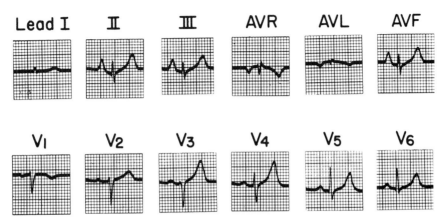

FIGURE 13–5. Chronic obstructive pulmonary disease simulating anterior myocardial infarction. The ECG shows P pulmonale and indeterminate QRS axis. The poor R-wave progression in V_1 through V_3, with R in V_3 smaller than R in V_2, suggests anterior myocardial damage. Autopsy showed no evidence of ventricular hypertrophy or myocardial infarction.

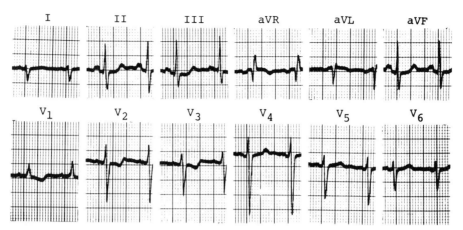

FIGURE 13–6. Chronic obstructive pulmonary disease with cor pulmonale. The patient is a 40-year-old man with clinical evidence of chronic cor pulmonale. The pulmonary arterial pressure was 29/12 mm Hg at rest and 54/24 mm Hg with mild exercise. The ECG shows abnormal P waves and a QRS axis of +120°. There is a monophasic R wave in lead V_1, suggesting right ventricular hypertrophy, and deep S waves, with an R/S ratio of less than 1, in V_5 and V_6. There are also ST-segment depression and T-wave inversion in leads V_1 through V_3.

enlargement also are present in the right precordial leads, when the frontal plane QRS axis is +110° or more, when an RSR' or a QR pattern is present in lead V_1, or when ST and T changes are present in the right precordial or inferior leads, right ventricular hypertrophy is most likely present (Fig. 13–6).

Kilcoyne and associates suggested the following transient ECG changes as early indications of cor pulmonale in patients with COPD who developed transient episodes of pulmonary insufficiency:

1. A rightward shift of the mean QRS axis of +30° or more
2. T-wave abnormalities in the right precordial leads
3. ST-segment depression in leads II, III, and aVF
4. Transient right bundle branch block

PNEUMOTHORAX

Both spontaneous and artificial pneumothorax may induce ECG changes in a significant number of patients.[1,25] In right-sided pneumothorax, there is often a rightward shift of the QRS axis and a decrease in the amplitude of the P, QRS, or T wave, mostly in lead I. In left-sided pneumothorax, similar changes are observed. In addition, there is a reduction of the QRS amplitude in the left precordial leads in most patients. Occasionally, QS deflections are present in many of the precordial leads (Fig. 13–7). The ST segment may be elevated. In one reported series, the T waves are inverted

in some of the precordial leads in almost all patients.[1] They are often symmetrical and resemble closely the ischemic type of T waves. Thus, the QRS, ST, and T-wave changes may mimic those of acute myocardial infarction. Some of these changes may be partially normalized when the ECG is recorded with the patient in the upright position.[8]

Although cardiac displacement, rotation, and interposition of air between the heart and the electrodes are responsible for some of the ECG changes, the exact mechanism is not entirely known. There is a rightward shift of the QRS axis regardless of whether the pneumothorax occurs on the left or right side. There also is no correlation between the amount of cardiac displacement and the degree of axis shift. The extent of other ECG changes is also not proportional to the degree of the lung collapse.

ACUTE PULMONARY EMBOLISM

The ECG changes in acute pulmonary embolism depend in large measure on the size of the embolus and the time of the recording in relation to the onset of the event. If the embolus is large and accompanied by a significant increase in the pulmonary arterial pressure, acute dilatation of the right ventricle may occur. This is often associated with a clockwise rotation of the heart along its longitudinal axis, a more vertical heart, and right ventricular conduction defect. The clockwise rotation of the heart is probably responsible for the S_1Q_3 pattern described by McGinn and

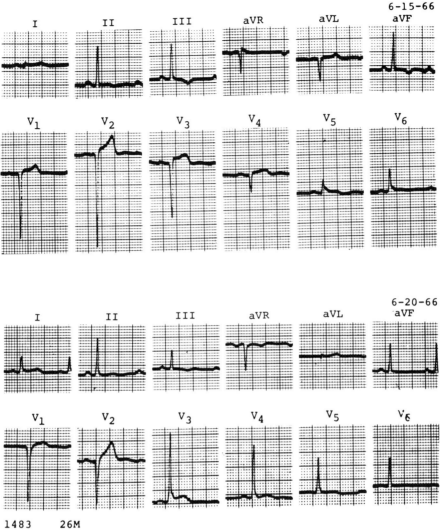

1483   26M

FIGURE 13–7. Spontaneous pneumothorax in a 26-year-old man. The tracing on 6-15-66 was recorded while the patient was having a massive left-sided pneumothorax, and that on 6-20-66 was recorded after the lung was reexpanded. Note the small QRS complex in lead I with a rightward shift of the QRS axis during pneumothorax. The changes in the precordial leads simulate acute myocardial infarction. There also is a reduction of the QRS voltage in the left precordial leads. (See Fig. 9–42 for the chest roentgenogram of this patient.)

White.[18] The initial left septal forces are now directed more superiorly, resulting in a q wave in lead III. The terminal QRS forces are displaced rightward and manifested as an S wave in lead I. The same mechanism also may explain the leftward displacement of the transitional zone in the precordial leads. The vertical position of the heart contributes further to the rightward shift of the frontal plane QRS axis. The right ventricular conduction defect secondary to the dilatation may present itself as incomplete or complete right bundle branch block.

Myocardial hypoxemia that results from sudden reduction of cardiac output and rela-

tive coronary insufficiency is probably responsible for the ST-segment and T-wave changes. Secondary repolarization abnormalities also occur when right ventricular conduction defect is present. Right atrial dilatation may explain the prominent P waves in the inferior leads. The same mechanism, perhaps with the addition of relative ischemia of the SA node and atrium, is the possible cause of atrial arrhythmias seen in some patients.

The term *acute right heart strain* is often used to describe the morphologic changes of the P, QRS, ST, and T waves secondary to pulmonary embolism and other causes of sudden increase of pulmonary vascular resistance.

Electrocardiographic Diagnostic Criteria

One of the most important diagnostic features in acute pulmonary embolism is the transient nature of the ECG changes. This characteristic also greatly influences the frequency that the various signs are observed.

FINDINGS GENERALLY CONSIDERED TYPICAL OF PULMONARY EMBOLISM

1. S_1Q_3 or $S_1Q_3T_3$ pattern[18]
2. Rightward shift of QRS axis[15]

3. Transient right bundle branch block, incomplete or complete[10]
4. T-wave inversion in the right precordial leads[32]

OTHER FINDINGS

1. Displacement of the transitional zone to the left (clockwise rotation)[19]
2. Left axis deviation[17]
3. QR pattern in V_1[9]
4. R>5 mm in V_1 or R/S in V_1>1[26]
5. "Staircase" ascent of ST segment in lead I or II[18]

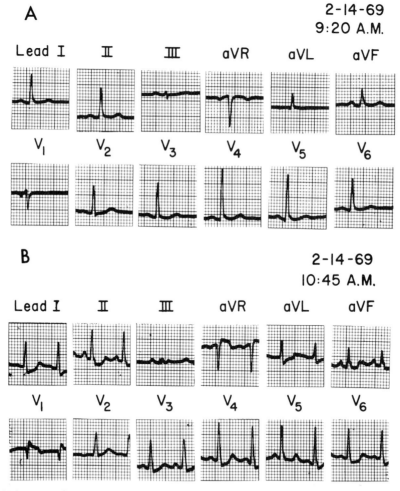

FIGURE 13–8. Acute pulmonary embolism proved by autopsy. The patient was a 59-year-old woman who had a hysterectomy. (A) The 9:20 A.M. tracing was recorded as a routine postoperative ECG. (B) Slightly more than an hour later, she developed symptoms consistent with pulmonary embolism. The ECG reveals sinus tachycardia with peaked P waves in the inferior leads. An S wave is present in lead I, and a Qr pattern has developed in lead V_1. There is ST-segment depression in leads I, II, and V_3 through V_6. ST-segment elevation with T-wave inversion is present in lead V_1. The patient died on the same day. At autopsy, there was a complete occlusion of the left pulmonary artery and the main branch of the right artery to the right lower lobe. There was mild right ventricular dilatation. Minimal coronary atherosclerosis was present, and there was no evidence of myocardial infarction.

6. ST elevation in lead III[31]

7. ST depression or elevation in right precordial leads

8. ST and T-wave changes in the left precordial leads[9]

9. P pulmonale pattern[32]

10. Sinus tachycardia and atrial arrhythmias, including atrial flutter, atrial fibrillation, atrial tachycardia, and atrial premature contractions.

11. First-degree AV block[34]

Figures 13–8 through 13–11 are examples of proven cases of pulmonary embolism illustrating many of the listed findings.

Clinical and Pathologic Correlation

SENSITIVITY AND SPECIFICITY

Because of the transient nature of the ECG changes in acute pulmonary embolism, the diagnostic sensitivity of the ECG depends a great deal on the frequency and time of the recording. The size of the embolus and its hemodynamic effect undoubtedly influences the incidence and severity of the various findings. The presence of preexisting pulmonary disease either accentuates or masks the changes. This is especially true if the ECG was abnormal before the onset of the acute event.

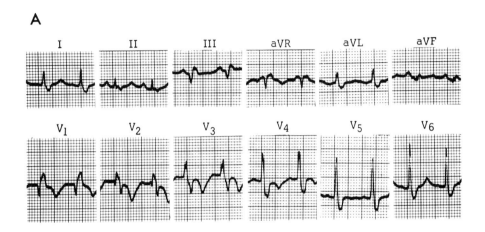

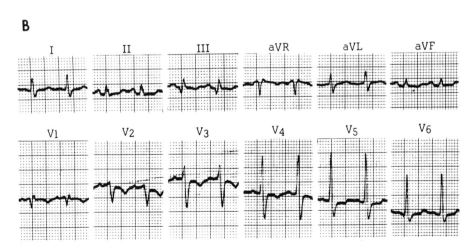

FIGURE 13–9. Massive pulmonary embolism confirmed by autopsy. The patient was a 61-year-old man who had dyspnea and dizziness 3 days before the tracing (A) was recorded. The tracing shows sinus tachycardia and complete right bundle branch block. Q waves are present in leads III, aVF, and V_1. There is rather deep T-wave inversion in the right and mid-precordial leads, suggesting additional primary T-wave changes. (B) The ECG recorded on the next day shows the $S_1Q_3T_3$ pattern. The complete right bundle branch block is no longer present, but lead V_1 reveals a Qr pattern. There is T-wave inversion in leads V_1 through V_5. The patient died the same day. At autopsy, there were large pulmonary emboli that almost totally occluded the lumen of both the left and right pulmonary arteries. No significant coronary artery disease or myocardial infarction was found.

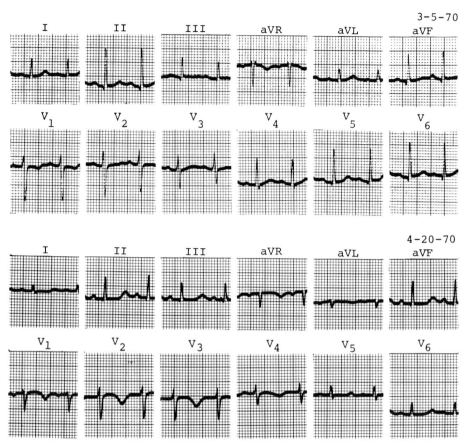

FIGURE 13-10. Pulmonary embolism proved by autopsy. The patient was a 20-year-old man with empyema. The tracing of 3-5-70 was recorded as part of a routine work-up. He had a sudden syncope episode on 4-20-70. The ECG taken immediately afterward reveals the development of a small S wave in lead I, with a rightward shift of the QRS axis of about +30°. The transitional zone is displaced to the left. The T waves are inverted in leads V_1 through V_4. The patient died on the same day. Autopsy confirmed the presence of bilateral multiple pulmonary emboli.

Table 13-1 summarizes the incidence of the individual ECG abnormalities reported in some of the larger series. There is a marked variation in the frequency of the findings in the different studies. Cutforth and Oram analyzed 50 cases of pulmonary embolism diagnosed by convincing clinical evidence.[9] In 11 of the patients, the diagnosis was verified at autopsy. Among the more typical signs, T-wave inversion in the right precordial leads was the most common finding. In their series, only 24 percent failed to show changes that are suggestive of pulmonary embolism. The duration of the various changes varied greatly. Generally, the right bundle branch block pattern was the most transient change and subsided within a few days. The S_1Q_3 pattern subsided in an average of 17 days, whereas the T-wave inversion in the right precordial leads was most persistent and lasted for an average of 41 days, varying between 16 and 120 days.

The ST-segment depression was more transient and lasted for an average of 9 days. Weber and Phillips studied 60 cases of acute pulmonary embolism, 26 of which had autopsy confirmation.[31] They observed a similar percentage of cases with the $S_1Q_3T_3$ pattern as in the previous study, but relatively more patients had right bundle branch block and fewer had T-wave inversion in the right precordial leads. They reported ST-segment elevation in lead III in 28 percent of the patients. Ten percent of the patients had ST-segment and T-wave changes in the left precordial leads. Twenty percent of the cases showed no significant change in the ECG.

Later studies indicate that the ECG is not a sensitive tool in the recognition of acute pulmonary embolism, as suggested by the previous series. Szucs and co-workers reported 58 patients in whom the diagnosis of acute pulmonary embolism was made by pulmonary ar-

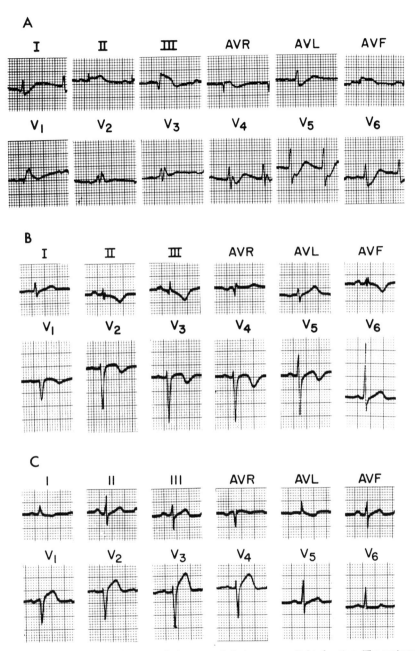

FIGURE 13–11. Acute pulmonary embolism simulating acute inferior myocardial infarction. The patient was a 67-year-old man who was brought into the hospital because of syncope and shock. (A) The ECG taken on arrival (4-3-73) shows complete right bundle branch block. A Q wave is present in lead III, with ST-segment elevation in all the inferior leads. ST-segment depression is present in leads I, aVL, and V₄ through V₆. The diagnosis of acute inferior myocardial infarction was made. On the same day, repeated ECGs show the disappearance of the right bundle branch block pattern. A definite Q wave also has developed in lead aVF, with T-wave inversion in the inferior leads. (B) The tracing recorded 2 days later (4-5-73) shows that the Q wave in lead III becomes smaller, and the Q wave in lead aVF is no longer present. In the precordial leads, there is a leftward displacement of the transitional zone, with T-wave inversion from leads V₁ through V₅. Radioisotope lung scan revealed large profusion defects. Serial enzymes were not consistent with myocardial infarction. The tracing gradually returned to normal. (C) The tracing made on 4-18-73 shows no Q wave in the inferior leads. The QRS complexes are within normal limits. The minor ST and T changes are consistent with digitalis effect.

TABLE 13–1. Frequency of ECG Changes in Patients with Acute Pulmonary Embolism

ECG Changes	Cutforth & Oram (1958)[9] 50 cases (% of cases)	Weber & Phillips (1966)[31] 60 cases (% of cases)	Szucs et al (1971)[28] 50 cases (% of cases)	Stein et al (1975)[26] 90 cases (% of cases)
S_1Q_3 or $S_1Q_3T_3$	28	27		12
Right axis shift		18	15	7
Right bundle branch block	14	25		15
Incomplete			8	6
Complete				9
T-wave inversion in right precordial leads	46	10		42*
Clockwise rotation	60	17		7
Left axis shift				7
Qr in V_1		17		
ST changes	18			
Depression in leads I or II		18		26*
Elevation in lead III		28		16*
ST, T changes in V_5, V_6		10		
P pulmonale	12	28		6
Sinus tachycardia	68	48		
Atrial arrhythmias	14	38	19	
Atrial fibrillation		10		
Atrial flutter		12		
Atrial tachycardia		2		
First-degree AV block		8		1
No significant abnormality	24	20		13

*Leads not specified.

teriogram.[28] An acute right axis shift was found in 15 percent, and incomplete right bundle branch block was observed in only 8 percent. Stein and associates analyzed 90 cases of massive or submassive pulmonary embolism documented by angiography that were included in the urokinase study.[26] None of the patients had evidence of preexisting cardiac or pulmonary disease. The embolism was regarded as massive if the obstruction involved two or more lobar pulmonary arteries, and submassive if it involved at least one segmental artery. The incidence of $S_1Q_3T_3$ pattern, right axis deviation, and complete and incomplete right bundle branch block was 12, 7, 9, and 6 percent, respectively. T-wave inversion in the various limb and precordial leads was present in 42 percent. Eleven percent of the patients displayed a pseudoinfarction pattern. Left axis shift was observed in 7 percent of the patients. ECGs were normal in 13 percent. During the follow-up period, by day 5 or 6 after the diagnosis was made, well over 50 percent of the QRS abnormalities and 22 percent of the T-wave inversion were no longer present. By 2 weeks, about half of the T-wave inversion subsided. The ST segment returned to normal sooner than did the T-wave changes. Atrial arrhythmias were uncommon, and the authors believed that they occurred mostly in patients with preexisting cardiac disease. In

both of these series, one or more of the classic signs of acute cor pulmonale ($S_1Q_3T_3$, right bundle branch block, right axis deviation) were observed in only 10 to 26 percent of the patients.[26,28] Because these studies included only patients with large-sized emboli, the results imply that the overall diagnostic sensitivity of the ECG in pulmonary embolism of all sizes is probably much lower. When pulmonary embolism is accompanied by the typical ECG evidence of right-sided heart strain, most of these patients have signs of acute right ventricular failure.[28] Pulmonary angiograms will likely demonstrate obstruction of more than 50 percent of the pulmonary vasculature.[28] Patients with normal ECGs generally have smaller perfusion defect and lower pulmonary arterial pressure.[26]

On the other hand, when pulmonary embolism is large enough to produce collapse, shock, or right-sided heart failure, ECG changes are seen in most such patients. In the 35 patients with these clinical presentations and with embolism involving at least half of the major pulmonary arterial branches, Sutton and associates reported ECG evidence of right-sided heart strain and T-wave inversion in the right precordial leads or right bundle branch block in 62 percent.[27] Only 3 patients had normal tracings.

In my experience, other than sinus tachycardia, T-wave inversion in the right precordial leads is the most common abnormality in acute pulmonary embolism. It is also the more persistent finding. Right bundle branch block, whether complete or incomplete, usually is transient, lasting only for a few hours or a few days. This is also true of atrial arrhythmias. The typical pattern of acute right ventricular strain is seen only in minority of the patients.

Information about the *specificity* of the ECG signs is quite limited. Hildner and Ormond evaluated the accuracy of the clinical diagnosis of pulmonary embolism in 78 patients by pulmonary angiography.[12] The clinical diagnosis was based on various combinations of symptoms, physical findings, ECG, enzymes, chest radiograph, and isotope lung scan. Pulmonary emboli were demonstrated in only 41 percent. The ECG was normal in 72 percent of the patients with pulmonary emboli and in 89 percent of those without. An $S_1Q_3T_3$ pattern and T-wave inversion in leads V_1 through V_3 were seen more frequently in patients with emboli than in those without (19 and 9 percent versus 8 and 4 percent, respectively). Right bundle branch block or right ventricular hypertrophy was present in similar number of both groups.

Although none of the individual signs is specific for acute right-sided heart strain, the presence of two or more of the classic abnormalities improves substantially the diagnostic accuracy. This is especially true when a prior ECG is available for comparison. Cutforth and Oram considered the combination of $S_1Q_3T_3$ plus right ventricular T-wave inversion, S_1T_3 plus right ventricular T-wave inversion, or $S_1Q_3T_3$ plus right bundle branch block as virtually diagnostic of pulmonary embolism.[9] As discussed later, many other conditions may present similar changes. Correlation with clinical and other laboratory data is therefore essential before a reasonable conclusion can be made.

Differential Diagnosis

NORMAL ELECTROCARDIOGRAM

An S wave in lead I and a Q wave in lead III are seen frequently in the normal individual, especially among younger subjects. The T wave in lead III also may be inverted, resulting in an $S_1Q_3T_3$ pattern. In young adults, the QRS axis may be vertical, the juvenile T-wave inversion in the right precordial leads may persist, and an r′ may even be present in lead V_1 as a normal variant. Therefore, all the typical signs of pulmonary embolism may be observed in a healthy person. If sinus tachycardia develops because of some other reasons, the P waves may become taller and peaked to mimic P pulmonale. Junctional ST-segment depression secondary to the tachycardia may further confuse the ECG presentation. If a previous tracing is not available for comparison, the differentiation could be difficult, especially if the clinical findings also mimic pulmonary embolism.

INFERIOR MYOCARDIAL INFARCTION

The differentiation of acute pulmonary embolism and inferior myocardial infarction is often one of the most difficult and yet important diagnostic problems. The clinical presentation is frequently similar. The appearance of new Q waves in leads III and sometimes aVF, with T-wave inversion in these leads, occurs in both conditions. Cutforth and Oram indicated that ST-segment elevation in the inferior leads was not found in acute pulmonary embolism.[9] This is contrary to my own experience as well as that of others,[31] and such ST-elevation further complicates the diagnostic dilemma. Figure 13–11 is an example in which an erroneous diagnosis of acute inferior myocardial infarction was initially made. In acute pulmonary embolism, however, Q waves usually do not appear in lead II. They are relatively small and narrow in lead aVF. They are transient. The simultaneous development of an S wave in lead I or right bundle branch block also is suggestive of pulmonary embolism, but S_1 may occasionally be seen in inferior myocardial infarction with left posterior hemiblock. If myocardial infarction is the cause of the right bundle branch block, the site of infarction is usually anterior rather than inferior except when inferior myocardial infarction is associated with right ventricular infarction. The appearance of P pulmonale also is more suggestive of embolism.

ACUTE ANTERIOR MYOCARDIAL INFARCTION OR ANTERIOR MYOCARDIAL ISCHEMIA

The Qr pattern in lead V_1, the occasional ST-segment elevation in V_1, the frequent T-wave inversion in the right precordial leads, and the clockwise rotation in acute pulmonary embolism often mimic acute anteroseptal myocardial infarction. The Q waves are usually confined to leads V_1 and occasionally V_2.

Sometimes, however, they may be more extensive. An example was given in Chapter 9 in the section on the pseudoinfarction pattern.

When T-wave inversion is observed in the right precordial leads without other abnormal findings, it is virtually impossible to determine whether the changes are related to right-sided heart strain or to coronary artery disease unless other clinical data are available. Even when the T-wave changes are extensive and involve the entire precordial leads, acute right-sided heart strain may be the sole responsible mechanism. In fact, ST-segment and T-wave changes in the left precordial leads are common in pulmonary embolism.[31]

CHRONIC COR PULMONALE

Chronic cor pulmonale secondary to COPD may present nearly all the ECG changes seen in pulmonary embolism. The P pulmonale, right axis deviation, Q waves with T-wave inversion in the inferior leads, clockwise rotation, Qr pattern, and T-wave inversion in the right precordial leads are commonly observed in both conditions. Again, the correct diagnosis often depends on the transient nature of the findings in pulmonary embolism. Patients with COPD may have temporary accentuation of ECG abnormalities during an acute respiratory distress. An increase in the T-wave inversion in the right and mid-precordial leads occurs frequently. Transient atrial arrhythmias also may be seen. On the other hand, patients with chronic cor pulmonale may have acute pulmonary embolism as a complication. Furthermore, cor pulmonale may be the result of recurrent pulmonary embolism.

OTHER CAUSES OF ACUTE RIGHT HEART STRAIN

Massive collapse of the lungs,[19] pneumothorax, pneumonectomy, massive atelectasis, extensive pneumonia, and large pleural effusion may result in right ventricular dilatation and the ECG findings of right ventricular strain, especially when there is preexisting pulmonary disease.

REFERENCES

1. Armen RN, Frank TV: Electrocardiographic patterns in pneumothorax. Dis Chest 15:709, 1949
2. Banta HD, Greenfield JC, Estes EH: Left axis deviation. Am J Cardiol 14:330, 1964
3. Burch GE, DePasquale NP: The electrocardiographic diagnosis of pulmonary heart disease. Am J Cardiol 11:622, 1963
4. Caird FI, Wilcken DEL: The electrocardiogram in chronic bronchitis with generalized obstructive lung disease. Am J Cardiol 10:5, 1962
5. Calatayud JB, Abad JM, Khoi NB, et al: P-wave changes in chronic obstructive pulmonary disease. Am Heart J 79:444, 1970
6. Chappel AG: The electrocardiogram in chronic bronchitis and emphysema. Br Heart J 28:517, 1966
7. Chou TC, Helm RA: The pseudo P pulmonale. Circulation 32:96, 1965
8. Copeland RB, Omenn GS: Electrocardiogram changes suggestive of coronary artery disease in pneumothorax. Arch Intern Med 125:151, 1970
9. Cutforth RH, Oram S: The electrocardiogram in pulmonary embolism. Br Heart J 20:41, 1958
10. Durant TM, Ginsburg IW, Roesler H: Transient bundle branch block and other electrocardiographic changes in pulmonary embolism. Am Heart J 17:423, 1939
11. Fowler NO, Daniels C, Scott RC, et al: The electrocardiogram in cor pulmonale with and without emphysema. Am J Cardiol 16:550, 1965
12. Hildner FJ, Ormond RS: Accuracy of the clinical diagnosis of pulmonary embolism. JAMA 202:567, 1967
13. Kamper D, Chou TC, Fowler NO, et al: The reliability of electrocardiographic criteria of chronic obstructive lung disease. Am Heart J 80:445, 1970
14. Kilcoyne MM, Davis AL, Ferrer MI: A dynamic electrocardiographic concept useful in the diagnosis of cor pulmonale: Result of a survey of 200 patients with chronic obstructive pulmonary disease. Circulation 42:903, 1970
15. Kuo PT, VanderVeer JB: Electrocardiographic changes in pulmonary embolism with special reference to an early and transient shift of the electrical axis of the heart. Am Heart J 40:825, 1950
16. Littman D: The electrocardiographic findings in pulmonary emphysema. Am J Cardiol 5:339, 1960
17. Lynch RE, Stein PD, Bruce TA: Leftward shift of frontal plane QRS axis as a frequent manifestation of acute pulmonary embolism. Chest 61:443, 1972
18. McGinn S, White PD: Acute cor pulmonale resulting from pulmonary embolism. Its clinical recognition. JAMA 104:1473, 1935
19. Phillips E, Levine HD: A critical evaluation of extremity and precordial electrocardiography in acute cor pulmonale. Am Heart J 39:205, 1950
20. Phillips JH, Burch GE: Problems in the diagnosis of cor pulmonale. Am Heart J 66:818, 1963
21. Simonson E: Differentiation Between Normal and Abnormal in Electrocardiography. St Louis, CV Mosby, 1961
22. Spodick DH: Electrocardiographic studies in pulmonary disease. I. Electrocardiographic abnormalities in diffuse lung disease. Circulation 20:1067, 1959
23. Spodick DH: Electrocardiographic studies in pulmonary disease. II. Establishment of criteria for the electrocardiographic inference of diffuse lung disease. Circulation 20:1073, 1959
24. Spodick DH, Hauger-Klevine JH, Tyler JM, et al: Electrocardiogram in pulmonary emphysema. Am Rev Respir Dis 88:14, 1963
25. Sreenivasan BR: The electrocardiogram in pneumoperitoneum, pneumothorax and phrenic crush. Br Heart J 18:226, 1956
26. Stein PD, Dalen JE, McIntyre KM, et al: The electrocardiogram in acute pulmonary embolism. Prog Cardiovasc Dis 17:247, 1975

27. Sutton GC, Honey M, Gibson RV: Clinical diagnosis of acute massive pulmonary embolism. Lancet 1:271, 1969
28. Szucs MM, Brooks HL, Grossman W, et al: Diagnostic sensitivity of laboratory findings in acute pulmonary embolism. Ann Intern Med 74:161, 1971
29. Thomas AJ, Valabhji P: Arrhythmia and tachycardia in pulmonary heart disease. Br Heart J 31:491, 1969
30. Wasserburger RH, Kelly JR, Rasmussen HK, et al: The electrocardiographic pentalogy of pulmonary emphysema. Circulation 20:831, 1959
31. Weber DM, Phillips JH: A re-evaluation of electrocardiographic changes accompanying acute pulmonary embolism. Am J Med Sci 251:381, 1966
32. Wood P: Pulmonary embolism: Diagnosis by chest lead electrocardiography. Br Heart J 3:21, 1941
33. Zuckermann R, Cabrera CE, Fishleder BL, et al: Electrocardiogram in chronic cor pulmonale. Am Heart J 35:421, 1948
34. Zuckermann R, Rodriguez MI, Sodi-Pallares D, et al: Electropathology of acute cor pulmonale. Am Heart J 40:805, 1950

Congenital Heart Disease in Adults

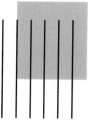

14

This chapter discusses the electrocardiographic (ECG) findings in a few selected congenital cardiac defects that are more likely to be seen in adult life. Emphasis is given to those lesions that are accompanied by characteristic ECG changes and to the changes that are helpful in the evaluation of the severity of the defect.

ATRIAL SEPTAL DEFECT

In atrial septal defect, the left-to-right shunting of the blood at the atrial level is accompanied by volume overloading and dilatation of the right atrium and ventricle. It is generally agreed that, in the uncomplicated cases, there is localized hypertrophy of the crista supraventricularis of the right ventricle. Activation of this area contributes to the late QRS vectors that are directed rightward and anteriorly and accounts for the appearance of the R' of the typical rSR' or RSR' pattern in lead V_1 seen in this condition[7] (Fig. 14–1). If pulmonary hypertension develops, pressure overloading of the right ventricle is superimposed on the volume overload. Hypertrophy of the free wall occurs in addition to that of the outflow tract. This may be associated with an increase in the amplitude of the R' in lead V_1 or a decrease of the S wave in V_1. An rR', a qR, or a monophasic R-wave pattern in lead V_1 and other signs of right ventricular hypertrophy may be recorded (Fig. 14–2). If a right ventricular conduction defect develops as a result of the ventricular dilatation, QRS prolongation and complete right bundle branch block pattern will appear.

Electrocardiographic Findings

RHYTHM

Most patients with atrial septal defect have normal sinus rhythms. The most common arrhythmia is atrial fibrillation, occurring in about 4 to 9 percent of the patients.[9,31,52] It is observed most often in older individuals (Fig.

14–3). In adults it is reported in 13 to 19 percent of the cases.[22,50] Some investigators believed that, in addition to advancing age, the elevation of left atrial pressure and left atrial enlargement in patients with large defects may be contributing factors.[50] Other less common arrhythmias that may occur include atrial flutter and atrial tachycardia. The experience in our institution as well as in that of others indicates that surgical correction of the defect does not necessarily have a favorable effect on the arrhythmias. Indeed, atrial fibrillation may appear in patients after surgery even though they had normal sinus rhythm preoperatively.[39,57]

P WAVE

In most patients with atrial septal defect, the P waves are normal. Signs of right atrial enlargement with tall P waves in the limb leads or right precordial leads are present in up to 36 percent of the patients[40,52] (Figs. 14–4 and 14–5). Abnormally wide P waves in lead II with slow upstroke were described by some investigators and were considered to be the result of volume overloading of the right atrium.[41]

PR INTERVAL

A PR interval greater than 0.20 second is observed in 6 to 19 percent of the patients with the ostium secundum defect[9,40] (see Figs. 14–2D and 14–6B). A higher incidence of 18 to 40 percent has been reported in the ostium primum type.[9,29,40] Second-degree and complete atrioventricular (AV) block are uncommon.

QRS COMPLEX

The frontal plane QRS axis is most helpful in the differentiation of the ostium primum and secundum types of defect. In the secundum

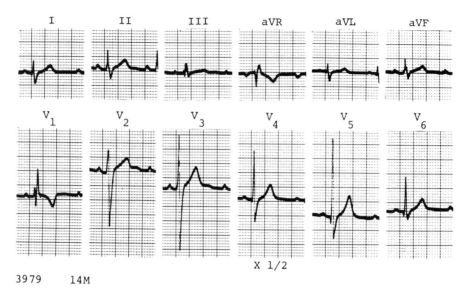

3979   14M

FIGURE 14-1. Atrial septal defect, ostium secundum type. The patient is a 14-year-old boy. The pulmonary-to-systemic flow ratio was 1.5:1, and the pulmonary arterial pressure was normal. In the ECG, the typical RSR' pattern is present in lead V_1. The frontal plane QRS axis is about +90°.

defect, the mean QRS axis is, with few exceptions, between 0° and +180°, most being to the right of +100°[40] (right axis deviation) (see Figs. 14-1 through 14-4). In the 910 patients with the secundum type of defect reported by Tan and associates, only 2.3 percent were found to have an axis between -10° and -160°.[49] Some of these patients had associated lesions, but others had only isolated defects. In the primum defect, the QRS axis is in the left superior quadrant, and most patients have true left axis deviation (a QRS axis superior to -30°) (see Figs. 14-5 and 14-6A). In the series of Prior and colleagues, 9 percent of the patients with primum defects had axes inferior to 0°, but none had true right axis deviation.[40] Figure 14-6B is an example of primum defect with normal QRS axis.

The genesis of the abnormal left axis deviation in ostium primum generally is attributed to the presence of left ventricular conduction defect. It is unchanged after surgical repair of the defect. Durrer and associates demonstrated in surgical patients early excitation of the posterobasal region of the left ventricle.[17] They suggested that the prominent leftward and superior forces originate from the anterolateral part of the left ventricle and are not opposed by the potential from the posterobasal wall that was depolarized prematurely.[17] This concept is supported by studies of serial histologic sections of the AV conduction system. Feldt and associates found in hearts with a partial or complete form of AV canal a marked posteroinferior displacement of the left bun-

dle branch system and relative hypoplasia of the anterior left bundle branches.[19] They believed that the anatomic configuration of the AV conduction system could result in relatively early impulse propagation to the posterior aspect of the left ventricle.

An rSR' or rSr' pattern in lead V_1 with a duration of 0.11 second or less is the most characteristic ECG finding in patients with atrial septal defect. In the 370 patients from four reported series,[9,31,40,52] such a pattern was observed in about 60 percent of the cases. It occurs more commonly in the ostium secundum than in the primum defect. Other less common morphologies include the RS, qR, qRS, monophasic R, or RSR'S' pattern. A normal rS or QS complex is seen in about 7 percent of the patients. Complete right bundle branch block with a QRS duration of 0.12 second or more occurs in 5 to 19 percent of cases.[22,40,52] It is more common in older individuals. Although the typical rSR' pattern in lead V_1 with a duration of less than 0.11 second often is interpreted as incomplete right bundle branch block, it is generally agreed that the pattern represents outflow tract hypertrophy. After surgical closure of the defect, the amplitude of the R' usually decreases after a few months. Failure of the regression may be an indication of incomplete closure of the defect or the presence of irreversible pulmonary vascular changes.

Most studies failed to demonstrate a definite relationship between the morphology of the QRS complex in lead V_1 and the hemody-

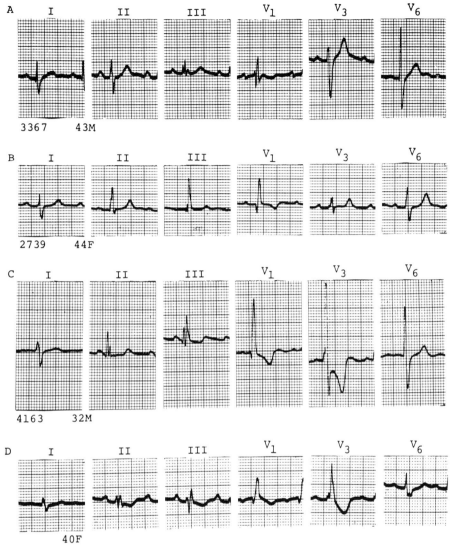

FIGURE 14–2. Four proved cases of ostium secundum atrial septal defect with different QRS morphology in lead V_1 and different hemodynamic findings. (A) The patient is a 43-year-old man with a small left-to-right shunt and normal pulmonary arterial pressure. He had paroxysmal atrial flutter. The ECG shows sinus rhythm and an rSR's' pattern in lead V_1. The frontal plane QRS axis is indeterminate. (B) The patient is a 44-year-old woman. Her pulmonary arterial pressure was moderately elevated, and there was a pulmonary-to-systemic flow ratio of 3:1. Lead V_1 shows a qR pattern. (C) The patient was a 32-year-old man with autopsy-proven ostium secundum atrial septal defect, anomalous pulmonary venous return to the right atrium, and severe pulmonary hypertension. In the ECG, there is abnormal right axis deviation, and an rsR' pattern in lead V_1 with tall R'. There are also secondary ST and T-wave changes in the right and mid-precordial leads. (D) The patient is a 40-year-old woman with a secundum-type defect proved at surgery. The pulmonary arterial pressure was normal. She had a large left-to-right shunt, with a pulmonary-to-systemic flow ratio of 6:1. In the ECG, the PR interval is 0.22 second. The frontal plane QRS axis is indeterminate. The QRS duration is 0.12 second, and there is an rsR' pattern in lead V_1 consistent with complete right bundle branch block. Some of the ST and T-wave changes probably are due to digitalis.

namic findings. Neither the pulmonary arterial pressure nor the size of the left-to-right shunt can be predicted from the ECG changes. Those patients with higher pulmonary arterial pressures, however, are likely to have tall R or R' waves or qR patterns in lead V_1.[29,31,52]

VENTRICULAR SEPTAL DEFECT

The ECG findings in isolated ventricular septal defect depend mainly on the hemodynamic consequence of the defect. The size of the defect, the amount of left-to-right shunt, and the

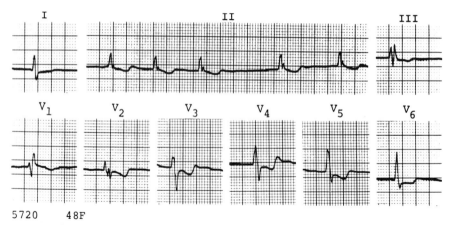

5720   48F

FIGURE 14–3. Atrial septal defect with atrial fibrillation. The patient is a 48-year-old woman, and the diagnosis of ostium secundum atrial septal defect was confirmed by cardiac catheterization. In the ECG, lead V_1 shows the typical rSR' pattern. Some of the ST and T-wave changes are due to digitalis effect.

response of pulmonary vasculature to the increased blood flow are the major determinants of the ECG manifestations. When the defect is small and hemodynamically insignificant, the ECG is normal (Fig. 14–7). Larger defects and left-to-right shunt cause increased pulmonary blood flow and volume overload of the left ventricle. The ECG usually displays left ventricular hypertrophy. When pulmonary hypertension develops as a result of increased pulmonary blood flow or increased pulmonary vascular resistance, right ventricular hypertrophy develops. The tracing may present signs of either left, right, or combined ventricular hypertrophy, depending on the degree of anatomic right ventricular hypertrophy (Fig. 14–8).

Electrocardiographic Findings in Isolated Ventricular Septal Defect

RHYTHM

Sinus rhythm is seen most often. Occasional AV junctional rhythm or premature ventricular contractions are observed.[51] Generally speaking, other causes should be searched for when either supraventricular or ventricular arrhythmia is present.

P WAVE

The P waves are normal in most patients. Signs of left atrial enlargement are found in 2 to 33 percent of the cases.[45] They are most com-

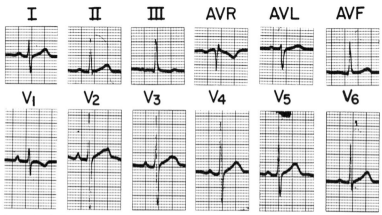

FIGURE 14–4. Ostium secundum atrial septal defect. The patient is a 17-year-old woman with a large left-to-right (2.2:1) shunt. The pulmonary arterial pressure was normal. The ECG shows tall, peaked P waves in the right precordial leads, suggesting right atrial enlargement. There is a borderline right axis deviation. Lead V_1 shows an RS pattern with the R/S ratio equal to 1, a borderline value for her age.

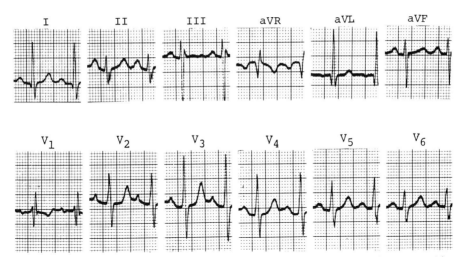

FIGURE 14–5. Ostium primum atrial septal defect. The patient is a 20-year-old woman with a pulmonary-to-systemic blood flow ratio of 2.5:1. The pulmonary arterial pressure was normal. The ECG shows a PR interval of 0.20 second. There is an abnormal left axis deviation. An rSR′s′ pattern is present in lead V_1. The S waves in the left precordial lead are deep. The P waves in lead V_2 are prominent, suggesting right atrial enlargement.

monly manifested by broad and notched P waves in leads I and II.[54] Evidence of right atrial enlargement is present in 10 to 25 percent.[45]

PR INTERVAL

Prolongation of the PR interval is uncommon,[8] but the PR interval was reported to be pro-longed in more than one third of the cases in one series.[51] Second- and third-degree AV blocks are rare.

VENTRICULAR COMPLEX

QRS AXIS. The frontal plane QRS axis is variable in isolated ventricular septal defect. It usually is directed leftward and inferiorly

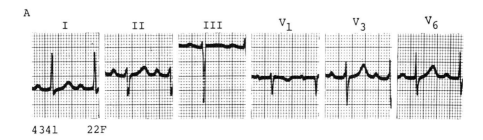

4341   22F

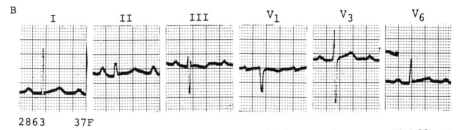

2863   37F

FIGURE 14–6. Two cases of ostium primum atrial septal defect proved at autopsy. (A) A 22-year-old woman with a large left-to-right shunt and normal pulmonary arterial pressure. The ECG shows marked abnormal left axis deviation. The morphology of the QRS complex in lead V_1 is normal and is not typical of atrial septal defect. (B) The patient was a 37-year-old woman. The tracing shows first-degree AV block. The frontal plane QRS axis is about +20°, which is atypical for ostium primum defect. Lead V_1 shows a normal rS complex.

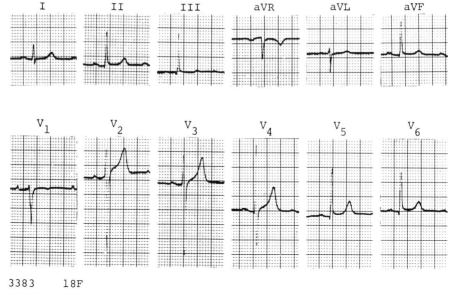

3383   18F

FIGURE 14–7. Small ventricular septal defect. The patient is an 18-year-old woman. Cardiac catheterization and angiography demonstrated a small ventricular septal defect in the membranous portion of the ventricular septum. The ECG is within normal limits.

except in patients with pulmonary hypertension and right ventricular hypertrophy. In about 4 percent of patients, the mean QRS axis is directed leftward and superiorly and the frontal plane QRS loop is inscribed in a counterclockwise direction.[35] Anatomically, the defect occupies a more posterior position, similar to that seen in patients with persistent common AV canal.

QRS-T MORPHOLOGY. The ventricular complex is normal in 10 to 15 percent of patients with isolated ventricular septal defect. It shows signs of isolated left ventricular hypertrophy in 2 to 10 percent.[8,37,54] The more

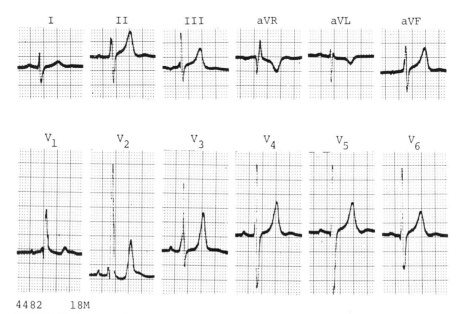

4482   18M

FIGURE 14–8. Ventricular septal defect with pulmonary hypertension. The patient is an 18-year-old man. The diagnosis was confirmed by cardiac catheterization. The pulmonary arterial pressure reached the systemic level. In the ECG, there is an $S_1S_2S_3$ pattern. There is an rSR' pattern in the right precordial leads. Because of the relatively tall R waves in the left precordial leads in the presence of right ventricular hypertrophy, left ventricular hypertrophy also may be present.

characteristic changes include deep Q waves, tall R waves with delay in the onset of the intrinsicoid deflection, and tall T waves in the left precordial leads. The deep Q waves are attributed to septal hypertrophy.

In 14 to 65 percent of patients, the tracing suggests right ventricular hypertrophy.[8,54] Lead V_1 may present an rR′, R, RS, rSR′, or qR pattern. Signs of both left and right ventricular hypertrophy are observed in 23 to 61 percent of cases. Many patients have large diphasic QRS complexes in the limb leads or mid-precordial leads, as described by Katz and Wachtel,[27] to suggest combined ventricular hypertrophy.[26]

Burch and DePasquale reported the frequent occurrence of an $S_1S_2S_3$ (35 percent) or S_1S_2 pattern (36 percent) in these patients.[8] Indeed, they noted that an $S_1S_2S_3$ or S_1S_2 pattern, an R′ in lead V_1, S waves of large magnitude in leads V_5 and V_6, and a deep Q wave in V_6 are the most characteristic findings in the 110 cases they examined. These investigators believed that the increased rightward terminal forces responsible for the $S_1S_2S_3$, R′ in V_1, and S waves in V_5 and V_6 are the result of hypertrophy of the crista supraventricularis due to volume overload of the right ventricle, as in the case of atrial septal defect.

Electrocardiographic and Hemodynamic Correlation

The ECG may provide a useful but imprecise estimation of the hemodynamic state in patients with isolated ventricular septal defect.[12,18,37,51,54,56] A normal ECG suggests a small defect. The pattern of isolated left ventricular hypertrophy usually indicates moderate shunt without increased pulmonary vascular resistance. A pure right ventricular hypertrophy pattern suggests the presence of pulmonary hypertension or Eisenmenger's syndrome. When the ECG is consistent with combined ventricular hypertrophy, there is usually a moderate or large defect, but the degree of pulmonary hypertension is variable. When large Q waves (greater than 4 mm) are present in the left precordial leads in association with either left or combined ventricular hypertrophy, the pulmonary vascular resistance is seldom increased.[56] In adults, a large uncomplicated ventricular septal defect is rare. Therefore, the ECG either is normal because the defect is small or is indicative of right ventricular hypertrophy because of the development of pulmonary hypertension.

PATENT DUCTUS ARTERIOSUS

In most patients who have patent ductus arteriosus, there is a left-to-right shunt from the aorta to the pulmonary artery. The increase in pulmonary blood flow is accompanied by an increase in pulmonary venous return to the left atrium and left ventricle. The ECG findings are the results of volume overload of the left-sided chambers. If pulmonary hypertension is present as a result of either developmental abnormalities or vascular changes secondary to high pulmonary blood flow, a reversal of the shunt may occur. Right ventricular hypertrophy may develop because of the increase in pressure overload of the right side of the heart.

Although the ECG contributes little in the diagnosis of patent ductus arteriosus, it is often helpful in the evaluation of the hemodynamic state of the patient. As a rule, the ECG is normal if the ductus is small and more marked changes are seen in patients with large ductus. When ECG changes of right ventricular hypertrophy are encountered, the presence of Eisenmenger's physiology can be assumed.

The rhythm is sinus in origin in practically all cases. Arrhythmias are rare. P-wave changes consistent with left atrial enlargement are seen in about 30 percent of patients.[6] The PR interval is increased in about 10 percent of cases.[33] The reason for the AV conduction delay is unclear, and the PR interval returns to normal after ligation of the ductus in most instances.

In most patients with left-to-right shunts, the ventricular complex reveals isolated left hypertrophy or, less often, combined ventricular hypertrophy.[8,30] Occasionally, an rSr′ pattern is seen in lead V_1, occurring in about 3 percent of the patients.[8,33] Although the typical left ventricular volume overload pattern usually is associated with ST-segment elevation and tall and peaked T waves in the left precordial leads, ST-segment depression or T-wave inversion may be seen in at least one third of the patients with patent ductus (Fig. 14–9). In adult subjects, however, the incidence of abnormal ECG is low. In 13 patients over the age of 30 described by Cosh, only 1 showed signs of left ventricular hypertrophy, whereas the ECG was normal in 11.[14]

In patients with pulmonary hypertension and right-to-left shunt, the ECG usually shows right atrial enlargement and right or combined ventricular hypertrophy (Fig. 14–10). According to Burch, the ECGs of such patients

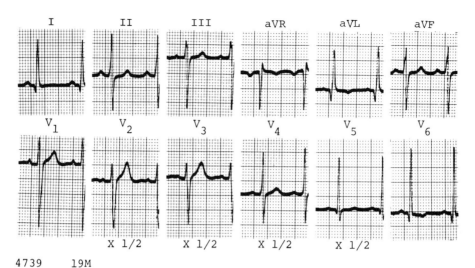

4739   19M

FIGURE 14-9. Patent ductus arteriosus. The patient is a 19-year-old man, and the diagnosis was proven at surgery. At cardiac catheterization, a 3:1 left-to-right shunt was demonstrated, and the pulmonary arterial pressure was normal. The ECG shows a frontal plane QRS axis of −15°. The QRS voltage and ST and T-wave changes are consistent with left ventricular hypertrophy.

differ from those with Eisenmenger's syndrome as a result of atrial septal defect or severe tetralogy of Fallot in that the R waves in the left precordial leads are relatively tall.[6]

COARCTATION OF THE AORTA

In coarctation of the aorta, the constriction is most commonly located just distal to the left subclavian artery. The site of the involvement sometimes is lower and may affect the abdominal aorta. Significant narrowing is accompanied by hypertension in the upper extremities and hypotension in the lower extremities. There is an increase in the pressure loading of the left ventricle. Left ventricular hypertrophy is therefore the ECG abnormality to be expected.

As a rule, there is normal sinus rhythm. The PR interval usually is within normal limits, but it was reported to be prolonged in 10 percent of one series.[6] In most patients, the P wave is normal. Signs of left atrial enlargement may be seen in about one fifth of the cases.[6] A small percentage of patients (15 percent) have left axis deviation. The incidence

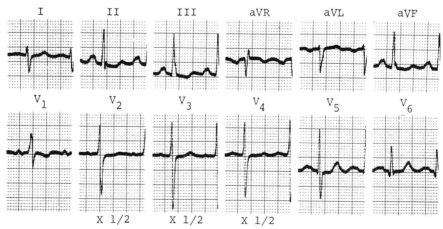

FIGURE 14-10. Patent ductus arteriosus with pulmonary hypertension. The patient is a 43-year-old woman. The diagnosis was confirmed by cardiac catheterization and angiography. The pulmonary and systemic arterial pressures were equal. In the ECG, there is abnormal right axis deviation. The R/S ratio in lead V_1 is greater than 1. There are large biphasic QRS complexes in leads V_2 through V_4. These findings are consistent with combined ventricular hypertrophy.

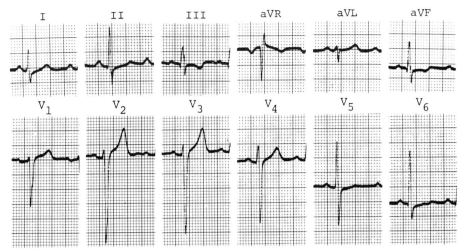

FIGURE 14–11. Coarctation of the aorta. The patient is a 19-year-old man. The coarctation is located just beyond the origin of the left subclavian artery. During catheterization, there was a gradient of 67 mm Hg across the area of constriction. In the ECG, ST and T-wave abnormalities are seen in the left precordial leads. A definite diagnosis of left ventricular hypertrophy could not be made, because the voltage of the QRS complex is within normal range for the patient's age.

of left ventricular hypertrophy in the ECG is variable in the different reports. In Wood's series of 200 cases, there was an increase in the QRS voltage with normal T waves in 22 percent.[58] Left ventricular strain pattern with inverted T waves in the leads with dominant R waves was present in 18 percent. Three fourths of those with inverted T waves had an additional cause of left ventricular overlaod, usually aortic valve disease but sometimes patent ductus arteriosus or ventricular septal defect. Only 4.5 percent of his series with uncomplicated coarctation displayed the typical left ventricular strain pattern. These patients had more severe hypertension than the average subjects of the series. Nearly half of their patients had normal ECGs. Other investigators reported left ventricular hypertrophy in about 60 percent of the patients.[6,48] Figures 14–11 and 14–12 are tracings recorded from patients with thoracic and abdominal coarctation, respectively. The changes are borderline for left ventricular hypertrophy.

Right or combined ventricular hypertrophy is seldom seen in adults with coarctation of the aorta unless other lesions coexist. An rSR′ pattern is observed in about 10 to 20 percent of the patients.[6,58] The pathogenesis of the

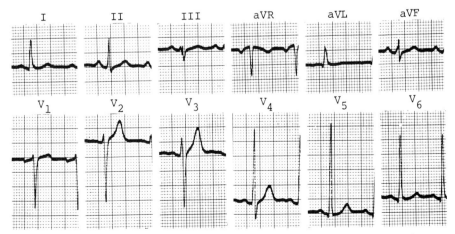

FIGURE 14–12. Coarctation of the abdominal aorta. The patient is a 22-year-old man with severe hypertension. The diagnosis of abdominal coarctation was confirmed at surgery. The ECG shows relatively high voltage of the QRS complex in the precordial leads. A definitive diagnosis of left ventricular hypertrophy could not be made, however, because of the age of the patient.

complete or incomplete right bundle branch block pattern is unclear. Some related it to involution of preexisting right ventricular hypertrophy in utero when the fetal ductus joined the aorta proximal to the stricture.[60] In a vectorcardiographic study, Gaum and asso-

ciates found prominent right posterior QRS forces in about half of the children with isolated coarctation.[23] They postulated that hypertrophy of the posterobasal region of the left ventricle may generate forces in this direction or that there is a left ventricular con-

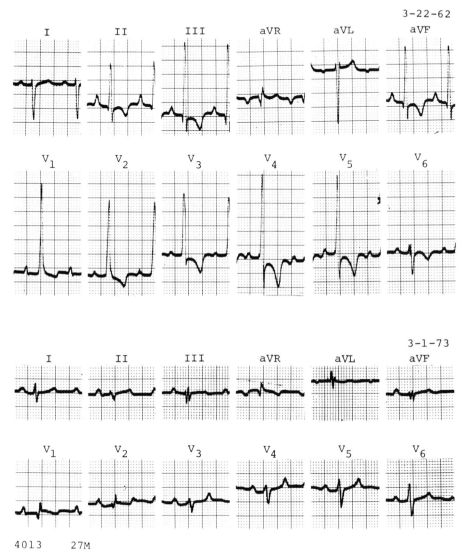

FIGURE 14-13. Valvular pulmonary stenosis. The patient was 16 years old when the 1962 tracing was obtained. Cardiac catheterization at that time demonstrated a right ventricular systolic pressure of 140 mm Hg, with a gradient of 120 mm Hg across the pulmonic valve. The ECG recorded on 3-22-62 shows right atrial enlargement with tall, peaked P waves in the inferior and right precordial leads. Marked abnormal right axis deviation is present. Tall monophasic R waves are present in the right precordial leads, and Rs deflections are present in the mid-precordial leads. In lead V_6, the R/S ratio is less than 1. ST and T-wave abnormalities are present in all the precordial leads and also in the inferior leads. A pulmonary valvulotomy was performed in that year. The bottom tracing was obtained about 11 years later. No clinical evidence of right ventricular hypertrophy was present at this time, but a repeat cardiac catheterization was not done. In the ECG, there is borderline first-degree AV block. The frontal plane QRS axis is indeterminate. The P waves in the right precordial leads are suggestive of right atrial enlargement. A QR pattern is present in lead V_1. The R/S ratio in lead V_5 is less than 1. The QRS changes are consistent with right ventricular hypertrophy. The abnormalities are, however, much less pronounced than those in the preoperative tracing.

duction defect that involves mainly the posterior division of the left bundle branch. It is possible that the abnormal rightward forces present themselves as an R' in the right precordial leads. Left bundle branch block also is occasionally seen.[6]

For a discussion of valvular aortic stenosis and idiopathic hypertrophic subaortic stenosis, see Chapters 3 and 12, respectively.

PULMONARY STENOSIS

In isolated pulmonary stenosis, there is an increase of the pressure overload of the right ventricle and right atrium. The characteristic ECG findings are therefore those of right ventricular hypertrophy and right atrial enlargement. The frequency and degree of the changes are, to a certain extent, related to the severity of the obstruction.

The ECG may be entirely normal in mild pulmonary stenosis. In one series, about half of the patients with a right ventricular systolic pressure below 60 mm Hg had normal tracings.[6] In all patients with pulmonary stenosis, sinus rhythm is the rule. Tall and peaked P waves, either in the limb leads or precordial leads, are present in about 10 to 50 percent of the patients.[11,42,59] Signs of right atrial enlargement are seen more frequently in patients with high right ventricular pressure. The PR interval is usually within normal limits. A prolonged PR interval is seen only occasionally in patients with extreme degrees of right ventricular hypertension.

The QRS axis in the frontal plane may be normal or displaced to the right. The incidence of abnormal right axis deviation generally increases with increased severity of the stenosis. When abnormal left axis deviation is observed, additional lesions should be suspected. The QRS duration is usually normal and seldom exceeds 0.11 second. In lead V_1, various QRS morphologies may be recorded. A monophasic R wave, a qR, or an Rs complex with ST-segment depression and T-wave inversion is most likely associated with severe lesion (Fig. 14–13). The less common rSR' pattern (11 percent in one series[42]) is encountered more often in patients with milder disease (Fig. 14–14). An rS pattern in lead V_1 rarely is seen in those with severe stenosis. In the 105 patients studied by Cayler and associates, those with R waves in V_1 greater than 20 mm almost always had systolic pressures in the right ventricle above 100 mm Hg, and patients with R waves in lead V_1 of less than 20 mm rarely had such pressures.[11] In other series, however, the correlation between the height of the R wave and the right ventricular pressure was not as clear-cut.[3,21]

In summary, the ECG in mild pulmonary stenosis may be normal, whereas changes of right ventricular hypertrophy are seen in most patients with moderate or severe elevation of the right ventricular systolic pressure. Although the trend is for prominent P waves, marked right axis deviation, and especially taller R waves in lead V_1 to be associated with increased severity of the stenosis, it is gener-

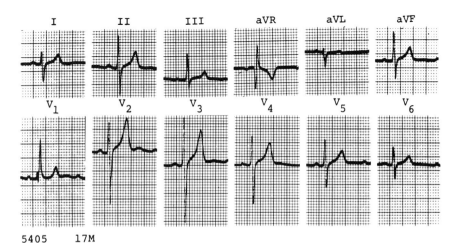

5405   17M

FIGURE 14–14. Pulmonary stenosis. The patient is a 17-year-old boy with isolated pulmonary stenosis of moderate severity. During cardiac catheterization, the right ventricular systolic pressure was 72 mm Hg, with a gradient of 57 mm Hg across the pulmonary valve. In the ECG, the frontal plane QRS axis is about +120°. The P waves are within normal limits. There is an rSR' pattern in lead V_1, with an upright T wave.

ally agreed that the ECG by itself cannot be relied on for an accurate estimation of the height of right ventricular systolic pressure.

TETRALOGY OF FALLOT

In its broad sense, the term *Fallot's tetralogy* encompasses a wide anatomic and physiological spectrum. The size and severity of the two major defects, namely ventricular septal defect and pulmonary stenosis, are variable. The size of the ventricular septal defect may be small or large. The pulmonary stenosis may be mild or severe, or the valve may even be atretic. The hemodynamic consequences of the various combinations of the malformation affect the degree of right ventricular pressure overloading and the development of the left ventricle. In most instances, the systolic pressure in the left and right ventricles are equal, but the flow resistance is greater in the right side of the heart. There is a right-to-left shunt, and the patient is cyanotic. Occasionally, when the pulmonary stenosis is mild and the ventricular septal defect is large, there is a left-to-right shunt, and the patient is acyanotic.

It is generally agreed that the ECGs of patients with tetralogy of Fallot show no specific signs to suggest the diagnosis. Sometimes, however, they give some indication of the hemodynamic status of this anomaly.

The electrocardiogram is abnormal in over 95 percent of patients with tetralogy of Fallot.[2] Arrhythmias are rare. P waves suggestive of right atrial enlargement are seen in about 30 to 50 percent of the patients.[2,15,38] In most of the patients, tall, peaked P waves are present in limb leads, but they may occasionally be limited to the right precordial leads. Prolongation of the PR interval is unusual, being observed in only 5 percent or less of the cases. The QRS duration is, as a rule, within normal limits. Right axis deviation and sign of right ventricular hypertrophy are the most common findings and are present in almost all patients with abnormal ECGs. In lead V_1 the QRS complex has an Rs configuration in about two thirds of the cases. An R or rR', rSR', rS or RS, and qR pattern are seen in descending order of frequency. The height of the R wave bears no apparent relationship to the height of the right ventricular pressure.[2] The rSR' pattern is said to occur mostly in patients with left-to-right shunt.[15] The presence of a left-to-right shunt also is suggested by the finding of prominent Q waves or a delay of the onset of intrinsicoid deflection in the left precordial leads (V_5 and V_6).[15,38]

In adult patients, the rSR' pattern in lead V_1 is seen more commonly, especially in cyanotic patients. In 25 adult patients reported by Higgins and Mulder, this pattern was present in 58 percent.[25] Signs of left ventricular hypertrophy also are seen frequently in older patients who have not undergone prior palliative or corrective surgery[10] (Fig. 14–15). In acyanotic patients, isolated right, left, or combined ventricular hypertrophy may be seen. The ECG changes occasionally are rather inconspicuous (Fig. 14–16).

Because an increasing number of children who have undergone corrective surgery for tetralogy of Fallot have now reached adulthood,

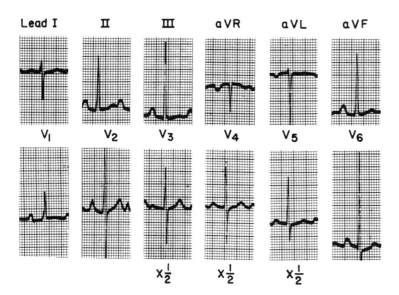

FIGURE 14–15. Tetralogy of Fallot with pulmonary atresia. The patient is a 19-year-old woman, and the diagnosis was confirmed at surgery. The ECG shows right atrial enlargement, abnormal right axis deviation, and biventricular hypertrophy. A monophasic R wave is seen in lead V_1. Large biphasic QRS complexes are present in the mid-precordial leads. Tall R waves are present in the left precordial leads.

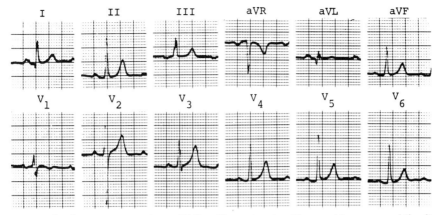

FIGURE 14–16. Acyanotic tetralogy of Fallot. The patient is a 21-year-old woman, and the diagnosis was supported by cardiac catheterization. There was a gradient of 55 mm Hg across the pulmonary outflow tract and a 1.7:1 left-to-right shunt at the ventricular level. The ECG is rather unremarkable. The R/S ratio in lead V_1 is about 1, which suggests the possibility of right ventricular hypertrophy.

the ECG findings in these postoperative patients deserve comment. One of the most common findings is right bundle branch block (Fig. 14–17). This may be the result of the injury either to the proximal right bundle branch during the repair of the ventricular septal defect[36] or to its more peripheral branches associated with right ventriculotomy.[28] In addition, about 10 percent of postoperative patients have left anterior hemiblock in addition to right bundle branch block.[16] Injury to the anterior division of the left bundle branch during the repair of ventricular septal defect is believed to be responsible for the bifascicular block.

EBSTEIN'S ANOMALY

The ECG is helpful in the clinical recognition of Ebstein's anomaly, a congenital lesion of the tricuspid valve. The anomaly often is suspected from the ECG alone. The downward displacement of the malformed leaflets is accompanied by the creation of an "atrialized" portion of the right ventricle and reduced pumping function of the right ventricle. There is tricuspid insufficiency, and the right atrium is markedly dilated. In most patients, there is a coexisting patent foramen ovale or an ostium secundum atrial septal defect. Fibrosis in the posterior and superior portion of

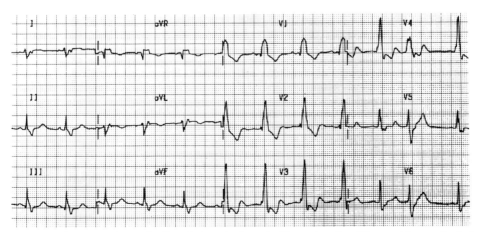

FIGURE 14–17. Tetralogy of Fallot after surgical repair. The patient is a 27-year-old man who had tetralogy of Fallot that was surgically repaired at the age of 6 years. The tracing shows complete right bundle branch block and one ventricular premature beat.

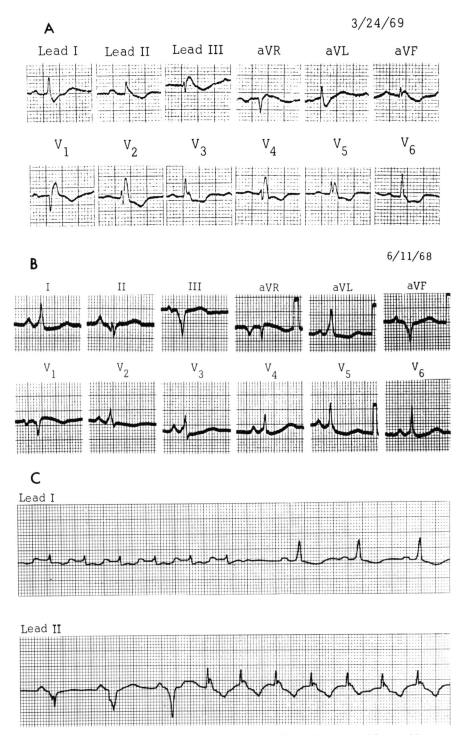

FIGURE 14–18. Ebstein's anomaly with WPW syndrome. The patient was a 35-year-old woman, and the diagnosis of Ebstein's anomaly was confirmed at surgery. (A) The PR interval is 0.20 second. There is a complete right bundle branch block with a QR pattern in lead V_1. Some of the ST and T-wave changes are probably due to digitalis. (B) The PR interval measures 0.15 second. Although the PR interval is within normal limits, it has shortened since the previous tracing. A delta wave is present and is directed downward in lead V_1. The right bundle branch block pattern is no longer observed. The tracing is consistent with type B WPW syndrome. The normal PR interval represents a variant form of the preexcitation syndrome. (C) Tracing demonstrates episodes of supraventricular tachycardia (orthodromic AV reentrant tachycardia) with a rate of 125 beats/min. The tracing shows the WPW pattern during sinus rhythm but right bundle branch block during tachycardia.

the interventricular septum, as well as in the free wall of the right ventricle, was found in some autopsied cases.[4]

Rhythm

The basic rhythm is usually sinus in origin, but paroxysmal supraventricular tachycardia occurs in 20 to 50 percent of the patients.[5,24,53] Atrial and AV junctional tachycardia are most common (Fig. 14–18), and atrial flutter and atrial fibrillation are occasionally observed. Ventricular arrhythmias also have been reported but are uncommon.

P Wave

Tall, peaked, or wide P waves are present in 60 to 95 percent of patients.[5,24,53] This can be explained by the usually dilated, thin, and occasionally hypertrophied right atrium, which requires longer duration for completion of excitation. The right atrial enlargement also was thought by some authors to be responsible for the appearance of Q waves in leads V_1 and V_2.[47] The dilated right atrium causes marked leftward displacement of the right ventricle, and the right precordial leads record the intraventricular potential of the right ventricle.

PR Interval

The AV conduction time is prolonged in 16 to 34 percent of patients.[5,6,32,53] Second- and third-degree AV block are uncommon.

Ventricular Complex

Complete or incomplete right bundle branch block is one of the most characteristic ECG findings in Ebstein's anomaly (Figs. 14–18 through 14–20). It occurs in 75 to 80 percent of cases.[24] In some cases, the initial tracing may be normal, but the typical changes appear during the follow-up period.[43] The right bundle branch block pattern is often atypical. The QRS morphology is frequently bizarre and polyphasic, especially in the right precordial leads (see Figs. 14–19 and 14–20). Leads V_1 and V_2 may record an RS, rSR', rR'S, rSr'S', or qRS pattern. A QR pattern with T-wave inversion in leads V_1 through V_4 was thought to be almost pathognomonic by some authors.[46] The amplitude of the QRS complexes in the right precordial leads may be small. Conspicuously deep Q waves are occasionally seen in the inferior leads.[6,13]

Of special interest is the presence of type B Wolff-Parkinson-White (WPW) syndrome in a number of patients with the Ebstein's anomaly (7 to 25 percent)[5,24,53] (see Fig. 14–18). The delta wave is inscribed downward in lead V_1. Ebstein's anomaly is the most common lesion in patients with WPW syndrome who have associated congenital heart disease. In a patient on whom I assisted in performing epicardial mapping during surgery, the accessory pathway was located at the lateral border of the right atrium and right ventricle (see Fig. 14–18).

Because preexcitation of the right ventricle tends to counterbalance the effect of right bundle branch block, their ECG changes are

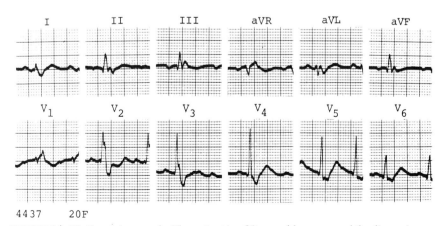

4437   20F

FIGURE 14–19. Ebstein's anomaly. The patient is a 20-year-old woman, and the diagnosis was supported by cardiac catheterization, angiography, and intracavitary electrogram. In the ECG, the P waves are abnormal, probably because of an ectopic atrial pacemaker. The QRS complexes show an atypical right bundle branch block pattern. The duration of the QRS complex is 0.16 second.

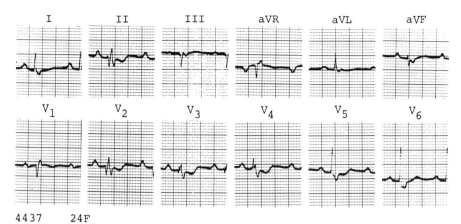

4437   24F

FIGURE 14–20. Ebstein's anomaly. The patient is a 24-year-old woman, and the diagnosis was confirmed by cardiac catheterization, angiography, and intracardiac electrogram. In the ECG, the tall P waves in leads V_2 and V_3 are suggestive of right atrial enlargement. The QRS complex shows an atypical right bundle branch block pattern, with an rSR′ pattern in lead V_1 and a rSr′S′ in lead V_2.

unlikely to be seen in a patient at the same time. Occasionally, however, such a rare combination of findings does occur. When present, it is virtually diagnostic of Ebstein's malformation (Fig. 14–21).

Intracardiac Electrogram

Although it is not the intention of this text to discuss invasive diagnostic methods, it should be mentioned that an intracavitary electrogram may be useful in confirming the diagnosis of Ebstein's anomaly. In the atrialized right ventricle, where the pressure pulse is similar to that of the right atrium, the electrogram resembles that of the right ventricle. Furthermore, ventricular extrasystoles and ST-segment displacement may be produced when the electrode catheter is pressed against the endocardial wall of the atrialized right ventricular chamber.[32] Watson, however, cau-

tioned that both false-positive and false-negative results have been encountered with these procedures.[55]

DEXTROCARDIA

In its broad sense, dextrocardia may be defined as a malposition of the heart in the right side of the chest. True dextrocardia also is referred to as mirror-image dextrocardia. The cardiac apex is pointed to the right and is formed by the left ventricle. The anatomic left atrium and left ventricle are to the right of the right-sided heart chambers. In most cases, there is a similar mirrorlike transposition of the other viscera, and the condition is called dextrocardia with situs inversus. This is the most common form of dextrocardia. The heart usually is normal other than for its malposition, but it may be associated with congenital heart disease or develop acquired heart dis-

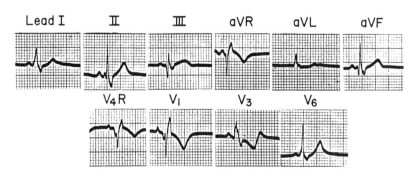

FIGURE 14–21. Ebstein's anomaly with type B WPW in a 7-year-old girl. The PR interval is 0.09 second. The QRS duration measures 0.12 second. Delta waves are present and are inscribed downward in leads V_{4R} and V_1. Signs of right bundle branch block are also present, with an R′ in leads V_{4R} and V_1. (Courtesy of Dr. Samuel Kaplan.)

ease as does the general population. When mirror-image dextrocardia is not accompanied by inversion of other viscera, it is called *isolated* dextrocardia. This type of dextrocardia is almost invariably associated with other serious and often complicated cardiac malformations and is rarely seen in adults.

The term *dextroversion* is used when the heart is rotated or swung to the right side of the chest. The interrelation between the various cardiac chambers is unchanged. The left atrium and ventricle remain to the left of the right chambers. Dextroversion also is almost always associated with other serious cardiac abnormalities and is rarely seen in adults.

If the heart is displaced to the right side of the chest because of disease of the lungs or other external causes the condition is called *dextroposition* of the heart.

A discussion of isolated dextrocardia and dextroversion and their various associated ab-

normalities is beyond the scope of this text. Only true dextrocardia with situs inversus is described. Because dextroposition of the heart usually is an acquired condition, it is discussed here mainly for the purpose of differential diagnosis. The reader is referred to the article by Neil and Mirowski[34] and to the text by Burch and DePasquale[6] for more detailed information.

Mirror-Image Dextrocardia with Situs Inversus

The most outstanding ECG changes in mirror-image dextrocardia are seen in lead I (Fig. 14–22). The P, QRS, and T waves are inverted or upside down. The negative P wave in lead I is particularly significant, since it seldom is seen in other conditions if the tracing is recorded correctly and the sinoatrial node is the pacemaker. Leads aVR and aVL are reversed,

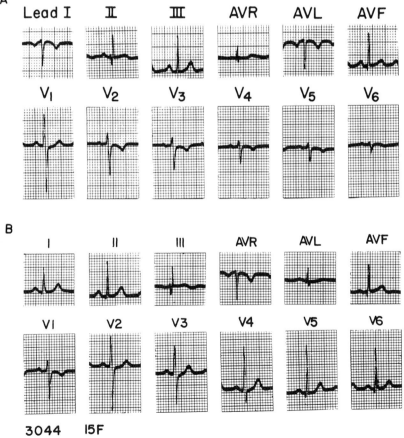

FIGURE 14–22. Mirror-image dextrocardia with situs inversus. The patient is a 15-year-old girl. There is no evidence of organic heart disease. (A) Tracing recorded with the conventional electrode placement. (B) Tracing obtained with the left and right arm electrodes reversed. The precordial lead electrodes also were relocated in the respective mirror-image positions on the chest. The tracing is within normal limits.

and prominent negative deflections are now seen in aVL rather than in aVR. Lead aVF is unaffected. Lead II represents the usual lead III and vice versa.

In the precordial leads, the usual lead V_1 to V_6 locations of the electrode will record complexes of decreasing amplitude. Lead V_1 is the equivalent of the usual V_2 and vice versa. Leads V_3 and V_4 are the equivalents of the usual V_{3R} and V_{4R}.

Although the interpretation of the limb leads can be accomplished by mental corrections, most of the information available from the precordial leads is missed. A repeat tracing with a reversal of the left and right arm electrodes and placement of the precordial leads in the equivalent positions on the right side of the chest are required for the proper interpretation of the ECG.

Differential Diagnosis

MISPLACED ELECTRODES

The most common error in the recording of the limb leads involves the reversal of the left and right arm electrodes. The changing polarity of lead I results in an inversion of the P, QRS, and T waves in this lead. The rest of the limb leads also are altered, mimicking mirror-image dextrocardia. Because, however, the sum of the limb lead potential remains at zero even though the electrodes are misplaced, the precordial leads are not affected. The marked dissimilarity of the morphology of the complexes in leads I and V_6 usually raises suspicion that the left and right arm electrodes are reversed.

DEXTROPOSITION

In dextroposition of the heart without intrinsic cardiac lesion, the morphology of the complexes in the limb leads closely resembles that of the normal ECG. The P waves in lead I are upright. In the precordial leads, left ventricular potential is recorded in the right as well as in the left precordial leads (Fig. 14–23).

ABNORMAL ELECTROCARDIOGRAM IN THE PRESENCE OF MIRROR-IMAGE DEXTROCARDIA

Figure 14–24 is an example of T-wave abnormalities consistent with myocardial ischemia in a patient with mirror-image dextrocardia and coronary artery disease. The dextrocardia was suspected because the P waves were inverted in lead I and misplacement of electrode was excluded. The proper interpretation was made after the electrodes were relocated.

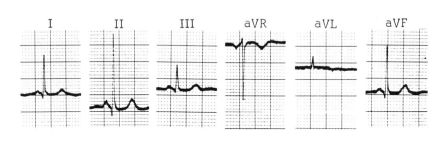

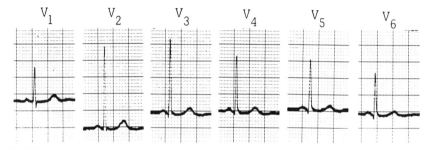

FIGURE 14–23. Dextroposition. The patient is a 40-year-old woman with hypoplastic right pulmonary artery and right lung, probably of congenital origin. The heart and mediastinum are displaced to the right chest. In the ECG, the limb leads are normal except for a relatively large R wave in lead II and S wave in lead aVR. The precordial leads show tall R waves in leads V_1 through V_3; the amplitude of the R waves decreases from V_2 to V_6.

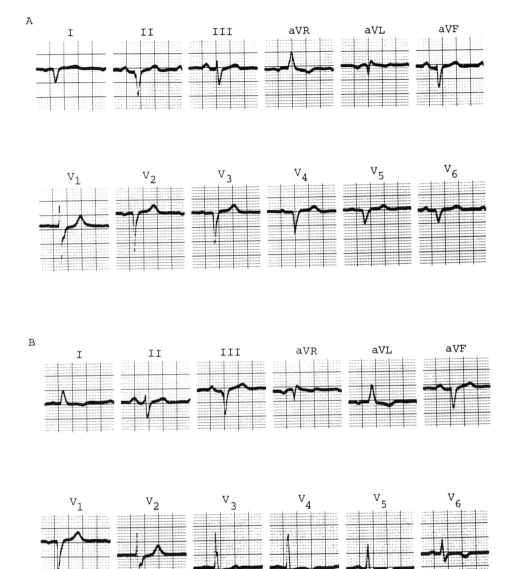

FIGURE 14–24. Mirror-image dextrocardia and coronary artery disease. The patient is a 72-year-old man with mirror-image dextrocardia and situs inversus. He also had coronary artery disease with angina pectoris. (A) Tracing showing an inverted P wave and QRS complex but an upright T wave in lead I. The precordial leads show diminishing amplitude of the QRS complex from leads V_1 through V_6. (B) Tracing recorded with the left and right arm electrodes reversed. The precordial lead electrodes also were relocated to the respective mirror-image positions on the chest. The tracing now shows abnormal left axis deviation consistent with left anterior hemiblock. Additional intraventricular conduction defect may be present because of the slurring of the QRS complexes in leads V_2 and V_3. The symmetrical T-wave inversion in leads I, aVL, and V_4 through V_6 is consistent with anterolateral myocardial ischemia.

CORRECTED TRANSPOSITION OF THE GREAT ARTERIES

This condition is also known as ventricular inversion or L-transposition. Systemic venous blood passes through a bicuspid AV valve into a "right-sided" ventricle that is structurally similar to that of the normal left ventricle. The venous blood is ejected into the lungs and returns to the left atrium, which empties through a tricuspid valve into a ventricle that is structurally similar to the right ventricle. The ascending aorta is more leftward and the pulmonary artery more posterior. Physiologi-

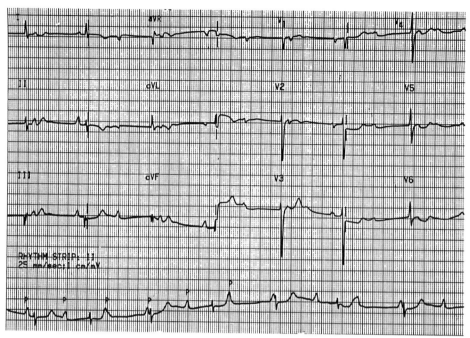

FIGURE 14–25. Corrected transposition of the great arteries. The patient is a 43-year-old woman. The diagnosis is supported by echocardiographic findings. No other anatomic cardiac lesion was found. The ECG shows complete AV block with junctional escape rhythm at the rate of 50 beats/min. A QS deflection is apparent in lead V_1, and an absence of Q waves can be seen in leads V_5 and V_6. Q waves are present in leads III and aVF. The P waves are abnormal.

cally, blood flow is normal, because systemic venous blood is oxygenated and arterialized blood is ejected in the normal manner. Commonly associated lesions are ventricular septal defect, pulmonary stenosis, and incompetence of the left AV valve due to Ebstein's anomaly of the left-sided tricuspid valve.

With the ventricular inversion, there is inversion of the ventricular conduction system. The AV node is situated in the anterior part of the right atrium.[1] From there, the His bundle descends into the morphologic left ventricle (right-sided) and encircles the anterolateral quadrant of the pulmonary outflow tract before its arrival at the anterior septum, where it bifurcates into the inverted bundle branches.[1]

In the ECG, AV conduction defect is common. Nineteen (32 percent) of the 60 patients reported by Friedberg and Nadas had some degree of AV block, 7 patients (12%) having complete AV block[20] (Fig. 14–25). The AV block may not be present at the first examination but may develop later in life. The excessive length of the abnormally located AV bundle and its subjection to considerable excursions during closure of the right-sided mitral valve have been proposed as the causes of fibrosis found at autopsy and AV conduction defect seen in these patients.[1]

The inversion of the bundle branches in L-transposition is accompanied by a reversal of the normal direction of the ventricular septal activation. The septal depolarization proceeds from right to left instead of left to right. The initial QRS forces are therefore directed leftward. They may be oriented posteriorly or anteriorly and superiorly or inferiorly. Q waves are present in lead V_1 and are absent in leads V_5 and V_6 in most patients.[44] The inferior leads may display abnormal Q waves that mimic inferior myocardial infarction. Figure 14–25 illustrates most of the ECG findings described here.

REFERENCES

1. Anderson RH, Becker AE, Arnold R, et al: The conducting tissues in congenitally corrected transposition. Circulation 50:911, 1974
2. Bender SR, Dreifus LS, Downing D: Anatomic and electrocardiographic correlation in Fallot's tetralogy. Am J Cardiol 7:475, 1961
3. Bentivoglio LG, Maranhao V, Downing DF: The electrocardiogram in pulmonary stenosis with intact septa. Am Heart J 59:347, 1960
4. Bialostozky D, Medrano GA, Munoz L, et al: Vectorcardiographic study and anatomic observations in 21 cases of Ebstein's malformation of the tricuspid valve. Am J Cardiol 30:354, 1972
5. Bialostozky D, Horwitz S, Espino-Vela J: Ebstein's

malformation of the tricuspid valve. Am J Cardiol 29:826, 1972

6. Burch GE, DePasquale NP: Electrocardiography in the Diagnosis of Congenital Heart Disease. Philadelphia, Lea & Febiger, 1967

7. Burch GE, DePasquale NP: Electrocardiogram and spatial vectorcardiogram of localized myocardial hypertrophy. Circulation 26:544, 1962

8. Burch GE, DePasquale N: The electrocardiogram, spatial vectorcardiogram, and ventricular gradient in congenital ventricular septal defect. Am Heart J 60:195, 1960

9. Burch GE, DePasquale N: The electrocardiogram and ventricular gradient in atrial septal defect. Am Heart J 58:190, 1959

10. Burch GE, DePasquale NP, Phillips JH: Tetralogy of Fallot associated with well developed left ventricular muscle mass and increased life span. Am J Med 36:54, 1964

11. Cayler GG, Ongley P, Nadas AS: Relation of systolic pressure in the right ventricle to the electrocardiogram. N Engl J Med 258:979, 1958

12. Char F, Adams P, Anderson RC: Electrocardiographic findings in one hundred verified cases of ventricular septal defect. Am J Dis Child 97:48, 1959

13. Chou TC, Helm RA, Kaplan S: Clinical Vectorcardiography, ed 2. New York, Grune & Stratton, 1974, p 346

14. Cosh JA: Patent ductus arteriosus: A follow-up study of 73 cases. Br Heart J 19:13, 1957

15. DePasquale NP, Burch GE: The electrocardiogram, vectorcardiogram, and ventricular gradient in the tetralogy of Fallot. Circulation 24:94, 1961

16. Downing JW, Kaplan S, Bove KE: Postsurgical left anterior hemiblock and right bundle branch block. Br Heart J 34:263, 1972

17. Durrer D, Roos JP, van Dam RTH: The genesis of the electrocardiogram of patients with ostium primum defects (ventral atrial septal defects). Am Heart J 71:642, 1966

18. DuShane JW, Weidman WH, Brandenburg RO, et al: The electrocardiogram in children with ventricular septal defect and severe pulmonary hypertension: Correlation with response to pulmonary arterial pressure to surgical repair. Circulation 22:49, 1960

19. Feldt RH, DuShane JW, Titus JL: The atrioventricular conduction system in persistent common atrioventricular canal defect: Correlations with electrocardiogram. Circulation 42:437, 1970

20. Friedberg DZ, Nadas AS: Clinical profile of patients with congenital corrected transposition of the great arteries. N Engl J Med 282:1053, 1970

21. Gamboa R, Hugenholtz G, Nadas AS: Corrected (Frank), uncorrected (Cube), and standard electrocardiographic lead systems in recording augmented right ventricular forces in right ventricular hypertension. Br Heart J 28:62, 1966

22. Gault JH, Morrow AG, Gay WA, et al: Atrial septal defect in patients over the age of forty years: Clinical and hemodynamic studies and effect of operation. Circulation 37:261, 1968

23. Gaum WE, Chou TC, Kaplan S: The vectorcardiogram and electrocardiogram in supravalvular aortic stenosis and coarctation of the aorta. Am Heart J 84:620, 1972

24. Genton E, Blount SG: The spectrum of Ebstein's anomaly. Am Heart J 73:395, 1967

25. Higgins CB, Mulder DG: Tetralogy of Fallot. Am J Cardiol 29:837, 1972

26. Hubbard TF, Angle WD: The electrocardiogram in ventricular septal defect: A correlative study of 50 cases. Am J Dis Child 94:20, 1957

27. Katz LN, Wachtel H: The diphasic QRS type of electrocardiogram in congenital heart disease. Am Heart J 13:202, 1937

28. Krongrad E, Hefler SE, Bowman FO, et al: Further observations on the etiology of the right bundle branch block pattern following right ventriculotomy. Circulation 50:1105, 1974

29. Kulbertus HE, Coyne JJ, Hallidie-Smith KA: Electrocardiographic correlation of anatomical and haemodynamic data in ostium primum atrial septal defects. Br Heart J 30:464, 1968

30. Landtman B: Postoperative changes in the electrocardiogram in congenital heart disease. II. Coarctation of the aorta and patent ductus arteriosus. Circulation 10:871, 1954

31. Lee YC, Scherlis L: Atrial septal defect. Electrocardiographic, vectorcardiographic and catheterization data. Circulation 25:1024, 1962

32. Lowe KG, Emslie-Smith D, Robertson PGC, et al: Scalar, vector, and intracardiac electrocardiogram in Ebstein's anomaly. Br Heart J 30:617, 1968

33. Mirowski M, Arevalo F, Medrano GA, et al: Conduction disturbances in patent ductus arteriosus: A study of 200 cases before and after surgery with determination of P-R index. Circulation 25:807, 1962

34. Neill CA, Mirowski M: Dextrocardia. In Cassels DE, Ziegler RF (ed): Electrocardiography in Infants and Children. New York, Grune & Stratton, 1966, p 324

35. Neufeld HN, Titus JL, DuShane JW, et al: Isolated ventricular septal defect of the persistent common atrioventricular canal type. Circulation 23:685, 1961

36. Okoroma EO, Guller B, Maloney JD, et al: Etiology of right bundle branch block pattern after surgical closure of ventricular septal defects. Am Heart J 90:14, 1975

37. Papadopoulos C, Lee YC, Scherlis L: Isolated ventricular septal defect: Electrocardiographic, vectorcardiographic and catheterization data. Am J Cardiol 16:359, 1965

38. Pileggi F, Bocanergra J, Tranchesi J, et al: The electrocardiogram in tetralogy of Fallot: A study of 142 cases. Am Heart J 59:667, 1960

39. Popper RW, Knott JMS, Selzer A, et al: Arrhythmias after cardiac surgery. I. Uncomplicated atrial septal defect. Am Heart J 64:455, 1962

40. Pryor R, Woodwork MB, Blount SG: Electrocardiographic changes in atrial septal defects: Ostium secundum defect versus ostium primum (endocardial cushion) defect. Am Heart J 58:689, 1959

41. Sanchez-Cascos A, Deuchar D: The P wave in atrial septal defect. Br Heart J 25:202, 1963

42. Scherlis L, Koenker RJ, Lee Y: Pulmonary stenosis: Electrocardiographic, vectorcardiographic and catheterization data. Circulation 28:288, 1963

43. Schiebler GL, Adams P, Anderson RC, et al: Clinical study of 23 cases of Ebstein's anomaly of the tricuspid valve. Circulation 19:165, 1959

44. Shem-Tov A, Deutsch V, Yahini JH, et al: Corrected transposition of the great arteries. Am J Cardiol 27:99, 1971

45. Scott RC: The electrocardiogram in ventricular septal defect. Am Heart J 62:842, 1961

46. Sodi-Pallares D: New Bases of Electrocardiography. St Louis, CV Mosby, 1956, p 270

47. Sodi-Pallares D, Marsico F: The importance of electrocardiographic patterns in congenital heart disease. Am Heart J 49:202, 1955

48. Sokolow M, Edgar AL: A study of the V leads in congenital heart disease. Am Heart J 40:232, 1950

49. Tan KT, Takao A, Hashimoto A, et al: Electrocardiogram of secundum type atrial septal defect simulating endocardial cushion defect. Br Heart J 37:209, 1975

50. Tikoff G, Schmidt AM, Hecht HH: Atrial fibrillation in atrial septal defect. Arch Intern Med 121:402, 1968

51. Toscano-Barboza E, DuShane JW: Ventricular septal defect: Correlation of electrocardiographic and hemodynamic findings in 60 proved cases. Am J Cardiol 3:721, 1959

52. Toscano-Barboza E, Brandenburg RO, Swan HJC: Atrial septal defect: The electrocardiogram and its hemodynamic correlation in 100 proved cases. Am J Cardiol 2:698, 1958

53. Vacca JB, Bussmann DW, Mudd JG: Ebstein's anomaly: Complete review of 108 cases. Am J Cardiol 2:210, 1958

54. Vince DJ, Keith JD: The electrocardiogram in ventricular septal defect. Circulation 23:225, 1961

55. Watson H: Electrode catheters and the diagnosis of Ebstein's anomaly of the tricuspid valve. Br Heart J 28:161, 1966

56. Witham AC, McDaniel JS: Electrocardiogram, vectorcardiogram and hemodynamics in ventricular septal defect. Am Heart J 79:335, 1970

57. Wolf PS, Vogel JHK, Pryor R, et al: Atrial septal defect in patients over 45 years of age. Br Heart J 30:115, 1968

58. Wood P: Disease of the Heart and Circulation, ed 3. Philadephia, JB Lippincott, 1968, p 379

59. Yahini JH, Dulfano MJ, Toor M: Pulmonic stenosis: A clinical assessment of severity. Am J Cardiol 5:744, 1960

60. Ziegler RF, Lam CR: Indications for the surgical correction of coarctation of the aorta in infancy. Am J Cardiol 12:60, 1963

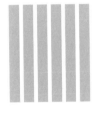

THE CARDIAC ARRHYTHMIAS

Sinus Rhythms

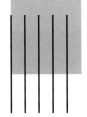

15

NORMAL SINUS RHYTHM

The sinoatrial (SA) node is an elongated comma-shaped structure measuring about 5 × 15 × 1 mm that is located at the junction of the superior vena cava and right atrium. Its arterial blood supply comes from a proximal branch of either the right or the left circumflex coronary artery. The SA node is richly innervated by both the vagal and sympathetic nerves. Its pacemaker cells are called the P cells. The sinus node electrogram recorded with transvenous electrodes shows two low-frequency, low-amplitude deflections that precede the P wave of the electrocardiogram (ECG).[22,27,42]

A normal sinus rhythm in an adult has a rate, by arbitrary definition, of between 60 and 100 beats/min. Considerably faster rates are seen in infants and young children, and slower rates are seen in many healthy adults. The P wave during sinus rhythm has an axis in the frontal plane, in the absence of atrial abnormalities, between +15° and +75°. An axis to the left of 0°, or to the right of +90°, is usually indicative of an ectopic atrial pacemaker. Therefore, during sinus rhythm, the P wave is always upright in leads I, II, and aVF and inverted in lead aVR. It is variable in leads III and aVL. In the precordial leads, the leftward orientation of the P axis results in an upright P wave in leads V_3 through V_6. The P wave in lead V_1 and, less commonly, V_2 is more variable in polarity. It may be upright, inverted, or biphasic. In sinus rhythm, the morphology of the P wave in the same lead usually remains the same from beat to beat. Minor changes related to the respiratory cycles may be seen, especially in leads III and aVF. The changes may be more pronounced if there is wandering of the pacemaker within the sinus node. Although normal sinus rhythm is a regular rhythm, minor variation of the PP interval exists in most patients. The differences between the longest and shortest intervals, however,

usually do not exceed 0.16 second except with sinus arrhythmia.

A sinus rhythm may be accompanied by atrioventricular (AV) conduction defect or ectopic impulse formation at the AV junction or the ventricle. Although by tradition such a rhythm is no longer called normal sinus rhythm, the sinus impulse formation per se may remain normal.

SINUS ARRHYTHMIAS

In sinus arrhythmia, the P-wave morphology is normal but the PP interval varies by more than 0.16 second. There are two types of sinus arrhythmia. The more common type is respiratory sinus arrhythmia in which the variation in heart rate is related to the respiratory cycle (Fig. 15–1). The sinus rate increases gradually during inspiration and decreases with expiration. The changes in vagal tone, as a result of reflex mechanisms arising from the pulmonary and systemic vascular systems during respiration, are probably responsible for the variation. The less common nonrespiratory form is unrelated to the phase of respiration. In many instances, the mechanism is unknown. Others appear to be associated with the administration of drugs, such as digitalis and morphine. This phenomenon is observed more often in patients who have diseased hearts.

Wandering of the pacemaker in the sinus node may be responsible for some cases of sinus arrhythmia (see Fig. 15–1). This is discussed in a later section of this chapter.

Sinus arrhythmia is seen more commonly when the sinus rate is slow. The rhythm tends to become regular when the rate is increased with exercise or atropine, a phenomenon that supports the diagnosis. It often is simulated by premature atrial beats, SA block, or sinus pauses. Its differentiation from the latter is sometimes difficult.

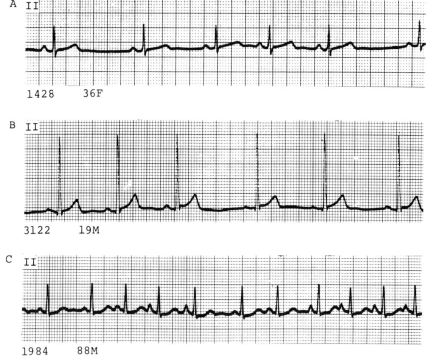

FIGURE 15–1. (A) Respiratory sinus arrhythmia. (B and C) Sinus arrhythmia with wandering pacemaker. In both cases, the amplitude of the P waves decreases as the rate is slower.

Clinical Significance

In most cases, sinus arrhythmia is a normal phenomenon, especially if it is related to the respiratory cycle. The arrhythmia is usually marked in infants and children and tends to decrease with age. The phenomenon is seen when there is an increase in vagal tone, such as during the administration of parasympathomimetic drugs, morphine, digitalis, and carotid sinus massage. Nonrespiratory sinus arrhythmia is more likely to be seen in older individuals and in those with heart disease. It is common after acute inferior myocardial infarction or during convalescence from an acute illness. It also is seen when there is an increase in the intracranial pressure.

Ventriculophasic Sinus Arrhythmia

Ventriculophasic sinus arrhythmia is seen in patients with partial or complete AV block. The PP interval that contains a QRS complex is shorter than the PP interval without it (Fig. 15–2). This phenomenon was reported in about 30 to 40 percent of cases of complete AV block and less often in second-degree AV block.[39,45,47] Various mechanisms have been proposed to explain this phenomenon, including the following:

1. Excitation of the Bainbridge reflex because of the slight increase in intraatrial pressure during ventricular systole. The resulting vagal inhibition accelerates the SA node.

2. An improved blood supply to the SA node after the ventricular systole, which results in a faster discharge rate from the SA node.

3. Traction on the atria by ventricular systole, which stimulates the SA node mechanically and increases its discharge rate.

Although ventriculophasic sinus arrhythmia is an interesting ECG finding, it is clinically insignificant.

Wandering of the Pacemaker Within the Sinus Node

The sinus pacemaker may shift location within the SA node from beat to beat.[6,24] As a result, there is a continual change in the amplitude and morphology of the P wave and sometimes in the duration of the PR interval. Atrial epicardial mapping during cardiac surgery has demonstrated that the pacemaker impulse may be initiated in the right atrium outside of the sinus node in some patients with

III

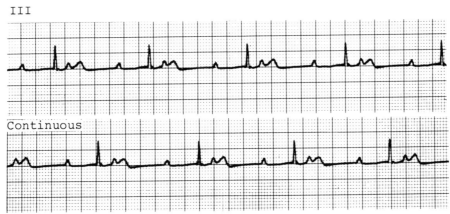

FIGURE 15–2. Ventriculophasic sinus arrhythmia. The patient is a 36-year-old man who has no symptoms. The rhythm strip shows a second-degree AV block with 2:1 conduction. The PP intervals that contain the QRS complexes are shorter than those without the QRS complexes. No other evidence of heart disease was found.

what appears to be sinus rhythm.[6] Shifting of the pacemaker from the sinus node to the right atrium also may be responsible for the P-wave changes. The term *wandering atrial pacemaker* often is used interchangeably with, or to include, wandering of the pacemaker within the sinus node. In view of the findings from the electrophysiologic studies, it is apparent that it is difficult to determine the precise location of the pacemaker from the body surface ECG.

With rare exceptions, wandering of the pacemaker in the SA node is seen only in patients with sinus arrhythmia. During faster rates, the P waves in the inferior leads are taller and the PR interval longer because the pacemaker is higher in location. The P waves in the inferior leads decrease in amplitude and the PR interval becomes shorter during slower rates as the pacemaker is shifted toward the tail of the SA node and is closer to the AV node. As long as the pacemaker is confined within the SA node, the P waves remain upright in leads I and II. This relationship between the location of the pacemaker and the morphology of the P waves is documented by

electrophysiologic studies during which the sinus node electrograms were correlated with the body surface ECGs.[6,24]

Wandering of the pacemaker may be simulated by respiratory variation of the P wave. In the latter case, the PR interval remains constant, and there is associated respiratory change of the QRS complex. The respiratory variation usually is limited to leads III and aVF.

The clinical significance of wandering pacemaker is the same as that of sinus arrhythmia.

SINUS BRADYCARDIA

By definition, sinus bradycardia indicates a sinus rate of less than 60 beats/min. A rate as slow as 35 beats/min or less may be seen, but the rate is usually above 40 beats/min in healthy individuals, especially during the waking hours. In the ECG, the P wave has a normal axis and the PR interval is at least 0.12 second. Sinus arrhythmia often coexists. If the sinus rate is less than 40 beats/min, the possibility of 2:1 SA block should be considered.

Sinus bradycardia is usually not considered

II

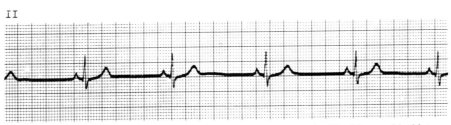

FIGURE 15–3. Sinus bradycardia with a rate of 45 beats/min in a healthy 30-year-old athlete.

clinically significant unless the rate is 50 beats/min or less. Such a rate, however, is frequently seen in healthy adults, especially athletes (Fig. 15–3). It occurs commonly during sleep when the rate may be in the mid-30s. Many elderly individuals have sinus bradycardia without apparent cause[2] (Fig. 15–4). Increased vagal tone is often responsible for the slowing of the sinus rate. Transient sinus bradycardia occurs with Valsalva maneuver, carotid sinus massage, or vomiting. Increased intracranial pressure may be accompanied by significant bradycardia. Commonly used drugs that cause sinus bradycardia include beta-adrenergic blocking agents, some calcium channel blocking agents such as verapamil and diltiazem, clonidine, digitalis, and occasionally quinidine, procainamide, and disopyramide. Electrolyte imbalance such as hyperkalemia may depress SA nodal function. Hypothyroidism and hypothermia are the well-known metabolic disorders associated with sinus bradycardia. Patients with Cheyne-Stokes respiration may have marked sinus bradycardia during the apneic phase[34] (Fig. 15–5).

Among organic heart diseases, sinus bradycardia is seen in 11 to 14 percent of patients with acute myocardial infarction.[36] Its incidence in the early phase of myocardial infarction is even higher, especially in inferior infarction.[1] It also is encountered in chronic coronary artery disease, myocarditis, and primary and secondary cardiomyopathy. In some elderly patients, symptomatic sinus bradycardia may occasionally result from idiopathic degeneration of the SA node.

SINUS TACHYCARDIA

In adults, when the rate of sinus impulse formation is greater than 100 beats/min, the rhythm is called *sinus tachycardia*. In most clinical conditions, the rate is between 101 and 160 beats/min, but a rate near 200 beats/min may be obtained during maximum exercise in young adults. The maximum sinus rate is slower in older individuals.

In the ECG, in addition to the increased heart rate, the P waves may increase in amplitude (Fig. 15–6). The PR interval usually is shortened but occasionally may be unchanged or lengthened. A junctional type of ST-segment depression may occur, part of which is the result of a larger atrial T wave. A previously upright T wave may become flattened or even inverted. Occasionally, the T wave increases in amplitude. An inconspicuous U wave may become prominent.[3] The QT interval is shortened. Most of the decrease of the RR interval, however, is at the expense of the TP segment. As the rate increases, the P wave may be superimposed on the preceding T wave, and it then becomes difficult to identify.

When the rate in sinus tachycardia is above 140 beats/min, it is often difficult to differentiate from paroxysmal supraventricular (atrial, junctional, or AV reentrant) tachycardia and atrial flutter with 2:1 conduction. In sinus tachycardia, the P waves are more likely to be better defined, whereas in paroxysmal atrial tachycardia, they are generally smaller and abnormal in configuration. In AV junctional tachycardia, either reentrant or auto-

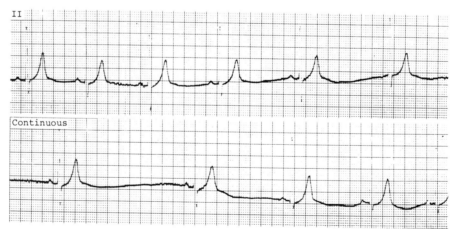

FIGURE 15–4. Symptomatic sinus bradycardia. The patient is a 75-year-old man with dizziness. The tracing was recorded during a dizzy spell. Considerable variation in heart rate is seen. The last complex in the upper strip is probably an ectopic atrial escape beat. Although sinus arrest or SA block cannot be excluded during the long pause in the bottom strip, sinus bradycardia is more likely because of the gradual change. The cause of the sinus bradycardia was unknown.

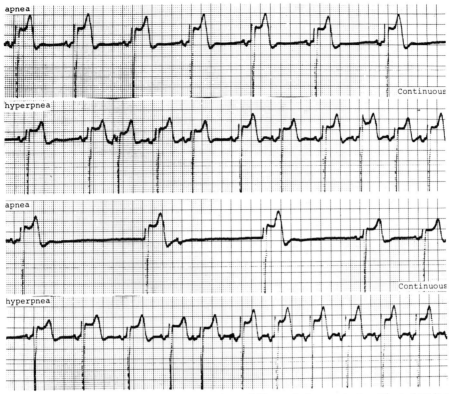

FIGURE 15–5. Bradycardia during the apneic phase of Cheyne-Stokes respiration. The patient is a 64-year-old man with chronic renal failure. Sinus bradycardia is present during apnea (first strip). In the third strip, there is sinus arrest or SA block with junctional escape beats.

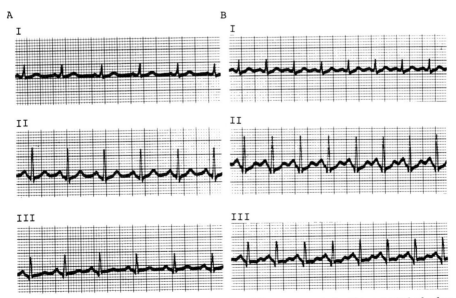

FIGURE 15–6. Sinus tachycardia. Both tracings A and B were recorded within a period of a few minutes from a 19-year-old man with considerable anxiety but no evidence of organic heart disease. (A) The rate is 108 beats/min; (B) the rate is 148 beats/min. There is a slight increase in the amplitude of the P waves when the heart rate is more rapid. There is also junctional ST-segment depression in tracing B. The T waves in lead III are biphasic during the more rapid rate.

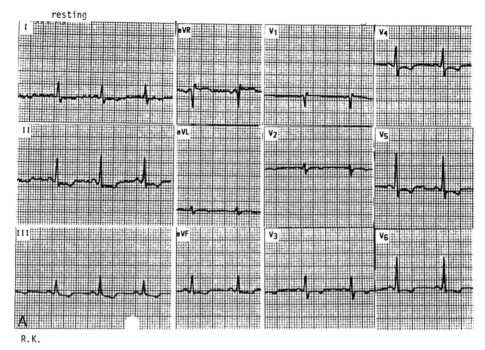

R.K.

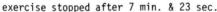

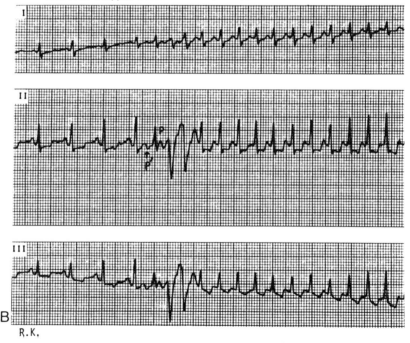

B

R.K.

FIGURE 15–7. Sinus node reentrant tachycardia. The patient is a 62-year-old woman with abnormal ST and T waves in her resting ECG (A). An exercise radionuclide venticulogram was performed. The patient developed sinus node reentrant tachycardia immediately after the exercise was stopped. (B) Tracing showing the initiation of the tachycardia by a premature atrial beat (P'). The three wide QRS complexes are due to aberrant ventricular conduction. The heart rate is 210 beats/min in the beginning of the tachycardia and gradually decreases to 134 beats/min 3 minutes after the exercise when the tachycardia terminates suddenly.

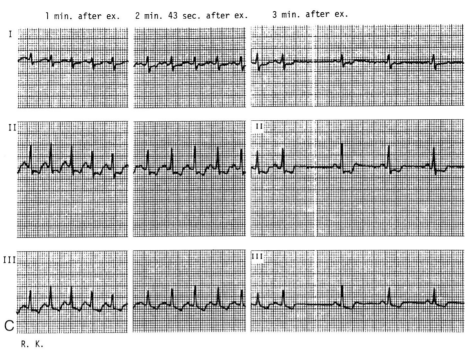

1 min. after ex.   2 min. 43 sec. after ex.   3 min. after ex.

C

R. K.

FIGURE 15–7. *Continued* (C). The appearance of the P waves in the three simultaneously recorded leads during the tachycardia is identical to that during normal sinus rhythm. The radionuclide ventriculogram revealed hypokinesis of the posterobasal wall of the left ventricle. The left ventricular ejection fraction was normal, however.

matic, the retrograde P waves are masked or closely follow the QRS complexes. In AV reentrant tachycardia using a bypass tract, the retrograde P waves are more clearly separated from the preceding QRS complexes. The heart rate in sinus tachycardia may change from time to time, but that of the paroxysmal supraventricular tachycardia and atrial flutter tend to be constant. With carotid sinus massage, there is a gradual slowing of the rate in sinus tachycardia during the procedure, and the rate returns to its previous level after it is discontinued. The maneuver, as a rule, either has no effect on paroxysmal supraventricular tachycardia or converts it to normal sinus rhythm. It may temporarily increase the AV block in atrial flutter and reveal the flutter waves. The differentiation of the various types of supraventricular tachycardia is discussed in further details in Chapters 16 and 17.

Sinus tachycardia may occur under a variety of circumstances. In healthy individuals, it may be induced by exercise and anxiety. Alcohol- or caffeine-containing beverages and drugs such as epinephrine and atropine are often the causes of sinus tachycardia. Among disease states, the common origins include fever, hypotension, hypoxia, congestive heart failure, high-output states such as anemia, hyperthyroidism, AV fistula, pheochromocy-

toma, and myocarditis. It is seen in about one third of patients with acute myocardial infarction.[13,31]

SINUS NODE REENTRANT TACHYCARDIA

Sinus node reentrant tachycardia is one of the uncommon types of paroxysmal supraventricular tachycardia.[22,28,53] There is a reentrant circuit that involves only the sinus node and perhaps some of the perinodal tissues. Because atrial depolarization is still initiated by impulses from the sinus node, the sequence of atrial activation remains normal. The morphology of the P waves is therefore identical to that of the common form of sinus tachycardia. The reentrant tachycardia, however, has sudden onset and termination. It often is initiated by a premature atrial beat and may be terminated by vagal maneuvers. Its rate varies from 100 to 160 beats/min with an average of 130 beats/min. It usually occurs in patients with organic heart disease. Figure 15–7 is an example of this tachycardia that developed during exercise.

SINUS PAUSE, SINUS ARREST

Sinus pause is the result of transient failure of impulse formation at the SA node. When the

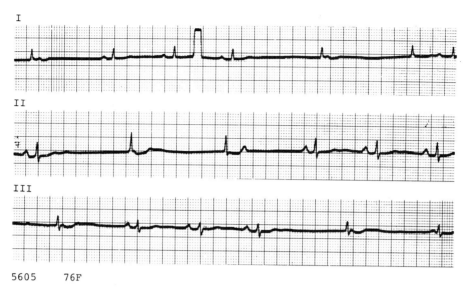

I

II

III

5605   76F

FIGURE 15–8. Sinus pauses. The tracing was recorded from a 76-year-old woman with coronary artery disease and near syncope. She was receiving digitoxin at the time, and the blood level was 24 mg/L (usual therapeutic range is 15 to 25 mg/L). Periods of sinus pauses with junctional escape beats are present in all three leads. Although the possibility of marked sinus bradycardia cannot be excluded, sinus pauses are more likely because of the sudden change in the PP interval. The possibility of digitalis toxicity is considered. The patient did not have any symptoms during the recording of this tracing.

sinus node inactivity is prolonged, the condition is called *sinus arrest*. There is no precise definition to separate these two entities. In either case, there is no P wave for the duration of the pause or arrest (Figs. 15–8 and 15–9).

Sinus pause should be differentiated from (1) SA block, (2) marked sinus arrhythmia, and (3) blocked premature atrial beats. In SA block, the long cycle is a multiple of the basic PP interval, but no such relationship is demonstrable in sinus pause. In sinus arrhythmia, the lengthening of the PP interval is usually gradual and phasic. With blocked premature atrial beats, an ectopic P wave often can be detected, distorting the preced-

ing T wave or the baseline, but this is not always the case. The premature P wave may be small in certain leads and is not recognized.

Depending on the duration of sinus inactivity, the pause may be terminated by a sinus beat or AV junctional or ventricular escape beat. If the sinus arrest is prolonged, a slow AV junctional or an idioventricular rhythm may be the presenting rhythm. Under such circumstances, it is impossible to determine whether the underlying mechanism is sinus arrest of SA block. When the ventricular rhythm is regular and the P wave is absent, the possibility of sinoventricular conduction should also be con-

Monitor lead

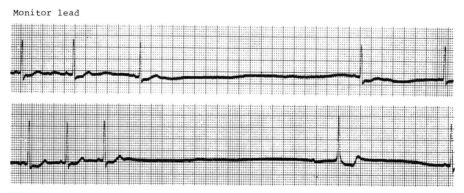

FIGURE 15–9. Sinus arrest. The patient is a 67-year-old man with recurrent syncope. The ECG shows prolonged periods of sinus arrest, but SA block cannot be excluded. In the bottom strip, evidence of AV block also is present.

sidered. In the latter case, impulse originated from the sinus node is transmitted to the AV junction through the internodal tracts while the atrial myocardium fails to depolarize.

Sinus pauses may occasionally be seen in normal individuals with increased vagal tone or a hypersensitive carotid sinus.[20] Sinus pauses or arrest may be caused by digitalis, quinidine, and other antiarrhythmic agents or antihypertensive drugs, especially when large dosage of these drugs is used. Various types of heart disease may be accompanied by sinus pauses or arrest. In patients with acute myo-

cardial infarction, sinus pauses or arrest usually are seen in those with infarction of the inferior wall. Further discussion of the various causes of sinus pause or arrest is presented later in this chapter in the section on sick sinus syndrome.

SINOATRIAL BLOCK (SA BLOCK)

In SA block, there is an interference of the transmission of the sinus impulse to the atrium. The SA conduction is either delayed or blocked. In first-degree SA block, the conduc-

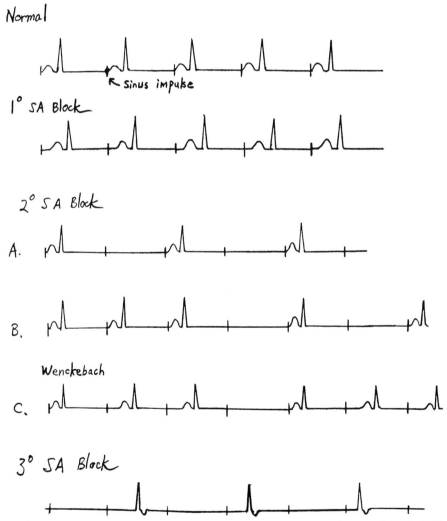

FIGURE 15–10. Diagram comparing normal sinus rhythm with various degrees of SA block. The sinus impulses that are not seen in the body surface ECG are represented by the vertical lines. In first-degree SA block, although there is a prolongation of the interval between the sinus impulse and the P wave, such a delay cannot be detected in the ECG. The diagnosis of second-degree SA block depends on the presence of pause or pauses that are the multiple of the basic PP interval (B). Persistent 2:1 SA block cannot be separated from marked sinus bradycardia (A). When there is a Wenckebach phenomenon, there is a gradual shortening of the PP interval before the pause (C). In third-degree SA block, the ECG records only the escape rhythm.

tion time is prolonged, but there is a 1:1 response. In second or partial SA block, some of the sinus impulses fail to capture the atria. In complete or third-degree SA block, there is a complete failure of SA conduction. Because SA electrograms are not available in most clinical settings, the existence of SA conduction defect can only be inferred indirectly from the P-wave activities. Figure 15–10 illustrates diagrammatically the assumed mechanism in the various types of SA block. In first-degree SA block, because the prolonged conduction time cannot be demonstrated by the body surface ECG, the conduction defect cannot be recognized. In the third-degree SA block, the survival of the patient depends on a subsidiary pacemaker, which is usually at the AV junction. This SA conduction abnormality cannot be differentiated from complete sinus arrest, since normal sinus P waves are not recorded in either case. It is only in second-degree SA block that the diagnosis can be made from the body surface ECG.

Electrocardiographic Findings

The ECG diagnosis of second-degree SA block is based on the presence of long cycle between the P waves, which is the multiple of the basic PP interval (Fig. 15–11). The duration of the long cycle may be the equivalent of two, three, or more beats. The long cycle

frequently has a duration of less than the exact multiple of the basic PP interval. This is especially true in patients who have sinus arrhythmia. The precise limit of the differences is difficult to define, but the interval of 0.10 second was suggested by one author.[41] In some cases, the Wenckebach phenomenon is observed, which was reported to occur in 17 percent of 219 examples of SA block reviewed by Greenwood and Finkelstein.[25] This phenomenon is similar to that of AV Wenckebach phenomenon, but there is progressive shortening of the PP interval instead of RR interval until the pause appears (Fig. 15–12).

Sinoatrial block is often intermittent. The patient may have normal sinus rhythm for days or weeks between episodes of SA block. The pause that results from SA block may be terminated by AV junctional escape beats. In many cases, the rather long duration of the pauses before the escape beats suggests a coexisting defect in the automaticity of the subsidiary pacemaker.[14] Occasionally, the escape beats may be atrial or ventricular in origin.

Patients with SA block often have additional rhythm disturbances. Supraventricular tachycardia, including paroxysmal atrial fibrillation, flutter, or atrial tachycardia is present in almost two thirds of these patients.[41,46] Such a combination is called the *bradycardia-tachycardia syndrome* and is discussed later in this chapter in the section on the sick sinus

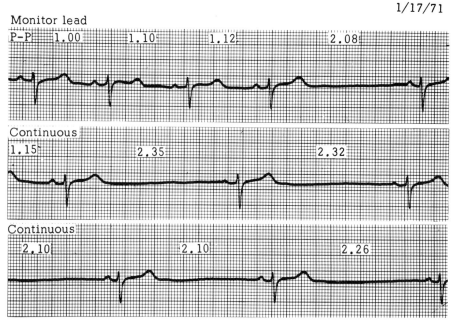

FIGURE 15–11. Second-degree SA block in an 84-year-old man with a history of syncope. The cause of the SA block in unknown. In the ECG, the long cycles have about twice the duration of the basic PP interval.

MCL$_1$

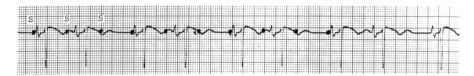

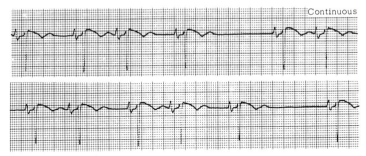

Continuous

FIGURE 15–12. Probable second-degree SA block with Wenckebach phenomenon. In the top strip, the hypothetical sinus impulses are represented by dots and labeled S. There is group beating. Using the hypothetical sinus rate, SA Wenckebach phenomenon can be demonstrated. Using the same method and the same sinus rate, the variation in the PP interval in the second and third strips also can be explained.

syndrome. Other associated arrhythmias include sinus bradycardia and AV block.

Sinoatrial block may be simulated by marked sinus bradycardia, sinus arrhythmia, and sinus pause or arrest. It is often impossible to separate SA block with 2:1 conduction from sinus bradycardia unless a period of 1:1 conduction and doubled atrial rate is recorded. SA block with the Wenckebach phenomenon may mimic marked sinus arrhythmia. The pause in SA block is longer, however, and occurs more suddenly. In sinus pause or arrest, the long cycle is usually not the multiple of the basic PP interval. If the long cycle is nearly the multiple of the basic PP interval, the separation of the two is impossible. As stated, prolonged sinus arrest and third-degree SA block cannot be differentiated.

Clinical Significance

Transient SA block is most commonly the result of digitalis toxicity (Fig. 15–13). It also may be caused by many of the other antiarrhythmic agents. It is seen in patients with acute myocardial infarction and acute myocarditis. It occasionally appears in an otherwise healthy individual, apparently as a result of increased vagal tone, since it has been observed during carotid sinus stimulation.[26]

In patients with chronic SA block, the cause often is obscured[41] (see Fig. 15–11). It is most commonly seen in elderly subjects. Id-

iopathic degeneration of the SA node may be the underlying mechanism. Chronic coronary artery disease and primary or secondary cardiomyopathy are additional common causes.

SICK SINUS SYNDROME

The sick sinus syndrome is caused by dysfunction of the sinus node in its impulse formation or its ability to transmit its impulse to the atrium.[5,14,18,30] It is usually manifested as bradycardia but often is associated with recurrent episodes of supraventricular tachycardia. In the latter case it is called *bradycardia–tachycardia syndrome*.[50]

In the ECG, the sick sinus syndrome may present itself as any of the following:

1. Severe sinus bradycardia
2. Sinus arrest
3. SA block
4. Bradycardia alternating with tachycardia
5. Chronic atrial fibrillation with failure of resumption of sinus rhythm after cardioversion
6. AV junctional escape rhythm

Many patients with the syndrome have more than one of the above mechanisms. In the series of 56 cases reported by Rubenstein and colleagues, sinus bradycardia with a heart rate of less than 50 beats/min was seen in 39 percent, sinus arrest or SA block in 60 percent, and bradycardia-tachycardia in 60 percent.[46]

310 THE CARDIAC ARRHYTHMIAS

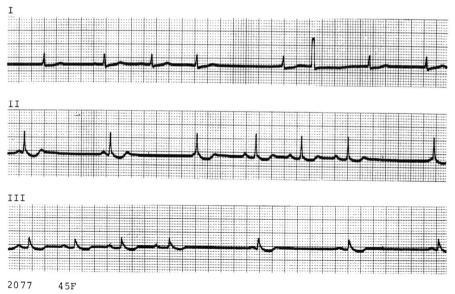

2077   45F

FIGURE 15–13. Second-degree SA block due to digitalis. The patient was a 45-year-old woman with coronary artery disease. The digoxin blood level was 2.8 ng/ml. In the ECG, there is intermittent SA block with 2:1 conduction. Junctional escape beats are present, with the QRS complex either superimposed on the P wave or following the P wave with short PR interval.

In the 46 patients with sinus bradycardia described by Eraut and Shaw, 35 percent also had sinus arrest or SA block and 76 percent had tachyarrhythmias.[16] On the other hand, all of these manifestations may be intermittent. The patient may have normal sinus rhythm for a long period between episodes of bradycardia (Fig. 15–14). Many patients with sick sinus syndrome have additional conduction defects, including AV block, intraventricular conduction defect, and bundle branch block. The reported incidence of such conduction defects is 50 percent or more.[37,46]

Detection of Sinus Node Dysfunction

Long-term ambulatory ECG monitoring is one of the most useful tools for evaluating patients suspected of having the sick sinus syndrome when the routine ECG fails to reveal diagnostic abnormalities. Sinus pauses longer than 2 seconds on the ambulatory ECG are generally considered to be abnormal and suggestive of sinus node dysfunction.[8,35,48] A definitive diagnosis can be made if the rhythm disturbances are observed during the time of the symptom.

Certain pharmacologic and electrophysiologic tests are used for the detection of sinus node dysfunction.[10] These include the administration of intravenous atropine,[32,44] the determination of sinus node recovery time (SNRT),[33,38] and SA conduction time

(SACT).[42,51,52] In the atropine test, the failure of the sinus rate to increase to a certain level after intravenous administration of atropine is considered an indirect sign of sinus node dysfunction. Rosen and co-workers suggested that the use of 1 mg atropine and an increase of heart rate to less than 90 beats/min was abnormal.[44] The SNRT or corrected SNRT is measured by using atrial stimulation. Normally, when the atrium is paced at a rapid rate (usually between 90 and 150 beats/min) and the pacing is abruptly stopped, there is a temporary pause before a sinus beat reappears as a result of overdrive suppression of the SA node pacemaker. In patients with SA node dysfunction, the pause is abnormally prolonged. The SACT is either estimated by using premature atrial stimulation or determined by directly recorded sinus node electrogram.[4,42] The reader is referred to the cited references for the details of these electrophysiologic tests and the criteria of an abnormal response. The sensitivity of the SNRT or corrected SNRT in the diagnosis of sick sinus syndrome appears to be low, mostly between 35 to 66 percent, but one report gave a value of 93 percent.[21,26,33,38,44] The wide discrepancy of the results is most likely due to the difference in the patient population studied. The test was shown to be highly (96 percent) specific by some investigators, however.[38] The indirectly estimated SACT also was found to be an insensitive indicator of sinus node dysfunction,

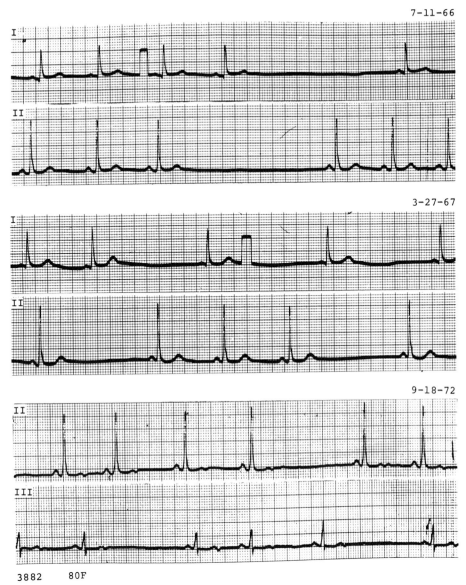

7-11-66

I

II

3-27-67

I

II

9-18-72

II

III

3882   80F

FIGURE 15–14. Intermittent second-degree SA block of many years' duration. The patient was an 80-year-old woman with heart disease of unknown cause. The diagnosis of second-degree SA block was first made in 1964. She has intermittent second-degree SA block with 4:1 or 2:1 conduction as illustrated. She remained symptom-free from the SA block in 1977.

being abnormal in only about 40 percent of patients with symptomatic sinus node dysfunction.[5,51] Crook and associates were not able to find significant difference in the conduction time between 14 patients with SA disease and 11 control subjects.[9] Data are insufficient in regard to the value of SACT measured from sinus node electrogram at this time.[4] In a consensus statement of the conference on the state of the art of electrophysiologic testing published by Rahimtoola and associates, the sensitivity of the SACT and SNRT combined in patients with symptomatic sinus

node disease was estimated to be about 68 percent and the specificity was 88 percent.[40]

Bradycardia–Tachycardia Syndrome

This particular manifestation of the sick sinus syndrome deserves special attention because of its therapeutic implication. If the patient is seen during the phase of paroxysmal tachycardia, the administration of suppressive drugs may result in worsening of the basic sinus node disease. The bradycardia–tachycardia syndrome is observed in 54 to 76 percent of patients with the sick sinus syndrome.[14,16,46] In 74 cases reviewed by Moss and Davis, sinus bradycardia was the most common type of bradyarrhythmia encountered (76 percent).[37] The tachyarrhythmias were mostly supraventricular and were paroxysmal atrial tachycardia in 40 percent, atrial flutter and atrial fibrillation in 38 percent, multiple supraventricular tachycardia in 12 percent, and ventricular tachycardia or fibrillation in 10 percent. Ventricular tachyarrhythmia was seen most often in patients with acute myocardial infarction.

In patients whose rhythm disturbance was documented during syncope, the major cause of syncope was prolonged asystole after the sudden cessation of the paroxysmal supraventricular tachycardia (Fig. 15–15). This phenomenon is a clinical manifestation of overdrive suppression of the SA node with prolonged sinus node recovery time. The mechanism was responsible for the symptom in 65 percent of 21 such patients, while bradycardia alone was responsible in 26 percent and tachycardia alone in 9 percent.[37]

Etiology of the Sick Sinus Syndrome

The causes of sick sinus syndrome may be summarized as follows[17,19,46]:

1. Idiopathic
2. Coronary artery disease
3. Idiopathic cardiomyopathy
4. Hypertensive heart disease
5. Rheumatic heart disease
6. Acute myocarditis
7. Secondary cardiomyopathies, including those resulting from connective tissue disease, metastatic tumor, amyloidosis, myxedema, hemochromatosis, Friedreich's ataxia, muscular dystrophy, scleroderma
8. Luetic aortic insufficiency
9. Mitral valve prolapse[11]
10. Congenital heart disease
11. Familial sinus node disease
12. Surgical injury to the SA node
13. Transient SA node dysfunction as a result of the administration of drugs such as beta-adrenergic blocking agents, digitalis, quinidine, calcium channel blockers such as verapamil and diltiazem, digitalis, quinidine,

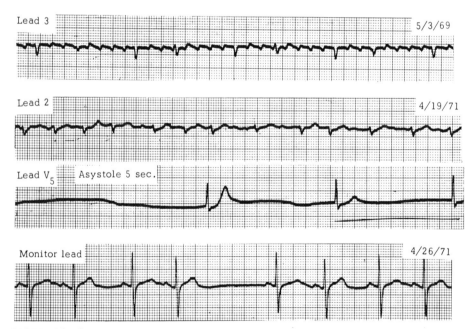

FIGURE 15–15. Bradycardia-tachycardia syndrome. The patient was a 75-year-old woman with a history of recurrent atrial flutter and atrial fibrillation, as illustrated in the top two strips of tracings, recorded in 1969 and 1971. While the ECG was being recorded on 4-19-71, she had atrial fibrillation with rapid ventricular response until lead V₅ was being recorded. She developed asystole for 5 seconds, followed by junctional escape rhythm. She complained of dizziness at that time. On 4-26-71, she had intermittent second-degree SA block. The pause was not the exact multiple of the basic PP interval because of sinus arrhythmia. The patient was not receiving digitalis at the time.

and other antiarrhythmic agents,[10] or electrolyte imbalance such as hyperkalemia.

In some reported series, patients without apparent cause constitute the largest group of cases,[19,46] while others found coronary artery disease in a larger number of patients.[14,29,37] Sinus node dysfunction occurred in about 5 percent of patients with acute myocardial infarction, but this is usually transient.[43] It is observed most often in patients with inferior infarction. Cardiomyopathies and hypertensive heart disease are the responsible causes in a significant but smaller group of cases, whereas rheumatic heart disease is only rarely associated with the sick sinus syndrome.

Anatomic Findings

Detailed pathologic studies of the SA node in patients with sick sinus syndrome have been carried out in only a limited number of cases.[29,41,46] Degenerative changes of the SA node were found. Kaplan and associates examined the entire conduction system of two patients with the bradycardia–tachycardia syndrome using serial sections.[29] Both patients had coronary atherosclerosis, and one also had atrial amyloidosis. There were degenerative changes and fibrosis of not only the SA node but also the AV junction and atria. Demoulin and Kulbertus reported the histologic findings of six cases of sick sinus syndrome. Total or subtotal destruction of the sinus node was seen in all and total or subtotal destruction of the areas of nodal atrial continuity in five of six cases.[12]

Engel and colleagues studied the angiographic findings of the sinus node artery in six patients with the sick sinus syndrome.[15] Although five of the patients had stenosis of one or more of the major coronary vessels, none of the six patients had evidence of involvement of the SA nodal artery. They concluded that the sick sinus syndrome is probably not related to coronary artery disease of the SA nodal artery. In a postmortem angiographic study of 25 patients with the sick sinus syndrome reported by Shaw and associates, reduced filling of the sinus node artery was, however, found in 5.[49]

REFERENCES

1. Adgey AAJ, Geddes JS, Webb SW, et al: Acute phase of myocardial infarction. Lancet 2:501, 1971
2. Agruss NS, Rosin EY, Adolph RJ, et al: Significance of chronic sinus bradycardia in elderly people. Circulation 46:924, 1972
3. Bellet S, Eliakim M, Deliyiannis S, et al: Radioelectrocardiographic changes during strenuous exercise in normal subjects. Circulation 25:686, 1962
4. Bethge C, Gebhardt-Seehausen U, Mullges W: The human sinus node electrogram: Techniques and clinical results of intra-atrial recordings in patients with and without sick sinus syndrome. Am Heart J 112:1074, 1986
5. Bigger JT, Reiffel JA: Sick sinus syndrome. Annu Rev Med 30:91, 1979
6. Boineau JP, Canavan TE, Schuessler RB, et al: Demonstration of a widely distributed atrial pacemaker complex in the human heart. Circulation 77:1221, 1988
7. Breithardt G, Seipel L, Loogen F: Sinus node recovery time and calculated sinoatrial conduction time in normal subjects and patients with sinus node dysfunction. Circulation 56:43, 1977
8. Brodsky M, Wu D, Denes P, et al: Arrhythmias documented by 24 hour continuous electrocardiographic monitoring in 50 male medical students without apparent heart disease. Am J Cardiol 39:390, 1977
9. Crook B, Kitson D, McComish M, et al: Indirect measurement of sinoatrial conduction time in patients with sinoatrial disease and in controls. Br Heart J 39:771, 1977
10. Crossen KJ, Cain ME: Assessment and management of sinus node dysfunction. Mod Concept Cardiovasc Dis 55:43, 1986
11. DeMaria AN, Amsterdam EA, Vismara LA, et al: Arrhythmias in the mitral valve prolapse syndrome. Ann Intern Med 84:656, 1976
12. Demoulin JC, Kulbertus HE: Histopathological correlates of sinoatrial disease. Br Heart J 40:1384, 1978
13. DeSanctis RW, Block P, Hutter AM: Tachyarrhythmias in myocardial infarction. Circulation 45:681, 1972
14. Easley RM, Goldstein S: Sino-atrial syncope. Am J Med 50:166, 1971
15. Engle TR, Meister SG, Feitosa GS, et al: Appraisal of sinus node artery disease. Circulation 52:286, 1975
16. Eraut D, Shaw DB: Sinus bradycardia. Br Heart J 33:742, 1971
17. Ferrer MI: The Sick Sinus Syndrome. Mt Kisco, NY, Futura Publishing, 1974
18. Ferrer MI: The sick sinus syndrome in atrial disease. JAMA 206:645, 1968
19. Fowler NO, Fenton JC, Conway GF: Syncope and cerebral dysfunction caused by bradycardia without atrioventricular block. Am Heart J 80:303, 1970
20. Gang ES, Oseran DS, Mandel WJ, et al: Sinus node electrogram in patients with the hypersensitive carotid sinus syndrome. J Am Coll Cardiol 5:1484, 1985
21. Gann D, Tolentino A, Samet P: Electrophysiologic evaluation of elderly patients with sinus bradycardia: A long-term follow-up study. Ann Intern Med 90:24, 1979
22. Gomes JA, Hariman RJ, Kang PS, et al: Sustained symptomatic sinus node reentrant tachycardia: Incidence, clinical significance, electrophysiologic observations and the effects of antiarrhythmic agents. J Am Coll Cardiol 5:45, 1985
23. Gomes JAC, Kang PS, El-Sherif N: The sinus node electrogram in patients with and without sick sinus syndrome: Techniques and correlation between di-

rectly measured and indirectly estimated sinoatrial conduction time. Circulation 66:864, 1982

24. Gomes JA, Winter SL: The origin of the sinus node complex in man: Demonstration of dominant and subsidiary foci. J Am Coll Cardiol 9:45, 1987
25. Greenwood RJ, Finkelstein D: Sinoatrial Heart Block. Springfield, IL, Charles C Thomas, 1964
26. Gupta PK, Lichstein E, Chadda KD, et al: Appraisal of sinus nodal recovery time in patients with sick sinus syndrome. Am J Cardiol 34:265, 1974
27. Hariman RJ, Krongrad E, Boxer R, et al: Method for recording electrical activity of the sinoatrial node and automatic atrial foci during cardiac catheterization in human subjects. Am J Cardiol 45:775, 1980
28. Josephson ME, Seides SF: Clinical Cardiac Electrophysiology. Philadelphia, Lea & Febiger, 1979
29. Kaplan BM, Langendorf R, Lev M, et al: Tachycardiabradycardia syndrome (so-called "sick sinus syndrome"). Am J Cardiol 34:365, 1974
30. Lown B: Electrical reversion of cardiac arrhythmias. Br Heart J 29:469, 1967
31. Lown B, Klein MD, Hershberg PI: Coronary and precoronary care. Am J Med 46:705, 1969
32. Mandel WJ, Hayakawa H, Allen HN, et al: Assessment of sinus node function in patients with the sick sinus syndrome. Circulation 46:761, 1972
33. Mandel W, Hayakawa H, Danzig R, et al: Evaluation of sinoatrial node function in many by overdrive suppression. Circulation 44:59, 1971
34. Massumi RA, Nutter DO: Studies on the mechanism of cardiac arrhythmias in Cheyne-Stokes respiration (Abstract). Circulation 31(Suppl II):II-146, 1965
35. Mazuz M, Friedman HS: Significance of prolonged electrocardiographic pauses in sinoatrial disease: Sick sinus syndrome. Am J Cardiol 52:485, 1983
36. Meltzer LE, Kitchell JB: The incidence of arrhythmias associated with acute myocardial infarction. Prog Cardiovasc Dis 9:50, 1966
37. Moss AJ, Davis RJ: Brady-tachy syndrome. Prog Cardiovasc Dis 16:439, 1974
38. Narula OS, Samet P, Javier RP: Significance of the sinus-node recovery time. Circulation 45:140, 1972
39. Parsonnet AE, Miller R: Heart block. The influence of ventricular systole upon the auricular rhythm in complete and incomplete heart block. Am Heart J 27:676, 1944

40. Rahimtoola AH, Zipes DP, Akhtar M, et al: Consensus statement of the conference on the state of the art of electrophysiologic testing in the diagnosis and treatment of patients with cardiac arrhythmias. Part 2. Mod Concept Cardiovas Dis 56:61, 1987
41. Rasmussen K: Chronic sinoatrial heart block. Am Heart J 81:38, 1971
42. Reiffel JA, Gang E, Gliklich J, et al: The human sinus node electrogram: A transvenous catheter technique and a comparison of directly measured and indirectly estimated sinoatrial conduction time in adults. Circulation 62:1324, 1980
43. Rokseth R, Hatle L: Sinus arrest in acute myocardial infarction. Br Heart J 33:639, 1971
44. Rosen KM, Loeb HS, Sinno MZ, et al: Cardiac conduction in patients with symptomatic sinus node disease. Circulation 43:836, 1971
45. Rosenbaum, MB, Lepeschkin E: The effect of ventricular systole on auricular rhythm in auriculoventricular block. Circulation 11:240, 1955
46. Rubenstein JJ, Schulman CL, Yurchak PM, et al: Clinical spectrum of the sick sinus syndrome. Circulation 46:5, 1972
47. Schamroth L: Ventriculophasic atrial extrasystoles associated with complete atrioventricular block. Am J Cardiol 21:593, 1968
48. Scheinman MM, Strauss HC, Abbott JA: Electrophysiologic testing for patients with sinus node dysfunction. J Electrocardiol 12:211, 1979
49. Shaw DB, Linker NJ, Heaver PA, et al: Chronic sinoatrial disorder (sick sinus syndrome): A possible result of cardiac ischaemia. Br Heart J 58:598, 1987
50. Short DS: The syndrome of alternating bradycardia and tachycardia. Br Heart J 16:208, 1954
51. Strauss HC, Bigger JT, Saroff AL, et al: Electrophysiologic evaluation of sinus node function in patients with sinus node dysfunction. Circulation 53:763, 1976
52. Strauss HC, Saroff AL, Bigger JT, et al: Premature atrial stimulation as a key to the understanding of sinoatrial conduction in man. Circulation 47:86, 1973
53. Wu D, Amat-y-Leon F, Denes P, et al: Demonstration of sustained sinus and atrial re-entry as a mechanism of paroxysmal supraventricular tachycardia. Circulation 51:234, 1975

Atrial Arrhythmias

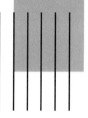

16

PREMATURE ATRIAL BEATS (PREMATURE ATRIAL CONTRACTIONS, ATRIAL EXTRASYSTOLES, PREMATURE ATRIAL DEPOLARIZATIONS)

In premature atrial beats, the premature impulse originates from an ectopic focus in the atrium. As the sequence of atrial activation is altered, the P wave not only appears early but also is abnormal in configuration. The P-wave axis, amplitude, and morphology in various leads depend mainly on the site of the ectopic atrial pacemaker.

Electrocardiographic Findings

1. The P (or P′) wave is premature in relation to the basic sinus rhythm.
2. The P (or P′) wave is abnormal and different in configuration from the sinus P wave.

The prematurity of the ectopic atrial beat varies. it may be early and superimposed on the ventricular complex of the preceding sinus beat or be late and occur just before the next sinus beat. In the latter instance, an atrial fusion beat may result if part of the atrial activation originates from the ectopic focus and part from the sinus node. Such a fusion beat has a morphology in between that of the sinus beat and the pure ectopic beat, but it is difficult to separate with certainty from an ectopic beat alone. When the premature atrial beats arise from the same focus, the coupling time is usually the same.

The morphology of the P wave depends on the location of the ectopic focus. If it is near the sinoatrial (SA) node, the P′ wave simulates the sinus P wave closely. If it is in the vicinity of the atrioventricular (AV) junction, the P′-wave axis is directed superiorly and the premature ectopic P wave is inverted in the inferior leads. It differs from premature AV junctional beat in that the PR interval is usually 0.12 second or longer. An ectopic right atrial focus is suggested if the P waves in the limb leads appear normal, but they are inverted in leads V_1 through V_4.[68] The P-wave axis is directed leftward, inferiorly, and posteriorly. In left atrial beats, the P vector is directed rightward and anteriorly. The P waves in leads I and V_6 are inverted, and the P wave in lead V_1 is upright. A "dome-and-dart" appearance of the P wave may be seen in lead V_1 in which the initial component of the upright P wave is rounded and the terminal part is sharp.[69] The results from electronic left atrial pacing suggested that the changes in lead V_1 are most important in the diagnosis of left atrial rhythm, whereas inversion of the P wave in leads I and V_6 is not an essential finding.[43] If the ectopic beats arise from more than one focus, the multifocal origin is indicated by the different configurations of the P waves.

Other Electrocardiographic Changes

PR INTERVAL

The PR interval of the premature atrial beat may remain unchanged, become shorter, or lengthen. It is usually similar to the PR interval of the basic sinus beat when the ectopic beat appears relatively late and the pacemaker is near the SA node. It becomes shorter if the focus is near the AV node. The PR interval tends to lengthen when the coupling time is short (Fig. 16–1). An early premature beat may not be conducted to the ventricles, and such an isolated P wave is called *blocked premature atrial beat* (see Figs. 16–1 and 16–2). A blocked premature atrial beat should not be mistaken for a second-degree AV block. In the latter case, the PP interval remains constant, and the P-wave morphology is unchanged.

QRS-T COMPLEX

Typically, the ventricular complex of a premature atrial beat is similar to that of the basic sinus beat. Because of the prematurity of the

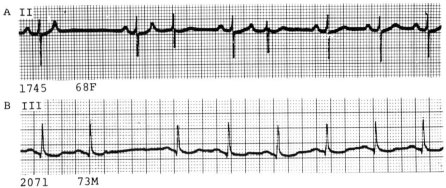

FIGURE 16–1. Premature atrial beats and the PR interval. (A) The relationship of the PR prolongation to the prematurity of the ectopic beats is shown. The first premature atrial beat is blocked. The second one has a longer PR interval than the third because of shorter coupling time. (B) There is a blocked premature atrial beat. The long pause may be mistaken as sinus arrest if the small ectopic P wave is not noticed.

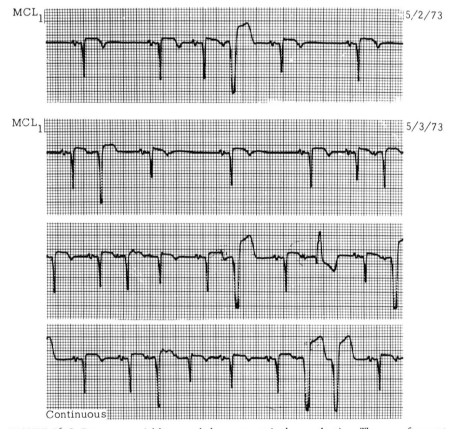

FIGURE 16–2. Premature atrial beats and aberrant ventricular conduction. There are frequent premature atrial beats, some of which are blocked, and others are followed by aberrant ventricular conduction. Both the type and the degree of aberrancy vary. Most of the abnormal QRS complexes have a left bundle branch block pattern. The QRS prolongation is more pronounced in some beats than in others, but the degree of aberrancy is unrelated to the prematurity of the ectopic beat in this patient. A right bundle branch block pattern is present in the second strip of 5-3-73. There is a couplet in the bottom strip.

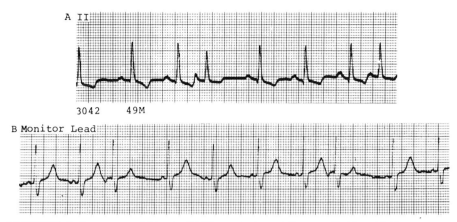

FIGURE 16-3. Premature atrial beats. (A) The postextrasystolic pause that is not fully compensatory. (B) An uncommon case of compensatory pause following premature atrial beats.

atrial impulse, however, it may find one of the bundle branches still refractory, resulting in an abnormal and wide QRS complex. In most instances, the aberrant ventricular conduction is represented by a right bundle branch block pattern because of the relatively longer refractory period of the right branch.[88] Left bundle branch block pattern may often be seen, however, especially in patients with heart disease, and different types of QRS morphology may be encountered in the same individual (see Fig. 16-2). As a rule, aberrancy is more likely to occur when the premature beat appears early.

POSTEXTRASYSTOLIC PAUSE

As the ectopic atrial impulse propagates and depolarizes the SA node, it resets the sinus cycle. Therefore, the cycle length after the premature atrial beat is longer than the basic sinus cycle. Furthermore, the premature discharge of the SA node tends to depress its rhythmicity temporarily and to increase further the cycle length.[80] In contrast to premature ventricular beats, however, the pause is not fully compensatory, that is, it is of insufficient duration to compensate completely for the shortened cycle of the premature beat (Fig. 16-3A). The only exception occurs when there is a retrograde SA block and the SA nodal rhythmicity is undisturbed (see Fig. 16-3B).

PATTERNS OF PRESENTATION

The premature atrial beats, either unifocal or multifocal, may present themselves at random intervals or after every one, two, or three sinus beats, resulting in a bigeminal, trigeminal, or quadrigeminal rhythm (Fig. 16-4). They may

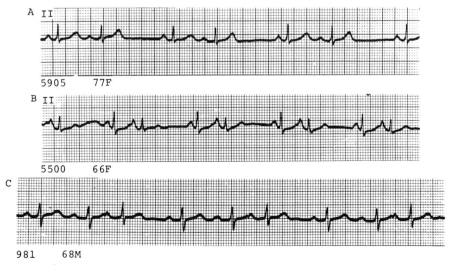

FIGURE 16-4. Premature atrial beats with bigeminal (A and B) and trigeminal (C) rhythm. (B) The QRS complex of the premature atrial beats shows aberrant ventricular conduction.

occur in pairs (see Fig. 16–2). Frequent premature atrial beats from multiple foci may cause a chaotic rhythm, which is discussed later in the chapter.

Clinical Significance

Most individuals with premature atrial beats do not have organic heart disease. In 100 healthy young men and women monitored by ambulatory electrocardiogram (ECG) for a 24-hour period, supraventricular ectopic beats were observed in 64 percent.[8,94] Less than 2 percent of these subjects, however, had more than 100 such ectopic beats in the 24-hour period. The frequency of the premature beats is higher in the older population.[83] In some patients without heart disease, the premature beats appear to be related to emotional stress, mental and physical fatigue, excessive smoking, or intake of alcohol or coffee.

The incidence of premature atrial beats is increased in patients with organic heart disease. The premature beats tend to occur more often when atrial disease or atrial enlargement is present. Patients with mitral stenosis or cor pulmonale commonly have frequent premature atrial beats that may lead to the development of atrial fibrillation or atrial flutter. On the other hand, no correlation has been found between premature atrial beats and increased incidence of coronary artery disease.[13,44]

ECTOPIC ATRIAL RHYTHM, ACCELERATED ATRIAL RHYTHM

In ectopic atrial rhythm (often called ectopic atrial pacemaker), the P-wave morphology is abnormal and different from that of the sinus P wave. The direction of the frontal plane P-wave axis varies, depending on the location of the ectopic focus. The atrial rate is less than 100 beats/min, and the PR interval is within the normal range. A left atrial origin of the rhythm (left atrial rhythm) is suggested when one or more of the following findings are present: (1) a frontal plane P-wave axis of +110° to +270°; (2) negative P waves in leads I and V_6; and (3) dome-and-dart P wave in lead V_1.[3,69] A dome-and-dart P wave consists of a rounded and broad first portion followed by a sharp and peaked late deflection.

Ectopic atrial rhythm is often transient. It can be easily recognized if the morphology of the P waves during sinus rhythm is known and compared. When the ectopic pacemaker is located in the lower atrium, the P waves in the

inferior leads are inverted and the rhythm may be mistaken as AV junctional. In the latter instance, the PR interval is less than 0.12 second unless there is antegrade AV conduction delay.

An ectopic atrial rhythm may be called accelerated atrial rhythm when the atrial rate is faster than the patient's sinus rate but is less than 100 beats/min. Accelerated atrial rhythm is most commonly recognized in ambulatory ECGs when the onset and termination of the ectopic rhythm can be identified. Ectopic and accelerated atrial rhythms are seen both in patients with organic heart disease and those without it.

PAROXYSMAL ATRIAL TACHYCARDIA

Paroxysmal atrial tachycardia may be divided into two groups depending on the mechanism by which the tachycardia is initiated and sustained. In intraatrial reentrant tachycardia, a reentry circuit consisting of two functionally distinct pathways with different conduction velocities and refractory periods is present and confined in the atrium.[22,39,49,72,106] (See Chapter 17 for further discussion of reentrant tachycardia). In automatic (or ectopic) atrial tachycardia, as the name implies, there is an increased automaticity of an ectopic focus in the atrium.[35,40,49] A third mechanism, triggered automaticity, has been suggested, but its role in tachycardia in humans has not been clearly defined.

In the past, paroxysmal atrial tachycardia was considered one of the most common forms of paroxysmal tachycardias. Electrophysiologic studies now suggest that many cases that were previously called paroxysmal atrial tachycardia were actually AV nodal reentrant tachycardia. Paroxysmal atrial tachycardia, as it is defined, is not seen frequently as a sustained (lasting more than 30 seconds) form of tachyarrhythmia. It accounts for about 10 percent of cases of paroxysmal supraventricular tachycardia.[48,107] In patients with paroxysmal supraventricular tachycardia without Wolff-Parkinson-White (WPW) syndrome, AV nodal reentry is the responsible mechanism in 60 to 70 percent of the cases, AV reentry using a concealed bypass tract is the cause in 13 to 30 percent, and SA nodal reentry, intraatrial reentry, and increased atrial automaticity are responsible in the remainder.[48,107]

With ambulatory (Holter) monitoring it has been found that short episodes of atrial tachycardia are common. In my experience, one or more episodes of nonsustained paroxysmal atrial tachycardia was observed in 582 (21.6 percent) of 2670 consecutive adult 12- to 24-hour ambulatory ECGs.[14] Most of these episodes have relatively slow rate, being less than 150 beats/min. This form of atrial tachycardia also has been called *benign slow paroxysmal atrial tachycardia.*[96]

Electrocardiographic Findings

1. Abnormal P waves that are different in morphology from the sinus P waves are seen.
2. The atrial rate is generally between 100 and 180 beats/min.
3. The rhythm is regular.
4. The paroxysm consists of three or more beats in succession.
5. There is a QRS complex after each P wave, and the QRS complex usually resembles that of the sinus beat but may be different because of aberrant ventricular conduction.
6. The PR interval may be within normal limits or prolonged.
7. Secondary ST-segment and T-wave changes may occur.

The morphology of the P waves in paroxysmal atrial tachycardia depends on the location of the ectopic atrial pacemaker and the pathway of the atrial activation. In many instances, the P waves are small and difficult to identify, since they are often superimposed on the preceding T waves (Fig. 16–5). The P waves in atrial tachycardia that result from increased automaticity are generally more clearly visible than those that result from reentrant mechanism.[35] The morphology of the first P wave of the tachycardia is the same as that of the subsequent beats in the automatic type, but this is not the case in the reentrant type.[35,49] In the latter, the P wave morphology during the episode also may vary, because the impulse exiting from the reentry circuit may be conducted in different pathways in the atria from beat to beat.[70] The heart rate is most commonly between 100 and 180 beats/min and usually does not exceed 150 beats/min in the reentrant variety.[70]

Although paroxysmal atrial tachycardia generally has a regular rhythm, in the automatic type there is often a gradual increase in the rate in the beginning of a paroxysm representing a warm-up period.[35,49] Some variation in the rate may occasionally be observed, even after the onset of tachycardia (Fig. 16–6).

Because of the rapid atrial rate, the AV junction may be only partially recovered when the successive atrial impulses arrive. The PR interval may, therefore, be longer than that of the sinus beat. If some of the P waves are not followed by a QRS complex, the rhythm is called *paroxysmal atrial tachycardia with block;* this is discussed later in the chapter.

The QRS complex in paroxysmal atrial tachycardia usually resembles that of the patient's sinus beat. If it has a normal duration,

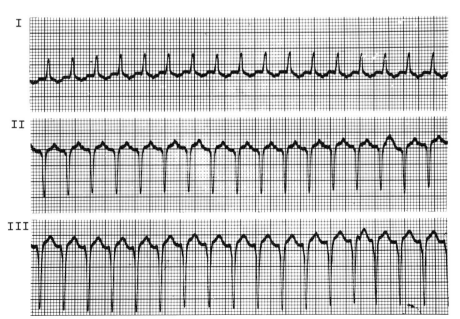

FIGURE 16–5. Paroxysmal atrial tachycardia in a 63-year-old man with coronary artery disease. The atrial rate is 188 beats/min. The small and abnormal P wave are superimposed on the T waves.

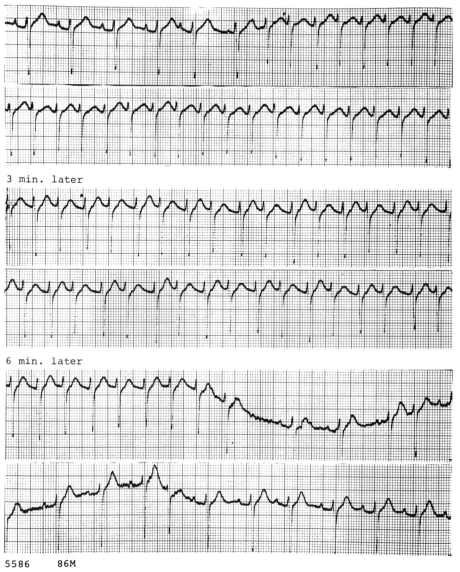

3 min. later

6 min. later

5586   86M

FIGURE 16–6. Paroxysmal atrial tachycardia of the automatic type in a patient with aortic valve disease. The rhythm is slightly irregular. Both the onset and termination of the paroxysm are illustrated. There is a variation of both the PP and RR intervals.

the supraventricular origin of the tachycardia can be easily assured. If it is abnormally wide and bizarre, it may be the result of aberrant ventricular conduction (Fig. 16–7). In most cases, the QRS complex has a right bundle branch block pattern, but a left bundle branch block pattern also is seen. Occasionally, aberrant ventricular conduction is present in the beginning part of a paroxysm and the intraventricular conduction becomes normal as the tachycardia continues (Fig. 16–8). The QRS complex may also be abnormal because of preexisting ventricular conduction defect. In either case, the rhythm may mimic paroxysmal ventricular tachycardia and present a difficult but important diagnostic problem.

As in sinus tachycardia, ST-segment depression and T-wave inversion may be seen during the tachycardia. Furthermore, ST-segment and T-wave abnormalities may be present for hours or even days after the conversion of the tachycardia to normal sinus rhythm. This phenomenon probably is related to the reduction of cardiac output and coronary blood flow and relative myocardial ischemia during tachycardia. It may be seen in patients without coronary artery disease and therefore should not be considered as an indication of such.

Atrial Arrhythmias

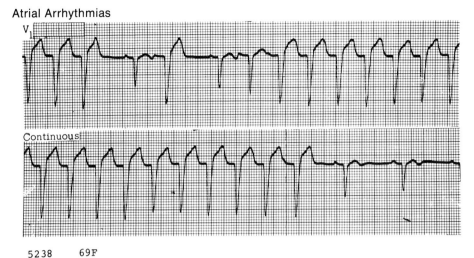

5238   69F

FIGURE 16–7. Paroxysmal atrial tachycardia with aberrant ventricular conduction. An isolated premature atrial beat with aberrant ventricular conduction is seen in the upper strip. During tachycardia, the rhythm simulates ventricular tachycardia.

Response to Vagal Stimulation

Vagal stimulation is a useful maneuver in the diagnosis and treatment of paroxysmal supraventricular tachycardia. The commonly used procedures such as carotid sinus massage and the Valsalva maneuver either have no effect on the tachycardia or convert it to normal sinus rhythm. Reentrant tachycardias that involve the SA or AV node are likely to be terminated by vagal maneuvers. Because the ectopic focus or the reentry circuit in paroxysmal atrial tachycardia is confined in the atria, the tachycardia is not affected by vagal stimulation, although the latter maneuver may produce AV block.[40,48,70]

Clinical Significance

Patients with sustained paroxysmal atrial tachycardia usually have evidence of organic

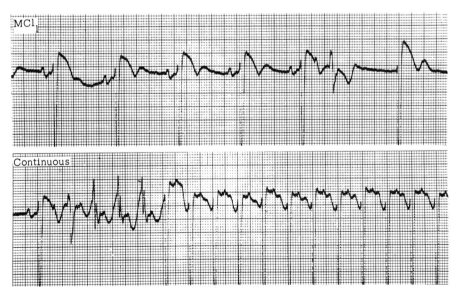

FIGURE 16–8. Paroxysmal atrial tachycardia. The top strip shows a premature atrial beat with aberrant ventricular conduction followed by a junctional escape beat. In the bottom strip, the onset of the paroxysmal atrial tachycardia is shown. There is aberrant ventricular conduction with a right bundle branch block pattern in the first four QRS complexes at the onset of the tachycardia, but the ventricular conduction becomes normal afterward.

heart disease.[48,107] Automatic atrial tachycardia often is precipitated by an acute event such as myocardial infarction, exacerbation of chronic obstructive pulmonary disease, alcohol ingestion, metabolic derangements, and drug toxicity (such as digitalis).[48] Nonsustained paroxysmal atrial tachycardia that usually lasts only for a few seconds is commonly seen in patients without organic heart disease.[14]

REPETITIVE PAROXYSMAL ATRIAL TACHYCARDIA

A variant of paroxysmal atrial tachycardia is repetitive paroxysmal atrial tachycardia. It is characterized by recurring short runs of atrial tachycardia almost constantly present for months or years and only occasionally interrupted by normal sinus rhythm[75] (Fig. 16–9). Using the more stringent definition, the individual paroxysms of this dysrhythmia should not be separated by more than two normal beats. The tachycardia often has a slightly irregular rhythm. Similar repetitive behavior also is seen in other types of tachycardias such as atrial flutter, atrial fibrillation, paroxysmal junctional tachycardia, and ventricular tachycardia.[60,75]

Repetitive atrial tachycardia is uncommon. A substantial number of patients with this rhythm have no evidence of heart disease (Fig. 16–10). Among those with organic heart disease, the causes include coronary artery, hypertensive, rheumatic, and various other types of heart disease.

PAROXYSMAL ATRIAL TACHYCARDIA WITH BLOCK

The clinical importance of paroxysmal atrial tachycardia with block was brought to attention mainly by Lown and associates.[64] Its ECG features (Fig. 16–11) include the following:

1. Abnormal P (or P′) waves that are different in morphology from the sinus P waves
2. Atrial rate of generally between 150 and 250 beats/min
3. Isoelectric intervals between P waves in all leads
4. AV block beyond a simple prolongation of the PR interval

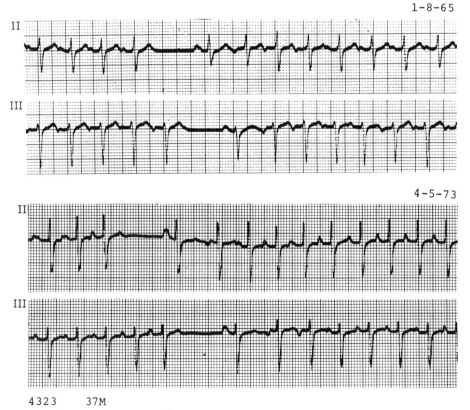

1-8-65

II

III

4-5-73

II

III

4323   37M

FIGURE 16–9. Repetitive paroxysmal atrial tachycardia. The patient is a 37-year-old man with probably idiopathic cardiomyopathy. Repetitive paroxysmal atrial tachycardia has been noted for at least 8 years.

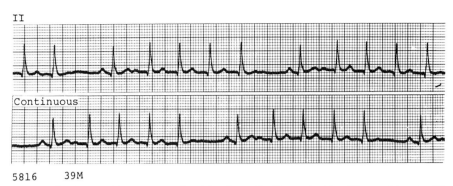

5816   39M

FIGURE 16–10. Repetitive paroxysmal atrial tachycardia. The patient is a 39-year-old man with no clinical evidence of organic heart disease.

As in other ectopic atrial rhythms the morphology of the P waves depends on the location of the ectopic atrial pacemaker. The P waves frequently are small and not easily identifiable. In some cases, lead V_1 may be the best lead to search for the blocked P waves. Although the atrial rate may range from 150 to 250 beats/min, it is less than 200 beats/min in most cases. Occasionally, the rate may be as low as 110 beats/min. The atrial rhythm is generally regular. Some variation of the PP interval, however, was seen in nearly half of the series reported by Lown.[64] In some of my cases, the variation was related to the QRS complex and was similar to that of ventriculophasic sinus arrhythmia. The PP interval containing the QRS complex is shorter than that without the QRS (Fig. 16–12).

In the typical cases of paroxysmal atrial tachycardia with block, there is an isoelectric

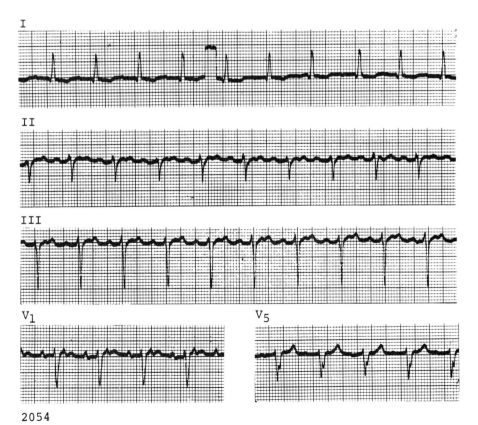

2054

FIGURE 16–11. Paroxysmal atrial tachycardia with block. The atrial rate is 200 beats/min, and there is 2:1 AV conduction. The P waves are seen best in lead V_1.

0.38   0.38
0.30   0.30

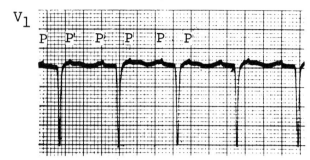

FIGURE 16–12. Paroxysmal atrial tachycardia with block. There is 2:1 AV conduction. There is a variation of the PP interval, which is ventriculophasic. The PP intervals that contain a QRS complex are shorter than those without.

baseline between the P waves. This finding is helpful in the separation of this arrhythmia from atrial flutter, in which there is a constant oscillation of the baseline.

The AV block in this dysrhythmia usually is manifested as second-degree AV block. More commonly, there is a 2:1 conduction, but a 3:1 conduction or Wenckebach phenomenon may be observed (Figs. 16–13 and 16–14). Complete AV block is uncommon. The diagnosis of paroxysmal atrial tachycardia with block cannot be made when there is 1:1 AV conduction with prolongation of the PR interval. The PR prolongation in such a case may be physiological because of the rapid atrial impulses. In some cases with 1:1 conduction, however, second-degree AV block may develop during carotid sinus massage. Such a response suggests the presence of latent AV block. An example of paroxysmal atrial tachycardia with latent block is given in Figure 16–15.

Differential Diagnosis

Because the P waves in paroxysmal atrial tachycardia with block are often small and su-

perimposed on the ventricular complexes, this rhythm frequently is mistaken for AV junctional tachycardia, paroxysmal atrial tachycardia without block, or sinus tachycardia. When there is varying block, the irregular ventricular rhythm may be mistaken for atrial fibrillation. The arrhythmia that most closely simulates paroxysmal atrial tachycardia with block is atrial flutter. Because paroxysmal atrial tachycardia with block is frequently the result of digitalis toxicity, and atrial flutter rarely is, the differentiation is clinically important. In atrial flutter, the atrial rate is usually greater than 250 beats/min. There is constant oscillation of the baseline because of the flutter waves. The diagnosis of atrial flutter is likely if the P-wave has a sawtooth appearance even though the atrial rate is less than 250 beats/min. Indeed, an atrial rate of 200 beats/min may be seen in atrial flutter if the patient is receiving quinidine or similar antiarrhythmic agents, or there is marked atrial enlargement. If the atrial rate is between 200 and 250 beats/min and the P waves are not typical for atrial flutter, the differentiation of these types of arrhythmias is often impossible from the ECG.

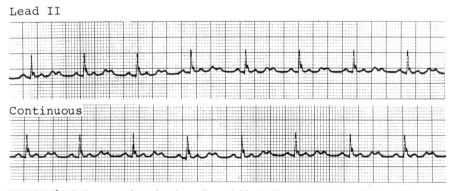

FIGURE 16–13. Paroxysmal atrial tachycardia with block. There is 3:1 AV conduction. The patient was not receiving digitalis.

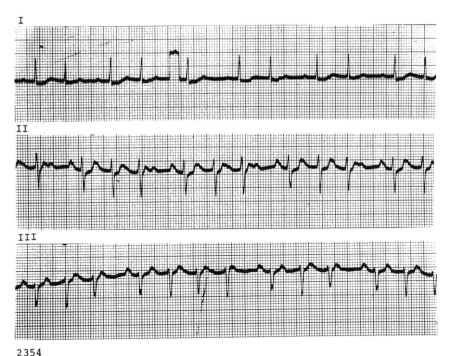

2354

FIGURE 16–14. Paroxysmal atrial tachycardia with block. A Wenckebach phenomenon is present. There is a gradual lengthening of the PR interval and shortening of the RR interval before the block occurs.

Clinical Significance

Digitalis intoxication is responsible for most cases of paroxysmal atrial tachycardia with block. In the 112 episodes of this arrhythmia reviewed by Lown and Levine in 1958, digitalis was the cause of 73 percent.[63] Other reports implicated digitalis toxicity in 40 to 82 percent of the cases.[26,32] In recent years, the dosage of digitalis used generally has been reduced. The incidence of this arrhythmia caused by the drug is probably lower. The rhythm was found most frequently in patients with advanced heart disease; depleted body potassium from diuretics was often the precipitating factor. The serum potassium level was not necessarily below the normal range, however. With potassium supplements, there is usually a slowing of the atrial rate followed by the resumption of 1:1 conduction. At a critical rate, generally ranging from 105 to 150 beats/min, there is an abrupt change in the site of the pacemaker with resumption of sinus rhythm.[64] In one reported series, chronic pulmonary disease was found in more than half of the patients who were receiving digitalis and who had this arrhythmia.[37] In patients who are not receiving digitalis, the etiology of this arrhythmia is diverse and covers that spectrum of heart diseases found in association with other types of atrial arrhythmias.

MULTIFOCAL ATRIAL TACHYCARDIA

Multifocal atrial tachycardia also is known as *chaotic atrial tachycardia* or *chaotic atrial mechanism*.[62,79,91] The characteristic ECG findings are as follows (Figs. 16–16 and 16–17):

1. P waves of varying morphology from at least three different foci demonstrated in the same lead
2. The absence of one dominant atrial pacemaker (in distinction to normal sinus rhythm with frequent multifocal premature atrial beats)
3. Variable PP, RR, and PR intervals

When the term *multifocal* or *chaotic atrial tachycardia* is used, it usually implies that the atrial rate is above 100 beats/min, whereas chaotic atrial mechanism includes both more rapid and slower atrial rates. In several reported series, multifocal atrial tachycardia was seen in 0.2 to 0.4 percent of the ECGs from the institutions where the studies were performed.[6,15,52,62,79,91] The rhythm is often pre-

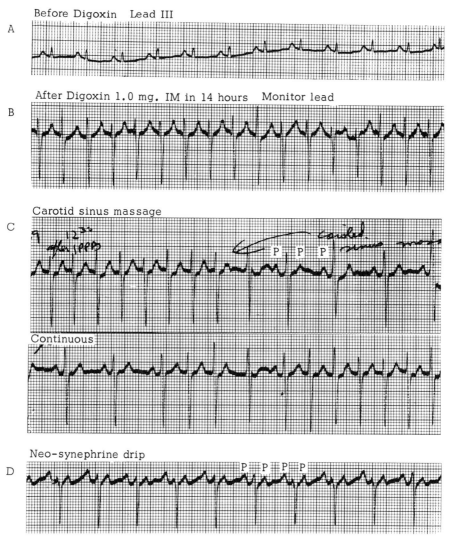

FIGURE 16–15. Paroxysmal atrial tachycardia with latent block. The patient has chronic obstructive lung disease with cor pulmonale and was receiving digitalis. Paroxysmal atrial tachycardia developed. AV block was induced during carotid sinus massage and intravenous infusion of Neo-Synephrine.

ceded or followed by frequent premature atrial beats, sinus tachycardia, atrial fibrillation, atrial flutter, paroxysmal atrial tachycardia, or paroxysmal atrial tachycardia with block (see Fig. 16–17A). In one series, it was preceded by or progressed to atrial fibrillation or flutter in 55 percent of the cases.[62] Because of the irregular irregularity of the rhythm, it is

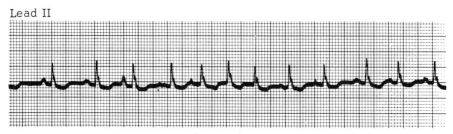

FIGURE 16–16. Multifocal atrial tachycardia.

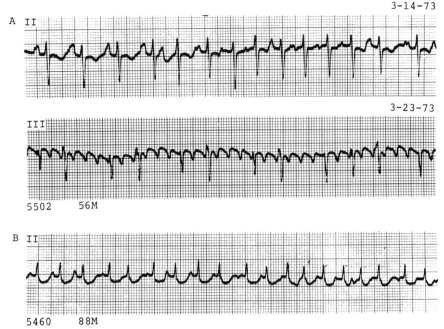

FIGURE 16–17. Multifocal atrial tachycardia. (A) The patient has chronic obstructive lung disease. The tracing on 3-14-73 shows multifocal atrial tachycardia. The rhythm changes to atrial flutter with varying AV conduction on 3-23-73. (B) Tracing obtained from an 88-year-old man with mitral insufficiency. The multifocal atrial tachycardia closely resembles atrial fibrillation with rapid ventricular response.

frequently mistaken as atrial fibrillation when the P waves are of lower amplitude (see Fig. 16–17B). The arrhythmia is usually transient, lasting no more than a few days, but recurrences are common.

Multifocal atrial tachycardia is mainly seen in elderly patients and in very ill patients. There is a high incidence of chronic obstructive pulmonary disease in patients with this arrhythmia, varying from 34 to 92 percent of some reported series. The higher incidence was observed mostly in the Veterans Administration hospitals. Coronary artery disease is also a common underlying clinical state. Other associated heart diseases include cor pulmonale, hypertensive cardiovascular disease, and occasionally, valvular heart disease. Of some interest is the fact that many of the patients had diabetes mellitus.[52,79] The role of digitalis as a cause of this rhythm has been debated.[15,62] Electrolyte imbalance such as hypokalemia and hypomagnesemia has been reported as the etiology of this arrhythmia.[97]

ATRIAL FLUTTER

The mechanism responsible for the genesis of atrial flutter has been a subject of controversy for many years. Electrophysiological studies during open chest surgery[85] and by means of intraatrial electrodes[34,101] suggest that the pathway of atrial activation in atrial flutter is consistent with a circus movement that incorporates most of atrial myocardium in some patients and with a focal origin in others. In the former cases, there is a cephalad activation of the left atrial wall followed by a caudad excitation of the right atrium. In cases thought to have a focal origin, the activation begins low in the left atrium, and the excitation spreads simultaneously through both atria in a general cephalad direction. The focus, however, is not necessarily a discrete point. It may encompass a circumscribed area and the tachyarrhythmia may be either the result of increased automaticity or reentry through a very small circuit.[34,103] Some investigators believed that intraatrial or interatrial conduction defect may be a prerequisite to the development of atrial flutter.[101]

Electrocardiographic Findings

1. The atrial deflections consist of rapid regular undulations (the F waves) that give rise to a sawtooth appearance in some leads.

2. The atrial rate is usually between 250 and 350 beats/min.

Lead II

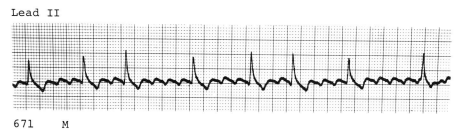

671   M

FIGURE 16–18. Atrial flutter with variable AV conduction in a patient with hyperthyroidism who was receiving digitalis.

3. The rate and regularity of the ventricular complexes are variable and depend on the AV conduction sequence.

4. The QRS complex may be normal or abnormal as a result of preexisting intraventricular conduction defect or aberrant ventricular conduction.

F WAVES

The flutter waves are generally best seen in leads II, III aVF, and V_1. In most cases, the F-wave axis is directed superiorly because of the cephalad direction of the atrial activation. The flutter waves are, therefore, inverted in the inferior leads (II, III, and aVF) (Fig. 16–18). In leads II, III, and aVF, the initial downward deflection of the F waves has a more gradual slope, followed by an abrupt upward inscription, giving rise to the typical sawtooth or "picket fence" appearance without an isoelectric line between the F waves. Such a morphology may not be seen in other leads that are more perpendicular to the F-wave axis. Thus, in lead I, the F waves are often small and difficult to identify. In lead V_1, the F waves sometimes consist of small diphasic complexes with an isoelectric baseline between them.

Occasionally, the flutter waves appear upright in the inferior leads (the so-called uncommon type), suggesting that the atrial acti-

Atrial flutter with 2:1 block   Atrial rate: 300

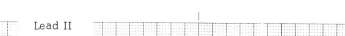

Lead II

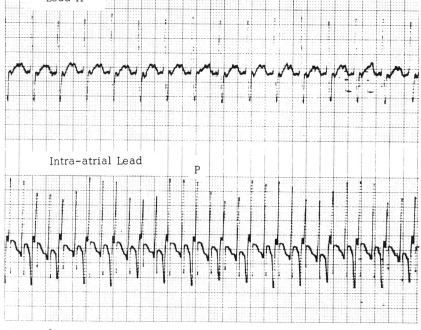

Intra-atrial Lead   P

FIGURE 16–19. Atrial flutter with 2:1 conduction. The atrial activity is not well documented in the conventional body surface leads. The intraatrial lead shows an atrial rate of 300 beats/min.

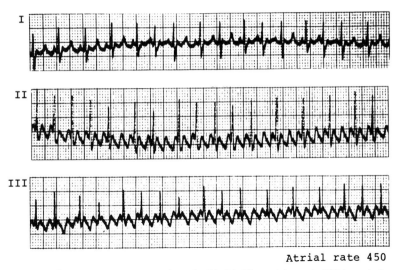

Atrial rate 450

FIGURE 16–20. Atrial flutter in a 6-week-old girl. The atrial rate is 450 beats/min. There is a varying degree of AV block.

vation has a caudal direction. On the other hand, because of the constant oscillation of the baseline, it is often difficult to be certain of the polarity of the deflections.

If the flutter waves have a gradual contour and they are superimposed on the QRS and T waves, the rhythm may be difficult to recognize. In many instances, the rather sharp but small deflections in lead V_1 are helpful in determining the atrial rate and leading to the correct diagnosis. Others require an intraatrial or esophageal lead to demonstrate the atrial rhythm (Fig. 16–19).

ATRIAL RATE

In adults, the atrial rate in atrial flutter usually ranges between 250 and 350 beats/min and is typically about 300 beats/min. In infants and children, the rate is often faster (Fig. 16–20). A rate slower than 250 beats/min is occasionally seen in adults. In 312 patients with atrial

Lead II   2/3/69

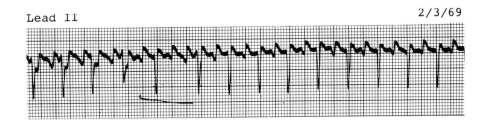

Lead II   2/5/69

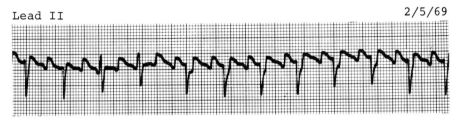

68M

FIGURE 16–21. Effect of quinidine on atrial rate in atrial flutter. The tracing on 2-3-69 was obtained before quinidine was given. The atrial rate is 300 beats/min, and there is 2:1 and occasionally 3:1 AV conduction. Two days after quinidine therapy, the atrial rate has slowed to 240 beats/min.

flutter analyzed by Rytand and associates, there was an apparent relation between the atrial size and the atrial rate.[86] The patients with markedly enlarged atria tended to have a slower rate than those without significant enlargement. Massive dilatation of the atria was accompanied by increased duration of the flutter cycle and a rate of less than 200 beats/min in some patients. The flutter rate also is influenced by certain drugs. Digitalis tends to increase the atrial rate as a result of its vagal effect, which decreases the atrial refractory period.[50] Quinidine and procainamide prolong the atrial refractory period and cause slowing of the atrial rate. An example of the effect of quinidine on the flutter rate is given in Figure 16–21. A flutter rate of 120 beats/min as a result of quinidine was described by Katz.[50]

Wells and associates described two types of atrial flutter in patients who exhibited the arrhythmia after open heart surgery.[103] Type I atrial flutter has atrial rates ranging from 240 to 338 beats/min. It is equivalent to the classic or common form of atrial flutter and can be interrupted by rapid atrial pacing. Type II atrial flutter has atrial rates ranging from 340 to 433 beats/min. It cannot be interrupted by rapid atrial pacing.

AV CONDUCTION

Ventricular Response. The most common mode of AV conduction in untreated cases of atrial flutter is 2:1. Therefore, a regular ventricular rhythm of about 150 beats/min is the typical presentation. A higher degree of AV block is usually the result of digitalis, propranolol, or other drug therapy. A 3:1 conduction is uncommon. In the untreated cases, a 4:1 conduction suggests the existence of AV conduction defect but also may result from concealed conduction. An atrial impulse may penetrate the AV junction but fail to reach the ventricles. The resulting partial depolarization of the AV junctional tissue increases its refractory period and blocks the next atrial impulse from its conduction to the ventricles. Atrial flutter may be associated with completed AV block[54] (Fig. 16–22). The RR interval is regular, but the F waves have no constant relationship to the QRS complexes. The ventricular rate is slow. The subsidiary pacemaker is located at the AV junction or in the ventricles. On the other hand, atrial flutter with AV block may be complicated by AV junctional tachycardia. There is a dissociation of the atrial and ventricular activities, but the ventricular rate is rapid.

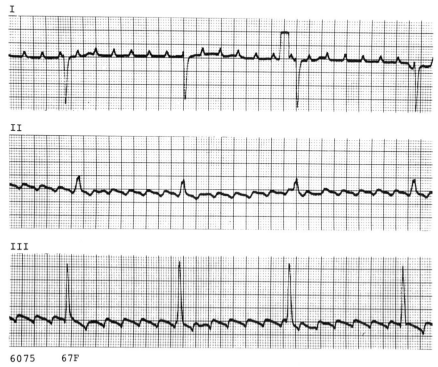

6075   67F

FIGURE 16–22. Atrial flutter with complete AV block. Variation of the FR interval and a constant RR interval are seen. The patient was receiving digitalis. The escape rhythm probably is idioventricular in origin.

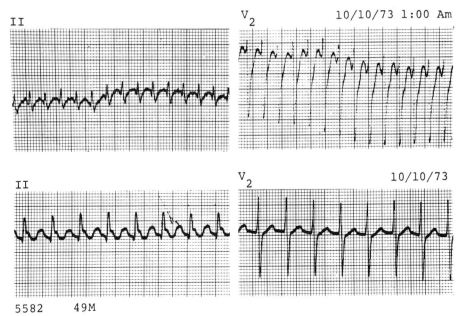

FIGURE 16–23. Atrial flutter in a 49-year-old man with chronic obstructive lung disease. The patient was not receiving digitalis or quinidine at the time. The tracing at 1:00 A.M. shows atrial flutter with 1:1 conduction. The atrial rate is 290 beats/min. The tracing recorded later in the day shows atrial flutter with 2:1 conduction with an atrial rate of 316 beats/min.

Atrial flutter with 1:1 conduction is rare. When it occurs, it constitutes a serious cardiac emergency because of the rapid ventricular rate (Fig. 16–23). The 1:1 conduction may be precipitated by excitement, exercise (Fig. 16–24), induction of anesthesia, or any state associated with increased sympathetic tone.[27]

It may occur in patients with the WPW syndrome when the atrial impulses are conducted antegrade through the bypass tract. In these cases, the QRS complexes are abnormal and wide. The administration of intravenous atropine in patients with atrial flutter and 2:1 AV conduction may result in 1:1 conduction.

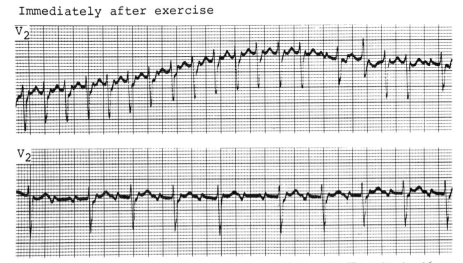

FIGURE 16–24. Atrial flutter with 1:1 conduction induced by exercise. The patient is a 16-year-old woman with congenital mitral insufficiency, and a mitral valve prosthesis was inserted 3 years previously. She was receiving digitalis and quinidine at the time this tracing was recorded. There is atrial flutter with 2:1 to 3:1 AV conduction at rest. The typical flutter wave morphology is seen in the inferior leads (not shown here). The atrial rate is 200 beats/min. The tracing taken immediately after exercise shows 1:1 AV conduction.

During the treatment of atrial flutter with quinidine or procainamide, the atrial rate may be decreased to facilitate 1:1 conduction (see Fig. 16–24).

The AV conduction in atrial flutter may be variable, resulting in irregular ventricular rhythm that resembles atrial fibrillation. A Wenckebach phenomenon is often seen in the presence of a basic 2:1 or higher degree of AV block. There is a gradual prolongation of the FR interval until the expected conduction fails to occur.

QRS COMPLEX

The QRS complex may be normal or abnormally wide. Abnormally wide QRS complexes may be due to preexisting intraventricular conduction defect or aberrant ventricular conduction. Atrial flutter with 2:1 conduction and wide QRS complexes closely mimic paroxysmal ventricular tachycardia. In such cases, flutter waves usually are masked by the ventricular complexes.

Atrial Flutter–Fibrillation

Atrial flutter–fibrillation also is known as impure atrial flutter. The flutter cycle is slightly irregular, with some variation of the morphology of the F waves. The atrial rate generally tends to be faster than the classical atrial flutter. At times, the atrial activities resemble atrial fibrillation. The ventricular rhythm is irregular unless complete AV dissociation or block exists. Intraatrial ECGs in patients with

atrial flutter–fibrillation suggest that dissimilar atrial rhythms, most commonly flutter of one atrium and fibrillation of the other, is responsible for the presentation.[58,107] Dissimilar rhythm also may occur within the same atrium.

Repetitive Atrial Flutter

Repetitive atrial flutter is an unusual form of atrial flutter in which short episodes of atrial flutter are interrupted by a few normal sinus beats (Fig. 16–25).

Relation of Atrial Flutter to Other Atrial Arrhythmias

Frequent premature atrial beats are seen in many patients who later develop atrial flutter. Atrial flutter and atrial fibrillation are often seen in the same patient (Fig. 16–26). In patients with atrial flutter treated with digitalis, the vagal effect of the drug tends to decrease the atrial refractory period and may convert the rhythm to atrial fibrillation in 70 to 80 percent of the cases.[4,29] Digitalization also converts most patients with atrial flutter to normal sinus rhythm with or without a transitional state of atrial fibrillation. In the 31 patients treated by Fowler and Gueron, 28 patients were converted to normal sinus rhythm with digitalis alone.[30] Conversely, in patients with atrial fibrillation, the administration of quinidine after digitalization is followed by the appearance of atrial flutter in about half of the patients.[12] Normal sinus rhythm may or

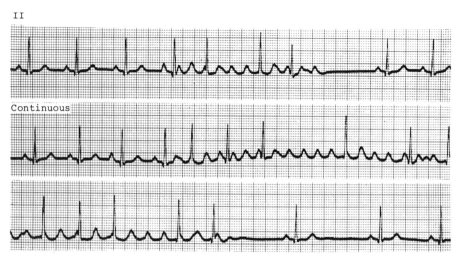

FIGURE 16–25. Repetitive atrial flutter. The patient is a 32-year-old woman who has no symptoms and shows no other evidence of organic heart disease. The flutter rate varies during different episodes.

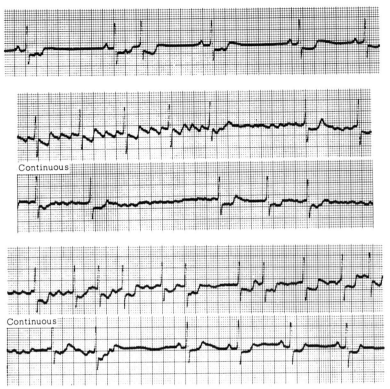

FIGURE 16–26. Atrial flutter and fibrillation. The tracing was recorded with a Holter monitor. It shows the change in atrial rhythm of different types during the period of recording. Sinus rhythm, premature atrial beats, atrial flutter, and atrial fibrillation are demonstrated.

may not follow. The occurrence of paroxysmal atrial tachycardia and atrial flutter in the same patient is much less common. Of special clinical importance is the association of atrial flutter and SA bradycardia in patients with the sick sinus syndrome and brady-tachyarrhythmia, which was described in Chapter 15 (see Fig. 15–15).

Response of Atrial Flutter to Vagal Stimulation

The application of vagal stimulation (e.g., carotid sinus massage) may increase the AV block but does not affect the atrial mechanism in atrial flutter. The ventricular rate is either unchanged or temporarily slowed during the

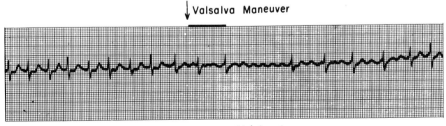

↓ Valsalva Maneuver

Ventricular rate
130/min.

Atrial rate
260/min.

39F. Atrial Septal Defect
Atrial Flutter with 2:1 A.V. Block   Lead II

FIGURE 16–27. Atrial flutter. The patient is a 39-year-old woman with atrial septal defect. In the beginning of the rhythm strip, the ventricular rate is 130 beats/min, but the atrial mechanism is not well demonstrated. With the Valsalva maneuver, there is an increase in the AV block to allow a better display of the flutter waves. (Reproduced from Fowler NO: Cardiac Diagnosis and Treatment. New York, Harper & Row, 1976, by permission.)

Control

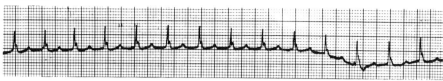

Carotid message

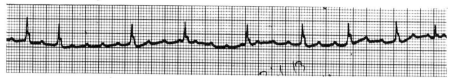

FIGURE 16–28. Atrial flutter with 2:1 conduction. The rhythm in the upper strip may be mistaken as paroxysmal supraventricular tachycardia with a rate of 133 beats/min. On carotid sinus massage, the flutter waves with a rate of 266 beats/min are demonstrated during the period of increased AV block.

procedure but returns immediately to its previous level when the vagal stimulation is stopped. The maneuver is often helpful in revealing the flutter waves (Figs. 16–27 and 16–28).

Differential Diagnosis

Because the AV conduction in atrial flutter is variable and the ventricular rhythm may be regular or irregular, the rhythm may simulate many other types of arrhythmias.

SINUS TACHYCARDIA

Sinus tachycardia with a rate between 120 and 180 beats/min may mimic atrial flutter with 2:1 conduction and vice versa. The alternate F waves in atrial flutter may be masked by the QRS-T complex. In sinus tachycardia, the heart rate may change from minute to minute. In atrial flutter, it tends to remain the same. With vagal stimulation, there is a gradual slowing of the heart rate if the tachycardia is sinus in origin. In atrial flutter, the rhythm is either unchanged or there is an increase in the AV block with temporary slowing of the ventricular rate. In most instances, the flutter waves are revealed.

PAROXYSMAL SUPRAVENTRICULAR TACHYCARDIA

Because atrial flutter with 2:1 conduction has a ventricular rate in a range similar to that of paroxysmal supraventricular (atrial or junctional) tachycardia, the two entities are often difficult to separate. In some cases, the flutter waves can best be seen in lead V_1 to indicate the atrial mechanism. Vagal stimulation may be helpful in other cases if it produces increased AV block in atrial flutter or paroxysmal atrial tachycardia or if it converts AV nodal reentrant tachycardia to normal sinus rhythm. Esophageal or intraatrial lead may be needed in occasional patients to demonstrate the atrial activity.

PAROXYSMAL ATRIAL TACHYCARDIA WITH BLOCK

The differentiation of atrial flutter and paroxysmal atrial tachycardia with block was discussed previously. In essence, the atrial rate in atrial flutter is usually above 250 beats/min, and that of paroxysmal atrial tachycardia with block is below 200 beats/min. Exceptions do occur, however, and the important finding is the characteristic morphology of the atrial deflection and the absence of an isoelectric line between the F waves in atrial flutter.

ATRIAL FIBRILLATION

Atrial flutter with variable AV conduction may resemble atrial fibrillation because of the irregular ventricular response. In most instances, the distinction can be made if care is taken in the identification of the atrial deflections. In some cases, however, the rhythm is consistent with atrial flutter–fibrillation or impure flutter.

PAROXYSMAL VENTRICULAR TACHYCARDIA

Atrial flutter with 2:1 or, rarely, 1:1 conduction may be accompanied by aberrant ventricular conduction, preexisting bundle branch block, or the WPW syndrome. The rapid and regular rhythm with wide QRS complexes may be mistaken for paroxysmal ventricular tachycardia. If previous ECGs are available and show the ventricular conduction abnormalities, the supraventricular origin of the tachycardia can be identified. Vagal stimulation does not affect the rhythm if it is ventricular tachycardia, but it may increase the AV block and reveal the flutter waves if the rhythm is atrial flutter. A more detailed discussion of the differential diagnosis of supraventricular and ventricular tachycardia is given in Chapter 18.

Clinical Significance

Among supraventricular tachyarrhythmias, atrial flutter is less common than atrial fibrillation and paroxysmal supraventricular tachycardia. It is seen most often in older individuals, although it may occur even in the very young (see Fig. 16–20). The arrhythmia may be transient, lasting for minutes or hours, or may persist for months or even years. In one series of 49 patients with atrial flutter, 55 percent of the episodes lasted less than 7 days and 10 percent lasted longer than 1 year.[11]

Most patients with atrial flutter have organic heart disease. The more common causes include coronary artery disease and rheumatic heart disease. In patients with acute myocardial infarction, continuous ECG monitoring revealed this arrhythmia in 0.8 to 5.3 percent.[25,51,65,66] In patients with rheumatic heart disease, especially mitral valve lesions, mitral stenosis is the most frequent finding. Other underlying causes include hypertensive heart disease, cardiomyopathy, chronic and acute cor pulmonale,[20,47] pulmonary diseases,[21] hyperthyroidism, and pericarditis. Atrial flutter is seen occasionally in older patients with

atrial septal defect[23] (see Fig. 16–27). It often occurs after cardiac surgery.[2,103] It may be a complicating arrhythmia in patients with the WPW syndrome. Patients with the sick sinus syndrome may have atrial flutter as a part of the brady-tachyarrhythmia. Although digitalis toxicity has been reported as a contributing cause,[24] it is uncommon. In a small percentage of patients, no evidence of organic heart disease was found.[30]

ATRIAL FIBRILLATION

Like that for atrial flutter, the basic mechanism responsible for the genesis of atrial fibrillation remains controversial. The proposed theories include the circus movement, unifocal or multifocal origin, and multiple reentry circuit theory. In either case, inhomogeneity of the responsiveness and conduction of the atrial tissue results in a chaotic sequence of atrial depolarization.[93] Multiple reentry circuits may be established to perpetuate the arrhythmia. The chaotic atrial impulse is conducted through the AV junction at random intervals, resulting in a totally irregular ventricular rhythm.

Electrocardiographic Findings

1. The P waves are absent. The atrial activity is represented by fibrillatory (f) waves of varying amplitude, duration, and morphology that cause random oscillation of the baseline.

2. The ventricular rhythm, in the absence of AV block, is irregularly irregular.

FIBRILLATORY WAVES

In atrial fibrillation the atrial rate is rapid and ranges from 400 to 700 beats/min. The duration, amplitude, and configuration of the f waves are variable. The f waves are best seen

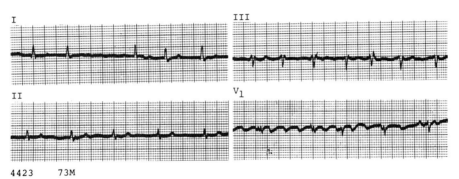

4423   73M

FIGURE 16–29. Atrial fibrillation with "flutter" waves in lead V_1.

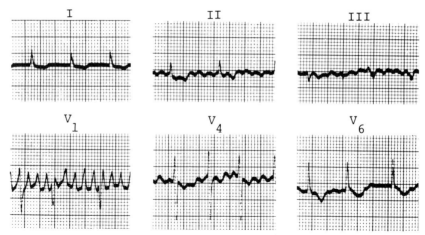

FIGURE 16–30. Atrial fibrillation with coarse fibrillatory waves in a patient with tight mitral stenosis.

in the right precordial and inferior leads. It is not uncommon to have a straight baseline in many of the limb leads, with the oscillation detected only in lead V_1. Occasionally, the tracing is typical of atrial fibrillation, but lead V_1 shows regular oscillation of the baseline suggestive of atrial flutter (Fig. 16–29). It is possible that this right precordial lead records the rhythmic activity of a localized area of the right atrium, whereas atrial fibrillation is present in a large part of the atrial chambers.

Depending on the size of the f waves, they may be called *fine* or *coarse* fibrillatory waves. Some authors consider f waves of greater than 0.5 mm as coarse,[99] others use 1 mm as the dividing value.[77] In 194 patients with atrial fibrillation, Thurmann and Janney found a significant relationship between the size of the fibrillatory waves and the cause of the heart disease.[99] Eighty-seven percent of the patients with f waves greater than 0.5 mm in lead V_1 had rheumatic heart disease, and 88

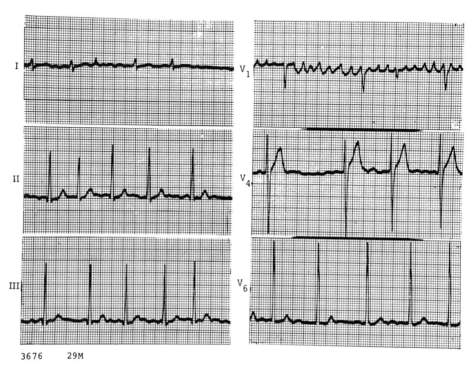

3676   29M

FIGURE 16–31. Atrial fibrillation with coarse fibrillatory waves, especially in lead V_1, in a patient with severe mitral and aortic insufficiency.

percent of the patients with f waves of less than 0.5 mm had arteriosclerotic heart disease. They also showed that coarse f waves in lead V_1 were associated with atrial enlargement. Figures 16–30 and 16–31 are examples of coarse fibrillatory waves associated with mitral valve disease. A significant correlation has been demonstrated between coarse fibrillatory waves and abnormal P terminal force in lead V_1 during sinus rhythm, suggesting left atrial enlargement.[71,77] A few cases of coarse atrial fibrillation also have been reported in patients with congenital heart disease and right atrial or biatrial enlargement.[98] Transient atrial fibrillation in patients with chronic cor pulmonale often is accompanied by coarse f waves in lead V_1. Several studies have shown that atrial fibrillation with fine fibrillatory waves from all causes are more difficult to convert to normal sinus rhythm.[41,42,73] In some cases, the f waves are not distinct in any of the leads, and the diagnosis of atrial fibrillation is based on the irregular irregularity of the ventricular rhythm. Confirmation of the atrial mechanism may be obtained by esophageal or intraatrial lead if necessary.

VENTRICULAR RESPONSE

In untreated cases of atrial fibrillation, the ventricular rate usually is between 100 and 180 beats/min (Fig. 16–32). Because the atrial rate is above 400 beats/min, a faster ventricular rate is expected in the absence of AV conduction abnormalities. The slower ventricular response seen clinically has been explained on the basis of concealed conduction.[57,81] There is a partial penetration of the AV junction by some of the atrial impulses rendering it refractory to the subsequent impulses. This concept is supported by the observation that long pauses often follow premature ventricular contractions in the presence of atrial fibrillation. They are attributable to prolonged refractoriness of the AV junction as a result of retrograde penetration by the ectopic ventricular impulse. In addition, with the development of atrial flutter or atrial tachycardia with slower atrial rate in such patients, there is an actual increase of the ventricular response[19,57] (Fig. 16–33).

If the ventricular rate in atrial fibrillation is greater than 200 beats/min, the possibility of WPW syndrome or its variants should be considered (Fig. 16–34). The presence of a bypass bundle allows the atrial impulses to avoid the longer refractory period at the AV junction, and the frequency of ventricular response is increased.

In the presence of AV junctional disease, the ventricular rate may be below 70 beats/min because of a high degree of AV block. A complete AV block is indicated by a slow ventricular rhythm with regular RR interval (Fig. 16–35). The escape pacemaker may originate from the AV junction or the His-Purkinje sys-

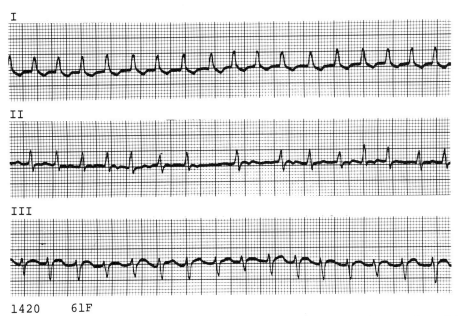

1420   61F

FIGURE 16–32. Atrial fibrillation with rapid ventricular response. The ventricular rate is about 180 beats/min. In leads I and III, the ventricular rhythm appears regular but is not.

Lead III   9:00 Am   2/3/69

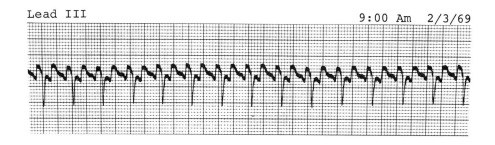

Monitor Lead   1:45 Pm   2/3/69

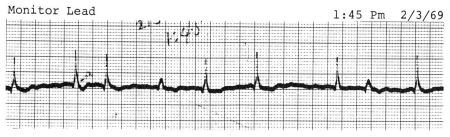

1714   68F

FIGURE 16–33. Atrial flutter and fibrillation from a 68-year-old woman. The upper strip shows atrial flutter with 2:1 conduction. The atrial rate is 300 beats/min, and the ventricular rate is 150 beats/min. Although no cardiac drug was given, the rhythm changed to atrial fibrillation a few hours later. The ventricular rate is much slower during atrial fibrillation. This decrease in ventricular rate probably is due to concealed conduction in atrial fibrillation. Ventricular extrasystoles also are present during atrial fibrillation. Because of the varying coupling time, the possibility of ventricular parasystole exists.

W.-P-W syndrome with atrial fibrillation
Lead II   Vent. rate 230

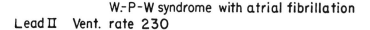

Simultaneous intracardiac lead and limb lead

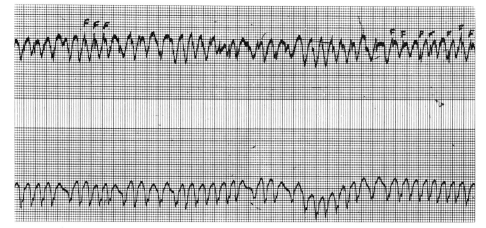

FIGURE 16–34. Atrial fibrillation in a patient with the WPW syndrome. The ventricular rate is 230 beats/min. The intracardiac electrogram shows the fibrillatory waves.

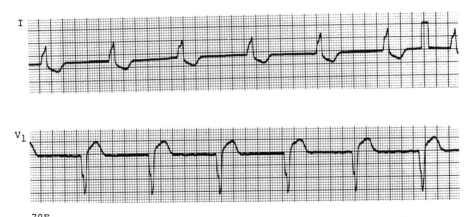

70F

FIGURE 16–35. Atrial fibrillation with complete AV block as a result of digitalis. The digoxin blood level was 3.4 µg/L. The lower pacemaker is junctional in origin, since the QRS morphology is the same as that before the development of complete AV block.

tem. An origin below the level of the His bundle is associated with abnormal and wide QRS complexes and slower ventricular rates. On the other hand, a rapid regular ventricular rhythm in the presence of atrial fibrillation may be due to AV junctional or ventricular tachycardia.

In most patients with atrial fibrillation, exercise accelerates the ventricular rate to a degree higher than that when the same patient is in normal sinus rhythm.[104] A dramatic example of such a response is given in Figure 16–36.

Ventricular Response in Patients Treated with Digitalis. In patients who have atrial fibrillation, digitalis increases the AV block and slows the ventricular response. There is a lack of correlation, however, between the blood level of the glycosides and the ventricular rate.[84] Generally speaking, the

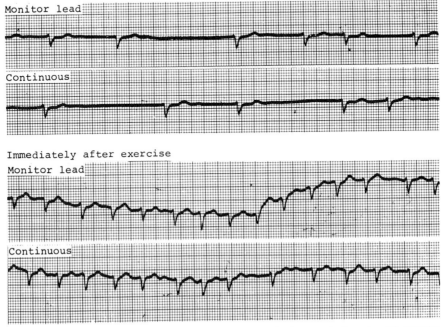

FIGURE 16–36. Atrial fibrillation with dramatic increase in the ventricular rate with exercise. The patient is a 29-year-old woman with no other evidence of organic heart disease. The control tracing shows atrial fibrillation with slow ventricular response. The ventricular rate increases from about 45 to 120 beats/min with mild exercise.

ventricular rate is easier to control in patients in clinically stable condition with chronic atrial fibrillation. The response is often unsatisfactory in patients in clinically unstable condition.[38] Postoperative patients and patients with fever, infection, pulmonary embolism, acute myocardial infarction, myocarditis, hypoxia, or thyrotoxicosis frequently maintain rapid ventricular response in spite of therapeutic or "toxic" blood level of the glycosides. Increased catecholamine release was thought to be responsible in these acutely ill patients.[38] As mentioned, patients with atrial fibrillation and the WPW syndrome or its variants may have a fast ventricular rate. Digitalis has no effect in the control of the ventricular rate, since the AV conduction is accomplished by the bypass fibers, which are not blocked by digitalis (Fig. 16–37). In some patients, the reason for the failure to control the ventricular rate is not apparent. In my experience, they constitute a major group of such resistant cases.

If the ventricular rhythm in patients who have atrial fibrillation and are receiving digitalis becomes regular, digitalis toxicity should be suspected. The regular ventricular rhythm,

depending on its rate, could be caused by (1) complete AV block with AV junctional escape rhythm, (2) complete AV block with idioventricular rhythm, (3) nonparoxysmal junctional tachycardia, (4) idioventricular tachycardia, or (5) paroxysmal ventricular tachycardia.

Differential Diagnosis

Atrial fibrillation may be simulated by the following arrhythmias:

1. Multifocal atrial tachycardia. In multifocal or chaotic atrial tachycardia, the varying morphology of the P wave and the changing PP, PR, and RR intervals without a dominant pacemaker result in a totally irregular rhythm. The identification of a P wave preceding each QRS complex avoids the error in diagnosis.
2. Paroxysmal atrial tachycardia with block.
3. Atrial flutter. In conditions 2 and 3, if the AV conduction is variable, the ventricular rhythm becomes irregular and mimics atrial fibrillation. In some patients with atrial fibrillation, however, lead V_1 shows a rather regular

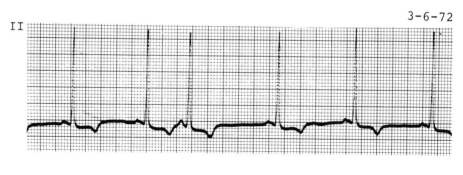

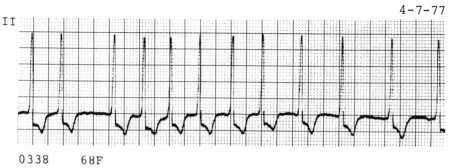

FIGURE 16–37. Atrial fibrillation with rapid ventricular response resistant to digitalis therapy. The patient had hypertensive and coronary artery disease. The tracing from 4-7-77 was recorded after large doses of digoxin were given and the digoxin blood level reached 4.6 μg/L. The ventricular rate remained above 120 beats/min. Previous tracing (3-6-72) shows a short PR interval of 0.11 second. The presence of an accessory pathway was suspected, which may account for the failure of digitalis to slow down the ventricular rate.

oscillation of the baseline. Furthermore, some patients may have atrial flutter–fibrillation or impure flutter as described previously.

4. Artifacts due to somatic tremors. This is particularly common in patients with parkinsonism. The frequency of the tremors is similar to the atrial rate in atrial fibrillation. The artifacts are most prominent in the limb leads. The sinus P waves usually can be identified in the precordial leads.

Clinical Correlation

Other than ventricular and atrial premature beats, atrial fibrillation is the most common ectopic arrhythmia.

The arrhythmia may be paroxysmal or established (chronic). In the paroxysmal variety, the episodes occur suddenly and last for seconds, minutes, or days. They terminate spontaneously but tend to recur and may ultimately become the established type. The duration of atrial fibrillation that is considered to represent the chronic variety varies from 1 or 2 weeks to a few months, depending on the authors.

Most patients with atrial fibrillation have other evidence of heart disease. In hospital populations, the most common cause is coronary artery disease, followed by rheumatic or hypertensive heart disease.[1] Atrial fibrillation is the most common type of supraventricular tachyarrhythmia in patients with acute myocardial infarction. Its reported incidence in this condition is about 7 to 16 percent when continuous monitoring is used.[25,66] Compromise of the SA node blood supply,[46] congestive heart failure, and cardiogenic shock have been proposed as the precipitating factors. One of the studies, however, showed that the incidence of this arrhythmia (and atrial tachyarrhythmias in general) was not related to the location of the infarction or the presence of power failure but was significantly higher in patients with pericarditis.[61] In patients with chronic coronary artery disease, atrial fibrillation is seen mostly in those with congestive heart failure. In the Coronary Artery Surgery Study (CASS), atrial fibrillation was found in 116 (0.6 percent) of the 18,343 patients with angiographically demonstrated coronary artery disease. The arrhythmia was seen more commonly in association with older age, male sex, the presence of mitral regurgitation, and congestive heart failure.[10] Atrial fibrillation and atrial flutter are observed frequently during the early postoperative period (mostly within the first 72 hours) in patients who underwent aortocoronary bypass surgery.[9,67] They occur in about 30 percent of these patients, atrial fibrillation accounting for most.

Atrial fibrillation is a common and characteristic arrhythmia in patients with rheumatic mitral valve disease. It is seen in about 33 to 42 percent of patients with mitral stenosis.[29,31] It has an apparent direct relationship to the size of the left atrium and the age of the patients (and presumably the duration of the disease) but not to the severity of the lesion.[31,82] In rheumatic mitral insufficiency, an incidence of up to 75 percent was reported in patients who required surgery or in whom the lesion was proved anatomically.[5,89] Mitral valve surgery itself seldom corrects the arrhythmia, and one third or more of patients with mitral valve disease and sinus rhythm preoperatively may have atrial fibrillation after surgery.[2,90] In acute mitral insufficiency of nonrheumatic origin (e.g., ruptured chordae tendineae, ruptured papillary muscle, and so forth), atrial fibrillation occurs in about 30 to 40 percent.[87,89] Aortic valve disease in general usually is not associated with atrial fibrillation until the disease is in its advanced stage with marked cardiomegaly.

The association of atrial fibrillation and hyperthyroidism is well known. It occurs in about 10 to 15 percent of the patients, many of whom have the paroxysmal variety.[92,105] It is seen predominantly in older patients with longer duration of the disease. Many of the patients have evidence of associated organic heart disease. It is uncommon in younger persons even if the hyperthyroidism is severe.

In 631 cases of idiopathic dilated cardiomyopathy reviewed by Flowers and Horan, 17.5 percent had either atrial fibrillation or flutter.[28] Atrial fibrillation was present in about one third of the patients seen by Fowler.[29] The frequency of this arrhythmia in the dilated type of cardiomyopathy is in contrast to the relatively low incidence of 3 to 10 percent seen in patients with the obstructive type of hypertrophic cardiomyopathy (idiopathic hypertrophic subaortic stenosis).[28,36] In hypertrophic cardiomyopathy, it is seen most often in the later phase of this disease. It is observed with variable frequency in the secondary cardiomyopathies.

In patients with chronic obstructive pulmonary disease with or without cor pulmonale, atrial fibrillation is usually a transient arrhythmia. It occurs mostly when there is intercurrent respiratory infections or respiratory failure. Transient atrial fibrillation also is seen in patients with acute pulmonary embolism. In one series of 60 proven cases, it occurred in 19 percent.[102]

Atrial fibrillation is relatively uncommon in acute pericarditis, especially in the absence of associated underlying heart disease. In the 100 consecutive patients studied by Spodick, 5 had atrial fibrillation and all had associated heart disease.[95] In contrast, it is common in patients with chronic constrictive pericarditis and occurred in 30 percent of a series of 67 patients reported by Levine.[59] Involvement of the SA node and the atrial musculature by the compression scar is believed to be responsible.

Among the congenital heart diseases, atrial fibrillation is seen primarily in patients with atrial septal defect, especially in older individuals. The overall incidence of this arrhythmia in this anomaly is about 4 to 9 percent, but it is 13 to 19 percent in the adult population.[100] Surgical correction of this defect does not necessarily have a favorable effect on the arrhythmia. Indeed, atrial fibrillation may appear for the first time after the surgery.

Although the most common arrhythmia in the WPW syndrome is AV reentrant tachycar-

dia, atrial fibrillation also occurs in a number of such patients. The AV conduction during the arrhythmia often is by way of the accessory bundle and is associated with abnormally wide QRS complex simulating ventricular tachycardia. The arrhythmia is usually more irregular, however, than that of paroxysmal ventricular tachycardia.

Atrial fibrillation may be the result of digitalis intoxication. Among the arrhythmias caused by digitalis, 10 percent is said to be atrial fibrillation.[45] In my experience, the incidence is much lower.

Paroxysmal atrial fibrillation may be the presenting arrhythmia in patients with the sick sinus syndrome. The latter should be suspected if the patients give a history of syncope. Treating the tachyarrhythmia without realizing the underlying problem may further increase the severity of the bradycardia.

Atrial fibrillation occasionally is seen in patients with the mitral valve prolapse syndrome (see Chapter 24).

IDIOPATHIC ATRIAL FIBRILLATION

Idiopathic atrial fibrillation also is called *lone* atrial fibrillation. It refers to those cases of

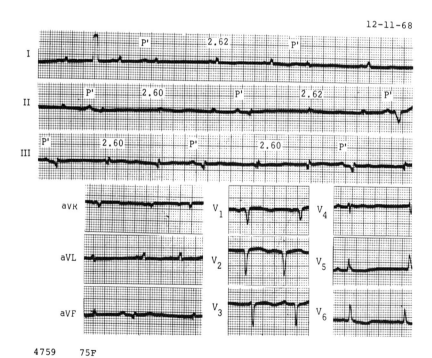

FIGURE 16–38. Atrial parasystole. The P's represent parasystolic atrial waves. They are all followed by a ventricular complex. The parasystolic rhythm has a rate of 23 beats/min. The voltage of the QRS complexes is small, and QS deflections are present in leads V_1 and V_2. The patient had myxedema with pericardial effusion. There was no evidence of myocardial infarction at autopsy.

ATRIAL DISSOCIATION

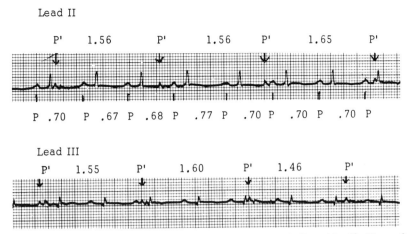

FIGURE 16–39. Atrial dissociation. The ectopic P waves are indicated by P′s. None of the P′ waves are conducted to the ventricle. The length of the P′P′ interval is more variable than that in atrial parasystole. The patient had an acute anterior myocardial infarction and died a few hours after this tracing was recorded.

atrial fibrillation that occur without any other evidence of organic heart disease.[56,74,76,78] In two population-based studies, 2.7 and 11.5 percent of the patients with atrial fibrillation belong to this group.[7,53] In one hospital-based report, 35 of 100 patients with atrial fibrillation did not have associated organic heart disease.[55] The arrhythmia is paroxysmal in most patients, often lasting for less than a day. It may be recurrent. The precipitating factors include heavy alcohol ingestion, nausea, vomiting, coughing, severe pain, physical exhaustion, or emotional disturbance. Indeed, heavy consumption of alcohol has been found to precipitate new-onset atrial fibrillation in patients with or without organic heart disease.[55]

ATRIAL PARASYSTOLE AND ATRIAL DISSOCIATION

Both atrial parasystole and atrial dissociation are rare. In atrial parasystole, the ectopic P waves (P′) are independent of the sinus activity (Fig. 16–38). The morphology of the ectopic P waves is often similar to that of the sinus beats. The coupling intervals vary. The interectopic (P′P′) intervals are mathematically related to each other. The atrial rate is usually slow and ranges between 35 and 55 beats/min. In most instances, the ectopic atrial impulse can be conducted to the ventricles whenever the latter are not in the refractory phase.[18,33] Atrial parasystole may be seen in individuals with or without heart disease.

In atrial dissociation, the ectopic impulse is

always limited to an area of one atrium. The ectopic P (P′) waves are small and bizarre and are never conducted to the ventricles (Fig. 16–39). The interectopic intervals are more variable than are those in atrial parasystole. It is always seen in patients with serious heart disease and often occurs a few hours before death.[16,17] One important exception is seen in patients who have had cardiac transplantation. A second set of P waves originated from the patient's own atrial remnant is dissociated from the P waves of the donor's heart. It also is important to exclude artifacts before the diagnosis of atrial dissociation is made.

REFERENCES

1. Aberg H: Atrial fibrillation. Acta Med Scand 184:425, 1968
2. Angelini P, Feldman MI, Lufschanowski R, et al: Cardiac arrhythmias during and after heart surgery: Diagnosis and treatment. Prog Cardiovasc Dis 16:469, 1974
3. Beder SD, Gillette PC, Garson A, et al: Clinical confirmation of ECG criteria for left atrial rhythm. Am Heart J 103:848, 1982
4. Bellet S: Clinical Disorders of the Heart Beat. Philadelphia, Lea & Febiger, 1971, p. 198
5. Bentivoglio LG, Uricchio JF, Waldow A, et al: An electrocardiographic analysis of sixty-five cases of mitral regurgitation. Circulation 18:572, 1958
6. Berlinerblau R, Feder W: Chaotic atrial rhythm. J. Electrocardiol 5:135, 1972
7. Brand FN, Abbott RD, Kannel WB, et al: Characteristics and prognosis of lone atrial fibrillation. JAMA 254:3449, 1985
8. Brodsky M, Wu D, Denes P, et al: Arrhythmias documented by 24 hour continuous electrocardio-

graphic monitoring in 50 male medical students without apparent heart disease. Am J Cardiol 39:390, 1977

9. Buxton AE, Josephson ME: The role of P wave duration as a predictor of postoperative atrial arrhythmias. Chest 80:68, 1981

10. Cameron A, Schwartz MJ, Kronmal RA, et al: Prevalence and significance of atrial fibrillation in coronary artery disease (CASS registry). Am J Cardiol 61:714, 1988

11. Castellanos A, Lemberg L, Gosselin A, et al: Evaluation of countershock treatment of atrial flutter. Arch Intern Med 115:426, 1965.

12. Cheng TO: Atrial flutter during quinidine therapy of atrial fibrillation. Am Heart J 52:273, 1956

13. Chiang BN, Perlman LV, Ostrander LD, et al: Relationship of premature systoles to coronary heart disease and sudden death in the Tecumseh epidemiological study. Ann Intern Med 70:1159, 1969

14. Chou TC, Ceaser JH: Ambulatory electrocardiogram: Clinical applications. Cardiovasc Clin 13:321, 1983

15. Chung EK: Appraisal of multifocal atrial tachycardia. Br Heart J 33:500, 1971

16. Chung EK: Parasystole, Prog Cardiovasc Dis 11:64, 1968

17. Chung KY, Walsh TJ, Massie E: A review of atrial dissociation, with illustrative cases and critical discussion. Am J Med Sci 250:72, 1965

18. Chung KY, Walsh TJ, Massie E: Atrial parasystole. Am J Cardiol 14:255, 1964

19. Cohen SI, Lau SH, Berkowitz WD, et al: Concealed conduction during atrial fibrillation. Am J Cardiol 25:416, 1970

20. Corazza LJ, Pastor BH: Cardiac arrhythmias in chronic cor pulmonale. N Engl J Med 259:862, 1958

21. Cosby RS, Herman LM: Atrial flutter and pulmonary disease. Geriatrics 21:140, 1966

22. Coumel P: Supraventricular tachycardias, In Kriker DM, Goodwin JF (eds): Cardiac Arrhythmias: The Modern Electrophysiological Approach. Philadelphia, WB Saunders, 1975, p 116

23. Craig RJ, Selzer A: Natural history and prognosis of atrial septal defect. Circulation 37:805, 1968

24. Delmar AJ, Stein E: Atrial flutter secondary to digitalis toxicity. Circulation 29:593, 1964

25. DeSanctis RW, Block P, Hutter AM: Tachyarrhythmias in myocardial infarction. Circulation 45:681, 1972

26. El-Sherif N: Supraventricular tachycardia with AV block. Br Heart J 32:46, 1970

27. Finkelstein D, Gold H, Bellet S: Atrial flutter with 1:1 conduction: Report of six cases. Am J Med 20:65, 1956

28. Flowers NC, Horan LG: Electrocardiographic and vectorcardiographic features of myocardial disease. In Flower NO (ed): Myocardial Diseases. New York, Grune & Stratton, 1973

29. Fowler NO: Atrial fibrillation. In Cardiac Arrhythmias: Diagnosis and Treatment, ed 2. New York, Harper & Row, 1977, p 65

30. Fowler NO, Gueron M: Conversion of atrial flutter with digoxin alone. Circulation 27:716, 1962

31. Fraser HRL, Turner RWD: Auricular fibrillation. Br Med J 17:1414, 1955

32. Freiermuth LJ, Jick S: Paroxysmal atrial tachycardia with atrioventricular block. Am J Cardiol 1:584, 1958

33. Friedberg HD, Schamroth L: Atrial parasystole. Br Heart J 32:172, 1970

34. Friedman PL, Brugada P, Kuck KH, et al: Inter- and intraatrial dissociation during spontaneous atrial flutter: Evidence for a focal origin of the arrhythmia. Am J Cardiol 50:757, 1982

35. Gilette PC, Garson A: Electrophysiologic and pharmacologic characteristics of automatic ectopic atrial tachycardia. Circulation 56:571, 1977

36. Glancy DL, O'Brien KP, Gold HK, et al: Atrial fibrillation in patients with idiopathic hypertrophic subaortic stenosis. Br Heart J 32:652, 1970

37. Goldberg LM, Bristow JD, Parker BM, et al: Paroxysmal atrial tachycardia with atrioventricular block: Its frequent association with chronic pulmonary disease. Circulation 21:499, 1960

38. Goldman S, Probst P, Selzer A, et al: Inefficacy of "therapeutic" serum levels of digoxin in controlling the ventricular rate in atrial fibrillation. Am J Cardiol 35:651, 1975

39. Goldreyer BN, Bigger JT: Site of re-entry in paroxysmal supraventricular tachycardia in man. Circulation 43:15, 1971

40. Goldreyer BN, Gallagher JJ, Damato AN: The electrophysiologic demonstration of atrial ectopic tachycardia in man. Am Heart J 85:205, 1973

41. Hall JI, Wood DR: Factors affecting cardioversion of atrial arrhythmias with special reference to quinidine. Br Heart J 30:84, 1968

42. Halmos PB: Direct current conversion of atrial fibrillation. Br Heart J 28:302, 1966

43. Harris BC, Shaver JA, Gray S, et al: Left atrial rhythm: Experimental production in man. Circulation 37:1000, 1968

44. Hinkle LE, Carver ST, Stevens M: The frequency of asymptomatic disturbance of cardiac rhythm and conduction in middle-aged men. Am J Cardiol 24:629, 1969

45. Irons GV, Orgain ES: Digitalis-induced arrhythmias and their management. Prog Cardiovasc Dis 8:539, 1966

46. James TN: The coronary circulation and conduction system in acute myocardial infarction. Prog Cardiovasc Dis 10:410, 1968

47. Johnson, JC, Flowers NC, Horan LG: Unexplained atrial flutter: A frequent herald of pulmonary embolism. Am J Cardiol 25:105, 1970

48. Josephson ME, Seides SF: Clinical Cardiac Electrophysiology. Philadelphia, Lea & Febiger, 1979

49. Josephson ME, Kastor JA: Supraventricular tachycardia: Mechanisms and management. Ann Intern Med 87:346, 1977

50. Katz LN, Pick A: Clinical Electrocardiography. Part I. The Arrhythmias. Philadelphia, Lea & Febiger, 1956

51. Kimball JT, Killip T: Aggressive treatment of arrhythmias in acute myocardial infarction: Procedures and results. Prog Cardiovasc Dis 10:483, 1968

52. Kones RJ, Phillips JH, Hersh J: Mechanism and management of chaotic atrial mechanism. Cardiology 59:92, 1974

53. Kopecky SL, Gersh BJ, McGoon MD, et al: The natural history of lone atrial fibrillation. N Engl J Med 317:669, 1987

54. Korst DR, Wasserberger RH: Atrial flutter associated with complete AV heart block. Am Heart J 48:383, 1954

55. Koskinen P, Kupari M, Leinonen H, et al. Alcohol and new onset atrial fibrillation: A case-control study of a current series. Br Heart J 57:468, 1987

56. Lamb LE, Pollard LW: Atrial fibrillation in flying personnel. Circulation 29:694, 1964

57. Langendorf R, Pick A, Katz LN: Ventricular response in atrial fibrillation: Role of concealed conduction in the AV junction. Circulation 32:69, 1965
58. Leier CV, Schaal SF: Biatrial electrograms during coarse atrial fibrillation and flutter-fibrillation. Am Heart J 99:331, 1980
59. Levine HD: Myocardial fibrosis in constrictive pericarditis: Electrocardiographic and pathologic observations. Circulation 48:1268, 1973
60. Levine HD, Smith C: Repetitive paroxysmal tachycardia in adults. Cardiology 55:2, 1970
61. Liberthson RR, Salisbury KW, Hutter AM, et al: Atrial tachyarrhythmias in acute myocardial infarction. Am J Med 60:956, 1976
62. Lipson MJ, Naimi S: Multifocal atrial tachycardia (chaotic atrial tachycardia). Circulation 42:397, 1970
63. Lown B, Levine HD: Atrial Arrhythmias, Digitalis and Potassium. New York, Landsberger Medical Books, 1958
64. Lown B, Wyatt NF, Levine HD: Paroxysmal atrial tachycardia with block. Circulation 21:129, 1960
65. Lown B, Vasaux C, Hood WB, et al: Unresolved problems in coronary care. Am J Cardiol 20:494, 1967
66. Meltzer LE, Kitchell JB: The incidence of arrhythmias associated with acute myocardial infarction. Prog Cardiovasc Dis 9:50, 1966
67. Mills SA, Poole GV, Breyer RH, et al: Digoxin and propranolol in the prophylaxis of dysrhythmis after coronary artery bypass grafting. Circulation 68(Suppl II):II-222, 1983
68. Mirowski M, Lau SH, Wit AL, et al: Ectopic right atrial rhythms: Experimental and clinical data. Am Heart J 81:666, 1971
69. Mirowski M, Neill CA, Taussig HB: Left atrial ectopic rhythm in mirror-image dextrocardia and in normally placed malformed hearts. Circulation 27:864, 1963
70. Morady F, Scheinman MM: Paroxysmal supraventricular tachycardia. Mod Conc Cardiovasc Dis 51:107, 1982
71. Morris JJ Jr, Estes EH, Whalen RE, et al: P-wave analysis in valvular heart disease. Circulation 29:242, 1964
72. Narula OS: Sinus node re-entry. A mechanism to supraventricular tachycardia in man. Circulation 50:1114, 1974
73. Oram S, Davies JPH: Further experience of electrical conversion of atrial fibrillation to sinus rhythm: Analysis of 100 patients. Lancet 1:1294, 1964
74. Orgain ES, Wolff L, White PD: Uncomplicated auricular fibrillation and auricular flutter. Arch Intern Med 57:493, 1936
75. Parkinson J, Papp C: Repetitive paroxysmal tachycardia. Br Heart J 9:241, 1947
76. Peter RH, Gracey JG, Beach TB: A clinical profile of idiopathic atrial fibrillation: A functional disorder of atrial rhythm. Ann Intern Med 68:1288, 1968
77. Peter RH, Morris JJ Jr, McIntosh HD: Relationship of fibrillatory waves and P waves in the electrocardiogram. Circulation 33:599, 1966
78. Phillips E, Levine SA: Auricular fibrillation without other evidence of heart disease. Am J Med 1:478, 1949
79. Phillips J, Spano J, Burch G: Chaotic atrial mechanism. Am Heart J 78:171, 1969
80. Pick A, Langendorf R, Katz LN: Depression of cardiac pacemakers by premature impulses. Am Heart J 41:49, 1951
81. Pritchett ELC, Smith WM, Klein GJ, et al: The "com-
pensatory pause" of atrial fibrillation. Circulation 62:1021, 1980
82. Probst P, Goldschlager N: Left atrial size and atrial fibrillation in mitral stenosis. Circulation 48:1282, 1973
83. Raftery EB, Cashman PMM: Long-term recording of the electrocardiogram in normal population. Postgrad Med J 52(Suppl 7):32, 1976
84. Redfors A: Plasma digoxin concentration: Its relation to digoxin dosage and clinical effects in patients with atrial fibrillation. Br Heart J 34:383, 1972
85. Rytand DA: The circus movement (entrapped circuit wave): Hypothesis and atrial flutter. Ann Intern Med 65:125, 1966
86. Rytand DA, Onesti SJ, Bruns DL: The atrial rate in patients with flutter: A relationship between atrial enlargement and slow rate. Stanford Med Bull 16:169, 1958
87. Sanders CA, Austen WG, Harthorne JW, et al: Diagnosis and surgical treatment of mitral regurgitation secondary to ruptured chordae tendineae. N Engl J Med 276:943, 1967
88. Sandler A, Marriott HJL: The differential morphology of anomalous ventricular complexes of RBBB-type in lead V_1. Circulation 31:551, 1965
89. Selzer A, Katayama F: Mitral regurgitation: Clinical patterns, pathophysiology and natural history. Medicine 51:337, 1972
90. Selzer A, Kelly JJ, Gerbode F, et al: Treatment of atrial fibrillation after surgical repair of the mitral valve. Ann Intern Med 62:1213, 1965
91. Shine KI, Kastor JA, Yurchak PM: Multifocal atrial tachycardia: Clinical and electrocardiographic features in 32 patients. N Engl J Med 279:344, 1968
92. Silver S, Delit C, Eller M: The treatment of thyrocardiac disease with radioactive iodine. Prog Cardiovasc Dis 5:64, 1962
93. Singer DH, Harris PD, Malin JR, et al: Electrophysiological basis of chronic atrial fibrillation (Abstract). Circulation 35–36 (Suppl II):239, 1967
94. Sobotka PA, Mayer JH, Bauernfeidn RA, et al: Arrhythmia documented by 24-hour continuous ambulatory electrocardiographic monitoring in young women without apparent heart disease. Am Heart J 101:753, 1981
95. Spodick DH: Arrhythmias during acute pericarditis: A prospective study of 100 consecutive cases. JAMA 235:39, 1976
96. Stemple DR, Fitzgerald JW, Winkle RA: Benign slow paroxysmal atrial tachycardia. Ann Intern Med 87:44, 1977
97. Strickberger SA, Miller CB, Levine JH: Multifocal atrial tachycardia from electrolyte imbalance. Am Heart J 115:680, 1988
98. Thurmann M: Coarse atrial fibrillation in congenital heart disease. Circulation 32:290, 1965
99. Thurmann M, Janney JG Jr: The diagnostic importance of fibrillatory wave size. Circulation 25:991, 1962
100. Tikoff G, Schmidt AM, Hecht HH: Atrial fibrillation in atrial septal defect. Arch Intern Med 121:402, 1968
101. Watson RM, Josephson ME: Atrial flutter. I. Electrophysiologic substrates and modes of initiation and termination. Am J Cardiol 45:732, 1980
102. Weber DM, Phillips JH: A re-evaluation of electrocardiographic changes accompanying acute pulmonary embolism. Am J Med Sci 251:381, 1966
103. Wells JL, MacLean WAH, James TN, et al: Characterization of atrial flutter: Studies in man after open

heart surgery using fixed atrial electrodes. Circulation 60:665, 1979

104. Wetherbee D, Brown M, Holzman D: Ventricular rate response following exercise during auricular fibrillation and after conversion to normal sinus rhythm. Am J Med Sci 223:667, 1952

105. Williams RH: Textbook of Endocrinology, ed 5. Philadelphia, WB Saunders, 1974, p 158

106. Wu D, Amat-Y-Leon F, Denes P, et al: Demonstration of sustained sinus and atrial re-entry as a mechanism of paroxysmal supraventricular tachycardia. Circulation 51:234, 1975

107. Wu D, Denes P, Amat-Y-Leon F, et al: Clinical, electrocardiographic and electrophysiologic observations in patients with paroxysmal supraventricular tachycardia. Am J Cardiol 41:1045, 1978

108. Zipes DP, DeJoseph RL: Dissimilar atrial rhythm in man and dogs. Am J Cardiol 32:618, 1973

Atrioventricular Junctional Rhythms

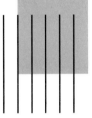

17

Electrophysiologically, the atrioventricular (AV) junction includes the specialized atrial fibers in the low right atrium or coronary sinus near the AV node, the AV node itself, and the bundle of His. The AV node can be divided into three regions: the AN (atrionodal), N (nodal), and N-H (nodal-His) regions. Evidence of automatic activity has been demonstrated from cells of the various parts of the AV junction except the N region of the AV node.[11,36] Because it is difficult to locate the exact site of the pacemaker in the different regions of the AV junction from the body surface electrocardiogram (ECG), and the N region does not contain pacemaker cells, the word *junctional* has now replaced *nodal* in the description of rhythms previously included under AV nodal rhythms.

The AV junction may become the site of impulse formation when there is depression of the SA node function or SA block and the effective sinus rate becomes slower than the inherent rate of the junctional pacemaker (35 to 60 beats/min). Such AV junctional rhythm represents an escape phenomenon and is called the *slow* or *passive* type of junctional rhythm. Similar escape mechanism also may occur when there is AV block. On the other hand, when there is an abnormal increase in the automaticity of the junctional pacemaker, the resultant rhythm usually has a rate faster than 60 beats/min. This is called the *active* type of AV junctional rhythm or junctional tachycardia.

When the ectopic pacemaker is junctional in origin, the activation of the atria proceeds in a retrograde direction unless there is AV dissociation or block. The P-wave axis is displaced superiorly, and inverted P waves are inscribed in the inferior leads II, III, and aVF. The ventricular depolarization usually is not altered unless aberrant conduction occurs. Because of the change in the temporal relation of the sequence of activation of the atria and ventricles, there is a change in the PR interval. The degree of the change depends on the lo-

cation of the pacemaker in the AV junction and the relative speed of antegrade and retrograde conduction.

ELECTROCARDIOGRAPHIC FINDINGS OF AV JUNCTIONAL BEATS (FIG. 17–1)

P Wave

The frontal plane axis of the P wave is generally between $-60°$ and $-80°$, in contrast to the normal axis of $0°$ to $+75°$. Therefore, the P waves are inverted in leads II, III, and aVF and are usually upright in leads aVR and I. In the precordial leads, the P-wave morphology is variable. Inverted P waves may be seen in none, some, or all of the precordial leads.

PR or RP Interval

The P wave of a junctional beat may precede, superimpose on, or follow the QRS complex. The terms *upper, middle,* and *lower* nodal beats were used to describe the above-mentioned P-QRS relationships respectively. The PR or RP interval, however, depends not only on the location of the pacemaker in the junction but also on the relative speed of conduction in the antegrade and retrograde direction. If the pacemaker is located at the upper part of the AV junction but is associated with retrograde conduction delay, the P wave may appear after, instead of before, the QRS complex. Therefore, these descriptive terms may be misleading as to the actual location of the pacemaker and should no longer be used in the interpretation of the body surface ECG.

In typical junctional beats the PR interval is less than 0.11 second. If the P wave comes after the QRS complex the RP interval varies and may be as long as 0.20 second. A PR interval of 0.12 second or longer may be seen if there is an antegrade conduction defect, and an excessive long RP interval is seen if there is a retrograde conduction delay. The P wave

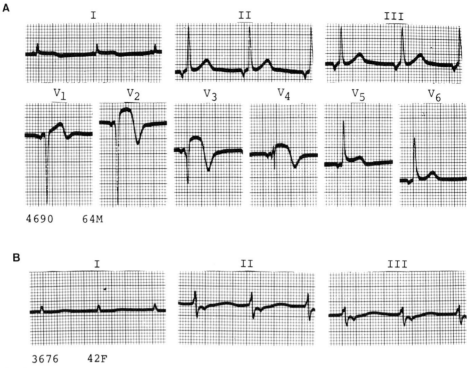

4690   64M

3676   42F

FIGURE 17–1. (A) AV junctional beats with retrograde P waves preceding the QRS complexes. The P waves are inverted in the inferior leads and all of the precordial leads. The PR interval is 0.10 second. The patient has an acute anterior myocardial infarction. (B) AV junctional beats with retrograde P waves following the QRS complexes.

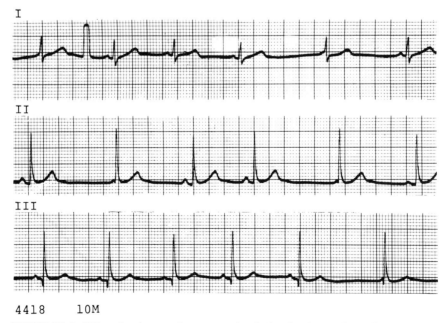

4418   10M

FIGURE 17–2. AV junctional escape beats occurring during the slower phase of sinus arrhythmia. The junctional QRS complexes are superimposed on the sinus P waves. The escape interval of the escape beats is 1.13 seconds.

may be absent when there is a retrograde block, and the QRS complex may be absent if there is a complete antegrade block. If there is a failure of conduction in both directions, no complex is recorded. In the absence of intracardiac electrograms, the presence of such a junctional impulse can be implied only by its effect on the impulse formation or conduction in the subsequent beat.

Ventricular Complex

In most instances, the sequence of activation of the ventricles is not altered in AV junction beats and the morphology of the QRS complex is unchanged from that of the sinus beat. Abnormal QRS complexes may be seen if there is preexisting intraventricular conduction defect, bundle branch block, or aberrant ventricular conduction. The latter may occur when there is junctional tachycardia or when the premature junctional beat has a short coupling interval.

PASSIVE AV JUNCTIONAL RHYTHMS

AV Junctional Escape Beats and Rhythm

AV junctional escape beats or junctional rhythm may occur under the following circumstances:

1. There is a decrease of the rate of impulse formation or conduction from the SA node. This is seen in patients with sinus arrhythmia (Fig. 17–2), sinus bradycardia (Fig. 17–3), sinus arrest, or SA block. Junctional escape beats may appear following the pause after cessation of supraventricular tachyarrhythmias.

2. There is a high-degree AV block at or proximal to the level of the bundle of His. The atrial mechanism may be sinus rhythm, paroxysmal atrial tachycardia, atrial fibrillation (Fig. 17–4), or atrial flutter.

3. Junctional escape beats may follow the postextrasystolic pause of an atrial or ventricular premature beat.

The morphology of junctional escape beats has been described previously. The retrograde P wave may precede, superimpose on, or follow the QRS complex (Figs. 17–5 and 17–6). If there is a slow sinus rhythm and the junctional impulse fails to be conducted retrograde to capture the atria, AV dissociation occurs (see Fig. 17–2). Occasionally, the sinus and AV junctional rates are similar, and the P and QRS waves are in proximity but unrelated to each other. This phenomenon is called *isorhythmic AV dissociation* (see Fig. 17–3).

The RR interval of the junctional escape beats is usually constant and varies less than

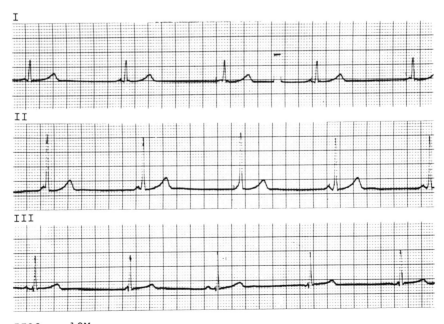

5792   18M

FIGURE 17–3. AV junctional escape rhythm in a healthy 18-year-old man with sinus bradycardia. The independent atrial and ventricular rhythms have similar rate. The rhythm is consistent with isorhythmic AV dissociation. In those beats with normal PR intervals, the possibility of sinus capture cannot be excluded.

II

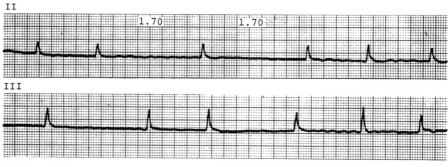

III

4665   31F

FIGURE 17–4. Atrial fibrillation in a 31-year-old woman with rheumatic mitral disease. The long pauses in lead II with identical cycle length suggest that the two ventricular complexes that terminate the pauses are junctional escape beats.

0.04 second. The rate of AV junctional rhythm is usually between 40 and 50 beats/min but may be as slow as 35 or as high as 60 beats/min (see Fig. 17–6). The ventricular rate in the same individual may or may not change. His bundle recordings in patients with complete AV block and narrow QRS complex demonstrated that the escape rate appeared to be related to the site of the junctional pacemaker.[32] In patients with heart rates between 45 and 60 beats/min, the impulses originated from the AV node. The ventricular rate increased with the administration of atropine. In patients with a rate between 35 and 45 beats/min, the pacemaker was located in the His bundle, and there was no significant response of the heart rate to atropine.

The morphology of the QRS complexes of AV junctional escape beats or rhythm is similar to that of the basic sinus or supraventricular beats. The QRS complex may be abnormal if there is preexisting intraventricular conduction defect. If the tracing during sinus rhythm is not available and the AV junctional rhythm is associated with an abnormally wide QRS complex, it may simulate idioventricular rhythm. Such a differentiation is often impossible from the body surface ECG alone unless some conducted supraventricular beats are recorded.

An interesting pattern of junctional escape is escape–capture bigeminy. The junctional beat is followed by a sinus capture that presents a group beating phenomenon.

I

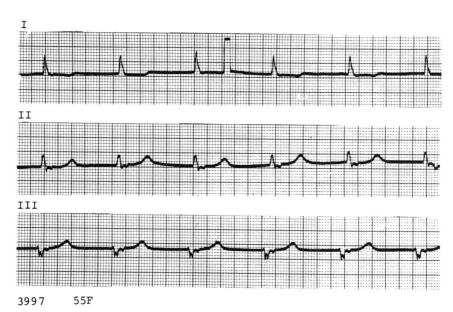

II

III

3997   55F

FIGURE 17–5. AV junctional rhythm with a rate of 53 beats/min. The retrograde P wave appears after the QRS complex.

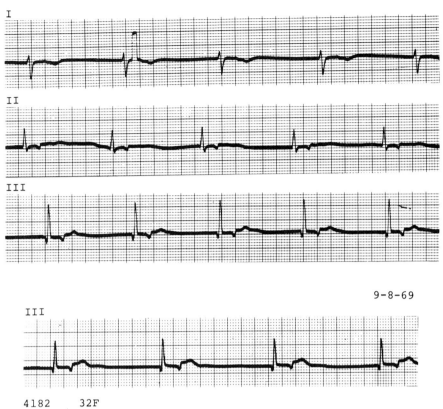

FIGURE 17–6. AV junctional rhythm in a patient with atrial septal defect of the secundum type. The RR interval in the tracing on 10-19-66 varies from 1.23 to 1.48 seconds. The tracing in 1969 shows longer RP interval and slower heart rate (36 beats/min).

Coronary Sinus Rhythm

Rhythm originated from the coronary sinus is characterized by retrograde P waves with normal PR interval. These findings have been reproduced experimentally in humans by pacing the interior of the coronary sinus.[16,17] Inverted P waves in leads II, III, and aVF with normal PR interval also can be produced by stimulation of the atrium at other sites.[35] Junctional impulse with antegrade conduction delay also may be accompanied by a normal PR interval. The term *coronary sinus rhythm* is no longer in common use and has been replaced by *low atrial rhythm* or *AV junctional rhythm.*[24]

Clinical Significance of AV Junctional Escape Beats and Rhythm

Because AV junctional escape beats or rhythm are a secondary phenomenon, they have the same clinical implication as that of the underlying primary rhythm disturbances. They often occur in a healthy person with sinus bradycardia (see Fig. 17–3). The ectopic rhythm is suppressed when the sinus rate is increased by exercise or other maneuvers. They may be seen in patients with various types of heart diseases that affect the SA or AV node (e.g., coronary artery disease). Drugs that suppress the SA node or impair the AV conduction may be accompanied by the appearance of junctional rhythm. Among the cardiac drugs, digitalis is the most common causative agent. In most instances, AV junctional rhythm is a transient phenomenon.

ACTIVE TYPE OF AV JUNCTIONAL RHYTHM AND JUNCTIONAL TACHYCARDIA

The following ectopic rhythms may be included in this group of junctional rhythm:

1. Premature junctional beats
2. Paroxysmal AV junctional tachycardia (AV nodal reentrant and automatic junctional tachycardia)

I

II

III

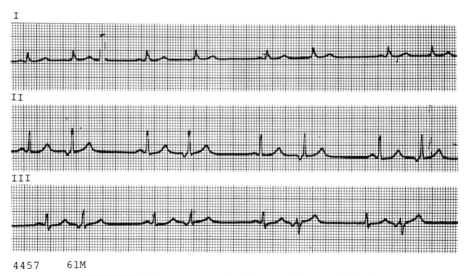

4457   61M

FIGURE 17-7. Premature junctional beats with bigeminal rhythm.

3. Nonparoxysmal junctional tachycardia (accelerated AV junctional rhythm)

Premature Junctional Beats (Premature Junctional Extrasystoles) (Fig. 17-7)

ELECTROCARDIOGRAPHIC FINDINGS

1. They are premature in relation to the basic cycle.

2. They have the morphologic characteristics of an AV junctional beat described in the beginning of this chapter.

3. They usually have a constant coupling interval. The premature junctional discharge is in some way related to, or precipitated by, the preceding sinus beat.

4. In most instances, the postextrasystolic pause is not fully compensatory. The retrograde conducted impulse discharges the SA node and resets its rhythmicity. The pause may be fully compensatory, however, if the SA node discharges its own impulse before the retrograde impulse from the AV junction arrives. If the sinus impulse occurs relatively early and depolarizes part of the atria before it meets with the junctional impulse, an atrial fusion beat is produced. The sinus node rhythm will, therefore, not be disturbed. Similarly, the sinus impulse may activate the entire atria and interfere with the junctional impulse at the AV junction. The junctional pacemaker, in fact, activates only the ventricles. Temporary AV dissociation occurs, and the sinus rhythm is not reset.

5. As in the case of premature atrial beats, premature junctional beats may occur at vari-

ous frequencies. They may appear in bigeminy, trigeminy, quadrigeminy, or in couplets.

DIFFERENTIAL DIAGNOSIS

PREMATURE ATRIAL BEATS. If the QRS complex is normal, the P waves are inverted in the inferior leads, and the PR interval is less than 0.12 second, the premature beat is, in all probability, junctional in origin. On the other hand, a retrograde P wave with normal PR interval may indicate either a low atrial or a junctional pacemaker. In the latter, the longer PR interval may be the result of antegrade conduction delay of the junctional impulse.

PREMATURE VENTRICULAR BEATS. Aberrant ventricular conduction may accompany premature junctional beats, and the resultant abnormal QRS complexes may resemble premature ventricular beats. If a retrograde P wave with short PR interval precedes the QRS complex, the diagnosis of junctional extrasystole can be made with a fair degree of certainty. If the retrograde P wave appears after the QRS and the RP interval is less than 0.11 second, the premature beat is unlikely to be ventricular in origin, since the interval is too short for ventriculoatrial (VA) conduction unless an accessory pathway is present. On the other hand, a longer RP interval does not exclude a junctional origin of the ectopic beat, because retrograde conduction delay may be present.

CLINICAL CORRELATION

Premature junctional beats are less common than are premature ventricular or atrial beats.

Lead II

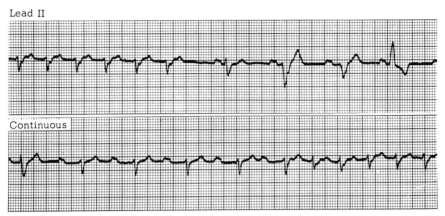

FIGURE 17–8. AV nodal reentrant tachycardia. The beginning of the rhythm strip shows paroxysmal junctional tachycardia with a rate of 132 beats/min. The retrograde P waves can be identified at the terminal portion of the QRS complexes. With carotid sinus massage, there is a temporary conversion of the tachycardia to sinus rhythm with abnormal P waves and first-degree AV block. The first five abnormal QRS complexes after the conversion are probably ectopic ventricular beats. AV nodal reentrant tachycardia reappears in the latter part of the bottom strip and is initiated by a premature atrial beat that is superimposed on the T wave of the preceding sinus beat.

They may be seen in normal subjects as well as in patients with organic heart disease. Isolated premature junctional beats usually do not have any significant hemodynamic effect.

Paroxysmal Junctional Tachycardia (AV Nodal Reentrant and Automatic Junctional Tachycardia)

Paroxysmal junctional tachycardia may be due to increased automaticity of a junctional pacemaker or AV nodal reentry. AV nodal reentrant tachycardia is the most common form of paroxysmal supraventricular tachycardia, whereas automatic junctional tachycardia is uncommon. Paroxysmal junctional tachycardia has the following ECG characteristics (Figs. 17–8 and 17–9):

1. Its onset and termination are abrupt. The episode may last for seconds, minutes, hours, or days.

2. The heart rate is usually between 140 and 220 beats/min, and the rhythm is regular.

3. The P-QRS complex has the morphologic characteristic of a junctional beat de-

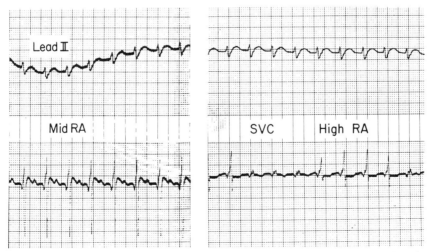

FIGURE 17–9. Paroxysmal AV junctional tachycardia. The P waves are superimposed on the QRS complexes. They are demonstrated by intraatrial electrogram taken simultaneously with lead II. Their amplitude is largest in the midright atrium. (Reproduced from Chou TC: Atrial and A-V junctional tachycardia. In Fowler NO [ed]: Cardiac Arrhythmias. New York, Harper & Row, 1977, by permission.)

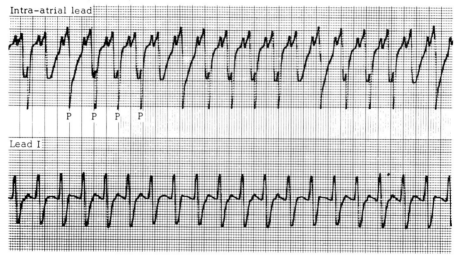

FIGURE 17–10. Paroxysmal AV junctional tachycardia with retrograde second-degree VA block and Wenckebach phenomenon. The gradual prolongation of the RP interval and shortening of the PP interval before block occurs are demonstrated by the simultaneously recorded intraatrial lead. Some of the P waves also can be seen, but less clearly, in lead I. The QRS complexes are wide, suggesting intraventricular conduction defect. The tachycardia is unlikely to be ventricular because of the short RP interval.

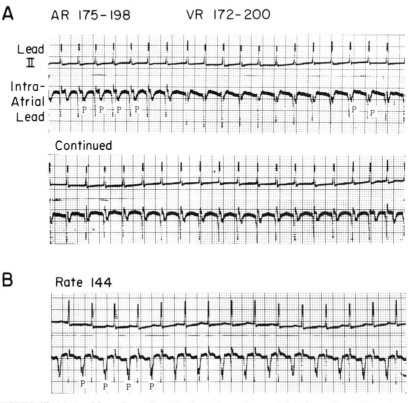

FIGURE 17–11. Double tachycardia. (A) The independent atrial tachycardia and junctional tachycardia are demonstrated by the intraatrial lead. (B) Paroxysmal atrial tachycardia only.

scribed previously. The P waves are inverted in leads II, III, and aVF. The P wave may precede, superimpose on, or follow the QRS complex. In most instances, the P waves cannot be identified, because they are masked by the QRS complexes or T waves (see Fig. 17–9). Partial antegrade or retrograde block may occur, usually presenting the Wenckebach phenomenon (Fig. 17–10). If there is a complete failure of retrograde conduction, AV dissociation occurs. If there is an atrial tachyarrhythmia coexisting with the junctional tachycardia and the two rhythms are independent of each other, the condition is called double tachycardia (Fig. 17–11).

4. The QRS complex may be normal or abnormally wide because of aberrant ventricular conduction or preexisting intraventricular conduction defect. A specific but uncommon type of paroxysmal junctional tachycardia is bidirectional tachycardia. Bidirectional tachycardia may be supraventricular or ventricular in origin.[1,2,23,28] In the former, the supraventricular impulses depolarize the ventricles

through alternate pathways (fascicles), resulting in QRS complexes of opposite polarities.

Although the mechanism of reentry in AV nodal reentrant tachycardia has been well documented by electrophysiologic studies,[9,13,15,22,40] the precise anatomic location of the reentrant circuit has not been delineated. Opinions differ as to whether the perinodal atrium is part of the circuit. The results of surgical treatment in some patients with AV nodal (or junctional) tachycardia suggest that one limb of the circuit connects the AV node or His bundle to the atrium.[4,29] The more prevailing view, however, is that only the AV node is involved. For the sake of simplicity, the latter view is presented here.

In patients with AV nodal reentrant tachycardia, there is functional longitudinal dissociation of the AV node into two pathways.[6,19,21] The two pathways, alpha and beta, have different conduction properties and refractory periods, but are linked by common pathways both proximally and distally[20] (Fig. 17–12).

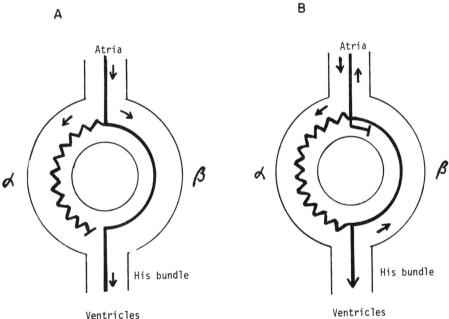

FIGURE 17–12. Mechanism for AV nodal reentrant tachycardia. (A) Diagram depicting the longitudinal dissociation of the AV node into two pathways, the slow alpha and the fast beta. A sinus impulse is conducted antegrade through the fast beta pathway to depolarize the ventricles. The impulse conducted slowly through the alpha pathway is blocked at the His bundle. (B) Diagram illustrating the conduction sequence when a premature atrial impulse arrives at a critical moment when the fast beta pathway is still refractory. It travels down the slow alpha pathway, which has a shorter refractory period, to depolarize the ventricles. As the impulse reaches the distal junction between the two pathways, the fast beta pathway is no longer refractory and is able to transmit the impulse retrograde and reexcite the atria. If it finds at the proximal junction of the two pathways that the alpha pathway is not refractory at this time, the impulse reenters and is conducted antegrade. A reentry circuit is established.

During sinus rhythm, the atrial impulse is conducted through the fast beta pathway to depolarize the ventricles. It also is conducted simultaneously through the slow alpha pathway but is blocked at the distal common pathway (His bundle), because the latter has already been depolarized and rendered refractory by the impulse transmitted through the fast pathway. AV nodal reentrant tachycardia may be initiated by a premature atrial or ventricular beat, the former being more common. If a premature atrial impulse arrives at the AV node when the fast beta pathway (with longer refractory period) is refractory, it is conducted slowly antegrade through the alpha pathway to activate the ventricles. Because of the prolonged antegrade conduction time in the slow pathway, the fast pathway is able to recover in the meantime and allows the excitation impulse to enter distally and be transmitted rapidly retrograde to depolarize the atria. If the retrograde impulse, on its arrival at the proximal common pathway, finds that the slow pathway is no longer refractory, it will travel antegrade and reexcite the ventricles. A reciprocal beat is produced (see Fig. 17–20). If such a sequence continues, a reentry circuit is established and a sustained tachycardia develops. The rapid retrograde conduction of the impulse results in almost simultaneous activation of the atria and ventricles. The retrograde P waves, which are inscribed as inverted P waves in the inferior leads, are superimposed or closely follow the QRS complexes. Therefore, in most cases of AV nodal reentrant tachycardia, the P waves cannot be clearly identified on the body surface ECG. Because the premature atrial beat initiating the tachycardia is conducted through the slow pathway, it has a prolonged PR interval.

In the uncommon and atypical form of AV nodal reentrant tachycardia, the excitation impulse is conducted antegrade through the fast pathway and retrograde, the slow pathway. Under such circumstance the retrograde P wave appears after the QRS complex with a long RP interval. Premature ventricular beat may initiate AV nodal reentrant tachycardia through such a mechanism.[12]

In both the common and uncommon types of AV nodal reentrant tachycardia, the arrhythmias may be terminated by carotid sinus massage (Fig. 17–13). The vagal stimulation causes further slowing and block of conduction in the slow alpha pathway. The reentry circuit is therefore interrupted.

Automatic junctional tachycardia also is called *junctional ectopic tachycardia*. Electrophysiologically documented cases of this arrhythmia are few in number.[8,40] Unlike AV nodal reentrant tachycardia, vagal stimulation has no effect on this rhythm. The rate of the tachycardia usually varies from minute to minute, whereas that of AV nodal reentrant tachycardia remains constant. AV dissociation is common in the automatic type. Ruder and colleagues described five cases of automatic junctional tachycardia in which the rhythm was grossly irregular, but His bundle potential was recorded preceding the QRS in each case.[30]

PAT Converted by Prostigmine and Left Carotid Massage

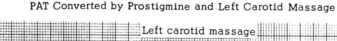

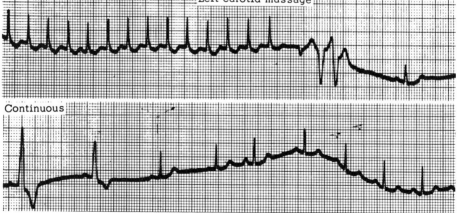

FIGURE 17–13. Termination of paroxysmal AV nodal reentrant tachycardia by carotid sinus massage. Note the appearance of ectopic ventricular triplet during the transitional period between the tachycardia and normal sinus rhythm. The reason for the first two abnormal QRS complexes in the bottom strip is unclear. It is possible that they are the result of bradycardia-related bundle branch block.

The arrhythmia may be mistaken as atrial fibrillation or multifocal atrial tachycardia.

CLINICAL CORRELATION

Paroxysmal junctional tachycardia, especially AV nodal reentrant tachycardia, is seen most often in healthy individuals without other evidence of heart disease. The rhythm also may be associated with coronary artery disease, hypertension, rheumatic heart disease, and hyperthyroidism, as well as with many other types of organic heart disease. Occasionally, it is associated with digitalis intoxication.

DIFFERENTIAL DIAGNOSIS

Paroxysmal AV junctional tachycardia should be differentiated from sinus tachycardia, other types of paroxysmal supraventricular tachycardia, atrial flutter with 2:1 conduction, and ventricular tachycardia. The subject was discussed briefly in the previous chapter under atrial flutter. The differentiation between paroxysmal junctional tachycardia with wide QRS complexes and ventricular tachycardia is often difficult. Additional discussion is given in the section on ventricular tachycardia. It is appropriate to summarize the various types of paroxysmal supraventricular tachycardia and their characteristics.

Paroxysmal Supraventricular Tachycardia

Paroxysmal supraventricular tachycardia is the most common type of paroxysmal tachyarrhythmia. It is usually so interpreted when the onset of the tachycardia is sudden, the rhythm is regular, the QRS complex is narrow and atrial flutter is excluded. Paroxysmal supraventricular tachycardia often is associated with wide QRS complexes due to aberrant ventricular conduction, preexisting bundle branch block, or ventricular preexcitation. For the sake of simplicity, the following discussion is limited to that with narrow QRS complexes.

Two basic mechanisms, namely reentry and abnormal automaticity, are generally recognized as being responsible for the genesis of paroxysmal supraventricular tachycardia. Electrophysiological studies in recent years[3,12,13,22,40] have demonstrated that paroxysmal supraventricular tachycardia may be produced by any of the following:

1. Sinus node reentry
2. Intraatrial reentry
3. AV nodal reentry
4. Reentry using an accessory pathway (the Wolff-Parkinson-White [WPW] syndrome)
5. Reentry using a concealed AV bypass tract
6. Enhanced automaticity of an atrial focus
7. Enhanced automaticity of an AV junctional focus

The recognition of the individual types of paroxysmal supraventricular tachycardia from the body surface ECG is usually difficult, but the separation is therapeutically important. Certain clues are, however, available. The morphology of the P wave, the relationship of the P wave to the QRS complex during the tachycardia, and the response to carotid sinus massage or other vagal maneuvers are often helpful in determining the underlying mechanism of the supraventricular tachycardia.

Sinus node reentry tachycardia is uncommon. It accounts for less than 5 percent of the cases of paroxysmal supraventricular tachycardia,[13] but an incidence of 17 percent was reported in one series.[10] It is suggested if the P waves during the paroxysmal tachycardia have identical morphology as those during normal sinus rhythm. Its rate is generally between 100 and 160 beats/min, with an average of 130 beats/min; this is slower than other forms of paroxysmal supraventricular tachycardia. The PR interval varies according to the rate and is usually longer when the rate is faster. Sinus node reentry tachycardia may be slowed and terminated by vagal maneuvers such as carotid sinus massage.[5,37,39]

Intraatrial reentry tachycardia is also uncommon and its incidence is similar to that of sinus node reentry tachycardia. Its rate is likewise relatively slow. The P waves have an abnormal morphology but are usually upright in the inferior leads. In contrast to sinus node reentry, it is not influenced by carotid sinus massage.

AV nodal reentrant tachycardia is responsible for about 60 percent of the cases of paroxysmal supraventricular tachycardia.[12,16] The P waves in AV nodal reentrant tachycardia are inverted in the inferior leads. In most instances (about two thirds) they are superimposed on the QRS complexes. In other cases, they appear immediately after the QRS complexes and rarely there is a long RP interval (see previous section). The rate of the tachycardia tends to be fast, ranging between 140 and 200 beats/min. As a rule, vagal maneuvers terminate the tachycardia.

In patients with the WPW syndrome and supraventricular tachycardia, the accessory pathway may serve as either the antegrade or the retrograde limb of the reentry circuit. In the former case, the ventricular preexcitation results in a wide-complex tachycardia. In the latter case (which is more common), the excitation impulse is conducted antegrade through the normal AV conduction system. The tachycardia has narrow QRS complexes. In patients with concealed AV bypass tract, the bypass tract is able to conduct impulses only retrograde. Therefore, the body surface ECG does not display any signs normally seen in the WPW syndrome (i.e., short PR interval, delta wave, and wide QRS complex). The QRS complex during supraventricular tachycardia is narrow. In supraventricular tachycardia associated with either the WPW syndrome or a concealed AV bypass tract, the P waves are inverted in the inferior leads and follow closely but are not superimposed on the QRS complexes. This relationship between the QRS and P waves is the most useful clue in the differentiation of tachycardia using a bypass tract from AV nodal reentrant tachycardia.[14] The rate of the tachycardia associated with a bypass tract is generally faster than that due to AV nodal reentry, ranging between 150 and 240 beats/min, but there is considerable overlap. Reentrant tachycardia using a bypass tract is often suspected when the rate exceeds 200 beats/min. Although supraventricular tachycardia is common in patients with the WPW syndrome, it is more frequently due to the presence of a concealed bypass tract. Concealed bypass tract is reported to be responsible for 15 to 30 percent of cases of supraventricular tachycardia.[7,38,39]

In paroxysmal tachycardia due to enhanced automaticity of an ectopic atrial focus, the morphology of the P wave depends on the location of the pacemaker. The abnormal P waves may be upright or inverted in the inferior leads, but they always precede the QRS complexes. The P wave that initiates the tachycardia has a morphology identical to that of the subsequent P waves, while it is not in reentry tachycardia. The rate of the automatic type of atrial tachycardia is relatively slow, usually ranging between 100 and 180 beats/min. There is often a warm-up period in the beginning of the tachycardia when, for several beats, the cycle length becomes progressively shortened until the ultimate rate is reached. The PR interval is greater than 0.12 second and may be lengthened, depending on the rate of the tachycardia. The tachycardia may be associated with AV block, commonly referred to

as paroxysmal atrial tachycardia with block. Although sustained paroxysmal atrial tachycardia due to increased automaticity is relatively uncommon and accounts for less than 5 percent of cases of supraventricular tachycardia,[13] short episodes of this tachyarrhythmia are frequently seen in the ambulatory (Holter) ECG. Vagal maneuvers do not terminate this type of supraventricular tachycardia even though they may produce AV block.

Paroxysmal supraventricular tachycardia due to increased automaticity of an AV junctional pacemaker is uncommon. A His bundle origin of an automatic ectopic tachycardia was identified in 2 of 79 patients with paroxysmal supraventricular tachycardia studied by Wu and co-workers.[40] The characteristics of the tachycardia are similar to those of ectopic atrial tachycardia.

Nonparoxysmal Junctional Tachycardia (Accelerated AV Junctional Rhythm)

The entity of nonparoxysmal junctional tachycardia was first described by Pick and Dominguez.[25] It also is often called accelerated AV junctional rhythm. There is an abnormal enhancement of impulse formation at the AV junction, but the arrhythmia differs from the more common paroxysmal variety in many aspects (Fig. 17–14).

1. The rate of the junctional discharge is only moderately increased, being about 70 to 130 beats/min instead of 140 to 220 beats/min.
2. The ectopic rhythm lacks the sudden onset and termination that are characteristic of the paroxysmal type.
3. Depending on the state of antegrade and retrograde conduction at the AV junction and the atrial and ventricular rates, various manifestations of rhythm disturbance may be observed. If retrograde activation of the atria occurs, a constant relationship will exist between the P wave and the QRS complex. If there is an impairment of the retrograde conduction, the atria will remain under the control of the sinus impulse. The independent atrial and ventricular activities result in AV dissociation. The ventricular rate is generally faster than the atrial rate except when nonparoxysmal AV junctional tachycardia develops in the presence of atrial tachycardia, atrial fibrillation, or atrial flutter.

Whereas paroxysmal junctional tachycardia is seen most often in patients without demonstrable heart disease, the reverse is true in the

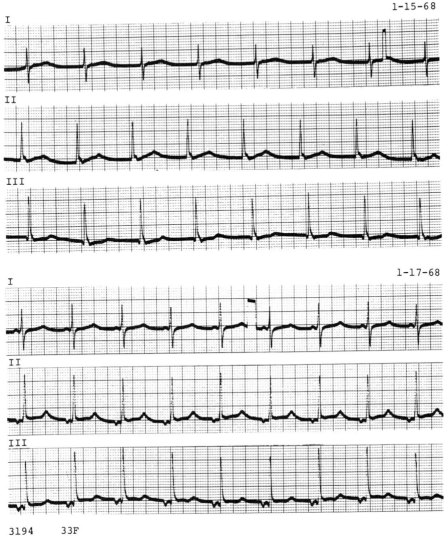

1-15-68

1-17-68

3194   33F

FIGURE 17–14. Nonparoxysmal AV junctional tachycardia related to surgery for the correction of atrial septal defect. The tracing on 1-15-68 shows the retrograde P waves appearing after the QRS complexes. The heart rate is 67 beats/min. The tracing of 1-17-68 shows the P waves appearing before the QRS complexes, and the heart rate is 77 beats/min.

nonparoxysmal form. The latter arrhythmia is most commonly the result of digitalis intoxication, acute myocardial infarction, intracardiac surgery, or myocarditis. Only in rare instances can the cause of the arrhythmia not be found. In the series described by Pick and Dominguez, digitalis was responsible for more than half of the cases.[25] Myocardial infarction and intracardiac surgery are probably the more common causes in recent years. The arrhythmia was reported in up to 10 percent of patients with acute myocardial infarction.[15] It is more commonly associated with inferior myocardial infarction, but it also occurs in anterior myocardial infarction. In the latter case, it is said to represent a poor prognostic sign.

Occasionally, there is antegrade exit block of the junctional impulse, and the ventricular rate becomes very slow. If there is a constant conduction ratio, the ventricular rhythm is regular and resembles the escape type of AV junctional rhythm. If the exit block is intermittent (Fig. 17–15), the duration of the long pause may be a multiple of that of the shorter RR interval, and the diagnosis of exit block can be deduced. In some instances, a Wenckebach phenomenon can be demonstrated, with progressive lengthening of the RR interval until pause occurs. Nonparoxysmal junctional tachycardia may resemble nonparoxysmal ventricular tachycardia if the QRS complex is wide and abnormal. In the latter case, the ec-

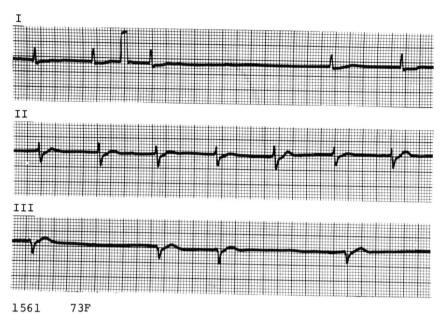

1561   73F

FIGURE 17–15. Nonparoxysmal junctional tachycardia resulting from digitalis toxicity. There is sinus arrest. The basic ventricular rate is 72 beats/min. The long pause in lead I has a duration approximately three times that of the basic RR interval. In lead III, the two long pauses have a duration of approximately twice that of the basic RR interval. These long pauses are probably due to antegrade exit block of the junctional impulse.

topic ventricular rhythm has a rate usually between 70 and 110 beats/min. The ventricular origin of the rhythm can be recognized if there are capture beats with narrow QRS or fusion beats (see Chapter 18).

AV DISSOCIATION

There is considerable disagreement and confusion about the definition of AV dissociation. In this text, the term *AV dissociation* indicates the following:

1. The atrial and ventricular activities are independent of each other.
2. The ventricular rate is faster than the atrial rate.
3. There is no retrograde conduction of the ventricular impulse to the atria.

Some authorities use the term in a broader sense to include also AV block, in which the ventricular rate is slower than the atrial rate.[24] Like others,[18] I prefer to separate AV dissociation and AV block into two distinct entities because the mechanisms involved are entirely different.

AV dissociation is always a secondary phenomenon that results from some other disturbances of cardiac rhythm. It may occur when there is a slowing of the sinus pacemaker or a failure of impulse formation or conduction from the sinus node. The atrial rate becomes slower than the inherent rate of the subsidiary pacemaker, which is usually the AV junction, but may occasionally be idioventricular in origin. AV junctional or ventricular escape rhythm develops. Alternately, there may be an increase in the automaticity of the subsidiary pacemaker, resulting in junctional or ventricular tachycardia. In either case, if there is retrograde block, the atria and ventricles become independent and AV dissociation is manifested.

AV dissociation may be complete or incomplete. The difference depends on whether there is antegrade conduction. In complete AV dissociation, both the atrial and ventricular rates (PP and RR intervals) remain constant, although the PR interval varies. None of the atrial impulses is conducted to the ventricles. In incomplete AV dissociation, some of the atrial impulses arrive at the AV junction at a time when the junction is no longer refractory and are conducted to the ventricles. Ventricular captures occur (Fig. 17–16). Premature ventricular complexes are present, and the basic ventricular rhythm is disturbed and reset. This phenomenon also has been called AV dissociation with interference, AV dissociation with ventricular capture, or interference dissociation.

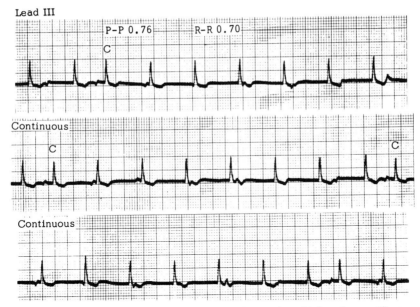

FIGURE 17–16. Incomplete AV dissociation or AV dissociation with interference. The ventricular rate is faster than the atrial rate. The RR interval remains constant except when ventricular captures occur (C).

Isorhythmic AV Dissociation

In isorhythmic AV dissociation, the rates of the dissociated pacemakers are nearly the same (Fig. 17–17). The P wave and QRS complex maintain a "flirtatious" relationship with each other.[18] When the relationship is persistent, it is called *synchronization;* if it is transient, it is called *accrochage.* The mechanism of the apparent synchronization is unclear. Based on experimental findings, it was proposed that the juxtaposition of the chambers may cause, by some undefined interaction, a synchronous discharge of impulse by the atrial and ventricular pacemakers.[33] Observation in patients with isorhythmic AV dissociation during surgery, however, suggested that

this phenomenon may be due to AV junctional rhythm with retrograde capture of the atria, but the retrograde P waves are not inverted in the inferior leads.[35]

Clinical Correlation

Because AV dissociation is always a secondary phenomenon, its clinical significance is determined by the primary disorder.

RECIPROCAL BEATS

Reciprocal beats (echo beats) occur when the impulse activates the chambers (either atria or ventricles), returns, and reactivates the same chambers again. The terms are used

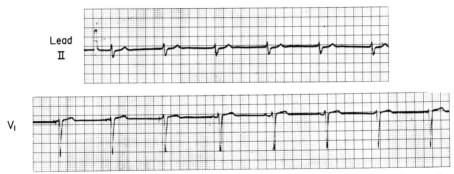

FIGURE 17–17. Isorhythmic AV dissociation. The nearly identical atrial and ventricular rates but unrelated P waves and QRS complexes are seen in lead V_1.

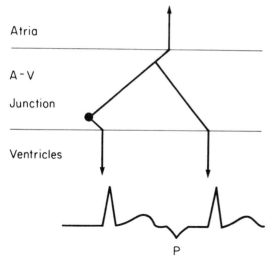

FIGURE 17–18. Ladder diagram illustrating the sequence of activation and the QRS-P-QRS pattern in reciprocal beat of junctional origin.

when the reentry phenomenon is limited to one or two beats. If the process continues, reentrant tachycardia develops. The impulses responsible for the appearance of reciprocal beats may originate from the atrium, AV junc-tion, or the ventricle. The fundamental requirement for the genesis of reciprocal beats is the existence of at least two pathways between the atria and ventricles. With the exception of the WPW syndrome, in which case an accessory bundle is present, the two pathways are located within the AV junction. They have different lengths of refractory period and speeds of conduction, resulting in longitudinal dissociation of the AV junctional issue.

Reciprocal Beats of Junctional Origin

The mechanism responsible for the development of reciprocal beats originating from the AV junction (Fig. 17–18) is similar to that of AV nodal reentrant tachycardia. The junctional impulse is conducted both antegrade and retrograde. The antegrade conduction results in ventricular depolarization and QRS complex. The retrograde impulse is blocked in one of the two junctional pathways and is conducted with considerable delay in the other pathway to activate the atria. During the course, it enters the previously unused pathway, which by now is able to conduct the impulse antegrade and activate the ventricles again, producing the reciprocal or echo beat.

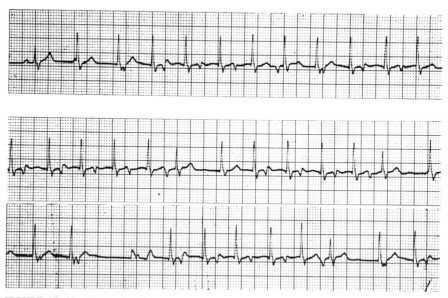

FIGURE 17–19. AV junctional tachycardia with retrograde Wenckebach and echo beats. The cause of the tachycardia is unknown. After the onset of the junctional tachycardia, there is a gradual prolongation of the RP interval. In the upper strip, the retrograde conduction is finally blocked following the eighth QRS complex. In the two lower strips, the gradual prolongation of the RP interval results in the appearance of reciprocal beats that are slightly aberrant. The slight variation in the RR interval in the tracing may be the result of some variation in the antegrade conduction time. The third complex in the bottom strip is a ventricular escape beat.

For the echo beat to occur, a long retrograde conduction time (RP interval) is necessary. Occasionally, a retrograde Wenckebach phenomenon with gradual prolongation of the RP interval occurs before the appearance of the reciprocal beat (Fig. 17–19).

ELECTROCARDIOGRAPHIC FINDINGS

1. The P wave is sandwiched between two closely grouped QRS complexes. It is inverted in the inferior leads.

2. The RP interval is longer than 0.20 second.

3. The PR interval (from the retrograde P wave to the second QRS) is variable but often prolonged.

4. The first QRS complex is the same as the basic QRS complex of the patient. The second QRS complex may be aberrantly conducted because of the relatively short RR interval.

Reciprocal Beats of Atrial Origin

The ECG shows a P-QRS-P pattern. The first P wave is the result of sinus or ectopic atrial impulse. The PR interval usually is prolonged. The second P wave or atrial echo is a retrograde P wave.[31] Ventricular echo may follow, and reciprocating (reentry) tachycardia may be initiated (Fig. 17–20).

Reciprocal Beats of Ventricular Origin
(Fig. 17–21)

The ECG of reciprocal beat originated from the ventricle reveals a QRS-P-QRS pattern. The first QRS complex is the result of an ectopic ventricular impulse and is, therefore, abnormal in duration and morphology. The P wave results from retrograde capture of the atria, and the RP interval is prolonged. The second QRS complex, the reciprocal beat (also called *return extrasystole*), is usually normal, because the return impulse follows the intraventricular conduction pathways. It may be ab-

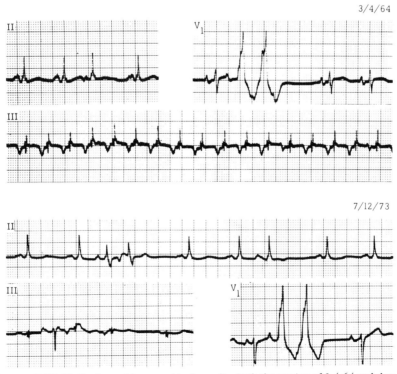

FIGURE 17–20. Reciprocal beats and tachycardia. Both the tracing of 3-4-64 and that of 7-12-73 demonstrate that the reciprocal beats originate from premature atrial contractions. The atrial echo in lead V₁ on 3-4-64 and all the leads on 7-12-73 are followed by a ventricular echo beat. Lead III of 3-4-64 probably represents reciprocating tachycardia, but its onset was not recorded. The ventricular complex of the echo beats is abnormal as a result of aberrant conduction.

#5059   9/29/70

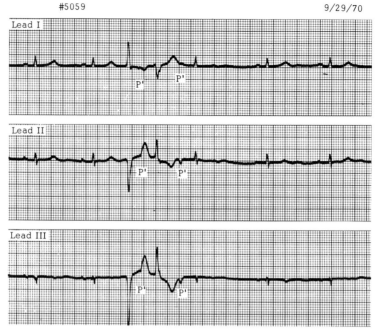

FIGURE 17–21. Reciprocal beat originated from the ventricle. The simultaneously recorded leads I through III show retrograde capture of the atria by the ectopic ventricular impulse, which returns to reactivate the ventricle, resulting in an abnormal QRS complex caused by aberrant ventricular conduction. Retrograde capture of the atria occurs again and is followed by another ventricular echo beat that is normal in morphology.

normal if there is aberrant ventricular conduction.

REFERENCES

1. Cohen SI, Deisseroth A. Hecht HS: Infra-His bundle origin of bidirectional tachycardia. Circulation 47:1260, 1973
2. Cohen SI, Voukydis P: Supraventricular origin of bidirectional tachycardia: Report of a case. Circulation 50:634, 1974
3. Coumel P: Supraventricular tachycardias. *In* Krikler DM, Goodwin JF (eds): Cardiac Arrhythmias: The Modern Electrophysiological Approach. Philadelphia, WB Saunders, 1975
4. Cox JL, Holman WL, Cain ME: Cryosurgical treatment of atrioventricular node reentrant tachycardia. Circulation 76:1329, 1987
5. Curry PVL, Evans TR, Krickler DM: Paroxysmal reciprocating sinus tachycardia. Eur J Cardiol 6:199, 1977
6. Denes P, Dhingra RC, Chuquimia R, et al: Demonstration of dual A-V nodal pathways in patients with paroxysmal supraventricular tachycardia. Circulation 43:549, 1973
7. Farshidi A, Josephson ME, Horowitz LN: Electrophysiologic characteristics of concealed bypass tracts: Clinical and electrocardiographic correlates. Am J Cardiol 41:1052, 1978
8. Garson A, Gillette PC: Junctional ectopic tachycardia in children: Electrocardiographic, electrophysiologic and pharmacologic response. Am J Cardiol 44:298, 1979
9. Goldreyer BN: Intracardiac electrocardiography in the analysis and understanding of cardiac arrhythmias. Ann Intern Med 77:117, 1972
10. Gomes JA, Hariman RJ, Kang PS, et al: Sustained symptomatic sinus node reentrant tachycardia: Incidence, clinical significance, electrophysiologic observations and the effects of antiarrhythmic agents. JACC 5:45, 1985
11. Hoffman BF, Cranefield PF: Physiological basis of cardiac arrhythmias. Am J Med 37:670, 1964
12. Josephson ME, Kastor JA: Supraventricular tachycardia: Mechanisms and management. Ann Intern Med 87:346, 1977
13. Josephson ME, Seides SF: Clinical Cardiac Electrophysiology, Philadelphia, Lea & Febiger, 1979
14. Kay GN, Pressley JC, Packer DL, et al: Value of the 12-lead electrocardiogram in discriminating atrioventricular nodal reciprocating tachycardia from circus movement atrioventricular tachycardia utilizing a retrograde accessory pathway. Am J Cardiol 59:296, 1987
15. Konecke LL, Knoebel SB: Nonparoxysmal junctional tachycardia complicating acute myocardial infarction. Circulation 45:367, 1972
16. Lancaster JF, Leonard JJ, Leon DF, et al: The experimental production of coronary sinus rhythm in man. Am Heart J 70:89, 1965
17. Lau SH, Cohen SI, Stein E: P waves and P loops in coronary sinus and left atrial rhythms. Am Heart J 79:201, 1970
18. Marriott HJL, Menendez MM: AV dissociation revisited. Prog Cardiovasc Dis 8:522, 1966
19. Mendez C, Moe GK: Demonstration of a dual A-V nodal conduction system in the isolated rabbit heart. Circ Res 19:378, 1966

20. Miller JM, Rosenthal ME, Vassallo JS, Josephson ME: Atrioventricular nodal reentrant tachycardia: Studies on upper and lower "common pathways." Circulation 75:930, 1987

21. Moe GK, Preston JB, Burlington H: Physiologic evidence for a dual A-V transmission system. Circ Res 4:357, 1956

22. Morady F, Scheinman MM: Paroxysmal supraventricular tachycardia. Part I. Diagnosis. Mod Cone Cardiovasc Dis 51:107, 1982

23. Morris SN, Zipes DP: His bundle electrocardiography during bidirectional tachycardia. Circulation 48:32, 1973

24. Pick A: AV dissociation. A proposal for a comprehensive classification and consistent terminology. Am Heart J 66:147, 1963

25. Pick A, Dominguez P: Nonparoxysmal AV nodal tachycardia. Circulation 16:1022, 1957

26. Pick A, Langendorf R: Recent advances in the differential diagnosis of AV junctional arrhythmia. Am Heart J 76:553, 1968

27. Rosen KM: Junctional tachycardia. Mechanisms, diagnosis, differential diagnosis and management. Circulation 47:654, 1973

28. Rosenbaum MB, Elizari MV, Lazzari JO: The mechanism of bidirectional tachycardia. Am Heart J 78:4, 1969

29. Ross DL, Johnson DC, Denniss AR, et al: Curative surgery for atrioventricular junctional ("AV nodal") reentrant tachycardia. J Am Coll Cardiol 6:1383, 1985

30. Ruder MA, Davis JS, Eldar M, et al: Clinical and electrophysiologic characterization of automatic junctional tachycardia in adults. Circulation 73:930, 1986

31. Schamroth L: The Disorders of Cardiac Rhythm. Oxford, Blackwell Scientific Publications, 1971

32. Scherlag BJ, Lazzara R, Helfant RH: Differentiation of "AV junctional rhythms." Circulation 48:304, 1973

33. Segers M, Lequime J, Denolin H: Synchronization of auricular and ventricular beats during complete heart block. Am Heart J 33:685, 1947

34. Waldo AL, Vitikainen KJ, Harris PD, et al: The mechanism of synchronization in isorhythmic AV dissociation. Circulation 38:880, 1968

35. Waldo AL, Vitikainen KJ, Kaiser GA, et al: The P wave and P-R interval: Effects of the site of origin of atrial depolarization. Circulation 42:653, 1970

36. Watanabe Y, Dreifus LS: Sites of impulse formation within the atrioventricular function of the rabbit. Circ Res 22:717, 1968

37. Weisfogel GM, Batsford WP, Paulay KL, et al: Sinus node re-entrant tachycardia in man. Am Heart J 90:295, 1975

38. Wellens JHH, Durrer D: The role of an accessory pathway in reciprocal tachycardia. Circulation 52:58, 1975

39. Wu D, Amat-y-Leon F, Denes P, et al: Demonstration of sustained sinus and atrial reentry as a mechanism of paroxysmal supraventricular tachycardia. Circulation 51:234, 1975

40. Wu D, Denes P, Amat-y-Leon F, et al: Clinical, electrocardiographic and electrophysiologic observations in patients with paroxysmal supraventricular tachycardia. Am J Cardiol 41:1045, 1978

Ventricular Arrhythmias

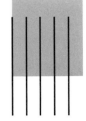

18

The ectopic location of the pacemaker in the ventricle alters the sequence of cardiac activation. The excitation impulse no longer follows the normal pathway of the intraventricular conduction network. There is asynchronous activation of the two ventricles. Consequently, the morphology of the QRS complex becomes abnormal, and the duration of the QRS complex is prolonged. ST-segment and T-wave abnormalities also occur as a result of secondary changes in the sequence of ventricular repolarization. The degree of the QRS, ST and T-wave changes depends, among other factors, on the location of the ectopic focus. A more bizarre ventricular complex is likely to be seen when the pacemaker is originated near the distal portion of the Purkinje network.

Atrial activation may or may not be disturbed, depending on whether ventriculoatrial (VA) conduction occurs. Retrograde P waves are seen if there is atrial capture. Otherwise, atrioventricular (AV) dissociation is the result.

Ventricular arrhythmias may develop as an escape phenomenon because of the failure of the sinus or supraventricular impulse to reach the ventricles at the expected time. The rate at which the impulse arrives at the ventricles is slower than the inherent rate of the ventricular pacemaker. These rhythms include ventricular escape beats and idioventricular rhythm. Ventricular arrhythmias also may appear as an active phenomenon because of enhanced ventricular activity. These include premature ventricular beats, paroxysmal ventricular tachycardia, ventricular flutter and fibrillation, nonparoxysmal ventricular tachycardia, and ventricular parasystole. The two suggested mechanisms responsible for this active type of ventricular arrhythmias are reentry and increased automaticity. The reentry theory proposes that there is a local area of impaired excitability and conductivity in the ventricular tissue (Fig. 18–1). The impulse of the basic rhythm is prevented from depolar-

izing this area temporarily but is able to activate the rest of the ventricles, resulting in a normal beat. Meanwhile, the previously refractory area has recovered and become responsive to the original impulse, which has now returned by a devious route. Its delayed activation generates an impulse that propagates and causes premature excitation of the rest of the ventricles with the appearance of premature ventricular beat. If the process repeats itself, ventricular tachycardia occurs. According to the theory of increased automaticity, there is an ectopic focus that contains pacemaker cells with subthreshold potential. The latter potential is enhanced by the impulse of the basic rhythm to reach threshold and precipitate an ectopic beat. The exact mechanism through which such an enhancement is accomplished is still not fully understood.

PREMATURE VENTRICULAR BEATS (PREMATURE VENTRICULAR CONTRACTIONS, PREMATURE VENTRICULAR DEPOLARIZATION, VENTRICULAR EXTRASYSTOLES, VENTRICULAR ECTOPIC BEATS)

Electrocardiographic Findings (Fig. 18–2 through 18–5)

1. They are premature in relation to the expected beat of the basic rhythm.
2. Ectopic beats from the same focus tend to have a constant coupling interval (the interval between the ectopic beat and the preceding beat of the basic rhythm).
3. The QRS complex is abnormal in duration and configuration. It is accompanied by secondary ST-segment and T-wave changes. The morphology of the complexes may vary in the same patient.
4. There is usually a full compensatory pause following the premature ventricular beats.

a.   b.   c.

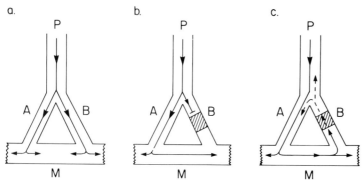

FIGURE 18–1. Diagrams illustrating the theory of reentry as a mechanism for the genesis of premature ectopic beat. (a) Activation impulse is conducted normally through the Purkinje fiber (P) and its branches (A and B) to depolarize the myocardium (M). (b) An area (hatched) of impaired conductivity and excitability in branch B, where the normal antegrade impulse is blocked. (c) This refractory area has recovered, however, when the impulse arrives later from the retrograde direction. Its activation generates an impulse that propagates (as indicated by the interrupted lines) and causes premature depolarization of the myocardium. Paroxysmal tachycardia occurs if the same process perpetuates.

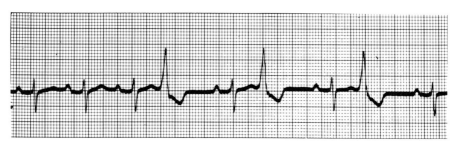

FIGURE 18–2. Premature ventricular beats. The tracing demonstrates the full compensatory pause after the premature ventricular beats. A short run of bigeminal rhythm is present.

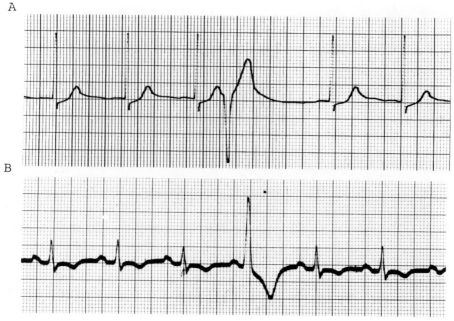

FIGURE 18–3. (A) Early premature ventricular beat with the R-on-T phenomenon. (B) Late or end-diastolic premature ventricular beat.

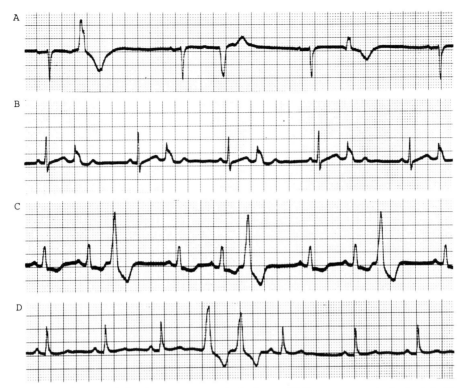

FIGURE 18–4. (A) Multifocal premature ventricular beats. (B) Premature ventricular beats in bigeminy. (C) Premature ventricular beats in trigeminy. (D) Premature ventricular beats in couplet.

5. Retrograde capture of the atria may or may not occur.

6. They may occur in various frequency and distribution pattern such as bigeminy, trigeminy, quadrigeminy, and couplets. Occasionally, they may be interpolated between two sequential normal sinus beats (see Fig. 18–5).

PREMATURITY AND COUPLING INTERVAL

The degree of prematurity of a premature ventricular beat is variable. It may be early and fall on the apex or descending limb of the preceding T wave. Such a presentation is called the *R-on-T phenomenon* (see Fig. 18–3A).

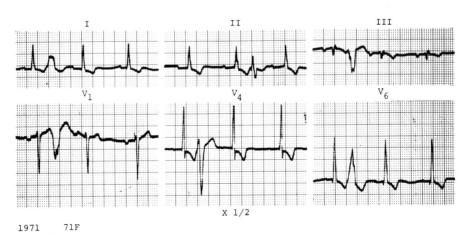

1971   71F

FIGURE 18–5. Interpolated premature ventricular beats. The premature ventricular beats have a left bundle branch block pattern, suggesting a right ventricular origin of the ectopic beats. The PR interval is prolonged after the premature ventricular beats, suggesting retrograde concealed conduction of the ectopic impulse in the AV junction.

The coupling interval of such a premature ventricular beat is short. A late premature ventricular beat may appear just before the next QRS complex of the basic rhythm. In patients with sinus rhythm, the premature ventricular beat may be inscribed after the P wave of the following beat, but they are unrelated to each other. Such a premature beat is often called an *end-diastolic premature ventricular beat* (see Fig. 18–3B).

The coupling interval of premature ventricular beats originating from the same focus (unifocal premature ventricular beats) generally remains constant. The variation usually does not exceed 0.08 seconds.[90] Premature ventricular beats with the same morphology but with marked variation of the coupling interval should make one suspect the possibility of a parasystolic mechanism (see the section on ventricular parasystole in the latter part of this chapter). Occasionally, the coupling interval may be influenced by the preceding cycle length.[141] A relatively long preceding RR interval is followed by a longer coupling interval. This phenomenon was attributed by Schamroth and Dolavo to a prolongation of the refractory period at the ectopic–ventricular junction, causing a delay in the exit of the impulse from the ectopic focus.[141]

QRS-T MORPHOLOGY

The altered sequence of ventricular activation due to the ectopic origin of the pacemaker changes the morphologic characteristics of the QRS, ST, and T complexes. The left and right ventricles are no longer being depolarized synchronously, and the QRS duration is, therefore, prolonged. If the ectopic pacemaker is right ventricular in origin, the ventricular complex has a configuration similar to that seen in left bundle branch block (see Fig. 18–5). A right bundle branch block pattern is seen when the ectopic focus is located in the left ventricle (Fig. 18–6). A superior frontal plane QRS axis under such circumference speaks for a location of the pacemaker in or near the posterior division of the left bundle branch and a rightward QRS axis in the anterior division of the left bundle branch. A basal location of the pacemaker is associated with essentially anterior QRS forces, and most or all of the precordial leads display an upright QRS complex.[133] An apical pacemaker gives rise to posteriorly oriented QRS forces and mostly negative QRS complexes in the precordial leads. If the ectopic focus is located high in the interventricular septum, the QRS complex is relatively narrow and simulates that of the sinus beat, since the ectopic impulse may

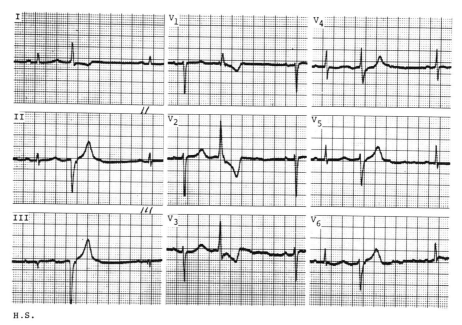

H.S.

FIGURE 18–6. Left ventricular premature beats. The ectopic ventricular beats have a right bundle branch block pattern.

enter the normal ventricular conduction pathway shortly after its origin (Fig. 18–7). Indeed, in patients with bundle branch block (especially left bundle branch block), premature ventricular beats often have a shorter QRS duration and more normal configuration than the basic complexes. This is probably because the ectopic focus is located distal to the area of block in the bundle branch. Its impulse is able to reach the conduction system of both ventricles in a shorter time. Electrophysiological studies using the technique of endocardial mapping in some patients with ventricular tachycardia have, however, cast some doubts as to the accuracy of predictions of the origin of the ectopic beats based on the body surface electrocardiogram (ECG), especially in patients with coronary artery disease.[71]

The duration of the QRS complex with ectopic ventricular beats is usually 0.12 second or longer, but a narrower QRS may be observed if the focus is high in the interventricular septum. Generally speaking, the complex is wide when the focus is near the peripheral part of the Purkinje network. It also tends to be wider when the coupling time is short, because the impulse conduction is likely to be more aberrant.

Premature ventricular beats with different QRS configurations usually indicate multifocal origin of the ectopic beats. Electronic pacing, however, has demonstrated that the QRS morphology may vary even though the site of stimulation is the same.[16] If the ectopic beats originate from different foci, their coupling intervals are usually different. If the premature contractions are late and end-diastolic, various degrees of fusion with the next sinus beat may occur because of the slight change in the sinus rate or coupling interval of the premature beats (Fig. 18–8). The changing morphology of the QRS complex naturally does not represent multifocal origin of the ectopic beat in such case. Another exception is when there are couplets. The morphology of the second QRS complex of the couplet may differ from that of the first because of the short RR interval resulting in additional aberrant conduction.

Secondary ST-segment and T-wave abnormalities occur in premature ventricular beats because of altered ventricular repolarization secondary to the abnormal depolarization process. The ST segment is depressed and the T wave is inverted if the major QRS deflection is upright. The ST segment is elevated and T wave upright if the QRS complex is essentially negative.

POSTEXTRASYSTOLIC PAUSE AND VENTRICULOATRIAL CONDUCTION

If the basic rhythm is sinus in origin, a premature ventricular beat is typically followed by a pause that is fully compensatory. The sum

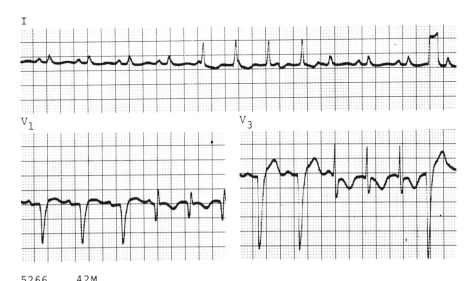

5266   42M

FIGURE 18–7. Ventricular ectopic beats with narrow QRS complex. The QRS complexes during sinus rhythm have a duration of 0.12 second and are consistent with left bundle branch block. During the short runs of ventricular tachycardia, the QRS complexes are narrow, with a duration of 0.08 second. The origin of the ectopic pacemaker is probably in the interventricular septum.

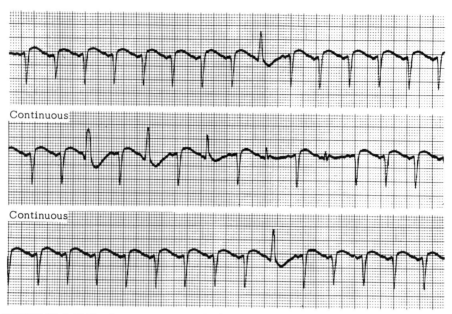

FIGURE 18–8. Unifocal premature ventricular beats with varying morphology owing to different degrees of fusion with the sinus beats. The varying morphology of the fusion beats simulates multifocal premature ventricular beats.

of the RR intervals that precede and follow the ectopic beat (or the RR interval that contains the premature ventricular beat) equals two RR intervals of the sinus beats. The fundamental requirement for a full compensatory pause to occur is that the sinus rhythmicity is undisturbed by the ectopic impulse. It is observed if one of the following conditions occur: (1) There is VA block. (2) There is a retrograde VA conduction and atrial capture, but the ectopic impulse is blocked at the sinoatrial (SA) junction. (3) The sinus impulse is discharged before the arrival of the ectopic impulse. The two excitation fronts may meet at the SA junction, in the atria, at the AV junction, or in the ventricles.

Because many patients have sinus arrhythmia, the RR interval that contains the premature ventricular beat may not be exactly twice the duration of the RR interval of the adjacent sinus beat, even though full compensatory pause does exist. If the ectopic impulse depolarizes the SA node and resets its rhythmicity, the postextrasystolic pause is no longer fully compensatory. Such depolarization of the SA nodal tissue by an extrinsic impulse may, however, temporarily depress its activity and a fortuitous "compensatory" pause may be observed.

In most instances, the P wave that occurrs during the time of ventricular premature beat cannot be clearly identified. It is masked by the QRS complex or T wave of the ectopic beat, which has a much larger amplitude (Fig. 18–9). The exact state of the VA conduction is therefore often difficult to determine by the routine ECG. With esophageal lead, retrograde VA conduction was demonstrated in 45 percent of patients with premature ventricular beats by Kistin and Landowne.[82] A much higher incidence of VA conduction (89 percent) was found during ventricular pacings in patients with normal antegrade AV conduction times.[55] Only 8 percent of patients with prolonged AV conduction time, however, showed VA conduction with pacing.

PATTERN OF PRESENTATION

Premature ventricular beats may occur in an isolated haphazard fashion. The frequency of the ectopic beats varies greatly not only among different individuals but also in the same subject at different periods of observation. Most authors use the adjective *frequent* when there are 5 or more premature ventricular beats per minute on the routine ECG but only 10 or 30 or more per hour by Holter monitoring.

Premature ventricular beats may appear in a pattern of bigeminy, trigeminy, or quadrigeminy (see Fig. 18–4). Langendorf and associates observed that, at times, the precipitation of a premature ventricular beat is

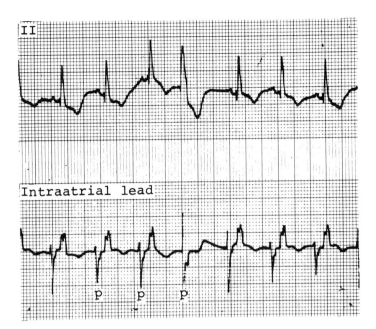

FIGURE 18-9. Premature ventricular beats (fourth complete complex) masking the P wave, which is revealed by the simultaneous intraatrial electrogram.

favored by a long preceding cycle (RR interval).[90] Furthermore, the compensatory pause of the premature ventricular beat, so precipitated, constitutes another long RR interval, which in turn favors the appearance of another premature ventricular beat. Therefore, there is a tendency for bigeminal rhythm to perpetuate itself. This phenomenon is called *the rule of bigeminy.*[90]

The term *complex premature ventricular beats* usually refers to premature ventricular beats that are frequent, or in bigeminy, trigeminy, couplets, multiforms, or on the preceding T waves (the R-on-T phenomenon).

Lown and Graboys proposed the following grading system for premature ventricular beats, which is commonly used for prognostic evaluation[98]:

Grade 0 = No premature ventricular beats
1 = Occasional (< 30 per hour)
2 = Frequent (> 30 per hour)
3 = Multiform
4 = Repetitive
A = Couplets
B = Salvos of ≥ 3
5 = R-on-T

Although higher grades of premature ventricular beats tend to imply more serious types of ectopic beats, the prognostic importance of the R-on-T phenomenon in relation to the other forms of presentation (e.g., repetitive beats) has been questioned.[11,24]

Interpolated Premature Ventricular Beat. An interpolated premature ventricular beat is sandwiched between two consecutive sinus beats without disturbing the sinus rhythm (see Fig. 18-5). It occurs mostly when the sinus rate is slow and the premature beat is early. The PR interval of the sinus beat following the premature ventricular beat is nearly always prolonged because of concealed retrograde conduction of the ectopic ventricular impulse, which renders the AV junction partially refractory to the closely following sinus impulse (see Chapter 19).

Differential Diagnosis

ABERRANT VENTRICULAR CONDUCTION

Aberrant ventricular conduction is a transient form of abnormal intraventricular conduction of a supraventricular impulse. It occurs when there is an unequal refractoriness of the bundle branches. A supraventricular impulse that arrives at an appropriate moment may find one of the bundle branches conductive and the other refractory. An abnormal ventricular complex is inscribed because of the resultant aberrant pathway. Because the right bundle branch has a longer action potential and therefore longer refractoriness, it is more vulnerable to conduction delay or failure than the left bundle branch. Aberrant ventricular conduction is usually seen when the supraventricular impulse arrives at the ventricular conduction system prematurely. Furthermore, the refractory period of the conduction pathway also is affected by the preceding cycle length. The refractory period is longer when there is a long preceding RR interval and vice versa.[110] Therefore, aberrant ventricular conduction is particularly favored when a premature impulse comes after a long preceding cycle length— the so-called Ashman's phenomenon.[57]

Aberrant ventricular conduction may occur with premature atrial beats, premature junctional beats, sinus tachycardia, and various forms of atrial and junctional tachyarrhythmias. For the reason stated previously, it may be expected that the QRS morphology has a right bundle branch block pattern in most instances. In patients with organic heart disease, however, left bundle branch block, as well as hemiblock patterns, are frequently observed. The various forms of aberrancy may be seen in the same individual (see Figs. 18–10 and 16–2). The degree of aberrancy also may vary. Different gradations of abnormalities may be seen in the same individual and are often related to the degrees of prematurity of supraventricular impulse. In an atrial pacing study of 52 subjects by Cohen and colleagues, multiple patterns of aberrant conduction were observed in 29 cases.[27] Right bundle branch block was in-

duced in 31 cases, right bundle branch block with left anterior hemiblock in 27, left anterior hemiblock in 14, left posterior hemiblock in 6, right bundle branch block with left posterior hemiblock in 7, and left bundle branch block in 6. In 40 cases of spontaneously occurring rate-dependent aberrancy reported by Fisch and co-workers, however, left bundle branch block patterns were observed in 32 patients, right bundle branch block in 4, and left anterior hemiblock in 3.[41] In 35 of the 40 patients, obvious organic disease was documented.

DIFFERENTIATION OF PREMATURE VENTRICULAR BEATS FROM PREMATURE SUPRAVENTRICULAR BEATS WITH ABERRANT VENTRICULAR CONDUCTION

If the basic rhythm is sinus in origin, the differentiation is easier but not always definitive. If the abnormal QRS complex is preceded by a *premature* P wave, the ectopic beat is supraventricular (either atrial or junctional) in origin. The absence of a fully compensatory pause further supports such a diagnosis. If no P wave can be identified, the ectopic focus may be located in the AV junction or ventricle. A fully compensatory pause following the pre-

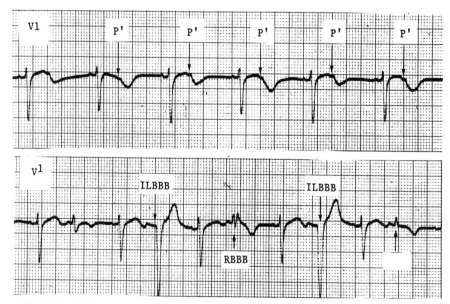

FIGURE 18–10. Bigeminal premature atrial beats, some of which are followed by aberrant ventricular conduction. In the upper strip, all the premature atrial beats are blocked. In the bottom strip, all the premature atrial beats are followed by aberrant ventricular conduction. Both left and right bundle aberrancies are present. The type of aberrancy in the second and last QRS complexes is uncertain. (Courtesy of Dr. Kenneth Gimbel.)

mature beat favors ventricular origin of the ectopic beat, but its absence does not exclude such a possibility, since retrograde depolarization of the SA node may have occurred. A normal sinus P wave may appear after the QRS complex in either premature junctional or ventricular beat if there is no retrograde atrial capture. If a retrograde P wave is identifiable after the QRS complex and the RP interval is less than 0.11 second, the premature beat is likely to originate from the AV junction, since the RP interval is too short for VA conduction unless an accessory pathway is present. A long RP interval of 0.20 second or longer is suggestive but not diagnostic of an ectopic ventricular beat, as the retrograde conduction time of a junctional beat is less likely to exceed this duration.[143]

The morphology of the QRS complex may be of some assistance in separating aberrant conduction from ventricular ectopy. The abnormal QRS complex is more likely to be due to aberrancy if its intitial forces are similar to those of the sinus beat and if it has a right bundle branch block pattern with an rSR' pattern in lead V$_1$.[139] On the other hand, if the QRS complexes in all precordial leads are either all positive or all negative, ventricular extrasystoles are more likely.[105] It should be emphasized, however, that, although these morphologic changes are helpful, exceptions occur frequently and the changes are not always dependable.

DIAGNOSIS OF PREMATURE VENTRICULAR BEAT IN THE PRESENCE OF ATRIAL FIBRILLATION

In the presence of atrial fibrillation, the differentiation of premature ventricular beats from aberrant conduction is more difficult and sometimes impossible from the body surface ECG alone. The absence of sinus P wave and the irregular RR interval of the basic ventricular rhythm are the obvious handicaps. In addition to the QRS morphology, the following findings may be useful:

1. A constant coupling time is suggestive of ventricular ectopy. Because the underlying ventricular rhythm is totally irregular, it is unlikely for all the aberrant beats to have the same RR interval from the preceding beats (Fig. 18–11).

2. The presence of the Ashman phenomenon is in favor of aberrancy. According to the rule of bigeminy,[90] however, a long cycle length also favors the precipitation of premature ventricular beats. Therefore, such a long–short cycle sequence is a useful, but not diagnostic, sign for aberrancy.

3. Ventricular ectopy is favored if the abnormal QRS complex terminates a short–long cycle sequence. It also is favored if, by comparison with the cycle sequence in the other part of the tracing, aberrancy is not expected.

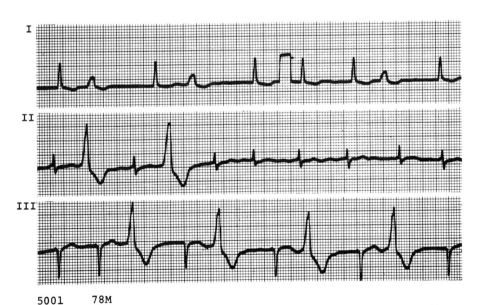

5001   78M

FIGURE 18–11. Atrial fibrillation and frequent premature ventricular beats with periods of bigeminal rhythm.

Clinical Correlation

APPARENTLY HEALTHY INDIVIDUALS

Premature ventricular beats are the most common arrhythmia in both normal subjects and patients with organic heart disease. They are less common in infants and children, but they increase with age. The reported incidence of this arrhythmia depends in large part on the method and length of the period of observation. Okajima and associates found premature ventricular beats in 2.8 percent of 715 normal adults by the conventional 12-lead ECG.[125] In 121,309 healthy men between the age of 16 and 49 years studied by Hiss and colleagues, premature ventricular beats were found in the routine ECGs of 0.77 percent of the subjects.[62] They are generally fewer in number and unifocal in origin. Only 3 of their 952 normal subjects with premature ventricular beats had multifocal beats, but it is well known that frequent and complex premature ventricular contractions may be seen in otherwise healthy subjects. According to Rosenbaum, premature ventricular beats in individuals with normal hearts almost always originate from the right ventricle.[133] They have a left bundle branch block pattern. The main QRS forces are directed inferiorly. In the horizontal plane vectorcardiogram, the QRS loop is inscribed counterclockwise, which is atypical for true left bundle branch block. He speculated that they may arise from the anterior papillary muscle of the right ventricle. In the 25 healthy subjects with frequent or complex premature ventricular beats examined by Kennedy and Underhill, a right ventricular origin of the ectopic beats was identified in 76 percent.[75] As mentioned, however, electrophysiological studies using endocardial mapping technique suggested that the determination of the site of origin of the ectopic beats by the body surface ECG may not be reliable.[69]

The prevalence of premature ventricular beats in otherwise healthy adults monitored with 24-hour ambulatory ECG ranged from 17 to 100 percent but most commonly from 40 to 55 percent[17,53,87] It increases with age. As a rule, the total number of premature ventricular beats is small. Complex ventricular ectopic beats may be present in 7 to 22 percent of the subjects and as high as 77 percent when older subjects were studied. A considerable variation in the number and complexity of the ectopic beats occurs from day to day and hour to hour in all age groups.

In normal individuals, premature ventricular beats may increase, decrease, or be totally suppressed by exercise.[67,75,107] They may be precipitated by exercise but not observed at rest. In the studies performed by McHenry and colleagues, 6 percent of clinically normal subjects had ventricular arrhythmias when they were exercised on the treadmill to increase their heart rate up to 130 beats/min.[108] The incidence of ventricular arrhythmias increased with increased degree of exercise, and 44 percent of the subjects developed arrhythmias when the heart rate was increased to more than 170 beats/min. The arrhythmias may appear during or immediately after exercise.

A relationship between premature ventricular beats and smoking or coffee, tea, or alcohol intake has not been established.[85] Generally, the frequency of premature ventricular beats decreases during sleep.[75,99] This is true for both normal subjects and patients who have heart disease.

CORONARY ARTERY DISEASE

Coronary artery disease is one of the most common causes of ventricular premature beats. The incidence of this arrhythmia in such patients differs at the various stages of the disease. It also varies depending on the length of the period of observation.

Chronic Coronary Artery Disease. Lown and co-workers found that in patients with chronic coronary artery disease without acute myocardial infarction, routine ECGs demonstrated premature ventricular beats in about 10 percent.[108] The incidence increased to 60 to 88 percent as the monitoring was increased to 12 and 24 hours, respectively. Other studies using 6- to 24-hour recordings showed similar results, the incidence varying between 75 and 90 percent.[11] In Lown's series of 184 patients with clinical evidence of coronary artery disease monitored for 24 hours, 17 percent had occasional isolated premature ventricular beats, 6 percent had premature ventricular beats of more than 1 beat/min, 25 percent had multifocal premature ventricular beats, and 27 percent had couplets. Salvos of 3 or more beats were observed in 14 percent.[96]

To study the relationship of ventricular arrhythmias and coronary angiographic results, Amsterdam and associates found frequent or complex ventricular ectopic beats in 11 percent of normal subjects but in 68 percent of those with significant coronary arterial lesions.[4] In 102 ambulatory patients with coronary artery disease, Amsterdam and associates found the frequency of complex premature ventricular beats increased as the number of significantly obstructed vessels increased.[3] Forty percent of patients with one-vessel, 53 percent of patients with two-vessel, and 78 percent with three-vessel disease had this type of ventricular arrhythmia.

Patients with coronary artery disease are more prone to develop ventricular arrhythmias with exercise. The incidence of such arrhythmias in these patients is more than four times that of the age-matched normal subjects when comparative heart rate is reached.[108] The incidence of complex ventricular arrhythmias also is higher in the patients with coronary artery disease. Patients with three-vessel disease and abnormal left ventricular wall motion have a significantly greater incidence of exercise-induced ventricular arrhythmias. Most investigators agree, however, that exercise-induced ventricular arrhythmias are of questionable value in the prediction of subsequent ischemic heart disease.[14,40,48]

Acute Myocardial Infarction. The reported incidence of premature ventricular contractions in acute myocardial infarction varies considerably. The variation probably results from the different methods of monitoring. With continuous recording, ventricular ectopic beats can be detected in all such patients.[115,132] In 32 patients, Romhilt and colleagues detected ventricular arrhythmias in 64.5 percent by the conventional oscilloscopic monitoring but in 100 percent with continuous recording and automated analysis system.[132]

In the prehospital phase of acute myocardial infarction, Pantridge and associates, using oscilloscopic monitoring in their mobile unit, detected ventricular ectopic beats in 58 percent of their 294 patients in the first hour and in 93 percent by 4 hours.[127] In the coronary care unit to which the patients were usually admitted several hours after the clinical onset of infarction, the reported incidence of premature ventricular beats ranged from 34 to 100 percent.[13] In Morgensen's series of 421 patients, all had some premature ventricular beats and 34 percent had complex ventricular arrhythmias, including frequent (more than 5 beats/min), paired, multifocal, or R-on-T premature ventricular beats by continuous oscilloscopic monitoring.[115] In 37 of their unselected patients with continuous ECG printout,

however, 81 percent had these types of ventricular arrhythmias.[115] After the initial 6 hours, the frequency of ventricular arrhythmias decreases.[11] The persistence of frequent and complex ventricular arrhythmias usually is associated with larger infarction size,[2] as determined by serial CPK enzyme measurements. Using radionuclide scanning technique for the determination of left ventricular function in patients 14 to 28 days after acute myocardial infarction, Schulze and co-workers reported a mean ejection fraction of about 50 percent in those patients with no or rare premature ventricular contractions and a value of about 30 percent in those with frequent or complex premature ventricular beats.[145]

OTHER ORGANIC HEART DISEASES

Premature ventricular beats also are commonly encountered in patients with other types of organic heart disease, including hypertensive and rheumatic heart disease and cardiomyopathies. In patients with rheumatic or valvular heart disease, ventricular arrhythmias are seen most often when there is cardiac enlargement or congestive heart failure. About 12 percent of patients with primary myocardial disease of the congestive variety display ventricular arrhythmias on their routine ECGs, whereas the arrhythmias occur only in about 1.6 percent of patients with obstructive cardiomyopathy.[43]

Premature ventricular beats are the most common arrhythmia in patients with the mitral valve prolapse syndrome. They are seen in about one third of the routine ECGs of these patients.[34] Ambulatory ECG monitoring by Winkle and associates revealed even higher incidence, with 50 percent of the patients showing frequent premature ventricular beats (defined by them as more than 425 beats in 24 hours) and another 25 percent exhibiting occasional premature ventricular beats.[172] Because these data were obtained from hospital-based studies and asymptomatic subjects are less likely to be included, the actual incidence of premature ventricular beats in this syndrome may be lower.

DRUGS

Frequent premature ventricular beats are also the most common arrhythmia in patients with digitalis excess. They account for about half of the arrhythmias induced by the drug.[23] They are often multifocal or bigeminal. Other drugs that may cause ventricular premature beats include quinidine, procainamide, disopyramide, other antiarrhythmic drugs, phenothiazine, and tricyclic antidepressants.

ELECTROLYTE IMBALANCE

Among electrolyte imbalances, hypokalemia is frequently associated with the appearance of ventricular arrhythmias. Although the arrhythmias occur most commonly in patients who also are receiving digitalis, they may be precipitated by hypokalemia alone.[63] Hypomagnesemia, which often is present in association with hypokalemia in patients receiving diuretic therapy, also may cause ventricular arrhythmias. Hypercalcemia also is known to induce ventricular ectopic beats as well as to potentiate the arrhythmogenic effect of digitalis.

Prognostic Significance

The prognostic significance of premature ventricular beats depends mainly on the type of population involved. Rodstein and others studied the mortality of 712 insured persons with extrasystoles in their routine ECGs who were followed for an average of 18 years.[131] There was no significant increase in the mortality of individuals with ventricular extrasystoles but without other evidence of cardiac abnormalities or hypertension. Their life expectancy was normal whether the subjects had simple or complex premature ventricular beats. There also was no appreciable difference in mortality when those under 40 and those 40 years of age and over at the time of discovery of the extrasystoles were compared. On the other hand, premature ventricular beats in the presence of other cardiac abnormalities or hypertension were associated with a mortality of more than twice that expected.

In the Tecumseh epidemiologic study, persons over the age of 30 years with premature ventricular beats on routine ECG had a significant increase in the incidence of sudden death.[21] A correlation also was noted, however, between the occurrence of premature beats and coronary artery disease in these individuals. It is, therefore, uncertain whether the premature ventricular beats can be considered an independent risk factor for sudden death.

Bleifer and co-workers studied 1281 consecutive unselected patients with symptoms of palpitations, weakness, syncope, seizures, and undiagnosed chest discomfort.[15] Ten-hour Holter monitoring was used, and the relation between the premature ventricular beats and the development of ventricular tachycardia was determined. The incidence of ventricular tachycardia was significantly higher in patients with unifocal premature ventricular beats of greater than 12 beats/min, couplets, and premature ventricular beats from multiple foci. This was particularly true when both couplets and R-on-T phenomenon occurred but not when the R-on-T phenomenon was present alone.

In patients with acute myocardial infarction, the association of frequent or complex premature ventricular beats and the development of ventricular tachycardia or fibrillation is well recognized.[97] Studies performed many years ago showed that the in-hospital mortality of patients with acute myocardial infarction and frequent or complex ventricular ectopic beats varied between 23 and 71 percent.[73,92,115] More recent observations indicate that the occurrence of complex ventricular ectopic beats in the acute phase of myocardial infarction does not appear to have any prognostic implications.[31] Their presence 2 or 3 weeks after the acute phase of myocardial infarction is, however, associated with increased risk of sudden death. In three large series of patients with acute myocardial infarction examined before their hospital discharge and followed for 1 to 3 years, the presence of complex ventricular arrhythmias increased the risk of sudden death by about threefold.[11,85,116]

The increased risk of sudden death also is found in patients who have the arrhythmias several months after their myocardial infarction.[87,137,163] In the Coronary Drug Project among 2035 survivors of myocardial infarction, 234 had one or more premature ventricular beats in their resting baseline 12-lead ECGs.[28] During a 3-year follow-up period, mortality was nearly twice as great among those with any premature ventricular beats (21.7 percent) compared with those with none (11.4 percent). The relation of premature ventricular beats to the risk of death, including sudden death, was independent of other clinical factors bearing on prognosis.

Ruberman and colleagues followed 416 men with effort angina but without recent or previous myocardial infarction for 5 years.[136] The mortality among those men with complex ventricular premature beats was about 30 percent, as compared with about 10 percent in those without arrhythmias. The mortality in men with simple premature ventricular beats also was increased but to a lesser extent.

VENTRICULAR PARASYSTOLE

In ventricular parasystole, there is an ectopic ventricular pacemaker that activates the ventricles concurrently with, but independent of, the impulse of the basic rhythm. The ectopic parasystolic focus is protected from the impulse of the basic rhythm because of the presence of an entrance block in its immediate vicinity. Its own impulse, however, is able to depolarize the ventricles whenever they are not refractory. Because its rhythmicity is unrelated to the basic rhythm, increased automaticity of an ectopic focus instead of reentry is the probable underlying mechanism.

Electrocardiographic Findings in Ventricular Parasystole (Fig. 18–12)

1. Varying coupling intervals
2. RR intervals of the ectopic beats being mathematically related to each other
3. The presence of fusion beats

VARYING COUPLING INTERVALS

The most prominent feature of ventricular parasystole is the variation of the coupling intervals. In the usual form of premature ventricular extrasystoles, the coupling intervals of the ectopic beats that have the same QRS morphology remain constant. In ventricular parasystole, such ectopic beats may appear early or late in the cycle. This finding usually alerts the interpreter and leads to the diagnosis of parasystole. The basic rhythm is usually sinus in origin but may be atrial fibrillation or, rarely, ectopic ventricular rhythm.

RR INTERVALS

The interectopic interval in ventricular parasystole is variable. Although the ectopic focus discharges its impulses regularly, only those that find the ventricles responsive are manifested electrocardiographically. Therefore, a mathematical relationship can be found between the longer and shorter intervals. The longer intervals are the multiples of the shortest interval, or a common denominator can be calculated between the various intervals. The ratio between the various intervals, however, is seldom in exact whole numbers (e.g., 2:1, 3:1, or 3:2). A difference of a few hundredths of a second is the usual finding, and the parasystolic cycle length, calculated by dividing the longer intervals, tends to be shorter than the basic interval measured directly.[25,142,166] Oreto and co-workers, noting that the interectopic intervals are more or less irregular in most cases of ventricular parasystole, suggested the following possible mechanisms responsible for the irregularity: (1) spontaneous variations of the parasystolic cycle, (2) autonomic nervous tone or hormonal factors that affect the ectopic cycle, (3) variation in the conduction time from the ectopic focus to

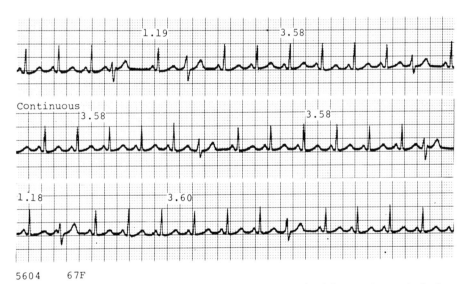

5604   67F

FIGURE 18–12. Ventricular parasystole. The coupling intervals of the ectopic ventricular beats vary. The longer RR intervals between the ectopic beats as indicated by the numerals are approximate multiples of the short RR intervals.

the surrounding myocardium, and (4) electrotonic modulation of the ectopic focus by the sinus beats.[126]

Parasystolic rates range between 20 and 400 beats/min.[25] In most patients, the rate is between 30 and 56 beats/min. Parasystolic ventricular tachycardia is present when the rate is greater than 70 beats/min. Occasionally, a parasystolic discharge may not be manifested even though it occurs at a time when the ventricles are not refractory. This phenomenon is explained by the presence of exit block.

FUSION BEATS

Because a parasystolic focus has an independent rhythm, it may discharge its impulse at about the same time when the impulse of the basic rhythm arrives at the ventricles. The ventricles are depolarized by two activation fronts, and a fusion beat is produced. The fusion beat has a morphology intermediate between the basic and parasytolic complexes. The morphology is variable depending on the proportion of the ventricles activated by the two separate impulses. Fushion beats are not a specific finding for ventricular parasystole. They are seen in all types of ventricular arrhythmias but occur more commonly with ventricular parasystole than with the ordinary ventricular extrasystoles.

Cinical Correlation

Ventricular paraystole is relatively uncommon. It is seen in 1 to 1.5/1000 ECGs.[25,73] Their presence in the routine ECG may be overlooked, because a long rhythm strip is required for the demonstration of the relationship between the interectopic intervals. Ventricular parasystole is seen more often than atrial or AV junctional parasystole. The most commonly associated heart diseases are coronary and hypertensive heart disease. In the 105 cases of ventricular parasystole reviewed by Chung, coronary artery or hypertensive heart disease was encountered in about 58 percent.[25] Some of them occurred during acute myocardial infarction. Other types of associated heart disease included rheumatic heart disease, chronic cor pulmonale, congenital heart disease, and cardiomyopathy. About 14 percent of the cases were not associated with any demonstrable heart disease. In another study, ventricular parasystole was found in 37 of 81 apparently normal individuals with ventricular ectopic beats.[118]

Although the ECG presentation and genesis of ventricular parasystole are different from those of the usual form of ventricular extrasystole, their clinical association appears similar. Whether there is a difference in their response to antiarrhythmic agents remains to be seen.

PAROXYSMAL VENTRICULAR TACHYCARDIA

In paroxysmal ventricular tachycardia, there is a rapid succession of three or more ectopic ventricular beats.[74] The tachycardia is called *sustained* if it lasts longer than 30 seconds and *nonsustained* if it lasts 30 seconds or less. It is described as incessant if the tachycardia is recurrent and the episodes are interrupted by only a few sinus beats. Its ECG diagnosis usually is based on the following changes, but some of the findings are often not observed. This is especially true in sustained ventricular tachycardia. Indeed, in most instances, its diagnosis by the routine ECG can be considered only as presumptive and not definitive (Figs. 18–13 through 18–17). Some of the morphologic changes of the QRS complexes that are helpful in the diagnosis are discussed later in the section on differential diagnosis of tachycardia with wide QRS complexes.

Electrocardiographic Findings

1. Abnormal and wide QRS complexes with secondary ST-segment and T-wave changes
2. A ventricular rate usually between 140 and 200 beats/min
3. A regular or slightly irregular rhythm
4. Abrupt onset and termination
5. AV dissociation
6. Capture beats
7. Fusion beats

VENTRICULAR COMPLEXES

The morphologic characteristics of the ventricular complexes are the same as those described under premature ventricular beats. The bizarre QRS complexes usually have a duration of 0.12 second or longer, but a shorter interval also is seen if the ectopic focus is located in the ventricular septum (see Fig. 18–18). The secondary ST-segment displacement and the T-wave polarity are usually in a direction opposite to the major deflection of the QRS complex.

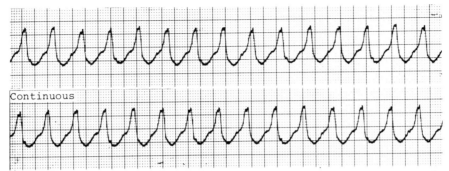

FIGURE 18–13. Probable ventricular tachycardia in a patient with coronary artery disease. The QRS complexes are abnormally wide and bizarre. Dissociation of the atrial and ventricular complexes can be seen. In the absence of other evidence, the possibility of junctional tachycardia with abnormal QRS complex and AV dissociation cannot be excluded.

VENTRICULAR RATE

Although the ventricular rate in paroxysmal ventricular tachycardia usually is between 140 and 200 beats/min, a rate as slow as 120 beats/min may occasionally be seen. An ectopic ventricular rhythm with a rate below 110 beats/min is generally referred to as *non-paroxysmal ventricular tachycardia.* When the ventricular rate is over 200 beats/min and the tracing resembles continuous sine wave, the rhythm is usually called *ventricular flutter.*

REGULARITY

The RR interval in paroxysmal ventricular tachycardia is constant. A slight variation of up to 0.03 second may be seen. Any gross irregularity should raise the suspicion of other mechanisms, such as atrial fibrillation with ventricular conduction defect.

ONSET AND TERMINATION

Paroxysmal ventricular tachycardia is initiated abruptly by a premature ventricular contrac-

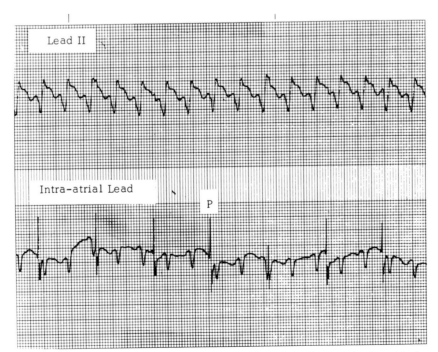

FIGURE 18–14. Probable ventricular tachycardia. The independent atrial and ventricular activities are demonstrated by the intraatrial lead. The possibility of junctional tachycardia with aberrant ventricular conduction or bundle branch block cannot be excluded.

A

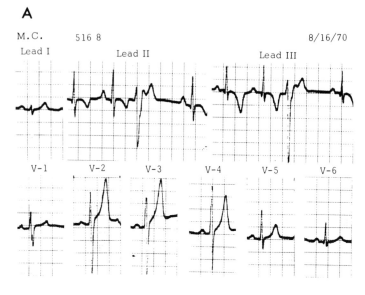

M.C.   516 8   8/16/70
Lead I   Lead II   Lead III

V-1   V-2   V-3   V-4   V-5   V-6

FIGURE 18–15. Ventricular tachycardia of undetermined cause in an 18-year-old man. (A) The tracing from 8-16-70 shows premature ventricular beats in leads II and III. (B) Paroxysmal ventricular tachycardia is present in the tracing of 8-18-70. The morphology of the QRS complexes is identical to that of the premature ventricular beats in the previous tracing. In lead II, there is a capture beat (C). In lead III, there is a fusion beat (F). AV dissociation also is demonstrated.

B

8/18/70
Lead II

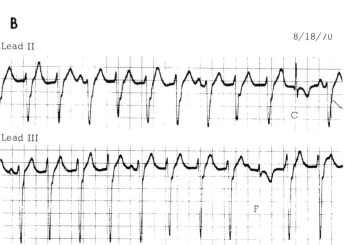

C

Lead III

F

tion. The degree of prematurity of the extrasystole is variable. Much emphasis has been given to the importance of R-on-T phenomenon in the genesis of ventricular tachycardia, especially in patients with acute myocardial infarction. In 44 unselected patients with ventricular tachycardia, including those with acute myocardial infarction, however, I observed the R-on-T phenomenon in only 14 percent of the cases. Many of the episodes of ventricular tachycardia were initiated by late diastolic premature beats that appeared at or shortly after the next sinus P wave[24] (Fig. 18–19). Similar findings were observed by other investigators.[56,161] Gomes and associates noted that a short–long cycle is often the sequence that precedes the onset of ventricular tachycardia.[56] The short cycle consists of a sinus beat followed by a premature ventricular beat.

The ensuing compensatory pause before the appearance of the next sinus beat represents the long cycle. Ventricular tachycardia initiated in such a manner (sinus–PVB–pause–sinus–VT) frequently is followed by polymorphic ventricular tachycardia and ventricular fibrillation.

AV DISSOCIATION

In patients with underlying sinus rhythm, the atria may remain under the control of the sinus impulse. The atrial and ventricular rhythms are independent of each other, and there is no demonstrable relation between the P waves and QRS complexes. The atrial rate is usually slower than the ventricular rate. However, retrograde impulse conduction to the atria from the ventricular focus often occurs

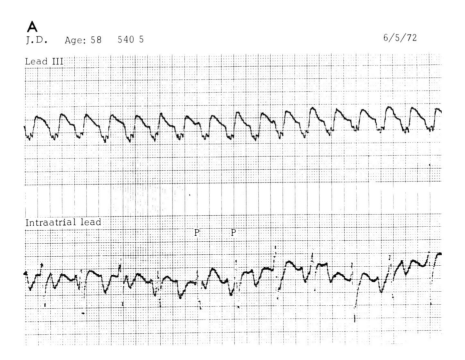

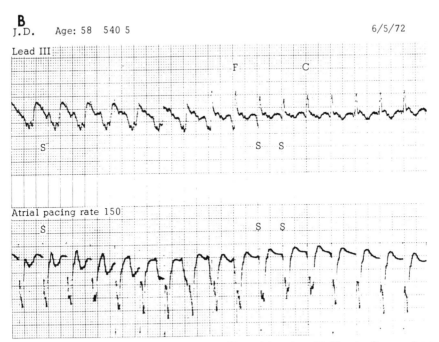

FIGURE 18–16. Ventricular tachycardia proved by atrial pacing. (A) The simultaneous intraatrial lead demonstrates the dissociation of atrial and ventricular complexes. (B) Tracing demonstrating atrial and ventricular captures by atrial pacing at the rate of 150 beats/min. S indicates pacemaker spike; F, fusion beat; and C, capture beat.

Ventricular Tachycardia

C. J. 4077614   10/2/68

Lead V 2

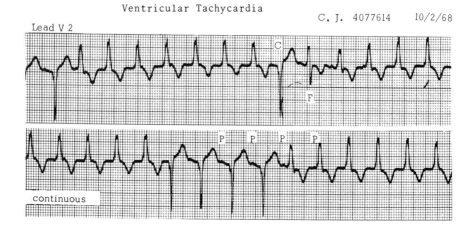

continuous

Intra-atrial Lead

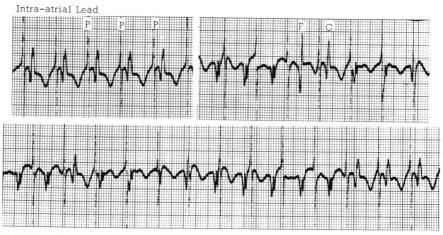

FIGURE 18–17. Intermittent ventricular tachycardia. The second strip shows four sinus beats. Capture (C) and fusion (F) beats are present. AV dissociation is demonstrated by the intraatrial lead.

in ventricular tachycardia, (Fig. 18–20). In 21 cases of ventricular tachycardia with esophageal lead studied by Kistin, 1:1 VA conduction was demonstrated in 10, VA conduction with variable block in 4, and independent atrial rhythm in 7.[79] The RP interval of the retrograde conducted beats is, as a rule, 0.11 second or longer. Wellens and Lie found 1:1 VA conduction in 29 (64 percent) of 45 consecutive patients with ventricular tachycardia in whom intracavitary atrial recordings were obtained.[171] Another 5 patients also had evidence of VA conduction but showed VA Wenckebach periods, 2:1 VA block, etc. VA conduction was uncommon when the ventricular rate was rapid, being seen in only 1 of 7 patients with a rate of 200 beats/min or more. In the 122 cases of ventricular tachycardia reported by Akhtar and co-workers 25 percent had 1:1 VA conduction and another 20 per-

cent had VA conduction but with varying degrees of VA block.[1]

In patients with supraventricular arrhythmia, such as paroxysmal atrial tachycardia, atrial flutter, and atrial fibrillation, AV dissociation usually occurs when ventricular tachycardia develops. Occasionally, however, retrograde atrial capture may be observed.

VENTRICULAR CAPTURE BEATS

Occasionally, early but normal QRS complexes appear during an episode of paroxysmal ventricular tachycardia (see Figs. 18–15 and 18–17). They are the result of ventricular captures by conducted supraventricular impulses. Their presence is helpful in confirming the ventricular origin of the ectopic tachycardia. Unfortunately, they are rare in the classical type of ventricular tachycardia.

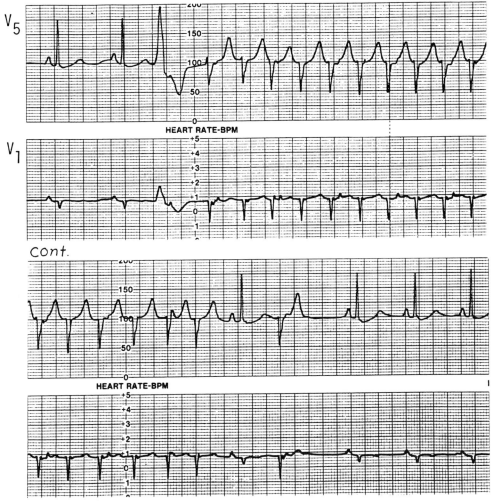

FIGURE 18–18. Nonsustained ventricular tachycardia with narrow QRS complexes. In this Holter recording, the first two beats are sinus beats. They are followed by a premature ventricular beat with retrograde atrial capture. A short epsiode of ventricular tachycardia follows. The QRS duration during the tachycardia is 0.08 second. There is 2:1 retrograde atrial capture during the tachycardia. After the tachycardia terminates, one sinus beat is followed by a premature ventricular beat with retrograde atrial capture (bottom strip). The morphology of this premature ventricular beat is similar to that of the QRS complexes during tachycardia.

FUSION BEATS (DRESSLER BEATS[36])

If ventricular capture by an atrial impulse occurs at about the same time when the ectopic ventricular impulse is activating the ventricles, a fusion beat may occur. The ventricles are depolarized partly by the atrial impulse and partly by the ventricular impulse. The resulting QRS complex has a morphology that is intermediate between the normal and ectopic beats (see Figs. 18–15 and 18–17). The presence of fusion beats also strongly supports the ventricular origin of the tachycardia. However, it is also rare in ventricular tachycardia with rapid rate.

Differential Diagnosis of Tachycardia with Wide QRS Complex

A regular tachycardia with a rate of 120 to 200 beats/min and a QRS duration of 0.12 second or longer may be due to one of the following rhythms:

1. Paroxysmal ventricular tachycardia
2. Supraventricular tachycardia with abnormally wide QRS complexes
   The supraventricular tachycardia may be:
   a. Sinus tachycardia
   b. SA nodal reentrant tachycardia
   c. Paroxysmal atrial tachycardia

Monitor lead

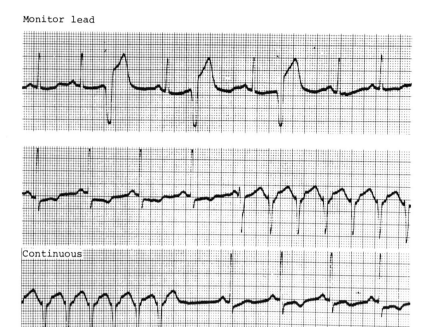

740   81F

FIGURE 18–19. Premature ventricular beats and nonsustained ventricular tachycardia. The top strip shows three premature ventricular beats with relatively short coupling time. The second and third strips illustrate an episode of ventricular tachycardia initiated by an end-diastolic premature ventricular beat. Retrograde atrial capture is present during ventricular tachycardia. (From Chou TC, Wenzke F: The importance of R-on-T phenomenon. Am Heart J 96:191, 1978, by permission.)

d. Intraatrial reentrant tachycardia
e. Atrial flutter with 2:1 conduction and occasionally 1:1 conduction (see Fig. 18–24)
f. AV nodal reentrant tachycardia
g. Automatic AV junctional tachycardia
h. AV reentrant tachycardia using a bypass tract

The abnormally wide QRS complexes may be due to:
a. Aberrant ventricular conduction (Fig. 18–21)
b. Preexisting left or right bundle branch block
c. Preexisting nonspecific intraventricular conduction defect
d. Antegrade conduction through the bypass tract in patients with the WPW syndrome (Fig. 18–22).

Occasionally, atrial fibrillation with rapid ventricular response may mimic ventricular tachycardia, but the correct diagnosis usually is not difficult to obtain if the rhythm is examined carefully (Fig. 18–23). In many cases of supraventricular tachycardia with wide QRS complexes, their differentiation from paroxysmal ventricular tachycardia by the body surface ECG is difficult or even impossible. The following discussion relates to the usefulness and limitations of some of the findings commonly used for the differential diagnosis.

MORPHOLOGY OF PREMATURE BEATS DURING SINUS RHYTHM

If a previous or subsequent tracing recorded during sinus rhythm is available, its usefulness in the recognition of preexisting intraventricular conduction defect is obvious. If premature ventricular beats are present and their morphology is identical to that of the complexes of the tachycardia, the ventricular origin of the ectopic rhythm can be assumed (see Fig. 18–15). On the other hand, the presence of premature atrial beats with aberrant ventricular conduction that have a similar QRS complex is suggestive of supraventricular tachycardia (see Fig. 18–21).

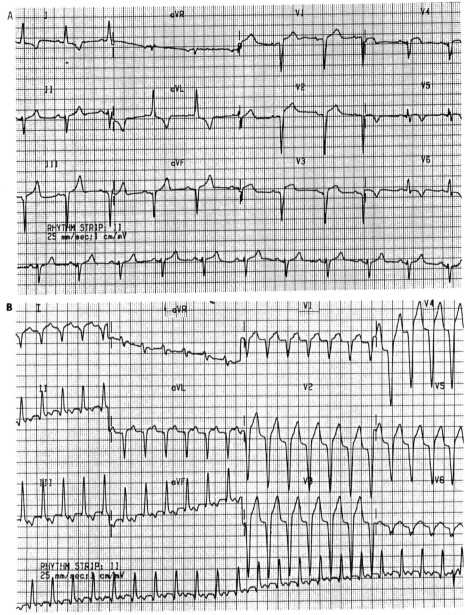

FIGURE 18–20. Probable ventricular tachycardia in a patient with acute anteroseptal myocardial infarction. Tracing A shows normal sinus rhythm with left anterior hemiblock and possible left ventricular hypertrophy based on the voltage in the limb leads. Changes in the precordial leads are consistent with acute anteroseptal myocardial infarction and anterolateral myocardial ischemia. An inferior myocardial infarction cannot be excluded. Serial cardiac enzyme levels supported the diagnosis of acute infarction. (B) The patient developed wide QRS complex tachycardia with a rate of 152 beats/min. The QRS morphology and axis are different from those during sinus rhythm. There is 1:1 VA conduction. With intravenous administration of lidocaine, the tachycardia was converted promptly to sinus rhythm. Although paroxysmal junctional tachycardia with aberrancy cannot be excluded, the response to lidocaine favors the diagnosis of ventricular tachycardia.

ONSET OF TACHYCARDIA

If the tachycardia is intermittent and its onset is recorded, the diagnosis of supraventricular tachycardia can be made if the episode is initiated by a premature P wave. On the other hand, if the paroxysm begins with a QRS complex, the tachycardia may be either ventricular or junctional in origin. If the first QRS complex of the tachycardia is preceded by a sinus

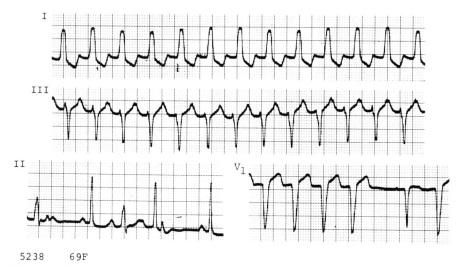

5238   69F

FIGURE 18–21. Paroxysmal atrial tachycardia with aberrant ventricular conduction. The supraventricular origin of the tachycardia is supported by the findings in leads II and V_1. Lead II shows three sinus beats and three premature atrial beats, two of which are blocked. One premature atrial beat is conducted with ventricular aberrancy (the third QRS complex). The first wide QRS complex also is an aberrantly conducted beat, but the preceding P wave is not shown in the tracing. The last complex in lead V_1 is a premature atrial beat with aberrant ventricular conduction. The QRS complex has the same morphology as that during tachycardia, which is shown in the first four complexes in lead V_1. The tachycardias shown in leads I and III have the same rate as that in lead V_1. The QRS morphology during the tachycardia has a left bundle branch block pattern.

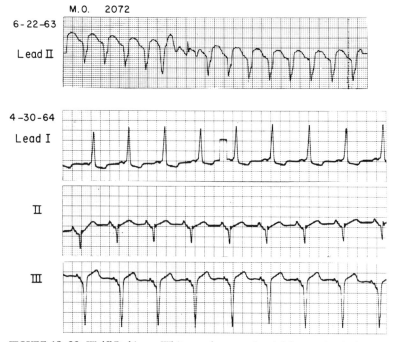

FIGURE 18–22. Wolff-Parkinson-White syndrome and atrial flutter simulating ventricular tachycardia. The short PR interval and delta wave of the WPW syndrome are demonstrated in the tracing of 4-30-64. The tracing (lead II) on 6-22-63 shows tachycardia with wide QRS complexes due to atrial flutter with 2:1 conduction through the accessory bundle. The flutter waves are seen transiently when normal AV conduction occurs for one beat.

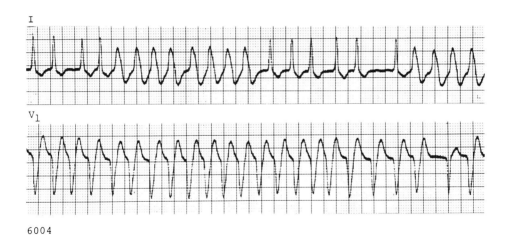

6004

FIGURE 18–23. Atrial fibrillation with rapid ventricular response. During the periods with aberrant ventricular conduction, the rhythm mimics ventricular tachycardia. Ashman phenomenon is demonstrated in the later part of both leads.

P wave with a PR interval shorter than that of the conducted sinus beats, the tachycardia is ventricular (see Fig. 18–19).

RATE OF THE TACHYCARDIA BEING IDENTICAL TO THE RATE OF PREVIOUSLY KNOWN SUPRAVENTRICULAR RHYTHM

The tachycardia is probably supraventricular in origin if such a relationship can be established (Fig. 18–24).

AV DISSOCIATION

Independent atrial and ventricular activities occur more commonly in ventricular tachycardia. Although its presence speaks heavily in favor of ventricular tachycardia, AV dissociation also may be seen in AV junctional tachycardia with retrograde block. On the other hand, a 1:1 atrial and ventricular relationship does not exclude ventricular tachycardia because of the frequent occurrence of atrial captures in ventricular tachycardia. If the RP interval is 0.10 second or less, the finding is in favor of junctional tachycardia, since the time interval is too short for VA conduction in the absence of a bypass pathway. A longer RP interval, however, does not exclude junctional rhythm, because retrograde conduction delay of the junctional impulse may exist.

MORPHOLOGY OF THE QRS COMPLEXES AND QRS AXIS

Although it has been estimated that about 80 to 85 percent of aberrant beats have a right bundle branch block pattern, ectopic beats that arise from the left ventricle have similar morphology. Therefore, the application of the RSR′ pattern in lead V_1 in the differential diagnosis is limited.[104] The finding of a positive or negative QRS complex in all precordial leads is in favor of ventricular ectopy.[105]

Wellens and associates examined the QRS morphology in 70 episodes of ventricular tachycardia from 62 patients and 70 episodes of supraventricular tachycardia with aberrant ventricular conduction from 60 patients.[170] The diagnoses were supported by His bundle electrograms in all patients. The findings that were suggestive of ventricular tachycardia were (1) a QRS width of more than 0.14 second, (2) left axis deviation, and (3) a monophasic or biphasic right bundle branch block type of QRS complex in lead V_1. As the authors properly emphasized, however, none of their patients with supraventricular tachycardia had preexisting bundle branch block. The clinical application of these findings in the differential diagnosis of tachycardia with wide QRS complex is, therefore, somewhat limited.

Akhtar and co-workers studied 150 patients with wide QRS complex tachycardia.[1] All of the patients had a QRS duration of 0.12 second[168] or longer. Based on electrophysiological studies, 122 patients had ventricular tachycardia and 21 had supraventricular tachycardia. They found that the following characteristics of the QRS complexes are highly reliable for the diagnosis of ventricular tachycardia:

1. The QRS duration is more than 0.14 second with a right bundle branch block pattern

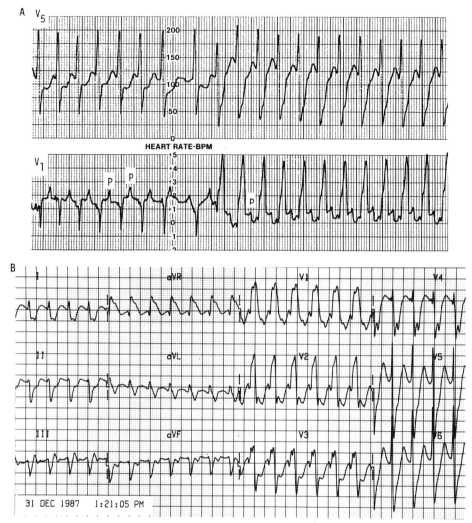

FIGURE 18–24. Atrial flutter with aberrant ventricular conduction. The patient was a 64-year-old woman with dilated cardiomyopathy. She was known to have recurrent atrial flutter occasionally with 1:1 conduction. She was maintained on digoxin and procainamide. (A) Tracing obtained with Holter monitor. The atrial rate is 192 beats/min. In the early part of the tracing, there is 1:1 AV conduction with narrow QRS complexes. After one blocked atrial impulse (the eighth P wave), 1:1 AV conduction resumes but there is aberrant ventricular conduction. The long–short cycle accounts for the development of aberrancy. The diagnosis of atrial flutter was based on many 12-lead ECGs that showed the typical flutter waves. The slow flutter rate probably was due to procainamide and large atrial size. (B) Atrial flutter with a very slow rate of 156 beats/min. The flutter waves can best be seen in lead aVF. There is 1:1 AV conduction with right bundle branch aberrancy. The QRS is wide, with a duration of 160 msec.

or more than 0.16 second with a left bundle branch block pattern.

2. All of the precordial leads (V_1 through V_6) show a positive deflection.

3. The QRS axis is in the right upper quadrant of the frontal plane between $-90°$ and $+180°$.

4. The QRS complexes have a left bundle branch block pattern, but the QRS axis is rightward.

5. In patients with preexisting bundle branch block, there is a change in the QRS pattern during the tachycardia.

Kindwall and associates analyzed the 12-lead ECGs of 118 patients with wide QRS complex tachycardia and a left bundle branch block morphology.[78] Ninety-one patients had ventricular tachycardia, and 27 had supraventricular tachycardia with aberration. All patients except 5 had electrophysiological studies. The authors concluded that, if the QRS complexes have a left bundle branch block morphology, the following changes are highly specific but not particularly sensitive for the diagnosis of ventricular tachycardia: (1) R wave in V_1 or V_2 greater than 30 msec in du-

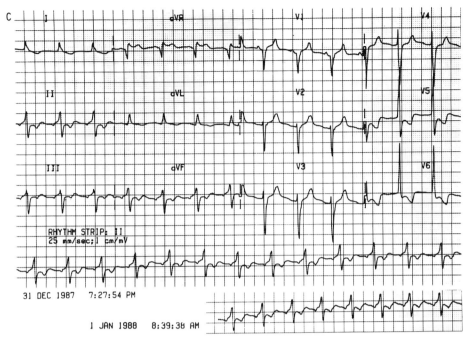

FIGURE 18–24. *Continued* (C) Tracing illustrating the variation of the atrial flutter rate in this patient. It is 176 beats/min at 7:27 P.M. on 12-31-87 and 200 beats/min on the next day. The typical flutter wave morphology is demonstrated in these tracings.

ration, (2) any Q wave in V_6, (3) a duration from the onset of the QRS to the nadir of the S wave in lead V_1 greater than 60 msec, and (4) notching on the downstroke of the S wave in lead V_1 or V_2. These investigators also found that left axis deviation was not helpful in the differentiation of ventricular and supraventricular tachycardia in their group of patients.

Based on these various characteristics of the QRS complexes and the presence of AV dissociation, a correct diagnosis of ventricular tachycardia can be made from the 12-lead ECG in about 90% of cases.[1,78,169] There are occasional cases of ventricular tachycardia, however, with a QRS duration of less than 0.12 second[168] (see Fig. 18–18). Such cases are not included in the reported series described here. Some patients with preexisting right bundle branch block may have a QRS duration of greater than 0.14 second during sinus rhythm and therefore also during supraventricular tachycardia. Even rate-related aberrancy may result in very wide QRS complexes as illustrated in Figure 18–24.

CAPTURE BEATS

Although capture beats are rarely seen, they are one of the strongest evidences for ventricular tachycardia. Because they are premature but normal in duration, their presence prac-

tically rules out aberrancy as the cause of the bizarre QRS complexes, since aberrancy rarely occurs in the beats following longer rather than shorter cycles.

FUSION BEATS

The presence of a fusion beat is also strongly suggestive of ventricular tachycardia. Rare exceptions are cases of AV junctional tachycardia with aberrant conduction through an anomalous pathway. Fusion may occur between these junctional beats and sinus beats that are transmitted through the normal AV pathway.[81]

RESPONSE TO VAGAL STIMULATION

Paroxysmal ventricular tachycardia is usually not affected by vagal stimulation, such as carotid sinus massage. Sinus tachycardia with wide QRS complex may be temporarily slowed by vagal stimulation. The procedure may, however, terminate SA nodal reentrant tachycardia. The atrial mechanism in paroxysmal (ectopic) atrial tachycardia and intra-atrial reentrant tachycardia is not affected by vagal stimulation, but the latter may cause AV block.

In AV nodal reentrant tachycardia, carotid sinus massage may not have an effect on the rhythm or the tachycardia may abruptly be converted to sinus rhythm. Automatic junctional tachycardia is not affected by it. In atrial flutter with 2:1 conduction, vagal stimulation may cause temporary increase of AV block and slowing of the ventricular rate. The atrial mechanism may be revealed during the slower ventricular response. AV reentrant tachycardia using a bypass tract may be terminated by increased vagal tone by interrupting the reentry circuit at the AV node. Vagal stimulation has no effect on supraventricular tachyarrhythmias in which the atrial impulses are conducted antegrade to the ventricles through a bypass tract and do not use the AV node as the returning limb of the circuit.

Waxman and Wald reported on four cases of well-documented ventricular tachycardia that was terminated by carotid sinus massage after pretreatment with large doses of edrophonium.[167] Such a response suggests that the conversion of a wide QRS complex tachycardia to sinus rhythm by vagal stimulation can usually but not always be considered as definitive evidence for supraventricular origin of the tachycardia.

ATRIAL PACING

Atrial pacing may provide confirmatory evidence for the diagnosis of ventricular tachycardia. The procedure involves the introduction of an electrode transvenously into the right atrium. The atrium is stimulated at a rate faster than that of the tachycardia. If ventricular captures occur and the QRS complex is normal in duration, one can exclude the possibility of aberrant conductions being responsible for the wide QRS complex during the tachycardia[38] (Fig. 18–16).

HIS BUNDLE RECORDING

In supraventricular tachycardia, each QRS complex is preceded by a His bundle potential. In ventricular tachycardia, the latter is absent (Fig. 18–25). The retrograde His deflection is usually obsured by the much larger QRS complex.[49] Although a definitive diagnosis can be made with His bundle recording or atrial pacing, the limitations of these invasive procedures in clinical practice are obvious.

SUMMARY OF DIFFERENTIAL DIAGNOSIS OF WIDE QRS COMPLEX TACHYCARDIA

Although a definitive diagnosis of the mechanism of a wide QRS complex tachycardia may require invasive electrophysiological studies, the presence of one or more of the following findings in the routine 12-lead ECG is in favor of ventricular tachycardia:

1. AV dissociation
2. Right bundle branch block QRS morphology with QRS duration longer than 0.14 second, or left bundle branch block QRS morphology with QRS duration longer than 0.16 second
3. QRS axis in the right upper quadrant between −90° and +180°

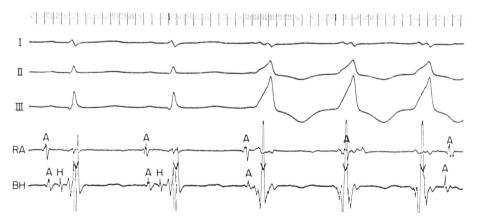

FIGURE 18–25. His bundle recording in a patient with ventricular tachycardia. Simultaneous leads I, II, and III and bipolar electrograms from high right atrium (RA) and bundle of His (BH) area are shown. In the two sinus beats (first and second complexes), His bundle potential (H) is present between the atrial (A) and ventricular (V) potentials. With the development of ventricular tachycardia, the bundle of His deflection is no longer seen before the ventricular deflection. (Courtesy of Dr. Winston Gaum.)

4. Positive QRS deflections in all of the precordial leads (V_1 through V_6)
5. Left bundle branch block QRS morphology with rightward QRS axis
6. Left bundle branch block QRS morphology with one of the following:
    a. R wave in V_1 or V_2 greater than 0.03 second
    b. any Q wave in V_6
    c. Onset of QRS to nadir of S wave in lead V_1 greater than 0.06 second
    d. Notching of downstroke of S wave in V_1 or V_2
7. Capture beats, fusion beats
8. QRS morphology identical to that of premature ventricular beats during sinus rhythm

Localizing the Origin of Ventricular Tachycardia

In most patients with sustained ventricular tachycardia, the responsible mechanism is microreentry. The reentrant circuit involves a relatively small area of ventricular myocardium and peripheral specialized conduction tissue. With the advent of surgical treatment for sustained ventricular tachycardia refractory to drug therapy, the site of origin of the tachycardia becomes important information. The ability of the 12-lead ECG to predict the site of origin is, however, limited in patients with coronary artery disease. Josephson and associates examined 34 patients with 41 episodes of ventricular tachycardia.[71] They found that, although all tachycardias with a right bundle branch block pattern originated within the left ventricle or septum, 16 of 19 ventricular tachycardias with left bundle branch block pattern also had their endocardial site of origin in the left ventricle on or adjacent to the septum. Only 3 patients without coronary artery disease who had left bundle branch block morphology had right ventricular origin of the tachycardia. They proposed the following possible explanations for a left ventricular site of origin of ventricular tachycardia with left bundle branch block configuration: (1) preferential left-to-right transseptal activation, (2) exit block from the reentrant site to the left ventricular free wall, and (3) underlying disease of the left ventricular muscle or conduction system that alters conduction patterns and makes it impossible to predict the QRS morphology on the basis of the site of impulse origin. Alteration of the conduction pathway also may explain the change in the morphology of the QRS complexes during the same episode of sustained ventricular tachycardia in some patients.[70] The 12-lead ECG is more reliable in differentiating anterior from posterior site of origin of the tachycardia.[71] The site is likely to be anterior if Q waves are present in leads I and V_6. The presence of R waves in lead I and all or almost all of the precordial leads is suggestive of a posterior origin of the tachycardia. More recently, investigators from the same institution correlated the findings in the 12-lead ECG during ventricular tachycardia with the endocardial site of origin obtained by mapping in 108 patients with prior myocardial infarction.[113] They found that the location of the infarct, the bundle branch block pattern, the QRS axis, and the precordial R-wave progression during the tachycardia are helpful in predicting the endocardial region of origin of the tachycardia. The readers are referred to this article for the details of the proposed criteria and their limitations.

In the absence of coronary artery disease, most of the ventricular tachycardias with left bundle branch block morphology have right ventricular origin.[129] Right ventricular tachycardia is seen in patients with arrhythmogenic right ventricular dysplasia[102,103,119] or Uhl's anomaly,[45] after surgical repair of tetralogy of Fallot[64] and in patients with no apparent associated heart disease.[18,92] Sustained ventricular tachycardia occasionally involve a macroreentrant circuit utilizing the bundle branches.[19] The tachycardia that results from bundle branch reentry usually has a left bundle branch block pattern. The QRS complexes during sinus rhythm frequently show nonspecific intraventricular conduction defect. Most of the patients have dilated cardiomyopathy. The ventricular tachycardia may be terminated by transcatheter electrical ablation of the right bundle branch.[159,160]

Clinical Correlation

Most patients with ventricular tachycardia have organic heart disease. Ventricular tachycardia may be associated with a variety of heart diseases. The most common cause is coronary artery disease. In the several series studied before continuous monitoring was available, more than 70 percent of patients with paroxysmal ventricular tachycardia had ischemic heart disease and about half of them had acute myocardial infarction.[5,61,101] The reported incidence of ventricular tachycardia in patients with acute myocardial infarction during continuous ECG monitoring is about 18.5

percent and varies between 6 and 40 percent.[13] In 289 survivors of myocardial infarction, Kleiger and associates observed ventricular tachycardia in 3 percent of the patients at 2 weeks and 11 percent at 1 month.[83] Among 820 patients monitored by 24-hour Holter recording for 8 to 14 days after acute myocardial infarction, Biggers and colleagues found nonsustained ventricular tachycardia in 11 percent and sustained ventricular tachycardia in 2 percent of the patients.[12] The presence of ventricular tachycardia nearly doubled the risk of death during an average follow-up period of 31 months. The increased mortality was independent of the state of ventricular function. Moller and others detected ventricular tachycardia in 19 percent of patients within the first 6 months after an acute myocardial infarction.[114] Ventricular tachycardia also was found by some investigators to be common during reperfusion in patients with acute myocardial infarction who were receiving thrombolytic therapy.[112] Accelerated idioventricular rhythm, however, is generally considered the more characteristic rhythm seen under such circumstances.

Ventricular tachycardia also may be seen in patients with hypertensive heart disease and especially idiopathic cardiomyopathy. The association between right ventricular tachycardia and arrhythmogenic right ventricular dysplasia was discussed previously.[103] Rheumatic heart disease was cited as one of the common causes of this arrhythmia in the past, but it is no longer one of its major causes in my experience. Only 1 of 44 consecutive unselected cases of ventricular tachycardia I reviewed had this disease.[24] Paroxysmal ventricular tachycardia and ventricular fibrillation occur occasionally in patients with mitral valve prolapse and may be responsible for syncope or sudden death in some patients.[68,148] Among the secondary cardiomyopathies, sarcoidosis is well known for its frequent association with arrhythmias, including ventricular tachycardia.[37,58]

Digitalis intoxication is a common cause of paroxysmal ventricular tachycardia. It was responsible for 25 percent of the cases in one study.[101] The incidence is much lower in recent years, because the dosage of digitalis used is generally lower. Many of the antiarrhythmic drugs such as quinidine, procainamide, disopyramide, mexiletine, flecainide, and encainide may cause ventricular tachycardia and ventricular fibrillation.[9,29,109,147] These arrhythmias also may be seen during the administration of psychotropic drugs, including the phenothiazines and tricyclic antidepressants, mostly when large doses are given.[46] We reported a case of recurrent ventricular tachycardia and torsades de pointes related to the use of pentamidine.[10] Patients with pheochromocytoma may develop ventricular tachycardia because of increased catechoamine blood level.[123] A similar mechanism is probably responsible for the development of ventricular tachycardia due to fright.[5]

Ventricular tachycardia may develop during cardiac catheterization and cardiac surgery because of mechanical irritation of the ventricles. It has been observed in patients after coronary artery bypass surgery when no such arrhythmia was seen preoperatively.[111] Ventricular tachycardia also may appear after direct-current countershock for the conversion of cardiac arrhythmias in patients who have received digitalis. The probable mechanism is that the electrical discharge affects myocardial cellular membranes, resulting in leakage of intracellular potassium. When a critical loss has occurred, toxic effects from the myocardium-bound glycoside ensue.[82]

Cases of ventricular tachycardia have been reported in the WPW syndrome, but they were not well documented. Gallagher and associates described seven convincing cases of ventricular fibrillation in patients with this syndrome.[50] Some of these patients exhibited this arrhythmia after atrial fibrillation.

Although ventricular tachycardia is relatively uncommon in patients with congenital heart disease, it may be responsible for sudden death in some of the patients years after corrective surgery such as repair of tetralogy of Fallot was performed.[66,89] It also is known to be associated with hereditary prolongation of the QT interval with or without congenital deafness[135] and with Uhl's anomaly.[45]

Ventricular tachycardia and other types of arrhythmias also have been implicated in "sudden sniffing death" as a result of inhalation of aerosols propelled by fluorinated hydrocarbons.[7,42]

Some patients with paroxysmal ventricular tachycardia have no identifiable cause (Fig. 18–26). Idiopathic ventricular tachycardia has been observed in families, but it occurs more commonly in sporadic fashion.[138] The reported incidence of idiopathic ventricular tachycardia varies between 5 and 12 percent.[5,61,101] The higher incidence was observed in studies done before many of the modern diagnostic procedures were available. Lesch and associates reviewed 35 cases of ventricular tachycardia in the absence of organic heart

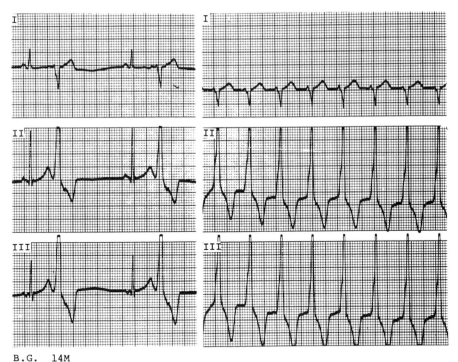

B.G.   14M

FIGURE 18–26. Paroxysmal ventricular tachycardia in a 14-year-old boy with no other evidence of organic heart disease. The ectopic ventricular beats are probably left ventricular in origin. Retrograde atrial capture is present.

disease reported in the literature.[93] The patients' ages at the onset of the tachycardia ranged between 10 and 38 years. In 29 cases, the arrhythmia appeared before the age of 30. The episodes often were precipitated by exercise or emotional stress. Some were apparently related to pregnancy. Buxton and coworkers reported on 30 patients with right ventricular tachycardia without associated heart disease.[18] In more than half of the patients, the tachycardia was probably provocable by exercise. Endocardial mapping of the patients suggested an origin of the tachycardia at the right ventricular outflow tract on the interventricular septum. In a small, but wellstudied series of 6 patients, Chapman and associates found that excessive consumption of alcohol, coffee, or tobacco may predispose to the arrhythmia.[20] In some cases, the tachycardia was abolished by exercise. Lemery and associates studied 52 patients with idiopathic ventricular tachycardia.[92] The mean age of the patients was 36 years. The ventricular tachycardia was sustained in 20 patients, incessant in 11, and nonsustained in 21. Electrophysiological studies of these patients showed that the ventricular tachycardia originated from the right ventricular outflow tract in more than half of the patients. Among the 33 patients who had a 12-lead ECG during ventricular tachycardia, left bundle branch block morphology was seen in 20 patients (61 percent) and all but 3 patients had right axis deviation.

Among cases of idiopathic ventricular tachycardia that originate from the left ventricle, one particular form is of special interest.[51,124,165] The patients are usually young, mostly between 20 and 30 years old. The QRS morphology typically has a right bundle branch block pattern and left axis deviation. The QRS duration is often less than 0.14 second. It is believed that the tachycardia originates from the posterior fascicle of the left bundle branch and the mechanism of the tachycardia is reentry. Most of these cases responded to the administration of verapamil.

Paroxysmal ventricular tachycardia is a life-threatening arrhythmia. This is particularly true when the episode is prolonged or when it occurs in the presence of acute myocardial infarction or serious heart disease. In one series, 59 of 114 patients with acute myocardial infarction and ventricular tachycardia developed ventricular fibrillation.[122]

A. McG.   #840   11/5/70
Monitor lead

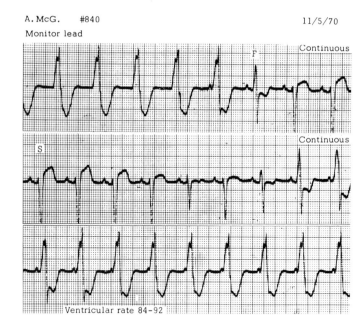

FIGURE 18–27. Nonparoxysmal ventricular tachycardia. The ectopic rhythm is intermittent. Fusion beats are present.

NONPAROXYSMAL VENTRICULAR TACHYCARDIA

Nonparoxysmal ventricular tachycardia also is called *idioventricular tachycardia* or *accelerated idioventricular rhythm*. It has the following ECG characteristics (Figs. 18–27 and 18–28):

1. The rhythm is regular and has a rate between 60 and 100 beats/min.
2. The QRS complexes are abnormal and wide.

3. The ventricular complexes are usually but not necessarily dissociated from the P waves.
4. Ventricular capture and fusion beats are common.

Nonparoxysmal ventricular tachycardia has most of the characteristics of paroxysmal ventricular tachycardia, but the ventricular rate is slower. Although the ventricular rate is 100 beats/min or less, the rhythm is called *tachycardia* because its rate is greater than the inherent rate of ventricular pacemakers. Be-

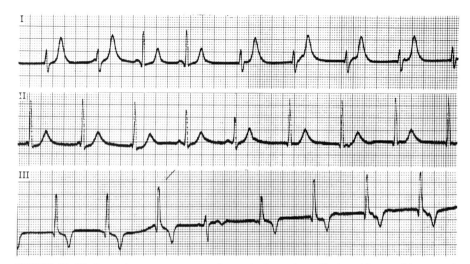

FIGURE 18–28. Intermittent nonparoxysmal ventricular tachycardia in a 19-year-old man with acute subdural hematoma. No evidence of organic heart disease was present. The third and fourth complexes in lead I, the fifth complex in lead II, and the fourth complex in lead III are sinus beats. The fourth complex in lead II and the fifth complex in lead III are fusion beats.

cause the rate is in the range of normal sinus rate and is, indeed, frequently almost identical to it, the term *accelerated isorhythmic ventricular rhythm* was suggested.[106] The slower ectopic ventricular rate also allows more opportunities for complete or partial activation of the ventricles by supraventricular impulses. Therefore, ventricular capture or fusion beats are seen much more commonly in this type of arrhythmia than in the paroxysmal variety.

Most of the episodes of nonparoxysmal ventricular tachycardia are transient, lasting for second or minutes. It is often suppressed or replaced by sinus rhythm when the sinus rate is increased. In patients with acute myocardial infarction, paroxysmal ventricular tachycardia with identical QRS morphology may occur in the same patient. In some cases, the RR interval of the nonparoxysmal ventricular tachycardia was the exact multiple of the RR interval of the rapid ventricular tachycardia. This relationship suggests that exit block of the rapid ventricular ectopic impulse is responsible for the appearance of nonparoxysmal ventricular tachycardia in some instances.[91]

Differential Diagnosis

Nonparoxysmal ventricular tachycardia may be simulated by nonparoxysmal junctional tachycardia with preexisting intraventricular conduction defect. Because of the frequent appearance of ventricular capture and fusion beats in the former, the differentiation usually is not difficult if a careful search is made for their existence.

Clinical Correlation

Nonparoxysmal ventricular tachycardia was first described by Rothfeld and associates in patients with acute myocardial infarction.[134] Its incidence in this disease was reported as varying between 8 and 36 percent.[94,134] It is seen in both anterior and inferior myocardial infarction. It is a common arrhythmia associated with reperfusion during intracoronary thrombolysis in patients with acute myocardial infarction.[54] Nonparoxysmal ventricular tachycardia usually occurs during sinus bradycardia. Because the ventricular rate is in a normal range and the rhythm causes little hemodynamic changes, it does not affect the prognosis adversely. Paroxysmal ventricular tachycardia often coexists in the same patient, however.

The arrhythmia also is seen in patients with other types of heart disease, such as hypertensive heart disease, primary myocardial disease, and rheumatic as well as congenital heart disease.[106] It also may be caused by digitalis.[146] Occasionally, no evidence of heart disease can be found. Such an example is given in Figure 18–29.

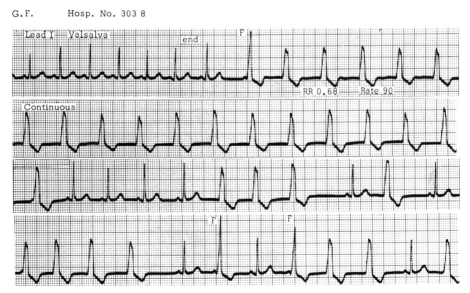

FIGURE 18–29. Nonparoxysmal ventricular tachycardia. The patient is a 15-year-old girl with no other evidence of organic heart disease. She has no symptoms. The ectopic rhythm is intermittent. It occurs when the sinus rhythm is slow. Fusion beats (F) are present.

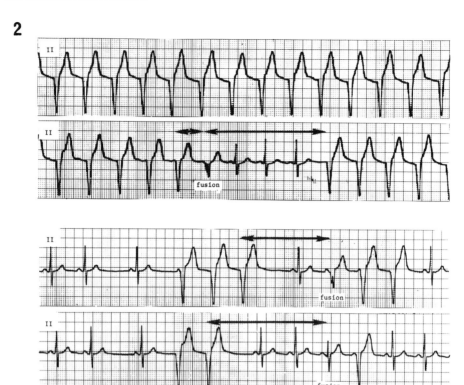

FIGURE 18–30. Parasystolic ventricular tachycardia. Note (1) the variation of the coupling intervals of the ectopic beats initiating the different episodes of ventricular tachycardia; (2) the mathematical relationship between the RR intervals of the ectopic beats; and (3) the presence of fusion beats. (Courtesy of Dr. Kenneth Gimbel.)

Parasystolic Ventricular Tachycardia

Ventricular tachycardia may originate from a parasystolic focus (Fig. 18–30). The ventricular rate is usually between 70 and 140 beats/min. Most of the patients have organic heart disease, especially coronary artery disease with myocardial infarction. Occasionally, it is seen in young and otherwise healthy individuals.[26] It may be diagnosed if the onset of recurrent episodes of the tachycardia is recorded. There is a variation of the coupling time of the ventricular ectopic beats initiating the tachycardias, but the tachycardias originate from the same focus.

TORSADES DE POINTES AND POLYMORPHOUS VENTRICULAR TACHYCARDIA

Torsades de pointes is an arrhythmia intermediary between ventricular tachycardia and ventricular fibrillation. It originally was described by Dessertenne and the term *torsades de pointes* (twisting of the points) was used to describe cycles of ventricular tachyarrhythmia with alternating electrical polarity and amplitude, such that the peaks of the QRS complexes appeared to be twisting around the isoelectric line of the recording.[32] The precise definition of torsades de pointes has been a matter of controversy. Most authors required the presence of prolonged QT interval in the baseline ECG in addition to the tachycardia for the diagnosis,[44,74,151,162] whereas others do not.[64] On the other hand, the term *polymorphous ventricular tachycardia* also has been used interchangeably with torsades de pointes. Because the presence or absence of QT prolongation may have significant therapeutic implications, the distinction of the two groups is essential, even though such an opinion is by no means unanimous.[119] I favor the inclusion of QT prolongation as part of the diagnostic criteria for torsades de pointes and use the term *polymorphous ventricular tachycardia* for those cases without QT prolongation but with the other characteristics of the tachyarrhythmia.

Electrocardiographic Findings in Torsades de Pointes (Figs. 18–31 through 18–33)

1. Paroxysms of ventricular tachyarrhythmias with irregular RR interval

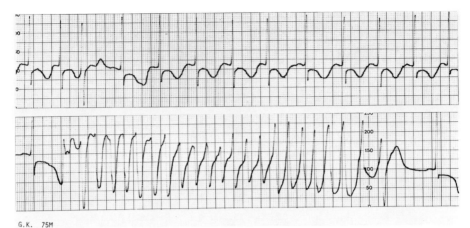

G.K. 75M

FIGURE 18–31. Torsades de pointes resulting from quinidine administration. The patient is a 75-year-old man who had syncope while receiving quinidine. The tracing shows a basic sinus rhythm. There is a marked prolongation of the QT interval, measuring 0.56 second. In the bottom strip, there is an ectopic ventricular beat falling on the T wave of the preceding sinus beat. The ectopic beat initiates an episode of ventricular tachyarrhythmia. The tachycardia has a rate of about 200 beats/min. The RR interval is irregular. The QRS complexes have a negative polarity in the first part of the episode and an upright polarity in the second part.

2. A ventricular rate usually between 200 and 250 beats/min

3. Two or more cycles of QRS complexes with alternating polarity

4. Changing amplitude of the QRS complexes in each cycle in a sinusoidal fashion

5. Prolongation of the QT interval

ONSET

Torsades de pointes is often initiated by premature ventricular beat with a long coupling interval. Because of the prolonged QT interval, however, the ectopic QRS complex usually falls on the T wave of the preceding beat. Kay and associates reported a characteristic

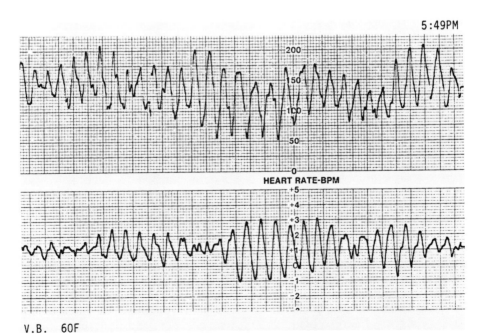

V.B. 60F

FIGURE 18–32. Torsades de pointes. The tracing illustrates an episode of tachycardia that is typical for torsades de pointes in one lead (bottom strip) but is less so in another lead recorded simultaneously (top strip).

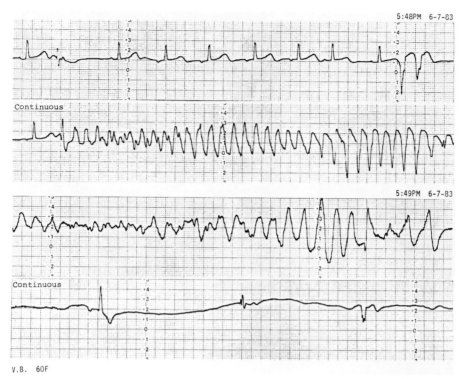

FIGURE 18–33. Torsades de pointes resulting from quinidine administration. The patient was a 60-year-old woman who had a previous myocardial infarction and was receiving digoxin and quinidine for the control of supraventricular and ventricular tachyarrhythmias. Because of recurrent dizziness, an ambulatory ECG was obtained. During the recording, she had a syncope episode. The tracing at the time of syncope (5:48 P.M.) shows torsades de pointes followed by ventricular fibrillation, sinus arrest with ventricular escape beats. Sinus rhythm returned in about 1 minute. Note the prolongation of the QT interval (0.48 second) in the top strip during sinus and ectopic atrial rhythm. There is a ventricular couplet followed by a pause and a supraventricular beat that falls on the terminal part of the T wave and initiates a 45-second episode of torsades de pointes. Thus, a long–short cycle initiating sequence is present (see text). The quinidine and digoxin levels were within therapeutic range. The patient did not have recurrence of syncope after quinidine administration was discontinued.

long-short ventricular cycle length sequence that preceded the onset of torsades de pointes[74] (see Fig. 18–33). The first ventricular complex of the sequence is a premature ventricular beat or the last beat of a salvo of premature ventricular beats. This is followed by a pause and a subsequent supraventricular beat. Then, another premature ventricular beat occurs at a relatively short cycle length and precipitates the torsades de pointes. Such a phenomenon was seen by these authors in 41 of the 44 episodes of torsades de pointes that occurred in 32 patients. The same sequence of cycle length was also noted frequently by Gomes and colleagues to trigger ventricular tachycardia and ventricular fibrillation.[56] The presence of severe bradycardia (as seen in complete AV block or SA block) in the basic rhythm before the onset of torsades

de pointes has been noted by some investigators.[117]

PAROXYSM

An episode of torsades de pointes consists of two or more cycles. Each cycle begins or ends at the point where the amplitude of the QRS complexes is the smallest and the polarity of the complexes changes. There are usually 5 to 20 complexes in each cycle. The rate of the tachycardia is generally between 200 and 250 beats/min but may range from 150 to 300 beats/min.[33,146] Because of the wide QRS complexes and rapid rate, it is often difficult to separate the QRS and T waves. In some instances, when multiple simultaneous leads are recorded, the tachycardia may appear to be monophasic in one lead but presents the typical torsades de pointes in another.[32] The rhythm is usually self-terminating but may degenerate into ventricular fibrillation. The attack also may end with sinus arrest with slow ventricular escape rhythm before the basal rhythm resumes (see Fig. 18–33).

QT PROLONGATION

To most investigators, prolongation of the QT interval in the basic rhythm is a prerequisite for the diagnosis of torsades de pointes. It is the finding that differentiates torsades de pointes from polymorphous ventricular tachycardia. Some authors suggest a QT interval of 0.60 second or more as a diagnostic criterion for torsades de pointes.[162] This limit was chosen arbitrarily and probably should be used only as a general guideline. Prominent U waves with varying amplitude and polarity in the basic complexes also have been described.[130]

Pathophysiology of Torsades de Pointes

The pathophysiology of torsades de pointes is not fully understood. In his original paper, Dessertenne proposed the theory that two competitive automatic ventricular pacemakers were alternatively controlling the heart.[32] Later, some authors believed that reentry is the responsible mechanism because they were able to induce this rhythm by ventricular pacing.[39,64] The presence of QT prolongation, which implies asynchrony of ventricular repolarization, also favors reentry. Other investigators, however, were not able to induce this arrhythmia by pacing.[44] The results of some experimental studies in dogs appear to support the theory of increased automaticity originally proposed by Dessertenne.[6] The reader is referred to a recent review article by Surawicz for more detailed discussion of this subject.[158]

Clinical Correlation

Torsades de pointes is generally seen in conditions that are associated with QT prolongation. The known predisposing factors of this arrhythmia are as follows:

1. Drugs
   Cardiac: quinidine, procainamide, disopyramide, amiodarone
   Psychotropic: phenothiazines, tricyclic antidepressants
   Pentamidine[10]
2. Electrolyte imbalances
   Hypokalemia, hypomagnesemia, hypocalcemia
3. Intrinsic heart disease
   Coronary artery disease, variant angina, myocarditis, mitral valve prolapse
4. Marked bradycardia due to complete or high-grade AV block or to SA node disease
5. Central nervous system disease
   Subarachnoid hemorrhage,[60] complications of air encephalogram studies[164]
6. Congenital QT prolongation syndrome
7. Hypothyroidism[47,128]
8. Liquid protein diet[65,163]
9. Organophosphorous insecticide poisoning[100]

Quinidine is by far the most common cause of torsades de pointes[74,151,152] (see Figs. 18–31 and 18–33). The arrhythmia often develops while the quinidine blood level is in the usual therapeutic range. In the 17 patients who received quinidine and developed torsades de pointes reported by Kay and colleagues, only 3 had quinidine levels that exceeded the therapeutic range.[74] Bauman and associates collected the data on 31 patients with torsades de pointes due to quinidine.[8] Quinidine was administered because of atrial fibrillation or flutter in 71 percent of the patients. The arrhythmia occurred within 1 week of initiation of the drug in 74 percent of the patients. Ninety percent of the 31 patients were also receiving digoxin and about two thirds had prolonged QT interval while not taking quinidine. Other class I antiarrhythmic drugs that prolong the QT interval and may cause torsades de pointes include procainamide,[159] disopyramide,[76,109,121] encainide, flecainide, and propafenone.[153] The percentage of patients who develop torsades de pointes while receiving the last three drugs is high, but the total number is relatively small because of their limited use.[153] This rhythm also may develop with the administration of class III antiarrhythmic drugs such as amiodarone[74,76] and sotolol.[155] Psychotropic drugs such as phenothiazine (especially thioridazine)[52,144] and tricyclic antidepressants[88] may occasionally cause torsades de pointes, mostly when there is an overdose. We have seen this rhythm in association with the use of pentamidine in a patient with the acquired immunodeficiency syndrome.[10]

The association of electrolyte imbalance and torsades de pointes is seen mostly in patients with hypokalemia,[30] hypomagnesemia,[95] and, rarely, hypocalcemia[77] (see Fig.

22–14). In Kay and colleagues' series of 32 patients with torsades de pointes, 14 had one of these electrolyte imbalances and all but 1 of the 14 patients were receiving one of the antiarrhythmic agents at the same time.[74]

Transient QT prolongation often occurs in the acute phase of myocardial infarction.[35] In a series of 771 consecutive patients with acute myocardial infarction, torsades de pointes was observed in 1.2 percent.[59] Drugs or electrolyte imbalance was not implicated in these patients. Torsades de pointes also was reported as isolated cases in patients with chronic stable coronary artery disease,[64] variant angina[22,150] and myocarditis.[88] Mitral valve prolapse may rarely cause torsades de pointes.[64] An illustrative example is given in Chapter 24, Figure 24–2.

Severe bradycardia in patients with high-grade AV block or sick sinus syndrome is believed by some investigators to be one of the important predisposing factors for torsades de pointes.[117] Asynchronization of ventricular activation may be the underlying mechanism responsible for the arrhythmia.[117]

It is generally known that ventricular tachyarrhythmia is the common cause of death in patients with the congenital prolonged QT syndrome with or without deafness. In some of the cases, torsades de pointes is the responsible arrhythmia.[107]

Torsades de pointes has been described in a few cases of hypothyroidism.[47,128] Bradycardia and prolonged QT interval also were noted in these patients.

Sudden death has been reported in patients on liquid protein reducing diet.[65,149] Prolongation of the QT interval and torsades de pointes were found in some of these patients. The cause of the ECG changes are not clear. Electrolyte imbalance does not appear to play an important role in the development of the arrhythmia.

VENTRICULAR FLUTTER AND FIBRILLATION

The ECG in ventricular flutter shows regular continuous waves, usually of large amplitude (Fig. 18–34). The tracing often resembles continuous sine wave, and no distinction between the QRS complex, ST segment, and T wave can be made. The rate of the undulations is usually above 200 per minute. The difference between ventricular tachycardia and ventricular flutter is based mainly on the morphology of the waveforms rather than on the rate. Ventricular flutter is diagnosed when the individual component of the ventricular complex can no longer be recognized.

In ventricular fibrillation, the rhythm is irregularly irregular (see Figs. 18–33 and 18–

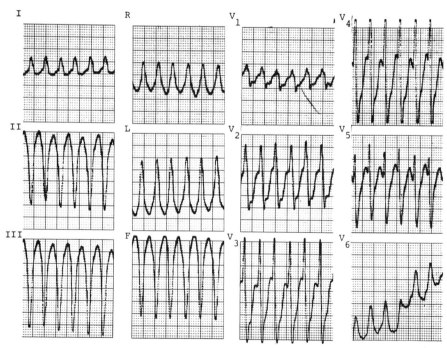

FIGURE 18–34. Ventricular flutter.

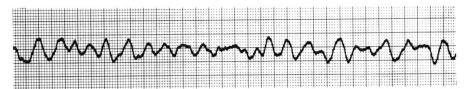

FIGURE 18–35. Ventricular fibrillation.

35). The ECG consists of chaotic deflections of varying amplitude and contour. No definite P waves, QRS complexes, or T waves can be recognized. The rate of the undulations varies between 150 and 500 per minute.

Both ventricular flutter and fibrillation usually lead to sudden death unless they are terminated promptly. Their cause or associated heart disease are similar to those of ventricular tachycardia.

VENTRICULAR ESCAPE BEATS AND IDIOVENTRICULAR RHYTHM

Ventricular escape beats occur when the rate of supraventricular impulses arriving at the ventricles is slower than the inherent rate of the ectopic ventricular pacemaker. They may be seen when there is sinus bradycardia, sinus arrest, SA block, or AV block. In the latter case, the atrial mechanism may be sinus or ectopic atrial in origin, including such atrial arrhythmias as premature atrial contractions (Fig. 18–36), atrial fibrillation, atrial flutter, or paroxysmal atrial tachycardia. In most instances, escape beats associated with bradyarrhythmias orginate from the AV junction unless there is an impairment of the automaticity of the junctional pacemaker. In AV block, ventricular escape also occurs when the block is at a level distal to the His bundle. When there are three or more consecutive ventricular es-

cape beats, the term *idioventricular rhythm* is used (Fig. 18–37).

The ventricular rate in idioventricular rhythm is usually between 30 and 40 beats/min, but may be as slow as 20 or as fast as 50 beats/min. This also is the equivalent rate of the escape interval of the isolated ventricular escape beats. The QRS-T morphology has the characteristics of ectopic ventricular escape beats described previously. The QRS complexes are abnormal and wide, but escape beats originated in the ventricular septum may have near-normal duration and configuration. Escape beats from the right bundle branch system generally have a QRS morphology similar to that seen in left bundle branch block. Escape beats from the left bundle branch block system usually have QRS complexes similar to those seen in right bundle branch block.

Idioventricular rhythm may be simulated by AV junctional escape rhythm with preexisting intraventricular conduction defect. The differentiation may sometimes be impossible from body surface ECG. The diagnosis of ventricular rhythm may be established if ventricular capture or fusion beats are observed.

Because ventricular escape beats and idioventricular rhythm are the results of other rhythm disturbances, their clinical significance also depends on the latter abnormalities.

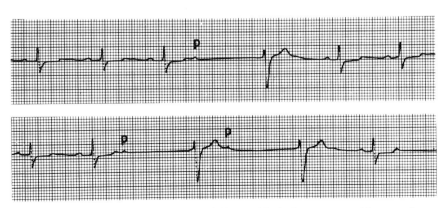

FIGURE 18–36. Ventricular escape beats following blocked premature atrial contractions.

E. C. 3001078

Monitor Lead

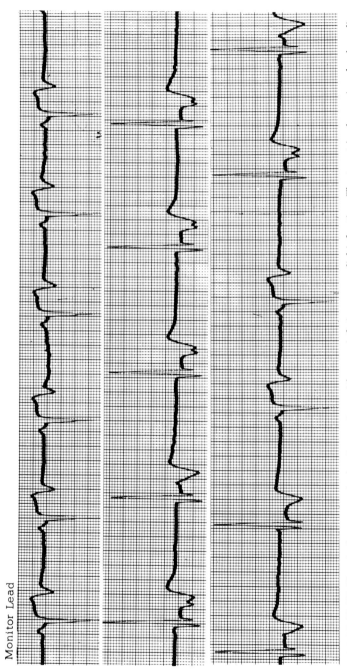

FIGURE 18–37. Ventricular escape rhythm in a patient with acute inferior myocardial infarction. The top strip shows sinus bradycardia. The middle strip shows idioventricular rhythm. Sinus bradycardia and ventricular escape beats are present in the bottom strip. Ventricular escape rhythm occurs when the sinus bradycardia is more pronounced.

REFERENCES

1. Akhtar M, Shenasa M, Jazayeri, et al: Wide QRS complex tachycardia. Ann Intern Med 109:905, 1988
2. Ambos HD, Roberts R, Oliver CG, et al: Infarct size: A determinant of persistence of severe ventricular arrhythmias. Am J Cardiol 37:116, 1976
3. Amsterdam EA, Brocchini R, Vismara LA: Sensitivity of portable monitoring and exercise stress in detection of ventricular arrhythmias in coronary patients. Circulation 49,50(Suppl III):213, 1974
4. Amsterdam EA, Vismara L, Brocchini R, et al: Ventricular ectopic beats: Relation to angiographically documented coronary artery disease. Clin Res 21:399, 1973
5. Armbrust CA, Levine SA: Paroxysmal ventricular tachycardia: A study of 107 cases. Circulation 1:28, 1950
6. Bardy GH, Ungerleider RM, Smith WM, et al: A mechanism of torsades de pointes in a canine model. Circulation 67:52, 1983
7. Bass M: Sudden sniffing death. JAMA 212:2075, 1970
8. Bauman JL, Bauernfeind RA, Hoff JV, et al: Torsade de pointes due to quinidine: observations in 31 patients. Am Heart J 107:425, 1984
9. Bellet S: Clinical Disorders of the Heart Beat. Philadelphia, Lea & Febiger, 1963
10. Bibler MR, Chou TC, Toltzis RJ, Wade PA: Recurrent ventricular tachycardia due to pentamidine-induced cardiotoxicity. Chest 94:1303, 1988
11. Bigger JT, Dresdale RJ, Heissenbuttel RH, et al: Ventricular arrhythmias in ischemic heart disease: Mechanism, prevalence, significance and management. Prog Cardiovasc Dis 19:255, 1977
12. Bigger JT, Fleiss JL, Polnitzky LM, et al: Prevalence, characteristics and significance of ventricular tachycardia detected by 24-hour continuous electrocardiographic recordings in the late hospital phase of acute myocardial infarction. Am J Cardiol 58:1151, 1986
13. Bigger JT, Weld FM, Rolnitzky LM: Which postinfarction ventricular arrhythmias should be treated? Am Heart J 103:660, 1982
14. Blackburn H, Taylor HL, Keys A: The electrocardiogram in prediction of five-year coronary heart disease incidence among men aged forty through fifty-nine. Circulation 41(Suppl I):154, 1970
15. Bleifer SB, Karpman HL, Sheppard JJ, et al: Relation between premature ventricular complexes and development of ventricular tachycardia. Am J Cardiol 31:400, 1973
16. Booth DC, Popio KA, Gettes LS: Multiformity of induced unifocal ventricular premature beats in human subjects: Electrocardiographic and angiographic correlations. Am J Cardiol 49:1643, 1982
17. Brodsky M, Wu D, Denes P, et al: Arrhythmias documented by 24 hour continuous electrocardiographic monitoring in 50 male medical students without apparent heart disease. Am J Cardiol 39:390, 1977
18. Buxton AE, Waxman HL, Marchlinski FE, et al: Right ventricular tachycardia: Clinical and electrophysiologic characteristics. Circulation 68:917, 1983
19. Caceres J, Jazayeri M, McKinnie J, et al: Sustained bundle branch reentry as a mechanism of clinical tachycardia. Circulation 79:256, 1989
20. Chapman JH, Schrank JP, Crampton RS: Idiopathic ventricular tachycardia: An intracardiac electrical, hemodynamic and angiographic assessment of six patients. Am J Med 59:470, 1975
21. Chiang BN, Perlman LV, Ostrander LD, Epstein FH: Relationship of premature systoles to coronary heart disease and sudden death in the Tecumseh epidemiologic study. Ann Intern Med 70:1159, 1969
22. Chiche P, Haiat R, Steff P: Angina pectoris with syncope due to paroxysmal atrioventricular block: Role of ischaemia. Report of two cases. Br Heart J 36:577, 1974
23. Chou TC: Digitalis-induced arrhythmias. In Fowler NO (ed): Treatment of Cardiac Arrhythmias, ed 2. New York, Harper & Row, 1977
24. Chou TC, Wenzke F: The importance of R on T phenomenon. Am Heart J 96:191, 1978
25. Chung EKY: Parasystole. Prog Cardiovasc Dis 11:64, 1968
26. Chung EKY, Walsh TJ, Massie E: Ventricular parasystolic tachycardia. Br Heart J 27:392, 1965
27. Cohen SI, Lau SH, Stein E, et al: Variations of aberrant ventricular conduction in man: evidence of isolated and combined block within the specialized conduction system. Circulation 38:899, 1968
28. Coronary Drug Project Research Group: Prognostic importance of premature beats following myocardial infarction. Experience in the Coronary Drug Project. JAMA 223:1116, 1973
29. Creamer JE, Nathan AW, Camm AJ: The proarrhythmic effects of antiarrhythmic drugs. Am Heart J 114:397, 1987
30. Curry P, Stubbs W, Fitchett D, et al: Ventricular arrhythmias and hypokalemia. Lancet 2:231, 1976
31. DeSoyza N, Bennett FA, Murphy ML, et al: The relationship of paroxysmal ventricular tachycardia complicating the acute phase and ventricular arrhythmia during the late hospital phase of myocardial infarction in long-term survival. Am J Med 64:377, 1978
32. Dessertenne F: La tachycardie ventriculaire a deux foyers opposes variable. Arch Mal Coeur 59:263, 1966
33. Dessertenne F, Coumel PH, Fabiato A: Fibrillation ventriculaire et torsades de pointes. Presse Med 77:193, 1969
34. Devereux RB, Perloff JK, Reichek N, et al: Mitral valve prolapse. Circulation 54:3, 1976
35. Doroghazi RM, Childers R: Time-related changes in the QT interval in acute myocardial infarction: Possible relation to local hypocalcemia. Am J Cardiol 41:684, 1978
36. Dressler W, Roesler M: The occurrence in paroxysmal ventricular tachycardia of ventricular complexes transitional in shape to sinoauricular beats. Am Heart J 44:485, 1952
37. Duvernov WFC, Garcia R: Sarcoidosis of the heart presenting with ventricular tachycardia and atrioventricular block. Am J Cardiol 28:352, 1971
38. Easley RM, Goldstein S: Differentiation of ventricular tachycardia from junctional tachycardia with aberrant conduction: The use of competitive atrial pacing. Circulation 37:1015, 1968
39. Evans TR, Curry PVL, Fitchett DH, et al: "Torsade de pointes" initiated by electrical ventricular stimulation. J Electrocardiol 9:225, 1976
40. Faris JV, McHenry PL, Jordan JW, et al: Prevalence and reproducibility of exercise-induced ventricular arrhythmias during maximal exercise testing in normal man. Am J Cardiol 37:617, 1976
41. Fisch C, Zipes DP, McHenry PL: Rate dependent aberrancy. Circulation 48:714, 1973
42. Flowers NV, Horan LG: Nonanoxic aerosol arrhythmias. JAMA 219:33, 1972
43. Flowers NV, Horan LG: Electrocardiographic and

vectorcardiographic features of myocardial disease. *In* Fowler NO (ed): Myocardial Disease. Orlando, Grune & Stratton, 1973

44. Fontaine G, Frank R, Grosgogeat Y: Torsades de pointes: Definition and management. Mod Conc Cardiovasc Dis 51:103, 1982

45. Fontaine G, Guiraudon G, Frank R, et al: Modern concepts of ventricular tachycardia. Eur J Cardiol 8:565, 1978

46. Fowler NO, McCall D, Chou TC, et al: Electrocardiographic changes and cardiac arrhythmias in patients receiving psychotropic drugs. Am J Cardiol 37:223, 1976

47. Fredlund BO, Olsson SB: Long QT interval and ventricular tachycardia of "torsade de pointe" type in hypothyroidism. Acta Med Scand 213:231, 1983

48. Froelicher VF, Thomas MM, Pillow C, et al: Epidemiologic study of asymptomatic men screened by maximal treadmill testing for latent coronary artery disease. Am J Cardiol 34:770, 1974

49. Gallagher JJ, Damato AN, Lau SH: Electrophysiologic studies during accelerated idioventricular rhythms. Circulation 44:671, 1971

50. Gallagher JJ, Gilbert M, Svenson RH, et al: Wolff-Parkinson-White syndrome: The problem, evaluation, and surgical correction. Circulation 51:767, 1975

51. German LD, Packer DL, Bardy GH, Gallagher JJ: Ventricular tachycardia induced by atrial stimulation in patients without symptomatic cardiac disease. Am J Cardiol 52:1202, 1983

52. Giles TD, Modlin RK: Death associated with ventricular arrhythmia and thioridazone hydrochloride. JAMA 205:98, 1968

53. Glasser SP, Clark PE, Appelbaum HJ: Occurrence of frequent complex arrhythmias detected by ambulatory monitoring: Findings in an apparently healthy asymptomatic elderly population. Chest 75:565, 1979

54. Goldberg S, Greenspon AJ, Urban PL, et al: Reperfusion arrhythmia: A marker of restoration of antegrade flow during intracoronary thrombosis for acute myocardial infarction. Am Heart J 105:26, 1983

55. Goldreyer BN, Bigger JT: Ventriculoatrial conduction in man. Circulation 41:935, 1970

56. Gomes JA, Alexopoulos D, Winters SL, et al: The role of silent ischemia, the arrhythmic substrate and the short-long sequence in the genesis of sudden cardiac death. J Am Coll Cardiol 14:1618, 1989

57. Gouaux JL, Ashman R: Auricular fibrillation with abberation simulating ventricular paroxysmal tachycardia. Am Heart J 34:366, 1947

58. Gozo EG, Cosnow I, Cohen HC, et al: Heart is sarcoidosis. Chest 60:379, 1971

59. Grenadier E, Alpan G, Maor N, et al: Polymorphous ventricular tachycardia in acute myocardial infarction. Am J Cardiol 53:1280, 1984

60. Grossman MA: Cardiac arrhythmias in acute central nervous system disease: Successful management with stellate ganglion block. Arch Intern Med 136:203, 1976

61. Hermann GR, Park HM, Hejtmancik MR: Paroxysmal ventricular tachycardia: A clinical and electrocardiographic study. Am Heart J 57:166, 1959

62. Hiss RG, Lamb LE: Electrocardiographic findings in 122,043 individuals. Circulation 25:947, 1962

63. Holland OB, Nixon JV, Kuhnert L: Diuretic-induced ventricular ectopic activity. Am J Med 70:762, 1981

64. Horowitz LN, Greenspan AM, Spielman SR, et al: Torsades de pointes: Electrophysiologic studies in patients without transient pharmacologic or metabolic abnormalities. Circulation 63:1120, 1981

65. Isner JM, Sours HE, Paris AL, et al: Sudden, unexpected death in avid dieters using the liquid-protein-modified-fast diet: Observations in 17 patients and the role of the prolonged QT interval. Circulation 60:1401, 1979

66. James FW, Kaplan S, Schwartz DC, et al: Response to exercise in patients after total surgical correction of tetralogy of Fallot. Circulation 54:671, 1976

67. Jelinek MV, Lwon B: Exercise stress testing for exposure of cardiac arrhythmias. Prog Cardiovasc Dis 16:497, 1974

68. Jeresaty RM: Sudden death in the mitral valve prolapse–click syndrome. Am J Cardiol 37:317, 1976

69. Josephson ME, Horowitz LN, Farshidi A, et al: Recurrent sustained ventricular tachycardia, 2. Endocardial mapping. Circulation 57:440, 1978

70. Josephson ME, Horowitz LN, Farshidi A, et al: Recurrent sustained ventricular tachycardia, 4. Pleomorphism. Circulation 59:459, 1979

71. Josephson ME, Horowitz LN, Waxman HL, et al: Sustained ventricular tachycardia: Role of the 12-lead electrocardiogram in localizing site of origin. Circulation 64:257, 1981

72. Julian DT, Valentine PA, Miller GG: Disturbances of rate, rhythm and conduction in acute myocardial infarction: A prospective study of 100 consecutive unselected patients with the aid of electrocardiographic monitoring. Am J Med 37:915, 1964

73. Katz LN, Pick A: Clinical Electrocardiography and the Arrhythmias. Philadelphia, Lea & Febiger, 1956

74. Kay GN, Plumb VJ, Arciniegas JG, et al: Torsades de Pointes: The long-short initiating sequence and other clinical features: Observations in 32 patients. J Am Coll Cardiol 2:806, 1983

75. Kennedy HL, Underhill SJ: Frequent or complex ventricular ectopy in apparently healthy subjects: A clinical study of 25 cases. Am J Cardiol 38:141, 1976

76. Keren A, Tzivoni D, Gavish D, et al: Etiology, warning signs and therapy of torsades de pointes: A study of 10 patients. Circulation 64:1167, 1981

77. Khan MM, Logan KR, McComb JM, et al: Management of recurrent ventricular tachyarrhythmias associated with Q-T prolongation. Am J Cardiol 47:1301, 1981

78. Kindwall KE, Brown J, Josephson ME: Electrocardiographic criteria for ventricular tachycardia in wide complex left bundle brach block morphology tachycardias. Am J Cardiol 61:1279, 1988

79. Kistin AD: Retrograde conduction to the atria in ventricular tachycardia. Circulation 24:236, 1961

80. Kistin AD: Problems in the differentiation of ventricular arrhythmia from supraventricular arrhythmia with abnormal QRS. Prog Cardiovasc Dis 9:1, 1966

81. Kistin AD, Landowne M: Retrograde conduction from premature ventricular contractions: A common occurrence in the human heart. Circulation 3:738, 1951

82. Kleiger R, Lown B: Cardioversion and digitalis. II. Clinical studies. Circulation 33:878, 1966

83. Kleiger RE, Miller JP, Thanavaro S, et al: Relationship between clinical features of acute myocardial infarction and ventricular runs 2 weeks to 1 year after infarction. Circulation 63:64, 1981

84. Kostis JB, Byington R, Friedman LM, et al: Prognos-

tic significance of ventricular ectopic activity in survivors of acute myocardial infarction. J Am Coll Cardiol 10:231, 1987

85. Kostis JB, McCrone K, Moreyra AE, et al: Premature ventricular complexes in the absence of identifiable heart disease. Circulation 63:1351, 1981

86. Kostis JB, Moreyra AE, Amendo MT, et al: The effect of age on heart rate in subjects free of heart disease: Studies by ambulatory electrocardiography and maximal exercise stress test. Circulation 65:141, 1982

87. Kotler MN, Tabatznik B, Mower MM, et al: Prognostic significance of ventricular ectopic beats with respect to sudden death in the late postinfarction period. Circulation 47:959, 1973

88. Krikler DM, Curry PVL: Torsades de pointes: an atypical ventricular tachycardia. Br Heart J 38:117, 1976

89. Kugler JD, Pinsky WW, Cheatham JP, et al: Sustained ventricular tachycardia after repair of tetralogy of Fallot: Electrophysiologic findings. Am J Cardiol 51:1137, 1983

90. Langendorf R, Pick A, Winternitz M: Mechanisms of intermittent ventricular bigeminy. I. Appearance of ectopic beats dependent upon length of cycle, the "rule of bigeminy." Circulation 11:422, 1955

91. Lawrie N, Greenwood TW, Goodard M, et al: A coronary-care unit in the routine management of acute myocardial infarction. Lancet 2:109, 1967

92. Lemery R, Brugada P, Bella PD, et al: Nonischemic ventricular tachycardia. Clinical course and long-term follow-up in patients without clinically overt heart disease. Circulation 78:990, 1989

93. Lesch M. Lewis E, Humphries JO, et al: Paroxysmal ventricular tachycardia in the absence of organic heart disease: Report of a case and review of the literature. Ann Intern Med 66:950, 1967

94. Lichstein E, Ribas-Meneelier C, Gupta PK, et al: Incidence and description of accelerated ventricular rhythm complicating acute myocardial infarction. Am J Med 58:192, 1975

95. Loeb HS, Pietras RJ, Gunnar RM, et al: Paroxysmal ventricular fibrillation in two patients with hypomagnesemia: Treatment by transvenous pacing. Circulation 37:210, 1968

96. Lown B, Calvert AF, Armington R, et al: Monitoring for serious arrhythmias and high risk of sudden death. Circulation 52(Suppl III):189, 1975

97. Lown B, Fakhro AM, Hood WB, et al: The coronary care unit: New perspectives and directions. JAMA 199:188, 1967

98. Lown B, Graboys TB: Management of patients with malignant ventricular arrhythmias. Am J Cardiol 39:910, 1977

99. Lown B, Tykocinski M, Garfein A, et al: Sleep and ventricular premature beats. Circulation 48:691, 1973

100. Ludomirsky A, Klein HO, Sarelli P, et al: Q-T prolongation and polymorphous ("torsades de pointes") ventricular arrhythmias associated with organophosphorus insecticide poisoning. Am J Cardiol 49:1654, 1982

101. Mackenzie GJ, Pascual S: Paroxysmal ventricular tachycardia. Br Heart J 26:441, 1964

102. Manyari DE, Klein GJ, Gulamhusein S, et al: Arrhythomogenic right ventricular dysplasia: A generalized cardiomyopathy? Circulation 68:251, 1983

103. Marcus FI, Fontaine GH, Guiraudon G, et al: Right ventricular dysplasia: A report of 24 adult cases. Circulation 65:384, 1982

104. Marriott HJL, Menendez MM: A-V dissociation revisited. Prog Cardiovasc Dis 8:522, 1966

105. Marriott HJL, Thorne DC: Dysrhythmic dilemmas in coronary care. Am J Cardiol 27:327, 1971

106. Massumi RA, Ali N: Accelerated isorhythmic ventricular rhythms. Am J Cardiol 26:170, 1970

107. McHenry PL, Fisch C, Jordan JW, et al: Cardiac arrhythmias observed during maximal treadmill exercise testing in clinically normal men. Am J Cardiol 29:331, 1972

108. McHenry PL, Morris SN, Kavalier M, et al: Comparative study of exercise-induced ventricular arrhythmias in normal subjects and patients with documented coronary artery disease. Am J Cardiol 37:609, 1976

109. Meltzer RS, Robert EW, McMorrow M, et al: Atypical ventricular tachycardia as a manifestation of disopyramide toxicity. Am J Cardiol 42:1049, 1978

110. Mendez C, Gruhzit CC, Moe GK: Influence of cycle length upon refractory period of auricles, ventricles and A-V node in the dog. Am J Physiol 184:286, 1956

111. Michelson EL, Morganroth J, MacVaugh H: Post-operative arrhythmias after coronary artery and cardiac valvular surgery detected by long-term electrocardiographic monitoring. Am Heart J 97:442, 1979

112. Miller FC, Krucoff MW, Satler LF, et al: Ventricular arrhythmias during reperfusion. Am Heart J 112:928, 1986

113. Miller JM, Marchlinski FE, Buxton AE, Josephson ME: Relationship between the 12-lead electrocardiogram during ventricular tachycardia and endocardial site of origin in patients with coronary artery disease. Circulation 77:759, 1988

114. Moller M, Nielsen BL, Fabricius J: Paroxysmal ventricular tachycardia during repeated 24-hour ambulatory electrocardiographic monitoring of postmyocardial infarction patients. Br Heart J 43:447, 1980

115. Morgensen L: A controlled trial of lignocaine prophylaxis in the prevention of ventricular tachyarrhythmias in acute myocardial infarction. Acta Med Scand 513:1, 1971

116. Moss AJ, Davis HT, DeCamilla J, et al: Ventricular ectopic beats and their relation to sudden and nonsudden cardiac death after myocardial infarction. Circulation 60:998, 1979

117. Motte G, Coumel P, Abitbol G, et al: Le syndrome de QT long et syncopes par "torsades de pointes." Arch Mal Coeur 63:831, 1970

118. Myburgh DP, Lewis BS: Ventricular parasystole in healthy hearts. Am Heart J 82:307, 1971

119. Nava A, Thiene G, Canciani B, et al: Familial occurrence of right ventricular dysplasia: A study involving nine families. J Am Coll Cardiol 12:1222, 1988

120. Nguyen PT, Scheinman MM, Seger J: Polymorphous ventricular tachycardia: Clinical characterization, therapy and QT interval. Circulation 74:340, 1986

121. Nicholson WJ, Martin CE, Gracey JG, et al: Disopyramide-induced ventricular fibrillation. Am J Cardiol 43:1053, 1979

122. Norris RM, Mercer CJ: Significance of idioventricular rhythms in acute myocardial infarction. Prog Cardiovasc Dis 16:455, 1974

123. Northfield TC: Cardiac complications of phaeochromocytoma. Br Heart J 29:588, 1967

124. Ohe T, Shimomura K, Aihara N, et al: Idiopathic sustained left ventricular tachycardia: Clinical and electrophysiologic characteristics. Circulation 77:560, 1988

125. Okajima M, Scholnerich P, Simonson E: Frequency of premature beats. Minn Med November, p 751, 1961

126. Oreto G, Satullo G, Luzza F, et al: "Irregular" ventricular parasystole: The influence of sinus rhythm on a parasystolic focus. Am Heart J 115:121, 1988

127. Pantridge JF, Adgey AAJ, Geddes JS, et al: The Acute Coronary Attack. Orlando, Grune & Stratton, 1975

128. Pechter RA, Osborn LA: Polymorphic ventricular tachycardia secondary to hypothyroidism. Am J Cardiol 57:882, 1986

129. Pietras RJ, Lam W, Bauernfeind R, et al: Chronic recurrent right ventricular tachycardia in patients without ischemic heart disease: Clinical, hemodynamic and angiographic findings. Am Heart J 105:357, 1983

130. Reynolds EW, Vander Ark CR: Quinidine syncope and the delayed repolarization syndromes. Mod Conc Cardiovasc Dis 45:117, 1976

131. Rodstein M, Wolloch L, Gubner RS: Mortality study of the significance of extrasystoles in an insured population. Circulation 44:617, 1971

132. Romhilt DW, Bloomfield SS, Chou T, et al: Unreliability of conventional electrocardiographic monitoring for arrhythmia detection in coronary care units. Am J Cardiol 31:457, 1973

133. Rosenbaum MB: Classification of ventricular extrasystoles according to form. J Electrocardiol 2:289, 1969

134. Rothfeld EL, Zucker IR, Parsonnet V, et al: Idioventricular rhythm in acute myocardial infarction. Circulation 37:203, 1968

135. Roy PR, Emanual R, Ismail SA, et al: Hereditary prolongation of the Q-T interval: Genetic observations and management in three families with twelve affected members. Am J Cardiol 37:237, 1976

136. Ruberman W, Weinblatt, E, Goldberg JD, et al: Ventricular premature complexes in prognosis of angina. Circulation 61:1172, 1980

137. Ruberman W, Weinblatt E, Goldberg JD, et al: Ventricular premature complexes and sudden death after myocardial infarction. Circulation 64:297, 1981

138. Sachs HS, Matisson R, Kennelly BM: Familial paroxysmal ventricular tachycardia in two sisters. Am Heart J 87:217, 1974

139. Sandler IA, Marriott HJL: The differential morphology of anomalous ventricular complexes of RBBB-type in lead V₁. Circulation 31:551, 1965

140. Schamroth L: Idioventricular tachycardia. J Electrocardiol 1:205, 1968

141. Schamroth L, Dolaro A: Paroxysmal ventricular tachycardia with rate-dependent coupling intervals. Circulation 36:255, 1967

142. Scherf D, Choi KH, Bahadori A, et al: Parasystole. Am J Cardiol 12:527, 1963

143. Scherf D, Cohen J: The Atrioventricular Node and Selected Cardiac Arrhythmias. Orlando, Grune & Stratton, 1964

144. Schoonmaker FW, Osteen RT, Greenfield JC: Thioridazine (Mellaril®)-induced ventricular tachycardia controlled with an artificial pacemaker. Ann Intern Med 65:1076, 1966

145. Schulze RA, Rouleau J, Rigo P, et al: Ventricular arrhythmias in the late hospital phase of acute myocardial infarction: Relation to left ventricular function detected by rated cardiac blood pool scanning. Circulation 52:1006, 1975

146. Sclarovsky S, Strasberg B, Lewin RF, et al: Polymorphous ventricular tachycardia: Clinical features and treatment. Am J Cardiol 44:339, 1979

147. Selzer A, Wray HW: Quinidine syncope. Paroxysmal ventricular fibrillation occuring during treatment of chronic atrial arrhythmias. Circulation 30:17, 1964

148. Shappel SD, Marshall CE, Brown RE, et al: Sudden death and the familial occurrence of the midsystolic click, late systolic murmur syndrome. Circulation 48:1128, 1973

149. Singh BN, Gaarder TD, Kanegae T, et al: Liquid protein diets and torsade de pointes. JAMA 240:115, 1978

150. Slama R, Motte G, Coumel PH, et al: Le syndrome "alongement de QT et syncopes par tosades de pointes." Laval Med 42:353, 1971

151. Smith WM, Gallagher JJ: "Les torsade de pointes": An unusual ventricular arrhythmia. Ann Intern Med 93:578, 1980

152. Soffer J, Dreifus LS, Michelson EL: Polymorphous ventricular tachycardia associated with normal and long Q-T intervals. Am J Cardiol 49:2021, 1982

153. Stanton MS, Prystowsky EN, Fineberg NS, et al: Arrhythmogenic effects of antiarrhythmic drugs: A study of 506 patients treated for ventricular tachycardia or fibrillation. J Am Coll Cardiol 14:209, 1989

154. Strasberg B, Sclarovsky S, Erdberg A, et al: Procainamide-induced polymorphous ventricular tachycardia. Am J Cardiol 47:1309, 1981

155. Stratmann HG, Kennedy HL: Torsades de pointes associated with drugs and toxins: Recognition and management. Am Heart J 113:1470, 1987

156. Surawicz B: Relationship between electrocardiogram and electrolytes. Am Heart J 73:814, 1967

157. Surawicz B: Role of electrolytes in etiology and management of cardiac arrhythmias. Prog Cardiovasc Dis 8:364, 1966

158. Surawicz B: Electrophysiologic substrate of torsade de pointes: Dispersion of repolarization or early afterdepolarization? J Am Coll Cardiol 14:172, 1989

159. Tchou P, Jazayeri M, Denker S, et al: Transcatheter electrical ablation of right bundle branch block: A method of treating macroreentrant ventricular tachycardia attributed to bundle branch reentry. Circulation 78:246, 1988

160. Touboul P, Kirkorian G, Atallah G, et al: Bundle branch reentrant tachycardia treated by electrical ablation of the right bundle branch. J Am Coll Cardiol 7:1404, 1986

161. Tye KH, Samant A, Desser KB, et al: R on T or R on P phenomenon? Relation to the genesis of ventricular tachycardia. Am J Cardiol 44:632, 1979

162. Tzivoni D, Keren A, Stern S: Torsades de pointes versus polymorphous ventricular tachycardia. Am J Cardiol 52:639, 1983

163. Van Durme JP, Pannier RH: Prognostic significance of ventricular dysrhythmias 1 year after myocardial infarction. Am J Cardiol 37:178, 1976

164. Vourc'h G, Tannieres ML: Cardiac arrhythmia induced by pneumoencephalography. Br J Anaesth 50:833, 1978

165. Ward DE, Nathan AW, Camm AJ: Fascicular tachycardia sensitive to calcium antagonists. European Heart J 5:896, 1984

166. Watanabe Y: Reassessment of parasystole. Am Heart J 81:451, 1971

167. Waxman MB, Wald RW: Termination of ventricular tachycardia by an increase in cardiac vagal drive. Circulation 56:385, 1977

168. Weiss J, Stevenson WG: Narrow QRS ventricular tachycardia. Am Heart J 112:843, 1986

169. Wellens HJJ: The electrocardiogram 80 years after Einthoven. J Am Coll Cardiol 7:484, 1986

170. Wellens HJJ, Bar FW, Lie KI: The value of the electrocardiogram in the differential diagnosis of a tachycardia with a widened QRS complex. Am J Med 64:27, 1978

171. Wellens HJJ, Lie KI: Ventricular tachycardia: The value of programmed electrical stimulation. *In* Krikler DM, Goodwin JF (eds): Cardiac Arrhythmias: The Modern Electrophysiological Approach. Philadelphia, WB Saunders, 1975, p 182

172. Winkle RA, Goodman DJ, Popp RL: Simultaneous echocardiographic-phonocardiographic recordings at rest and during amytal nitrate administration in patients with mitral valve prolapse. Circulation 51:522, 1975

Atrioventricular Block; Concealed Conduction

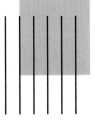

19

Atrioventricular (AV) conduction defect traditionally is divided into incomplete and complete block. Incomplete AV block includes first-degree, second-degree, and advanced AV block. Complete AV block also is called third-degree AV block. With the advent of the technique of His bundle recording, a more precise localization of the block became feasible.[40] The block may be located proximal to, in, or distal to the His bundle.[34] When it is proximal to the His bundle, the block may be in the atrium or AV node. Some investigators classify AV block into intraatrial, AV nodal, and infranodal (which includes intrahisian and infrahisian) blocks.[15,29,33] In intraatrial block, there is a prolongation of the PA time (normal range, 25 to 45 msec), which represents the interval between the onset of the P wave in the surface electrocardiogram (ECG) and the deflection A recorded by the intracardiac electrode at the low right atrium (Fig. 19–1). This is an uncommon condition and is responsible only for occasional cases of PR prolongation in the surface ECG. In AV nodal block, there is an increase of the AH interval (normal range, 60 to 140 msec), which is the interval between deflection A from the low right atrium to the onset of the first rapid deflection of the His bundle electrogram (H). In intrahisian block (or block within the His bundle itself), there is an increase in the duration of His bundle potential or BH time, to exceed the upper limit of 20 msec (normal range, 15 to 20 msec). The His bundle potential is "split." In infrahisian block, the conduction defect is at the level of the bundle branches and there is a prolongation of the HV time (normal range, 35 to 55 msec), which is the interval between the onset of His bundle potential and the onset of ventricular depolarization recorded on the intracardiac electrogram (V) or any of the surface leads.

Although His bundle recording often gives more precise and additional useful information about AV conduction, it is not routinely obtained in clinical practice. Furthermore, in most instances, a reasonable therapeutic decision may be made, even though His bundle recording is not available. In the following discussion, the traditional classification of first-, second-, and third-grade AV block is used. Attempts are made to correlate the findings in the surface ECG with those from the His bundle recordings.

All degrees of AV block may be intermittent or persistent. The degree of the conduction defect also may change from time to time. It is not uncommon for a patient to have a normal PR interval with 1:1 AV conduction for days or weeks but develop transient complete AV block resulting in a syncope episode.

AV CONDUCTION DEFECT WITH NORMAL PR INTERVAL

Conduction delay in a part of the AV conduction system may not be sufficient to prolong the PR interval beyond the upper limit of normal, which is 0.20 second in adults. In some patients, a comparison with previous ECGs may reveal an increase in the duration of the PR interval, even though it is still within the normal range.

In 96 patients with normal PR interval and abnormally wide QRS complex studied by Puech, 53 percent were found to have prolongation of the HV interval to greater than 55 msec.[33] The HV prolongation was more common in patients with left bundle branch block or right bundle branch block with left hemiblock.[8,33] In these patients, conduction delay in the other fascicle, resulting in a mild degree of bilateral bundle branch block, may be implicated as the cause of the HV prolongation.

FIRST-DEGREE AV BLOCK

Electrocardiographic Findings
(Fig. 19–2)

1. The PR interval is greater than 0.20 second.

411

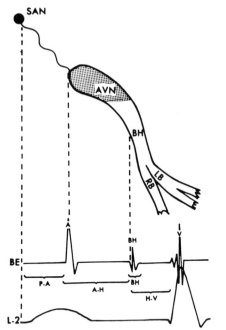

FIGURE 19-1. Diagram of the AV conduction system and the corresponding bipolar intracardiac electrogram (BE) and standard surface electrocardiogram (L-2). SAN = sinoatrial node; AVN = atrioventricular node; BH = bundle of His; RB and LB = right and left bundle branches, respectively; A-H = conduction time through the AVN; H-V = conduction time through the His Purkinje system; A = bipolar atrial electrogram; V = bipolar ventricular electrogram recorded from the area of the A-V junction. (Adapted from Narula OS, Schlerlag BJ, Samet P, et al: Atrioventricular block: Localization and classification by His bundle recordings. Am J Med 50:146, 1971, with permission of author and American Journal of Medicine.)

2. Each P wave is followed by a QRS complex.

The range of PR prolongation is usually between 0.21 and 0.40 second. Occasionally, an interval greater than 0.60 second may be seen (Fig. 19-3). When the prolongation is marked, the P wave may be masked by the preceding T wave or simulate a U wave. The degree of prolongation may change in the same individual (see Fig. 19-3). The interval may be shortened when the heart rate increases and lengthened when there is an increase in vagal tone. Marked spontaneous fluctuation in the PR interval is seen most often in individuals with no clinical evidence of heart disease, whereas the interval is more likely to be constant in those with organic heart disease.

Electrophysiological Correlation

In patients with first-degree AV block associated with a narrow QRS complex, the conduction delay is most commonly in the AV node with prolongation of the AH time.[6] Only occasionally is prolongation of the PA or BH time responsible; even less often is prolonged HV time the reason for the PR prolongation.[29] In patients with first-degree AV block and bundle branch block, the conduction delay may occur in any of the various regions of the conduction system. Prolongation of the HV time is most common in those patients with left bundle branch block.

SECOND-DEGREE AV BLOCK

In second-degree AV block, there is an intermittent failure of the supraventricular impulse to be conducted to the ventricles. Some of the P waves are not followed by a QRS complex. The conduction ratio (or P/QRS ratio) varies. It may be 2:1, 3:1, 3:2, 4:3, and so forth, or it may vary from time to time in a haphazard fashion. In the description of the conduction sequence, it is important to specify whether the ratio refers to conduction or block. For example, if only every third P wave is followed by a QRS complex, there is a 3:1

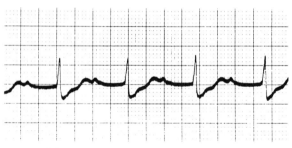

FIGURE 19-2. First-degree AV block.

PR 0.36

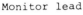

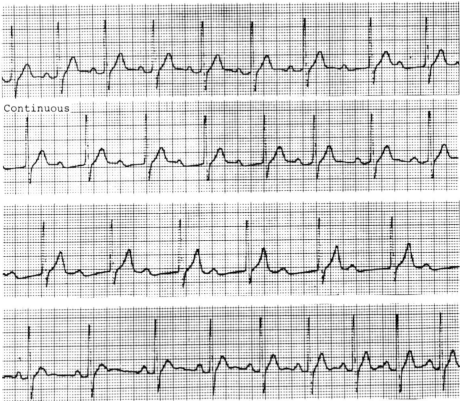

FIGURE 19–3. First-degree AV block with marked variation of the PR interval in an apparently healthy individual. The PR interval varies from 0.18 to 0.66 second. The shorter PR interval is associated mostly with more rapid heart rate.

conduction or 3:2 block. Much confusion may result if the words *conduction* and *block* are used interchangeably.

There are two types of second-degree AV block, namely types I and II. Type I also is called *Wenckebach phenomenon* or *Mobitz type I* and is the common type. Type II also is called *Mobitz type II* and is the uncommon type.

Type I Second-Degree AV Block: The Wenckebach Phenomenon

ELECTROCARDIOGRAPHIC
FINDINGS (Fig. 19–4)

1. Progressive lengthening of the PR interval until a P wave is blocked

2. Progressive shortening of the RR interval until a P wave is blocked

3. The RR interval containing the blocked P wave is shorter than the sum of 2 PP intervals

In the typical case of type I second-degree AV block, the increase of the PR prolongation is longest in the second conducted beat after the pause. This is probably related to the marked increase in the refractory period of the AV junction following the pause. In the subsequent beats, the PR interval continues to increase, but the degree of the increment decreases. This phenomenon may be explained by the balancing effect of the shorter preceding cycle length (which shortens the refractory period) on the increasing refractoriness of the junctional tissue due to the previously conducted impulse.

The progressive shortening of the RR interval until a blocked P wave occurs is the result of the decrease in the increment of PR prolongation. The following example serves to illustrate this finding (Fig. 19–5). Assuming the PP interval is 1.0 second, the PR interval increases stepwise from 0.20 to 0.30 to 0.36 and 0.40 second, following which the P wave is blocked. There is, therefore, a 5:4 conduction. The increments of the PR interval of the

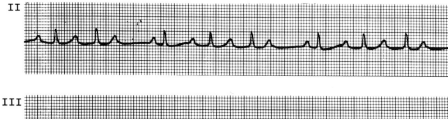

5476   76M

FIGURE 19–4. Type I second-degree AV block with typical Wenckebach phenomenon.

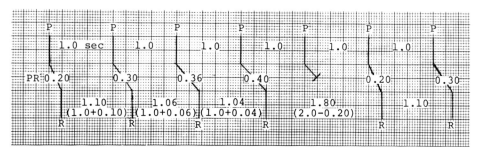

FIGURE 19–5. Diagram illustrating and explaining the progressive shortening of the RR interval during a typical Wenckebach period. Although there is progressive prolongation of the PR interval, the increment of the increase decreases.

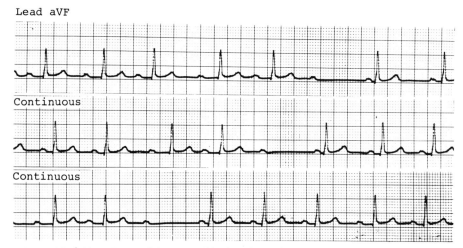

FIGURE 19–6. Type I second-degree AV block without the typical Wenckebach phenomenon. Note the random variation of the PR and RR intervals, except that the PR interval that follows the blocked P waves is always short. The QRS complexes that terminate the pauses may be junctional escape beats.

II

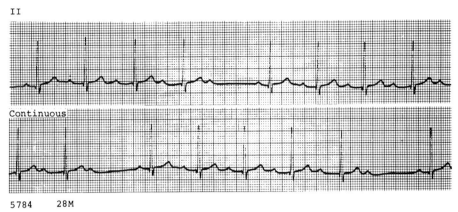

Continuous

5784   28M

FIGURE 19-7. Type I second-degree AV block without the typical Wenckebach phenomenon. There is no progressive shortening of the RR interval before the block.

conducted beats are 0.10, 0.06, and 0.04 second, respectively. The RR intervals are 1.0 + 0.10 (1.10), 1.0 + 0.06 (1.06), and 1.0 + 0.04 second (1.04), respectively.

Using the same diagram, the reason that the RR interval that contains the blocked P wave is shorter than two PP intervals also can be visualized. The marked shortening of the PR interval after the pause results in earlier appearance of the QRS complex than does the one before the pause.

Because of the periodic pauses, the rhythm shows "group beating," a finding that frequently leads to the diagnosis of Wenckebach phenomenon. The sequence between one pause to the next is referred to as a *Wenckebach period.*

Contrary to the generally held impression, the typical Wenckebach phenomenon is not seen frequently in type I second-degree AV block. The prolongation of the PR interval may not be progressive, neither is the shortening of the RR interval (Fig. 19–6). The largest increment of the PR interval sometimes is seen just before block occurs (Fig. 19–7). The most common reason for the atypical findings is sinus arrhythmia, which alters the RR interval, which in turn affects the RP and PR intervals of the subsequent beats. Fluctuation of vagal tone also may affect both the sinus rate and the PR interval. When the Wenckebach period is long, many successive cycles may not show any measurable change in the PR interval.

ELECTROPHYSIOLOGICAL CORRELATION

In patients with type I block and narrow QRS complexes, the block is usually located in the AV node.[28,33] There is a progressive prolongation of the AH interval until the blocked P wave occurs. The latter is not followed by a His bundle potential. Occasionally, the block is in the His bundle, with progressive prolongation of the interval between the split His potentials. In the blocked beat, the A potential is followed by the first but not the second part of the split H. Intrahisian block may often be distinguished from intranodal block in the body surface ECG in that the AV conduction ratio becomes worse with atropine administration (which increases the sinus rate) and improves with carotid sinus massage (which decreases the sinus rate) if the block is intrahisian.[24] The opposite effects are observed if the block is intranodal. When type I second-degree AV block is associated with bundle branch block, the block may occur in the AV node, His bundle, or the contralateral bundle branch. In about 75 percent of the cases, the block is in the AV node; in 25 percent it is infranodal.[27,33]

Type II Second-Degree AV Block: Mobitz Type II

ELECTROCARDIOGRAPHIC FINDINGS (Figs. 19–8 and 19–9)

1. There are intermittent blocked P waves.
2. In the conducted beats, the PR intervals remain constant.

The PR interval of the conducted beats may be normal or prolonged. It remains constant, except that slight shortening may occur in the first beat after the blocked cycle. This is the result of improved conduction following block. In some cases, this shorter interval is

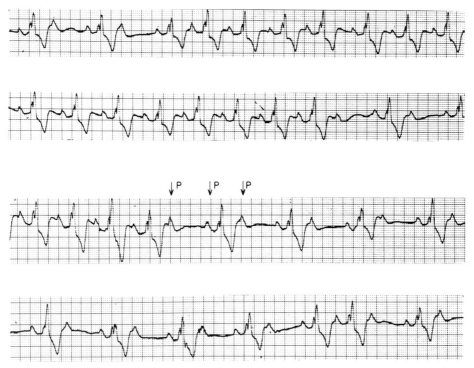

FIGURE 19–8. Mobitz type II second-degree AV block. Note the constant PR interval before block occurs. The QRS complex has right bundle branch block morphology. (Demonstrated by the 12-lead ECG, which is not shown here.)

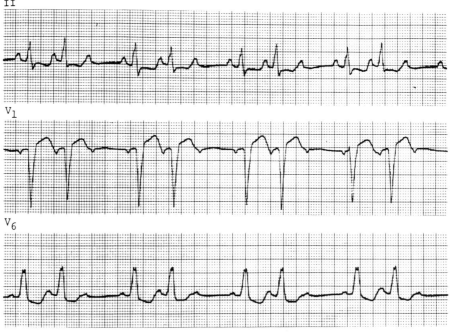

FIGURE 19–9. Mobitz type II second-degree AV block. There is a 3:2 conduction. The QRS complex has a left bundle branch block morphology.

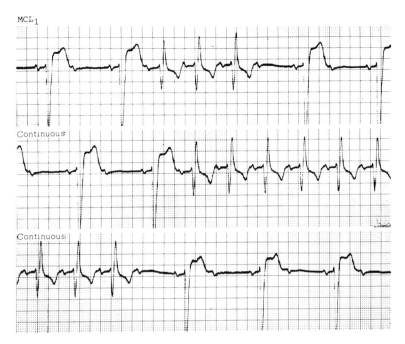

FIGURE 19–10. Mobitz type II second-degree AV block resulting from bilateral bundle branch block. The monitor lead shows alternating left and right bundle branch block patterns. A His bundle recording demonstrated that the block was distal to the His bundle.

due to an escape beat but it may occur in its absence.[17] Therefore, in a patient with 3:2 conduction, it may be difficult to determine whether the block is type I or II. Some investigators insist on a strict diagnostic criterion for Mobitz type II block, namely that the PR interval of all beats be the same.[2]

ELECTROPHYSIOLOGICAL CORRELATION

Most patients with type II second-degree AV block have associated bundle branch block (see Figs. 19–8 and 19–9). In these patients,

the block is usually located distal to the His bundle (Fig. 19–10).[47] In about 27 to 35 percent of Mobitz type II blocks, the lesion is in the His bundle itself[27,33] and a narrow QRS complex may be inscribed[28] (Fig. 19–11). Rarely, the block may be AV nodal in origin.[35]

2:1 AV BLOCK

When the AV conduction ratio is 2:1, it is often impossible to determine whether the second-degree AV block is type I or II. A long rhythm strip may record an episode of chang-

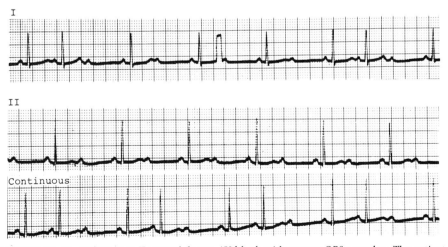

FIGURE 19–11. Mobitz type II second-degree AV block with narrow QRS complex. The patient had recurrent episodes of syncope. Because of the narrow QRS complex the block is probably at the level of the His bundle.

II

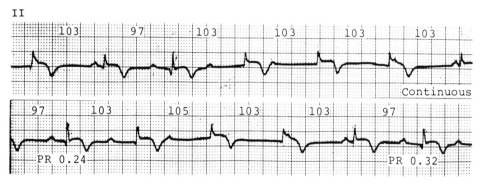

0201   44M

FIGURE 19–12. Advanced AV block. The captured ventricular beats are represented by the premature QRS complexes, which have a more prominent Q wave than the escape beats. In the bottom strip, the first captured beat has a PR interval of 0.24, and the second captured beat has a PR interval of 0.32 second. The shorter PR interval is preceded by a longer RP interval and vice versa. The patient had an acute inferior myocardial infarction.

ing conduction ratio, and the behavior of the PR interval may be observed. When the atrial rate is increased by exercise or atropine, the AV block in type I tends to decrease and that in type II tends to increase.[17,24]

HIGH-GRADE OR ADVANCED AV BLOCK

When the AV conduction ratio is 3:1 or higher, the rhythm is called *advanced* AV block (Fig. 19–12). In some cases, only occasional ventricular captures are observed, and the dominant rhythm is maintained by a subsidiary pacemaker. Identification of the type of the second-degree block in such instances is also difficult. Comparison of the PR intervals of the occasional captured beats may provide a clue. If the PR interval varies and its length is inversely related to the interval between the P wave and its preceding R wave

(RP), type I block is likely (see Fig. 19–12). A constant PR interval for all the captured beats suggests type II block.[17]

DIFFERENTIAL DIAGNOSIS OF SECOND-DEGREE AV BLOCK

Second-degree AV block may be simulated by blocked premature atrial beats (Fig. 19–13). This occurs especially when the premature atrial impulse has a relatively long coupling time with the preceding cycle. A careful measurement of the PP cycle length and examination of the P-wave morphology will avoid the erroneous diagnosis. Conversely, in some cases of second-degree AV block, ventriculophasic sinus arrhythmia is present. The PP intervals that contain the QRS complexes are shorter than those without. The blocked P waves may be mistaken for blocked premature atrial beats.

Monitor lead

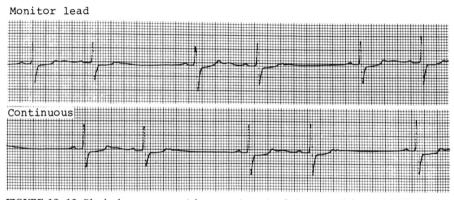

FIGURE 19–13. Blocked premature atrial contractions simulating second-degree AV block with 3:2 conduction.

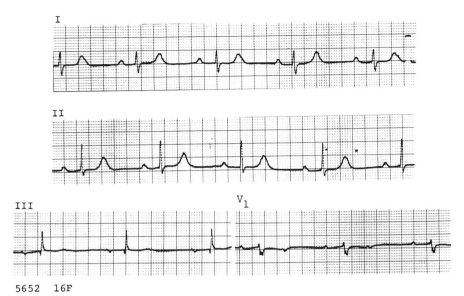

5652 16F

FIGURE 19-14. Second-degree AV block with 2:1 conduction simulating sinus bradycardia with first-degree AV block. The blocked P waves can best be seen in lead V$_1$. They are masked by the preceding T waves, especially in leads I and II.

An AV conduction ratio of 2:1 may simulate or be simulated by sinus bradycardia. The P waves of the nonconducted beats may fall on the preceding T waves and are not recognized (Fig. 19-14). If they occur right after the T waves, they may be mistaken for U waves. On the other hand, the U waves in patients with sinus bradycardia may be mistaken for blocked P waves and second-degree AV block diagnosed.

COMPLETE (THIRD-DEGREE) AV BLOCK

In third-degree AV block, there is a complete failure of the supraventricular impulses to reach the ventricles. The atrial and ventricular activities are independent of each other. The ventricular excitation is initiated by a subsidiary pacemaker distal to the site of block, which may be in the AV node, His bundle, or bundle branches. If the block is in the main bundle branches, it is called *bilateral bundle branch block*. If it involves the right bundle branch and two divisions of the left bundle branch, it is called *trifascicular block*.

Electrocardiographic Findings
(Figs. 19-15 and 19-16)

1. There is an independence of the atrial and ventricular activities.

2. The atrial rate is faster than the ventricular rate. The atrial rhythm may be sinus or ectopic in origin.

3. The ventricular rhythm is maintained by either a junctional or an idioventricular pacemaker.

In patients with sinus rhythm and complete AV block, the PP and RR intervals are regular, but the P waves bear no constant relation to the QRS complexes. The PR interval varies. The PP intervals may be slightly irregular because of sinus arrhythmia. In about 30 to 40 percent of patients with complete AV block, ventriculophasic sinus arrhythmia can be demonstrated.[39]

When the atrial mechanism is atrial fibrillation, the presence of complete AV block is recognized by the regularity of the ventricular rhythm. This is also true in atrial flutter or paroxysmal atrial tachycardia, but, in addition, the flutter or ectopic P waves should have no demonstrable relation to the QRS complexes.

There is considerable confusion about the use of the terms *complete AV block* and *AV dissociation*. In this text, the term *complete AV block* is used when the atrial rate is faster than the ventricular rate, whereas the reverse is true in AV dissociation. In AV block, there is a failure of impulse conduction even though the ventricles are receptive. In AV dissociation, there is an increase in the automaticity of the subsidiary pacemaker, which ren-

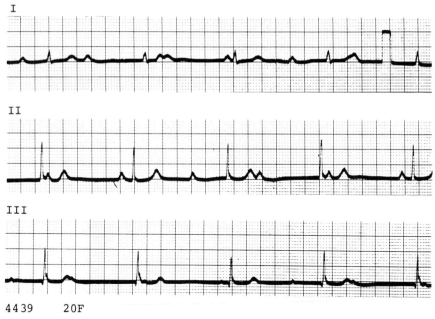

4439   20F

FIGURE 19–15. Congenital complete AV block. The narrow QRS complexes suggest that the escape pacemaker is junctional in origin. No other associated congenital defects were found.

ders the ventricles functionally refractory to the slower atrial impulses.

The morphology of the QRS complexes depends mainly on the location of the block. The escape pacemaker usually originates from a site just distal to the region of the block. If the block is proximal to the bifurcation of the

His bundle, the escape pacemaker is likely to be AV junctional in origin, and the QRS complexes are narrow unless bundle branch block coexists (see Fig. 19–15). If the block is below the bifurcation of the His bundle, the escape rhythm is idioventricular in origin and the QRS complexes are wide and bizarre (see

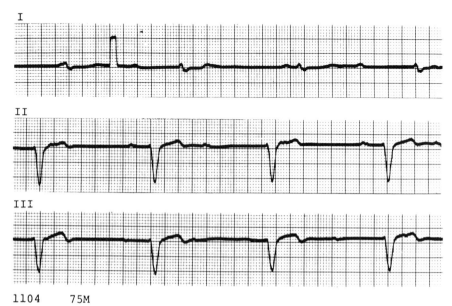

1104   75M

FIGURE 19–16. Complete AV block with idioventricular rhythm. The QRS complexes are abnormally wide and are different from those seen during sinus rhythm. The ventricular rate is 36 beats/min.

Fig. 19–16). Therefore, in the presence of complete AV block, narrow QRS complexes indicate a junctional location of the block (AV node or His bundle), but wide QRS complexes may be the result of either bilateral bundle branch block, trifascicular block, or AV junctional block with unilateral bundle branch block. This relationship between the duration of the QRS complexes and the location of the block was demonstrated by histologic studies of the conduction system in a limited number of patients from whom His bundle records were obtained.[31]

The ventricular rate in complete AV block is usually also related to the location of the block and origin of the escape pacemaker. AV junctional escape rhythm generally has a rate between 40 and 60 beats/min. Idioventricular rhythm usually has a rate between 30 and 40 beats/min but may be as slow as 20 beats/min or as high as 50 beats/min. If the pacemaker is high in the AV junction, the ventricular rate may be increased by exercise or vagolytic agents[41] (Fig. 19–17). An escape rhythm from the ventricle or low AV junction is not affected by such maneuvers.

Electrophysiological Correlation

His bundle recordings indicate that the site of block in patients with complete AV block may be proximal to, within, or distal to the His bundle. In chronic acquired complete AV block, most cases (about 50 to 60 percent) have block located distal to the His bundle and the QRS complexes are wide.[33,34] Those with block proximal to or in the His bundle have either narrow or wide QRS complexes, the former being more common. In acute heart block resulting from inferior myocardial infarction, infections, or drugs, the site of the block is usually proximal to the His bundle. In complete AV block associated with acute anterior myocardial infarction, the block is usually distal to the His bundle.

CLINICAL CORRELATION OF AV BLOCK

Normal Subjects

A PR interval of greater than 0.20 second occasionally is seen in apparently healthy individuals. In the 67,375 male pilots without symptoms who were examined by Johnson and associates, this was found in 0.52 percent.[13] The PR interval ranged from 0.21 to 0.39 second but most often did not exceed 0.28 second. The occurrence of first-degree AV block in normal subjects is higher when 24-hour ambulatory ECG is obtained.[3,42] Longer PR intervals may be seen. An example of a healthy person with a PR interval of 0.66 second is illustrated in Figure 19–3. Second-degree AV block with Wenckebach phenomenon also may be seen, mostly during sleep, in younger individuals.[3,42] It also was reported in routine ECGs of trained athletes.[46] In a small series of 16 subjects with prolonged PR intervals among 1000 healthy young aviators, none had clinical evidence of heart disease during 10 years of follow-up.[32]

Vagal Stimulation

Transient AV block may be produced by vagal stimulation, such as carotid sinus massage and Valsalva maneuver. It may be the responsible mechanism for syncope in patients with hypersensitive carotid sinus reflex,[12] but it has been suggested that the symptom is most

II

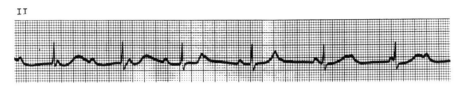

After Exercise

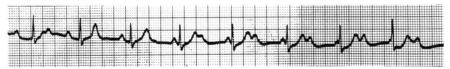

FIGURE 19–17. Effect of exercise on ventricular rate in a patient with congenital complete AV block. The QRS complexes are narrow and the ventricular rate increases after exercise. The escape pacemaker probably is located in the proximal part of the AV junction.

likely caused by asystole that results from vagal effect on the sinus node.[45]

Coronary Artery Disease

AV block in patients with coronary artery disease may be acute or chronic, transient or permanent. In acute myocardial infarction, various degrees of AV conduction defect occur in about 16 to 21 percent of patients; first-degree AV block develops in 8 to 13 percent; second-degree block in 3.5 to 10 percent; and complete AV block in 2.5 to 8 percent.[25,43] The ECG manifestations are closely related to the location of the infarct. AV block is more common in patients with inferior myocardial infarction (Fig. 19–18); it is observed in up to one third of such patients.[30] In 90 percent of human hearts, the inferior wall is supplied by the right coronary artery, which also gives off the branch to the AV node. Therefore, in inferior myocardial infarction, there is often ischemia of the AV node, resulting in AV conduction disturbances. The block is proximal to the His bundle.[33] If the block is complete, the escape rhythm is usually junctional in origin, with narrow QRS complexes unless there is coexisting bundle branch block. First-degree or type I second-degree AV block often precedes the complete block. As a rule, the AV block is transient, and normal conduction resumes within a week of the acute episode.[5,30,43] Structural damage of the AV node is usually not seen.[23,44]

Some degree of AV block may be seen in up to 21 percent of patients with acute anterior myocardial infarction.[37] The reported incidence of second-degree and third-degree AV block is between 5 and 7 percent.[30,43] It is the result of extensive damage of the interventricular septum, which is supplied by the anterior descending branch of the left coronary artery. There is involvement of the bundle branches either in the form of bilateral bundle branch block or trifascicular block.[44] Right bundle branch block, right bundle branch block with left anterior or left posterior hemiblock, or left bundle branch block often appears before the development of AV block. The PR interval is usually normal or minimally prolonged before the sudden onset of second- or third-degree AV block. Although the AV block is mostly transient, there is a relatively high incidence of recurrence of the high-degree AV block after the acute event.[11]

In chronic AV block resulting from coronary artery disease, in addition to ischemia, fibrosis and calcification of the summit of the ventricular septum that involve the branching part of the AV bundle and left bundle branch play an important role in the genesis of the conduction defect. Although coronary artery disease was previously thought to be the most important cause of chronic complete AV block,

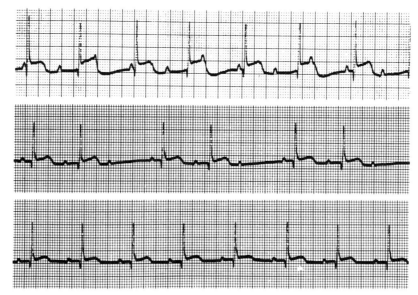

FIGURE 19–18. AV block resulting from acute inferior myocardial infarction. The upper strip shows complete AV block with junctional escape rhythm. The middle and lower strips show type I second-degree and first-degree AV block, respectively. All the rhythm strips were recorded on the same day.

TABLE 19–1. Cause of Chronic AV Block (100 Autopsied Cases)*

Idiopathic bilateral bundle branch fibrosis	46
Ischemic coronary artery disease	
Destruction of both bundle branches	14
Destruction of AV node	1
Cardiomyopathy	13
Calcific valve disease	8
Myocarditis	4
Connective tissue disorder	3
Amyloidosis	3
Transfusion siderosis (only AV node affected)	2
Congenital heart block (only main bundle affected)	3
Gumma of interventricular septum	3
Total	100

*Adapted from Davies MJ: Pathology of Conducting Tissue of the Heart. New York, Appleton-Century-Crofts, 1971, by permission.

more recent pathologic studies have shown that this is not the case (Table 19–1).[7] Only 15 of 100 cases of chronic complete AV block examined by Davies were caused by coronary artery disease.[7]

Degenerative Diseases

Lenegre first described sclerodegenerative lesions of the bundle branches as a cause of chronic complete AV block.[19] The pathologic process is also called *idiopathic bilateral bundle branch fibrosis,* and the heart block is called *primary heart block.* It is generally agreed that idiopathic bilateral bundle branch fibrosis is the most common cause of chronic AV block. In the 100 autopsied cases of complete AV block examined by Davies, such a process was found in 46.[7]

Lev described similar degenerative lesions, which he referred to as sclerosis of the left side of the cardiac skeleton.[20] There is progressive fibrosis and calcification of the mitral annulus, the central fibrous body, the pars membranacea, the base of the aorta, and the summit of the muscular ventricular septum. Various portions of the His bundle or the bundle branches may be involved, resulting in AV block.

Hypertension

The chronic AV block seen in patients with hypertension is thought to be due to coronary arteriosclerosis or sclerosis of the left side of the cardiac skeleton exacerbated by hypertension.[22] The bifurcation of the His bundle or the bundle branches are usually involved.

Myocardial Diseases

AV conduction defect is seen in both idiopathic and secondary cardiomyopathies, particularly the former (see Table 19–1). Various degrees of heart block are observed in about 15 percent of patients with the dilated type of idiopathic cardiomyopathy, but they are less common in the hypertrophic variety (about 3 percent).[10] Among secondary cardiomyopathies, myocardial sarcoidosis is well known for its frequent association with AV block. Other causes include infiltrative diseases, such as amyloidosis and hemachromatosis; neuromuscular diseases, such as progressive muscular dystrophy; and connective tissue diseases, such as systemic lupus erythematosus, dermatomyositis, and scleroderma. AV block also has been described in rheumatoid heart disease but is rare[22]; it is more common in ankylosis spondylitis. Tumors, either primary or metastatic, may involve the AV node. His bundle, or bundle branches to produce AV block.

AV block may occur in all types of acute myocarditis. Prolongation of the PR interval is a common finding in patients with acute rheumatic fever. Its incidence varies considerably (from 25 to 95 percent) among different reported series. Type I second-degree AV block also may occur, but complete AV block is uncommon.[4] AV block in acute rheumatic fever is not specific for rheumatic carditis, however. In 508 patients with acute rheumatic fever reviewed by Clark and Keith, no significant difference in the PR interval was found between patients with and without carditis.[4] The PR prolongation also is not significantly related to severity of carditis or subsequent cardiac damage.[9]

Incomplete AV block is not uncommon in patients with viral infections, many of which (such as infectious mononucleosis) are known to be accompanied by myocarditis. Among bacterial infections, diphtheria was once a well-known cause of heart block but is no longer an important factor. The conduction defect in myocarditis is usually transient and disappears when the patient recovers. Chronic AV block is uncommon except in Chagas' disease.

Valvular Heart Diseases

Calcific aortic stenosis may be accompanied by chronic partial or complete AV block. There is an extension of the calcification process to involve the main bundle or its bifurcation, resulting in degeneration and necrosis of the conduction tissue.[7] Similar consequences may be observed in rheumatic mitral valve disease but are uncommon. Occasionally, massive calcification of the mitral annulus as an aging process may cause AV block.[38] This entity is probably related to the degenerative lesions described by Lev.[21] AV block also may be seen in patients with bacterial endocarditis, especially on the aortic valve. Extension of the infectious process to the adjacent AV conduction tissue is responsible for the conduction defect (Fig. 19–19).

Drugs

Digitalis is one of the most common causes of reversible AV block. Its vagal effect on the AV node is used in the treatment of various types of supraventricular tachyarrhythmias to reduce the ventricular response. In patients with sinus rhythm, slight prolongation of the PR interval is often seen, even though the dosage of the drug is in the therapeutic range. A PR interval of greater than 0.24 second generally should raise the possibility of digitalis toxicity. When second-degree AV block is induced by the drug, it is always of the type I variety (Fig. 19–20). When complete AV block occurs, the QRS complexes are narrow because the block is at the AV node. The ventricular rate is usually more rapid than that due to organic lesions. Increased automaticity of the AV junctional escape pacemaker may be partly responsible.

Quinidine and procainamide may produce slight prolongation of the PR interval as a result of their direct action on the AV junction. AV block may occur in association with the use of beta-adrenergic blocking agents. Among the calcium-channel blocking agents, verapamil and diltiazem are known to cause

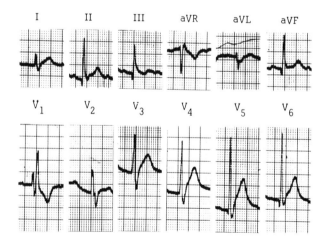

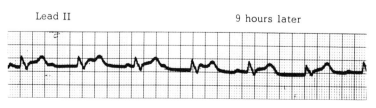

FIGURE 19–19. Complete AV block in a patient with bacterial endocarditis of the aortic valve. Autopsy showed an extension of the destructive infectious process to involve the AV conduction system. The 12-lead ECG shows complete right bundle branch block. Although there is rather diffuse ST-segment elevation, no evidence of pericarditis was found at autopsy. There was minimal coronary atherosclerosis. Complete AV block developed 9 hours later. The morphology of the QRS complex suggests that the block is distal to the bifurcation of the His bundle, and the escape rhythm is idioventricular in origin. The QRS complex is different from that seen during sinus mechanism in the same lead.

Age: 14

Lead II

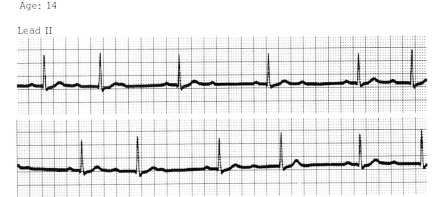

FIGURE 19–20. Type I second-degree AV block due to digitalis intoxication.

AV conduction delay and PR interval prolongation.[1]

Congenital Heart Disease

Congenital AV block occurs most commonly in the absence of other evidence of organic heart disease. As a rule, the site of the block is proximal to the bifurcation of the His bundle mostly in the AV node, and the QRS complex is narrow. In children the ventricular rate is usually above 40 beats/min. In one study, a persistent heart rate at rest of 50 beats/min or less was significantly correlated with the incidence of syncope.[14] Among patients who also have other congenital cardiac defects, AV block is frequently seen in those with corrected transposition of the great vessels. In adult patients with congenital heart disease, AV block, usually incomplete, is seen more commonly in cases of atrial septal defect and Ebstein anomaly.

Trauma

AV block may be induced during open heart surgery in the area of the AV conduction tissue. It is seen in patients operated on for the correction of ventricular septal defect, tetralogy of Fallot, and endocardial cushion defect.

The conduction defect may be the result of edema, transient ischemia, or actual disruption of the conduction tissue. The AV block may, therefore, be transient or permanent.

Complete AV block also has been reported in patients who sustained nonpenetrating or penetrating trauma of the chest.[21]

CONCEALED CONDUCTION

In the body surface ECG, the state of AV conduction usually is implied by the relationship between the P wave and QRS complex. The electrical potential generated by the AV junctional tissue itself cannot be identified because of its low amplitude. Consequently, partial penetration of a supraventricular impulse into the AV conduction system may have occurred but is not recognized because there is no ventricular response. This type of incomplete conduction of an impulse is called *concealed conduction*.[16,18] Its presence may be implied by its effect on subsequent impulse conduction or impulse formation or both. It may be suspected when there is an unexpected prolongation of conduction time or block or unexpected delay of an otherwise regular rhythm. The concept of concealed conduction is helpful in the interpretation of many phenomena seen in cardiac arrhythmias.

FIGURE 19–21. Concealed conduction associated with interpolated premature ventricular beat. The prolongation of the PR interval following the premature ventricular beat is due to retrograde concealed conduction of the ectopic ventricular impulse in the AV junction.

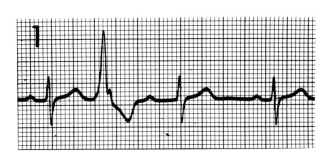

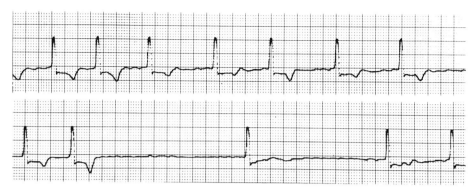

FIGURE 19–22. Concealed conduction in atrial fibrillation. The unexpected marked prolongation of the RR interval in the bottom strip can best be explained by repeated concealed conduction in the AV junction and concealed discharge of the junctional pacemaker. The RR intervals are longer than the expected junctional escape interval.

Its actual existence has been confirmed by His bundle recordings. In addition to the AV junction, concealed conduction also may occur at the SA junction or at one of the bundle branches, but it is most common at the AV junction.

The effect of concealed conduction on impulse conduction may be best exemplified when it is seen in association with premature ventricular beats. If the premature ventricular beat is interpolated, retrograde conduction of the impulse may penetrate into the AV junction and reset its refractory period. The conduction of the postextrasystolic sinus impulse is delayed and the PR interval prolonged (Fig. 19–21).

If a premature ventricular impulse is conducted retrograde and partially penetrates the AV junction but fails to excite the ventricles, no recognizable deflection is present in the ECG, but the next PR interval may be prolonged or the P wave blocked. An erroneous diagnosis of second-degree AV block may be made. Similarly pseudo-AV block may be the result of nonpropagated premature His bundle depolarization.[36]

In atrial fibrillation, the irregular ventricular response is probably the result of varying depth and frequency of concealed conduction into the AV junction.[26] This mechanism also may be responsible for the unexpected excessively long RR intervals in some patients with atrial fibrillation. The RR interval may be longer than the expected junctional escape interval because of the concealed discharge of the junctional pacemaker (Fig. 19–22).

The effect of concealed conduction on impulse formation can be illustrated in patients with AV dissociation. In Figure 19–23, the regular junctional impulse is delayed in the sixth beat of the bottom strip. This is probably due to partial penetration of the AV junction

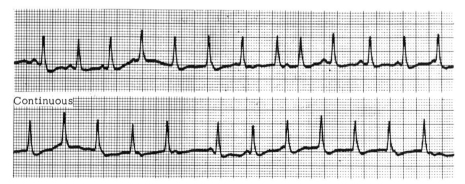

FIGURE 19–23. Concealed conduction. The basic rhythm is accelerated AV junctional rhythm with AV dissociation. In the upper strip, the ninth QRS complex is premature and represents a capture beat. In the bottom strip, the long RR interval following the fifth QRS complex can best be explained by concealed conduction. The atrial impulse represented by the P wave following the fifth QRS complex partially penetrates the AV junction and causes premature discharge of the junctional pacemaker. The rhythmicity of the junctional pacemaker is reset.

by the atrial impulse represented by the preceding P wave, which resets the rhythmicity of the junctional pacemaker.

REFERENCES

1. Antman EM, Stone PH, Muller JE, et al: Calcium channel blocking agents in the treatment of cardiovascular disorders. Part I. Basic and clinical electrophysiologic effects. Ann Intern Med 93:875, 1980
2. Barold SS, Friedberg HD: Second degree atrioventricular block: A matter of definition. Am J Cardiol 33:311, 1974
3. Brodsky M, Wu D, Denes P, et al: Arrhythmia documented by 24 hour continuous electrocardiographic monitoring in 50 male medical students without apparent heart disease. Am J Cardiol 39:390, 1977
4. Clarke M, Keith JD: Atrioventricular conduction in acute rheumatic fever. Br Heart J 34:472, 1972
5. Courter SR, Moffat J, Fowler NO: Advanced atrioventricular block in acute myocardial infarction. Circulation 27:1034, 1963
6. Damato AN, Lau SH, Helfant R, et al: A study of heart block in man using His bundle recordings. Circulation 39:297, 1969
7. Davies MJ: Pathology of Conducting Tissue of the Heart. New York, Appleton-Century-Crofts, 1971
8. Dhingra RC: His bundle recording in acquired conduction disease. Arch Intern Med 135:397, 1975
9. Feinstein AR, Wood HF, Spagnuolo M: Rheumatic fever in children and adolescents: A long term epidemiologic study of subsequent prophylaxis, streptococcal infections and clinical sequelae. VII. Cardiac changes and sequelae. Ann Intern Med 60(Suppl 5):87, 1964
10. Flowers NV, Horan LG: Electrocardiographic and vectorcardiographic features of myocardial disease. In Fowler NO (ed): Myocardial Diseases. Orlando, Grune & Stratton, 1973
11. Hindman MC, Wagner GS, JaRo M, et al: The clinical significance of bundle branch block complicating acute myocardial infarction. 2. Indications for temporary and permanent pacemaker insertion. Circulation 58:689, 1978
12. Hutchinson EC, Stock JTT: Carotid sinus syndrome. Lancet 2:445, 1960
13. Johnson RL, Averill KH, Lamb LE: Electrocardiographic findings in 67,375 asymptomatic subjects. VII. Atrioventricular block. Am J Cardiol 6:153, 1960
14. Karpawich PP, Gillette PC, Garson A, et al: Congenital complete atrioventricular block: Clinical and electrophysiologic predictors of need for pacemaker insertion. Am J Cardiol 48:1098, 1981
15. Kastor JA, Josephson ME: Treatment of atrioventricular block. In Fowler NO (ed): Cardiac Arrhythmias, Diagnosis and Treatment, ed 2. New York, Harper & Row, 1977, p 118
16. Langendorf R: Concealed AV conduction: The effect of blocked impulses on the formation and conduction of subsequent impulses. Am Heart J 35:542, 1948
17. Langendorf R, Cohen H, Gozo EG: Observations on second degree atrioventricular block, including new criteria for the differential diagnosis between type I and type II block. Am J Cardiol 29:111, 1972
18. Langendorf R, Pick A: Concealed conduction: Further evaluation of a fundamental aspect of propagation of the cardiac impulse. Circulation 31:381, 1956
19. Lenegre J: Etiology and pathology of bilateral bundle branch block in relation to complete heart block. Prog Cardiovasc Dis 6:409, 1964
20. Lev M: Anatomical basis for atrioventricular block. Am J Med 37:742, 1964
21. Lev M: The pathology of atrioventricular block. Cardiovasc Clin 4:159, 1972
22. Lev M, Bharati S: Atrioventricular and intraventricular conduction disease. Arch Intern Med 135:405, 1975
23. Lev M, Kinare SG, Pick A: The pathogenesis of atrioventricular block in coronary disease. Circulation 42:409, 1970
24. Mangiardi LM, Bonamini R, Conte M, et al: Bedside evaluation of atrioventricular block with narrow QRS complexes: Usefulness of carotid sinus massage and atropine administration. Am J Cardiol 49:1136, 1982
25. Meltzer LE, Kitchell JB: The incidence of arrhythmias associated with acute myocardial infarction. Prog Cardiovas Dis 9:50, 1966
26. Moore EN, Knoebel SB, Spear JF: Concealed conduction. Am J Cardiol 28:406, 1971
27. Narula OS: Wenckebach type I and type II atrioventricular block (revisited). In Fisch C, Brest AN (eds): Complex Electrocardiography, vol 6. Philadelphia, FA Davis, 1974, p 1
28. Narula OS, Samet P: Wenckebach and Mobitz type II AV block due to block within the His bundle and bundle branches. Circulation 41:947, 1970
29. Narula OS, Scherlag BJ, Samet P, et al: Atrioventricular block: Localization and classification by His bundle recordings. Am J Med 50:146, 1971
30. Norris RM: Heart block in posterior and an anterior myocardial infarction. Br Heart J 31:352, 1969
31. Ohkawa S, Sugiura M, Itoh Y, et al: Electrophysiologic and histologic correlations in chronic complete atrioventricular block. Circulation 64:215, 1981
32. Packard JM, Graettinger JS, Graybiel A: Analysis of the electrocardiograms obtained from 1000 young healthy aviators: Ten year follow-up. Circulation 10:384, 1954
33. Puech P: Atrioventricular block; the value of intracardiac recordings. In Krikler DM, Goodwin JF (eds): Cardiac Arrhythmias: The Modern Electrophysiological Approach. Philadelphia, WB Saunders, 1975, p 81
34. Rosen KM, Dhingra RC, Loeb HS, et al: Chronic heart block in adults: Clinical and electrophysiological observations. Arch Intern Med 131:663, 1973
35. Rosen KM, Loeb HS, Gunnar RM, et al: Mobitz type II block without bundle branch block. Circulation 44:1111, 1971
36. Rosen KM, Rahimtoola SH, Gunnar RM: Pseudo AV block secondary to premature non-propagated His bundle depolarizations: Documentation by His bundle electrocardiography. Circulation 42:367, 1970
37. Rotman W, Wagner GS, Wallace AG: Bradyarrhythmias in acute myocardial infarction. Circulation 45:703, 1972
38. Rytand DA, Lipsitch LS: Clinical aspects of calcification of mitral annulus fibrosis. Arch Intern Med 78:544, 1946
39. Schamroth L: Ventriculophasic atrial extrasystoles associated with complete atrioventricular block. Am J Cardiol 21:593, 1968
40. Scherlag BJ, Lau SH, Helfant RH, et al: Catheter technique for recording bundle activity in man. Circulation 39:13, 1969
41. Scherlag BJ, Lazzara R, Helfant RH: Differentiation of "A-V junctional rhythms." Circulation 48:304, 1973
42. Sobotka RA, Mayer JH, Bauernfield RA, et al: Arrhythmias documented by 24-hour continuous ambulatory

electrocardiographic monitoring in young women without apparent heart disease. Am Heart J 101:753, 1981

43. Stock RJ, Macken DL: Observations on heart block during continuous electrocardiographic monitoring in myocardial infarction. Circulation 38:993, 1968

44. Sutton R, Davies M: The conduction system in acute myocardial infarction complicated by heart block. Circulation 38:987, 1968

45. Walter PF, Crawley IS, Dorney ER: Carotid sinus hypersensitivity and syncope. Am J Cardiol 42:396, 1978

46. Zeppilli P, Fenici R, Sassara M, et al: Wenckebach second-degree A-V block in top-ranking athletes: An old problem revisited. Am Heart J 100:281, 980

47. Zipes DP: Second-degree atrioventricular block. Circulation 60:465, 1979

Wolff-Parkinson-White Syndrome and Its Variants

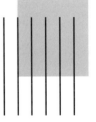

20

The syndrome of short PR interval with abnormal QRS complex and paroxysmal tachycardia was first described by Wolff, Parkinson, and White in 1930.[96] It also is called the ventricular preexcitation syndrome, the bundle of Kent syndrome, or anomalous atrioventricular (AV) excitation syndrome. The term Wolff-Parkinson-White (WPW) *pattern* or ventricular preexcitation is used when the abnormal PR interval and QRS complex are not associated with the occurrence of tachycardias[91] (Fig. 20–1). In the classic form of the syndrome, there is an accessory AV pathway or bundle of Kent, which allows the atrial impulse to bypass the AV node and activates the ventricle prematurely[93] (Fig. 20–2A). The accessory pathway may be located between the free wall of the left or right atrium and the corresponding ventricle or between the atrial and ventricular septa.[5,76] Because the normal delay at the AV node is avoided, the PR interval is shortened. The abnormal preexcitation of an area of the ventricle distorts the initial part of the QRS complex, which is the delta wave. The abnormal sequence of ventricular activation results in a prolongation of the QRS duration and is associated with secondary ST-segment and T-wave abnormalities. Depending on the degree of prematurity of atrial impulse arriving at the ventricle, ventricular depolarization may depend partly or entirely on the impulse transmitted through the bypass. When the ventricles are depolarized by both the impulse conducted through the accessory bundle and that through the normal AV conduction system, the QRS complex represents a fusion beat.

An alternative mechanism has been proposed that is based on the bypass fibers described by James[43] and Mahaim and Winston[57] (see Fig. 20–2B). The pathway of James is a paranodal pathway that bypasses the upper and central AV node, where normal AV conduction delay occurs, to connect with the lower third of the node or directly with the bundle of His. The PR interval is therefore shortened when the impulse is conducted through the James fibers. The bypass fibers of Mahaim are a short, direct connection between the lower AV node or His bundle and the ventricular septum. Excitation through these fibers results in preexcitation of the ventricular septum, resulting in a delta wave. Such a combination of connections has been demonstrated anatomically in a patient with the typical WPW syndrome.[52] These bypass fibers also may serve to explain some of the variants of the WPW syndrome. In the Lown-Ganong-Levine (LGL) syndrome, the PR interval is shortened, but the QRS complex is normal.[55] The accelerated AV conduction may be the result of AV nodal bypass through the James fibers. In some patients, the PR interval is normal but a delta wave is present. Under these circumstances, the atrial impulse may travel through the AV node in the normal fashion, but abnormal ventricular excitation occurs because of the presence of Mahaim fibers. Whether these are the mechanisms responsible for most of the variant forms of ventricular preexcitation syndrome is, however, open to question. Data that correlate structure and function in such cases are scanty.[5,8]

Another variant of the syndrome is called *concealed* WPW syndrome. There is an accessory pathway that is capable of conducting impulse only in the retrograde (ventriculoatrial) direction. During sinus rhythm, the electrocardiogram (ECG) shows normal PR interval and QRS complex.

Because of the presence of the accessory pathway, a reentry circuit is established (Fig. 20–3). Paroxysmal tachycardia occurs frequently in patients with ventricular preexcitation and is an essential part of the WPW syndrome. Depending on whether the normal AV bundle or the accessory bundle is used in the antegrade conduction, the QRS complex during tachycardia may be normal or wide and bizarre. The former is more common and is

V₃

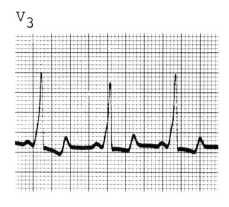

3754   24F

FIGURE 20–1. Typical WPW pattern showing the short PR interval, delta wave, wide QRS complex, and secondary ST and T-wave changes.

called *orthodromic reentrant tachycardia.* Wide QRS complex tachycardia that results from antegrade conduction through the accessory bundle is less common and is called *antidromic tachycardia.*[83]

WOLFF-PARKINSON-WHITE ELECTROCARDIOGRAPHIC PATTERN

1. A PR interval of less than 0.12 second, with normal P wave
2. Abnormally wide QRS complex with a duration of 0.11 second or more

3. The presence of an initial slurring of the QRS complex, the delta wave
4. Secondary ST-segment and T-wave changes
5. The frequent association of paroxysmal tachycardia

In many patients with the WPW pattern, the characteristic ECG changes appear only intermittently. Such an intermittent finding is seen in about 50 percent of the cases.[7,48] In some cases, the change from the preexcitation pattern to normal AV conduction, and vice versa, occurs in the same tracing (Figs. 20–4 and 20–5). In other cases, there may be a progressive shortening of the PR interval, with a corresponding widening of the QRS complex and vice versa. The phenomenon is called the *concertina effect.* It is related to the degree of ectopic ventricular preexcitation. In a longitudinal electrophysiological study of patients with the WPW pattern but without symptoms, Klein and Gulamhusein found that a considerable number of patients (9 of 29) lost their capacity for antegrade conduction over the accessory pathway when they were examined again after 36 months.[48]

PR Interval

The length of the PR interval in the WPW pattern is affected by the time required for impulse conduction in the atria and in the nor-

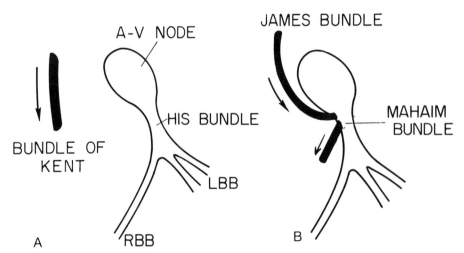

FIGURE 20–2. Schematic diagrams illustrating the possible anatomic findings associated with the WPW pattern. (A) An accessory AV bypass or the bundle of Kent is responsible for premature activation of the free wall of the left or right ventricle or the interventricular septum. (B) The James fibers bypass the AV node to avoid the normal AV conduction delay. The Mahaim fibers serve as a short direct connection between the lower AV node or His bundle and the ventricular septum.

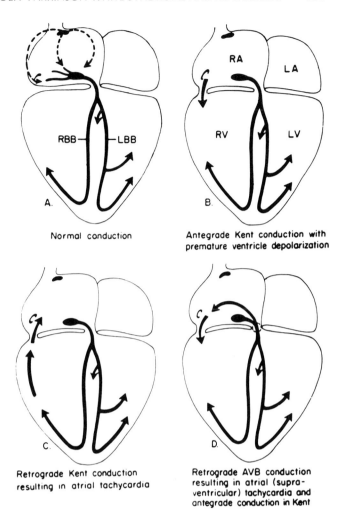

FIGURE 20-3. Schematic diagram depicting the most common mechanism responsible for the development of paroxysmal tachycardia in the WPW syndrome. (A) Normal conduction pathways of atria and ventricles. (B) Antegrade Kent conduction with premature ventricular depolarization. (C) The excitation impulse is conducted antegrade through the normal AV conduction system and returns to the atrium by retrograde conduction through the accessory bundle. A circus movement is therefore established, resulting in reentrant tachycardia. (D) The exciting impulse is conducted antegrade through the Kent bundle and retrograde through the AV bundle. The reentrant supraventricular tachycardia has wide QRS complexes stimulating ventricular tachycardia. (Reproduced from Dreifus LS, Nichols H, Morse D, et al: Control of recurrent tachycardia of Wolff-Parkinson-White syndrome by surgical ligature of the A-V bundle. Circulation 38:1030, 1968, by permission of the American Heart Association, Inc.)

Normal conduction

Antegrade Kent conduction with premature ventricle depolarization

Retrograde Kent conduction resulting in atrial tachycardia

Retrograde AVB conduction resulting in atrial (supraventricular) tachycardia and antegrade conduction in Kent

mal AV conduction system in relation to that in the accessory pathway. In typical cases, the PR interval is less than 0.12 second. In my experience, an interval of 0.12 second is common. In most instances, it is between 0.08 and 0.11 second, but a value as low as 0.06 second may be encountered. About 12 percent of the cases may have an interval greater than 0.12 second, and a value of up to 0.20 second has been reported.[17,94,95] They may be considered as variant forms of the WPW pattern, some of which are associated with Mahaim bypass fibers. When the PR interval is within normal range, the diagnosis of preexcitation can be confirmed if the tracing during normal AV conduction is available for comparison. If the baseline PR interval is relatively long, considerable shortening of the interval may occur but the duration remains in the normal range.

In the absence of coexisting cardiac disease,

the P wave is normal. The diagnosis of WPW pattern cannot be made with certainty if there is a superior displacement of the P-wave axis with P-wave inversion in the inferior leads. Under such circumstances, the shortened PR interval may be the result of an ectopic pacemaker located at the AV junction.

QRS Complex

In typical cases, the QRS duration is increased to 0.11 second or more. The duration may range between 0.08 and 0.16 second, however, with almost one third of the cases in some series having a value of 0.10 second or less.[17,38] As mentioned, the duration of the QRS complex is often inversely proportional to the PR interval and depends on the degree of preexcitation. When the ventricles are depolarized entirely by the impulse conducted

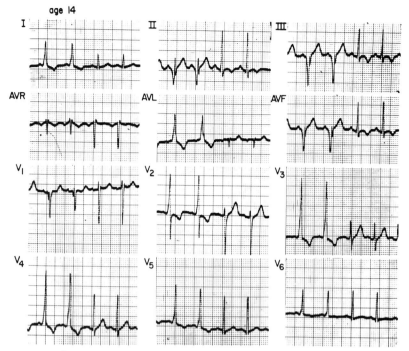

FIGURE 20–4. Intermittent WPW pattern. The tracing was obtained from a 14-year-old boy with no other evidence of heart disease. The first two complexes in each lead are the WPW complexes, and the last two are normally conducted beats. Note the pseudoinfarction pattern in the WPW complexes in the inferior leads. The delta wave and the major part of the QRS complex in lead V_1 are downward, consistent with type B WPW pattern.

through the accessory pathway, the QRS complex is wider and more bizarre. The sum of the PR and QRS intervals usually remains within the normal range.

Delta Wave

The initial slurring of the QRS complex, the delta wave, is the most important finding in the WPW pattern. The duration of the delta wave varies between 0.02 and 0.07 second but is usually between 0.03 and 0.06 second. Theoretically, the delta wave should be present in all leads. In the leads with the lead axis nearly perpendicular to the initial QRS forces, however, the delta wave may become isoelectric and be easily overlooked.

Using the morphology of the QRS complex in the precordial leads, Rosenbaum and associates classified the WPW pattern into type A and type B.[71] In type A, the delta wave and the remainder of the QRS complex are primarily upright in all the precordial leads (Fig. 20–6). Generally, lead V_1 shows either a notched R wave or RS or RSr′ deflections. The pattern superficially resembles that of right bundle

branch block. In type B, which is more common, the delta wave and the remainder of the QRS complex are negative in V_1 and V_2 but are upright in the left precordial leads (Figs. 20–7 and 20–8). The changes may closely resemble those of left bundle branch block (see Fig. 20–8). Although most patients can be classified into types A and B, there are many patients who present intermediate changes. Type C preexcitation also has been described.[29,52] In type C WPW pattern, the delta wave is negative in leads V_5 and V_6 but is positive in leads V_1 through V_4. It is, however, rare.

When the delta wave is negative, the downward deflection may resemble the abnormal Q wave associated with myocardial infarction (see Figs. 20–4, 20–5, and 20–7). Such a pseudoinfarction pattern may be seen in up to 70 percent of patients with the WPW pattern.[65] In type B WPW pattern, the erroneous diagnosis of anterior myocardial infarction may be made because of the negative delta waves in the right precordial leads. In both types A and B, abnormal Q waves may be seen in leads II, III, and a VF to mimic inferior myocardial infarction. Furthermore, the tall R

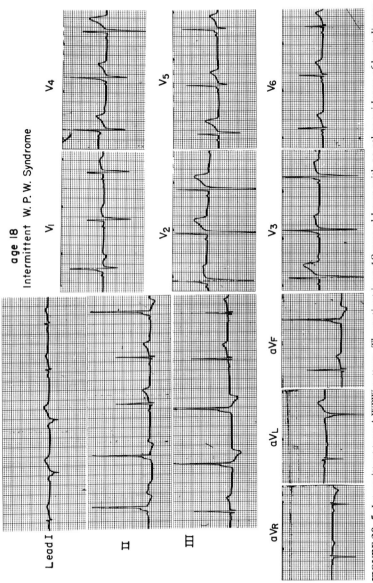

age 18
Intermittent W. P. W. Syndrome

FIGURE 20–5. Intermittent type A WPW pattern. The patient is an 18-year-old man with no other evidence of heart disease. The delta wave and the major part of the QRS complex in lead V_1 are upright. Leads I and aVL show a pseudoinfarction pattern.

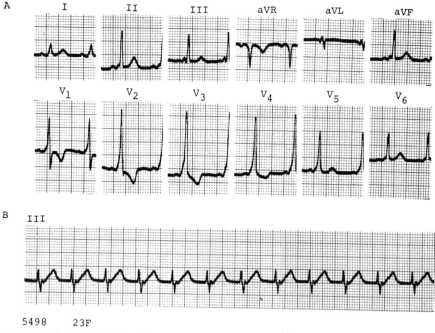

5498   23F

FIGURE 20–6. Type A WPW syndrome. The patient is a 23-year-old woman with no other evidence of organic heart disease. (A) The delta wave and the major part of the QRS complex in lead V_1 are upright. The QRS complexes in the rest of the precordial leads are also upright. The patient has recurrent episodes of paroxysmal supraventricular tachycardia. (B) The QRS complexes are normal during the tachycardia, suggesting normal antegrade AV conduction (orthodromic reentrant tachycardia). Negative P waves are superimposed on the terminal part of the QRS complexes.

wave in lead V_1 in type A WPW pattern often simulates true posterior myocardial infarction. As mentioned, type A resembles right bundle branch block and is often so interpreted. The tall R wave in V_1 also may be mistaken for a sign of right ventricular hypertrophy.

ST-Segment and T-Wave Changes

The altered sequence of ventricular activation in patients with the WPW pattern results in secondary repolarization abnormalities. Most commonly, the direction of the ST-segment displacement and the T-wave polarity are op-

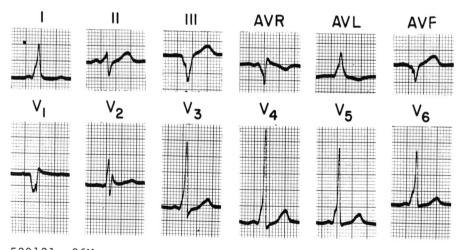

529121   26M

FIGURE 20–7. Type B WPW pattern in a 26-year-old woman with no other evidence of organic heart disease. The delta wave and the major portion of the QRS complex in lead V_1 are downward. A pseudoinfarction pattern is present in leads III and aVF.

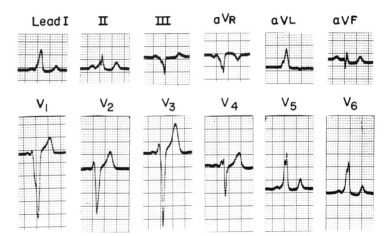

FIGURE 20–8. Type B WPW pattern in a 35-year-old healthy man. The tracing resembles closely that of complete left bundle branch block.

posite to the direction of the delta wave and the major deflection of the QRS complex. In type A WPW pattern, ST-segment depression and T-wave inversion are usually seen in the right precordial leads. In type B, they are present in the left precordial leads. The changes are similar to those of right and left bundle branch block. In some cases, however, no apparent ST-segment and T-wave abnormalities are seen (Fig. 20–9).

Tachyarrhythmias

Paroxysmal tachycardias are the most important clinical manifestations in patients with the WPW *syndrome*. They were reported in 13 to 80 percent of the patients with the WPW pattern. The incidence is closely related to the population sampled. It was low (13 percent) when the WPW pattern was diagnosed from routine ECGs among clinically healthy population.[7] In hospitalized or cardiac clinic patients with this pattern, paroxysmal tachycardias occurred in 40 to 80 percent.[17,65] In many cases, it is the tachyarrhythmia that first leads to the diagnosis of the preexcitation syndrome.

Paroxysmal supraventricular tachycardia is the most common form of tachyarrhythmia seen in patients with the WPW syndrome and is responsible for 75 to 80 percent of all paroxysmal tachycardia in such patients.[16,83] The tachycardia is a reciprocating or reentrant tachycardia and is called *AV reentrant tachycardia*. It is often initiated by premature atrial or ventricular beats[25] (Fig. 20–10). The impulse of excitation usually is conducted antegrade through the normal AV conduction system and returns to the atrium through the accessory pathway in a retrograde fashion. A circus movement is therefore established (see Fig. 20–3). In such patients, the delta wave is not observed during the tachycardia, and the QRS complex is normal in duration (narrow) (see Figs. 20–6B and 20–11). The heart rate usually ranges between 140 and 250 beats/min. It is generally faster than the rate of tachycardia due to reentry in the AV node.[33] The supraventricular tachycardia may occasionally lead to the development of atrial fibrillation.[30]

Atrial fibrillation and flutter are less common than paroxysmal supraventricular tachycardia in the WPW syndrome (Figs. 20–11 through 20–14). Atrial fibrillation was reported in 20 to 35 percent of those patients

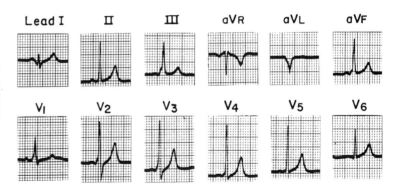

FIGURE 20–9. Type A WPW pattern in a 21-year-old woman with no other evidence of heart disease. Note that the secondary ST and T-wave changes are not evident in this tracing.

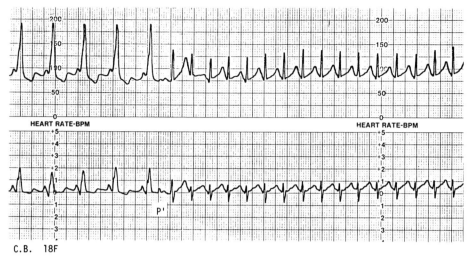

C.B. 18F

FIGURE 20–10. Orthodromic AV reentrant tachycardia initiated by a premature atrial beat. The first five beats of the simultaneously recorded leads show sinus rhythm with ventricular preexcitation. A premature atrial beat (P') initiates the narrow QRS complex tachycardia (orthodromic AV reentrant tachycardia) with a rate of 186 beats/min. During the tachycardia, the retrograde P waves can be seen after the QRS complexes, especially in the bottom strip.

who have tachyarrhythmias.[10,16,33,83] Atrial flutter is uncommon.[17] In most cases, the atrial impulses in atrial fibrillation and atrial flutter are conducted to the ventricles through the accessory pathway. The QRS complexes are wide and bizarre as a result of preexcitation, and additional aberrant ventricular conduction often is present because of the rapid ventricular rate. The ventricular rate may be as rapid as 220 to 360 beats/min (see Fig. 20–13). Such a rapid rate is possible because of the shorter effective refractory period of the accessory bundle. In atrial flutter, the regular rhythm with wide QRS complexes is often mistaken for paroxysmal ventricular tachycardia (see Fig. 20–14). The AV conduction ratio may be 2:1 or 1:1. Indeed, atrial flutter with 1:1 conduction is rare in the absence of the WPW syndrome unless the atrial rate is relatively slow owing to antiarrhythmic therapy (such as quinidine and precainamide).

In atrial fibrillation, the erroneous diagnosis of ventricular tachycardia can often be avoided because of the gross irregularity of the ventricular response (see Fig. 20–13). In fact, the presence of the WPW syndrome often can be suspected from the rhythm strip alone if the atrial fibrillation is accompanied by a ventricular rate greater than 200 beats/min. Such a rapid ventricular response would be highly unusual if the conduction is by way of the normal AV conduction system.

Because of the rapid ventricular response,

patients with the WPW syndrome and atrial fibrillation may have ventricular fibrillation that results in sudden death.[22,32] Klein and coworkers found that patients with shorter RR interval during atrial fibrillation of 250 msec or less are more likely to develop ventricular fibrillation than those with longer intervals.[47] The presence of multiple accessory pathways also renders the patient more susceptible to the development of this lethal arrhythmia. Although cases of ventricular tachycardia have been reported in the WPW syndrome, they were not well documented. In all likelihood, most of them were supraventricular tachyarrhythmias with wide QRS complexes.

DIFFERENTIAL DIAGNOSIS

The typical WPW pattern with short PR interval, delta wave, and abnormally wide QRS complex usually is not difficult to recognize. As described previously, however, the following misinterpretations may occur:

1. Type A WPW pattern
   a. Right bundle branch block
   b. Right ventricular hypertrophy
   c. True posterior myocardial infarction
   d. Inferior myocardial infarction
2. Type B WPW pattern
   a. Left bundle branch block
   b. Anterior myocardial infarction
   c. Inferior myocardial infarction

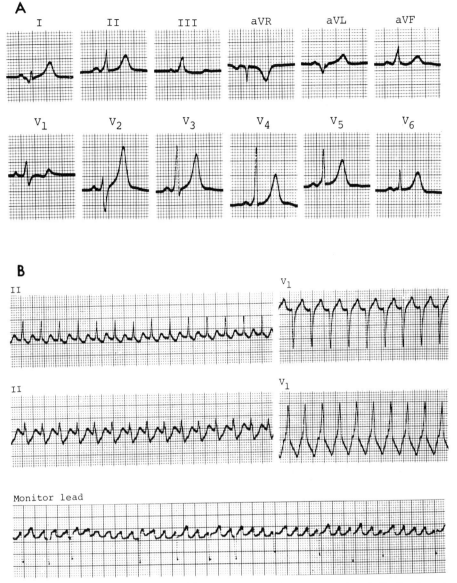

FIGURE 20–11. WPW syndrome in a 46-year-old man with recurrent tachyarrhythmias since the age of 15 years. (A) Type A WPW pattern with upright delta wave in lead V_1. (B) Tracings showing the forms of tachyarrhythmias observed. They include paroxysmal supraventricular tachycardia with normal QRS complexes, as well as wide QRS complexes due to aberrant ventricular conduction. The latter simulates paroxysmal ventricular tachycardia. The atrial origin of the tachyarrhythmias was verified by other tracings showing premature atrial beats with and without aberrant ventricular conduction having similar QRS morphologies. Atrial flutter with variable AV conduction was also observed and is demonstrated in the monitor lead.

3. WPW pattern and atria flutter:
Paroxysmal ventricular tachycardia or flutter

Intermittent WPW pattern may simulate or be simulated by late-diastolic premature ventricular beats (Figs. 20–15 and 20–16). When the ectopic ventricular beat appears after the succeeding P wave, the unrelated atrial and ventricular complexes have a short PR interval. The ectopic ventricular complex usually has a slurred initial deflection that simulates the delta wave. Therefore, the diagnosis of intermittent WPW pattern (although it may exist) should not be made unless two successive complexes with short PR interval and abnormal QRS complex are present.

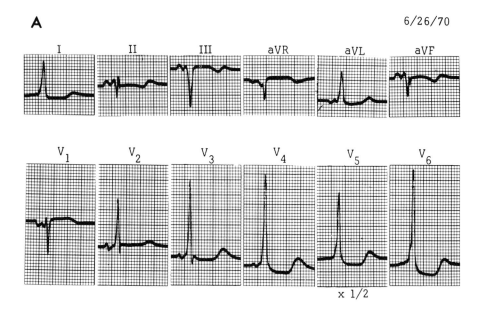

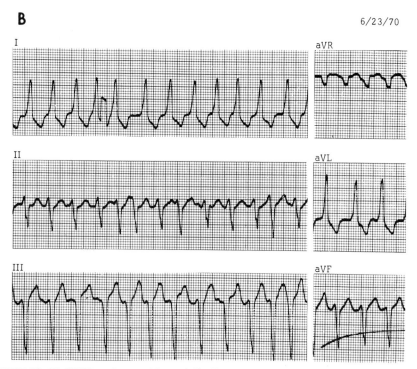

FIGURE 20–12. WPW syndrome with atrial fibrillation. The patient was a 44-year-old man with rheumatic mitral and aortic valve disease. (A) Normal sinus rhythm with type B WPW pattern. (B and C) Tracings recorded during atrial fibrillation. The ventricular response is rapid. The morphology of the QRS complexes is similar to that during sinus rhythm, suggesting that the antegrade AV conduction was by way of the accessory bundle.

C

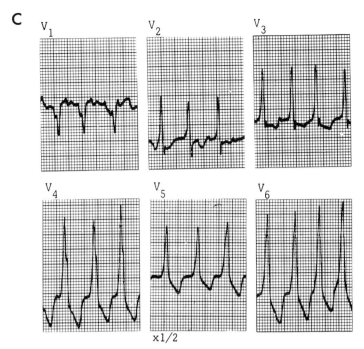

x1/2

FIGURE 20–12. *Continued*

CLINICAL SIGNIFICANCE

It has been estimated that the WPW pattern is present in 0.15 to 0.2 percent of the general population.[17] Most (about two thirds) patients with the WPW pattern have no associated organic heart disease.[17,40,92] In older individuals, the presence of coronary, hypertensive, or rheumatic heart disease in such patients is, in most instances, a coincidental finding. There is a higher incidence of this pattern in patients with primary myocardial disease, however, both the congestive and obstructive types. In patients with idiopathic hypertrophic subaortic stenosis, the typical form of the pattern was reported in 4 percent.[31] Many of these patients have the atypical form of the pattern with either the delta wave or short PR interval only, the former being more common. In the congestive type of primary myocardial disease, WPW pattern is more often seen in the familial variety.[30] Patients with hyperthyroidism are said to have a higher incidence of the WPW pattern.[16] In one series of WPW pattern, 6 percent of the patients had this endocrine abnormality. Twelve of the 163 patients reported by Gallagher and associates had the mitral valve prolapse syndrome.[33] All but one had type A WPW pattern.

Among patients with congenital heart disease, the WPW pattern is seen most commonly in patients with Ebstein's anomaly (Fig. 20–17). In the series of 83 patients with congenital heart disease and WPW pattern reported by Schiebler and co-workers, 24 had such anomalies.[75] About 5 to 10 percent of patients with the anomaly have the pattern.[53] Type B morphology is seen in practically all such patients.[32] Other associated congenital heart diseases include atrial septal defect (see Fig. 20–14), tricuspid atresia, corrected transposition of the great vessels, ventricular septal defect, tetralogy of Fallot, and coarctation of the aorta.[36,74,80]

Anatomic and Electrophysiological Correlations

Ventricular preexcitation was once believed to be the result of congenital clefts in the fibrous AV ring that are occupied by muscular bridges serving as accessory pathways. Later anatomic studies at autopsy and surgery indicate that the accessory pathways (Kent bundles) skirt but do not perforate the fibrous annulus.[5,76] They may be found in the right (tricuspid) or left (mitral) side of the AV ring as well as in the interventricular septal area.[29] Lev and associates reviewed the anatomic findings in 17 reported cases of ventricular preexcitation in which serial sections of the AV ring and the conduction system were performed.[52] The bundle of Kent or AV nodal bypass fibers

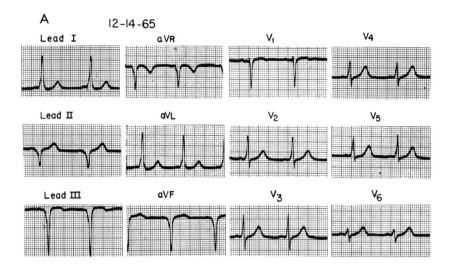

FIGURE 20–13. Wolff-Parkinson-White syndrome with atrial fibrillation. The patient is a 53-year-old woman with no other evidence of heart disease. (A) The 12-lead electrocardiogram shows type B pattern. (B) During atrial fibrillation, the atrial impulses are conducted through the accessory bundle with extremely rapid ventricular response. The very rapid ventricular rate by itself should raise the suspicion of anomalous AV conduction.

of James and Mahaim fibers were found in most of the cases. In general, the cases with type A WPW pattern were associated with left-sided accessory bundles, whereas cases with type B were associated with right-sided accessory pathways. The pathways may be multiple. Most of the cases examined had the type B variety. Occasionally, AV nodal bypass fibers with Mahaim fibers were found in patients with the type B variety. Becker and associates correlated the histopathology with ECG findings in seven cases of WPW pattern.[5] Accessory AV connections were found in all. The sites predicted by the ECG were correct in four cases.

With the advent of surgical treatment of refractory tachyarrhythmias in patients with the WPW syndrome, precise localization of the site of the accessory pathway becomes important. The extensive surgical experience from Duke University indicated that the routine ECG was useful in giving an approximate site of the accessory pathway in most cases[32,33,82] (Fig. 20–18). Type A WPW was generally associated with left-sided accessory bundle, whereas type B was associated with right-sided accessory pathway.[33,82] The ECG, however, was unable to discriminate between free wall and septal accessory pathways. The only exception was when the delta waves were negative in leads V_5 and V_6 (type C WPW pattern). The area of preexcitation was always found in the lateral free wall of the left ventricle.[33] The limited ability of the ECG in predicting the site of the bypass was attributed to (1) alteration of the QRS complex due to other coexisting cardiac abnormalities; (2) existence of multiple accessory pathways; (3) variable degrees of fusion over the normal and accessory pathways; (4) superimposition of the terminal part of P wave on the initial part of the delta wave; and (5) possible endocardial instead of epicardial location of the accessory pathway.

The World Health Organization task force, based on some of the published reports, listed the following criteria for locating the site of ventricular preexcitation[91]:

1. Anterior right ventricular preexcitation
   Delta wave—positive in lead I, isoelectric in lead V_1
   Main QRS—negative in leads III and V_1
2. Posterior right ventricular preexcitation

A

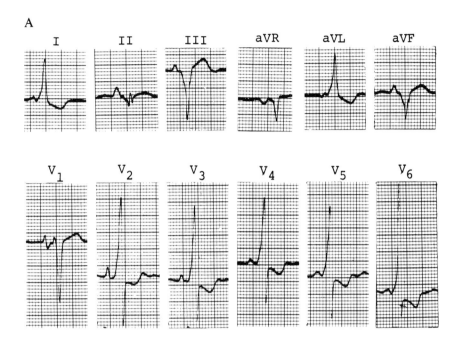

B

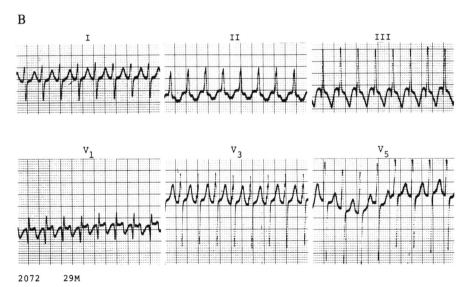

2072   29M

FIGURE 20–14. Wolff-Parkinson-White syndrome in a 28-year-old man with ostium secundum type of atrial septal defect. (A) During sinus rhythm, the P waves are suggestive of biatrial enlargement. The QRS complex is consistent with the type B WPW pattern with a pseudoinfarction pattern in the inferior leads. (B) During paroxysmal supraventricular tachycardia, the QRS complex is narrow and the delta wave is no longer present, suggesting normal antegrade AV conduction (orthodromic tachycardia). The morphology of the QRS complexes is consistent with right ventricular hypertrophy.

C

Lead
I

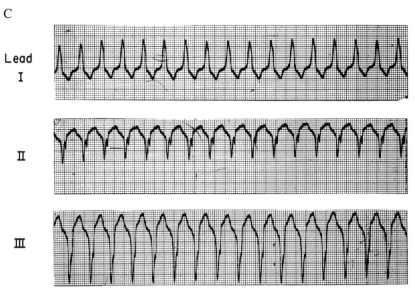

II

III

FIGURE 20–14. *Continued* (C) On another occasion, the patient developed tachycardia with wide QRS complexes, which are similar to those during sinus rhythm, suggesting anomalous antegrade AV conduction through the bypass (antidromic tachycardia). The rhythm was later proved to be atrial flutter with 2:1 conduction.

8/11/70

I

II

8/28/70

I

II

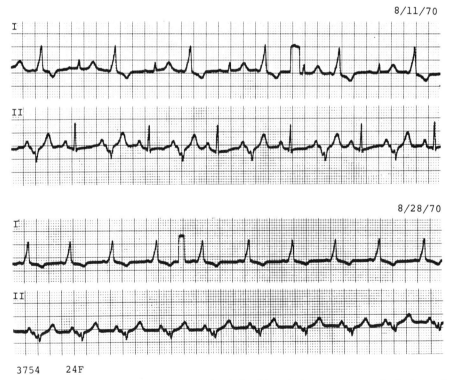

3754   24F

FIGURE 20–15. Intermittent WPW pattern simulating bigeminal premature ventricular beats. In the tracing on 8-11-70, the alternate abnormal QRS complexes may be interpreted as late end-diastolic premature ventricular beats. However, the tracing on a later date (8-28-70) indicates that the abnormal QRS complexes are due to preexcitation.

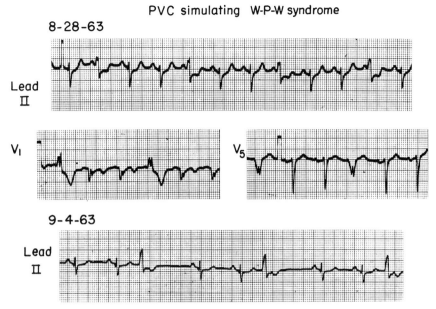

FIGURE 20–16. Premature ventricular beats simulating WPW pattern. In lead II of the tracing on 8-28-63 the abnormal beats with short PR interval and abnormal and wide QRS complex may be interpreted as intermittent WPW pattern. However, leads V_1, V_5, and later tracings (9-4-63) confirm that the abnormal beats are premature ventricular beats occurring in a trigeminal rhythm.

Delta wave—negative in leads III and V_1
Main QRS—negative in leads III and V_1
3. Posterior left ventricular preexcitation
   Delta wave—positive in leads I and V_1, negative in lead III, negative or isoelectric in V_6
   Main QRS—negative in lead III, positive in lead V_1
4. Lateral left ventricular preexcitation
   Delta wave—negative in leads I and V_6, positive in lead V_1
   Main QRS—positive in lead III
5. Anterior paraseptal preexcitation
   Delta wave—positive in leads I, II, and aVF, positive or isoelectric in lead III, isoelectric in lead V_1
6. Posterior paraseptal preexcitation
   Delta wave—positive in lead I, negative in leads II, III, aVF, positive in leads V_2 through V_6
   Main QRS—rS in lead V_1, Rs in lead V_2

Lemery and associates examined the usefulness of the criteria suggested by the Duke group and World Health Organization in 47 patients in whom the location of the accessory pathway was determined by electrophysiological studies and surgery.[51] In only 15 (32 percent) of the patients was the location of the bypass correctly identified by either set of these criteria. Lindsay and associates, however, using slightly different criteria, were able to predict correctly in 60 (91 percent) of 66 patients the location of the accessory pathway as determined by electrophysiological studies.[54] In 45 patients, intraoperative mapping also was performed.

As was mentioned, the presence of multiple accessory AV pathways often complicates the diagnosis and renders it difficult to determine accurately the locations of the pathways. Its recognition is obviously essential, especially in patients considered for surgical ablation. Fifty-two (13 percent) of 388 patients with accessory pathways studied at Duke University were found to have multiple pathways by electrophysiological studies and intraoperative mapping.[19] It was noted that right free wall and posteroseptal accessory pathways were more common in patients with multiple AV pathways and that they were frequently associated.

To localize the accessory bundle accurately, the following electrophysiological studies are usually performed.[32]

Atrial Pacing

A comparison of the degree of preexcitation during left and right atrial pacing may be helpful in determining the approximate site

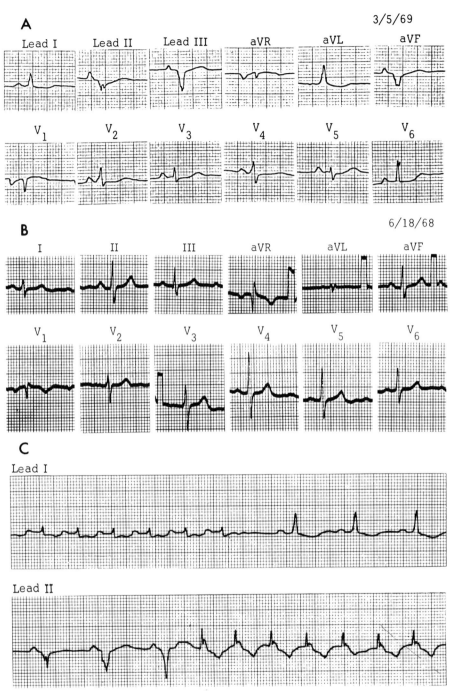

FIGURE 20–17. Ebstein's anomaly with right lateral bypass demonstrated by epicardial mapping. The patient was a 35-year-old woman with Ebstein's anomaly and recurrent episodes of paroxysmal supraventricular tachycardia. (A) Abnormal P waves; the QRS morphology is consistent with ventricular preexcitation. The PR interval is, however, within normal limits (0.14 second). (B) Tracing recorded during normal AV conduction. The PR interval is longer. There is borderline abnormal right axis deviation. Lead V_1 shows a QR pattern. (C) Tracing demonstrating intermittent paroxysmal supraventricular tachycardia. Note the change in morphology of the QRS complexes during tachycardia. Epicardial mapping during sinus rhythm with the WPW pattern revealed early ventricular excitation at the lateral border of the right ventricle near the AV groove. During orthodromic supraventricular reentrant tachycardia, the same area became the latest among the mapping sites to be activated. The findings suggest the right lateral location of the bypass.

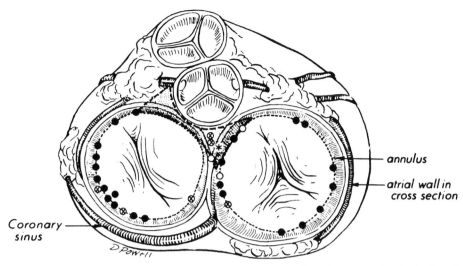

FIGURE 20–18. Schematic diagram depicting the presumptive sites of preexcitation in the first 29 patients with the WPW syndrome who were operated on and reported on by the Duke University group. Pathways are located on the mitral and tricuspid annuli as well as in the septum between the atrium and ventricle. Thirty-two pathways are illustrated because of the presence of two separate pathways in three patients. (Reproduced from Gallagher JJ, Gilbert M, Svenson RH, et al: Wolff-Parkinson-White syndrome: The problem, evaluation, and surgical correction. Circulation 51:767, 1975, by permission of the American Heart Association, Inc.)

of bypass.[32,88] In patients with type B WPW syndrome and right ventricular bypass, the degree of anomalous excitation is usually greater with right atrial pacing than with left atrial pacing. In patients with type A WPW pattern, it is possible to enhance the degree of preexcitation by left atrial pacing, suggesting that the accessory pathway is on the left side. In cases of septal bypass, however, changing the site of atrial pacing does not significantly alter the degree of preexcitation.[33]

Recording Electrogram from the Distal Coronary Sinus

In patients with type A WPW pattern and left ventricular preexcitation, the electrogram reveals left ventricular activity closely coinciding with the onset of the delta wave recorded in the body surface ECG. In patients with type B WPW pattern and right ventricular preexcitation, the left ventricular electrogram is recorded after the initiation of the delta wave and usually during the terminal part of the QRS complex.

Atrial Electrogram During Supraventricular Tachycardia

Since most patients with the WPW syndrome and supraventricular tachycardia have retrograde VA conduction by the accessory path-

way, identification of the earliest point of the retrograde atrial activation may give a presumptive location of the pathway. This may be accomplished by simultaneous recording of the electrogram from the right and left atria.

Epicardial Mapping

Epicardial mapping at the time of surgery provides the most direct means of locating the site of preexcitation and accessory pathway.[9,18,23,26] The point of earliest epicardial activation can be identified.

In the first 30 patients studied by Gallagher and associates,[32] it was found that patients whose ECGs presented predominantly anteriorly directed forces in lead V_1 during maximum preexcitation were found to have an area of epicardial preexcitation in the left ventricular free wall or just to the left of the crux. Those patients whose ECGs showed predominant negative complexes in lead V_1 were found to have an area of epicardial preexcitation on the right ventricle overlying the anterior interventricular septum, the free wall, or just to the right of the crux posteriorly. Patients who show similar ECG findings were found to have similar areas of epicardial preexcitation. Correlation between the timing of the earliest epicardial activation and the delta wave in the conventional ECG is also useful in the differentiation between free wall and septal bypass. In patients with free wall AV bypass, the earliest epicardial activation occurs before the onset of the delta wave. In patients with septal bypass, the area of earliest epicardial activation occurs 5 to 15 msec after the onset of the delta wave.[32]

Other invasive procedures, including His bundle recording, also have been used for localization of the site of the accessory pathway. The discussion of these procedures is beyond the scope of this text.

DIAGNOSIS OF VENTRICULAR HYPERTROPHY, BUNDLE BRANCH BLOCK, AND MYOCARDIAL INFARCTION IN THE PRESENCE OF WOLFF-PARKINSON-WHITE PATTERN

Because of the altered sequence of ventricular activation, the usual diagnostic criteria for left and right ventricular hypertrophy can no longer be applied in patients with the WPW pattern. In type A WPW pattern, there is an exaggeration of the anterior QRS forces, and in type B, of leftward QRS forces. Therefore, both false-positive and false-negative diagnoses of either left or right ventricular hypertrophy may be made. In patients with right bundle branch block during normal AV conduction, the appearance of type B WPW pattern masks the evidence of bundle branch block because the effect of the block is counterbalanced by preexcitation of the right ventricle. Similarly, left bundle branch block is masked when the patient has type A WPW pattern. Exceptional cases have been reported.[13,69] When changes of type B WPW pat-

ter and right bundle branch block coexist, the findings are highly suggestive of Ebstein's anomaly (Fig. 20–19).[69]

The frequent occurrence of the pseudoinfarction pattern in the WPW syndrome has been emphasized. In addition, preexcitation usually obscures the abnormal Q waves of true myocardial infarction (Fig. 20–20). An interesting example is illustrated in Chapter 9 (see Fig. 9–61), in which the sign of old anterior myocardial infarction is no longer seen with the appearance of the WPW pattern but is replaced by a pseudoinfarction pattern in the inferior leads. In patients with the WPW pattern and acute myocardial infarction, ST-segment elevation suggestive of myocardial injury may be seen in leads that normally would display isoelectric or depressed ST segment (see Figs. 20–21 and 9–62).

The usefulness of the ECG stress test for the diagnosis of ischemic heart disease also is limited in patients with the WPW pattern (see Chapter 10). In 14 subjects under the age of 30 years studied by Sandberg, 9 showed ischemic type of ST-segment changes after exercise.[73] An example of a false-positive exercise response in a patient with this syndrome is given in Chapter 10.

EFFECT OF PHYSIOLOGICAL MANEUVERS AND DRUGS ON THE IMPULSE CONDUCTION THROUGH THE ACCESSORY PATHWAY

Table 20–1 gives the effect of various maneuvers and drugs on the impulse conduction through the accessory pathway and the normal AV conduction system. Vagal stimulation,

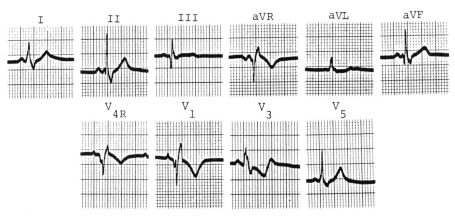

FIGURE 20–19. Ebstein's anomaly with WPW pattern. The presence of both WPW pattern and right bundle branch block pattern is highly suggestive of Ebstein's anomaly. (Courtesy of Dr. Samuel Kaplan.)

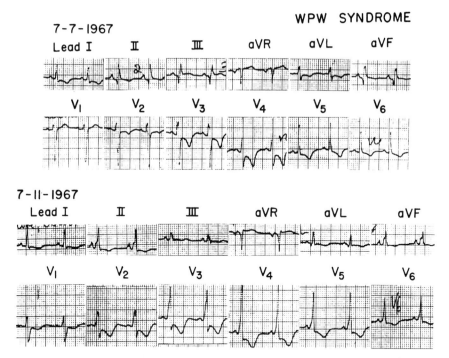

FIGURE 20–20. Myocardial infarction masked by WPW pattern. The tracing on 7-7-67 shows evidence consistent with recent inferior myocardial infarction and anterior and lateral myocardial ischemia. The appearance of the WPW pattern on 7-11-67 masked the signs of inferior myocardial infarction.

parasympathomimetic drugs, beta-adrenergic blocking agents, digitalis, and verapamil depress normal AV conduction and therefore favor conduction through the accessory pathway and the appearance of the WPW pattern.[16,20,68,70,81,87,97] Digitalis and verapamil also have been shown to shorten the refractory period of the accessory pathway and facilitate its

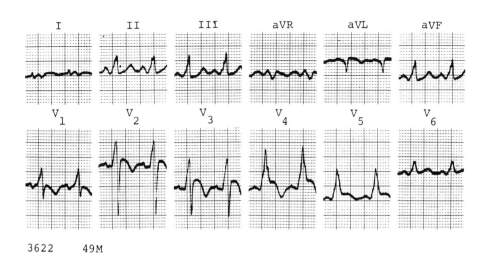

3622   49M

FIGURE 20–21. Acute myocardial infarction in the presence of WPW pattern. The patient is a 49-year-old man with typical symptoms and enzyme changes of acute myocardial infarction. The tracing shows type A WPW pattern. The presence of acute injury is indicated by the ST segment elevation in leads V_3 through V_5. In uncomplicated cases of WPW pattern, the ST segment is either isoelectric or depressed in leads with essentially upright QRS complex.

TABLE 20–1. Effect of Various Maneuvers and Drugs on the Impulse Conduction in the Accessory Pathway and Normal AV Conduction System

Agent/Maneuver	Accessory Pathway	AV Conduction
Vagal stimulation	0	Depress
Parasympathomimetic drugs	0	Depress
Exercise	0	Enhance
Sympathomimetic drugs	0 or enhance	Enhance
Atropine	0	Enhance
Digitalis	0 or enhance	Depress
Quinidine	Depress	0, enhance, or depress
Procainamide	Depress	0
Disopyramide	Depress	0
Lidocaine	Variable	0
Phenytoin	0	0
Beta-adrenergic blockers	0	Depress
Encainide	Depress	Depress
Flecainide	Depress	Depress
Propafenone	Depress	Depress
Amiodarone	Depress	Depress
Verapamil	0 or enhance	Depress

impulse conduction.[39,78,86] Sellers and associates studied 21 patients with the WPW pattern during atrial fibrillation. They found that digitalis increased the ventricular rate and decreased the cycle length of the shortest preexcited RR interval in 6, decreased the ventricular rate in 7, and had no or uncertain effect on the rate in 8.[77] Nine of the 21 patients had histories of ventricular fibrillation while taking digitalis. Gulamhusein and colleagues administered verapamil intravenously to 8 patients with the WPW syndrome and atrial fibrillation.[39] In four patients with predominantly preexcited ventricular complexes during atrial fibrillation, the ventricular rate accelerated and the shortest RR interval decreased after verapamil. Two of the patients required cardioversion because of hemodynamic deterioration.

Procainamide, quinidine, and disopyramide usually increase the effective refractory period of the accessory pathway and, therefore, favor normal AV conduction.[45,46,50,58,70,78,87] The effect of lidocaine on the accessory pathway is variable. Although studies suggest that it lengthens the refractory period of the bypass,[45,70] a more recent report indicates that it has either no significant effect or may shorten the refractory period and cause acceleration of the ventricular response in patients with atrial fibrillation.[1] The difference in the results may be partly related to the initial length of the effective refractory period. If it is relatively short, it is unlikely to be prolonged by the administration of the drug. Such a relation

between the refractory period and the effectiveness of the drug also has been seen with procainamide and quinidine.[84] The effects of various drugs on antegrade and retrograde conduction through either the accessory or normal pathway also may not be the same.[84]

Normal AV conduction may be enhanced by exercise, sympathomimetic drugs, and atropine. However, isoproterenol has also been found to shorten the antegrade refractory period of the accessory pathway and increase the ventricular rate in atrial fibrillation.[35,67,85] This finding suggests that beta adrenergic stimulation induced by hypotension or anxiety may have a similar undesirable effect.[85]

Flecainide, encainide, propafenone, and amiodarone prolong the refractory period of the AV node and the accessory pathway, both antegrade and retrograde.[24,28,63,66,84]

The effect of these maneuvers and drugs has important implications in the management of tachyarrhythmias in these patients. The conversion of the WPW pattern to normal AV conduction also may help to uncover changes associated with the underlying heart disease if it is present.

LOWN-GANONG-LEVINE SYNDROME[55]

Electrocardiographic Findings
(Fig. 20–22)

1. PR interval of less than 0.12 second (in adults), with normal P wave

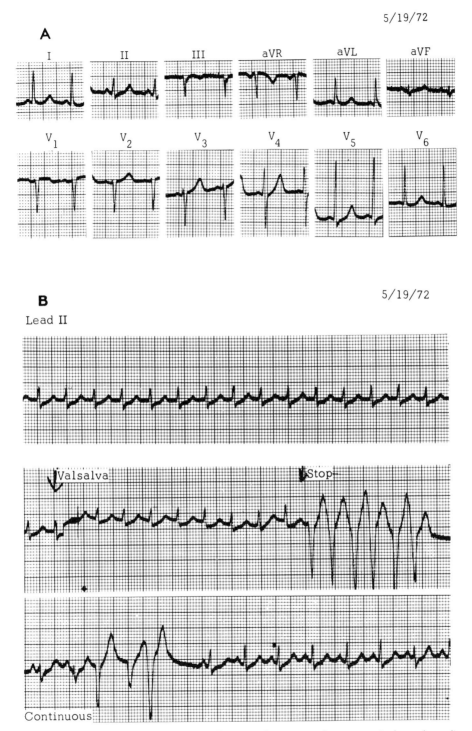

FIGURE 20–22. Lown-Ganong-Levine syndrome with paroxysmal supraventricular tachycardia. (A) A short PR interval of 0.11 second, but the QRS complex is within normal limits. (B) Tracing illustrating an episode of paroxysmal supraventricular tachycardia that was terminated by Valsalva maneuver. A short episode of ventricular tachycardia occurs before the conversion.

2. Normal QRS duration
3. Paroxysmal tachycardia

The term *Lown-Ganong-Levine syndrome* also has been used to describe the ECG findings of short PR interval, normal QRS, but no history of paroxysmal tachycardia. I agree with those who believe that it should be restricted to patients with tachycardia as it was described originally.[60] Such a definition excludes many normal subjects with clinically insignificant short PR intervals. During routine ECG interpretation, I have used the term *accelerated AV conduction* when the history of tachycardia is unknown.

The short PR interval has been attributed to the presence of paranodal fibers described by James.[43] The sinus impulse is conducted through these fibers and bypasses most or all of the AV node, thereby avoiding the normal delay at the AV node. The excitation impulse enters the His bundle and is conducted in a normal fashion through the rest of the AV conduction system. The QRS complex is therefore normal in duration and morphology. Other explanations for the short PR interval have been suggested. They include a small, underdeveloped AV node,[11,14] a preferential fast pathway or unusually rapid conduction in an anatomically normal AV node.[21,33,41,90] The term *enhanced AV nodal conduction* has been used to describe an electrophysiological syndrome with the findings of short AH interval (60 msec or less), 1:1 AV conduction with atrial pacing rate above 200 beats/min, and abnormally small increase in the AH interval as atrial pacing rate is increased.[4,6,41] Patients with enhanced AV nodal conduction, however, often do not have an ECG clue (short PR interval) to its presence and patients with the LGL syndrome often do not show enhanced AV nodal conduction by electrophysiologic studies. Indeed, the existence of such a syndrome as a distinct entity was questioned.[42]

Paroxysmal supraventricular tachycardia is the most common arrhythmia in patients with the LGL syndrome.[6,55] The mechanism in most of the cases is AV nodal reentry.[44] In some, the AV node is used for antegrade conduction and a bypass tract for retrograde conduction.[90] Atrial fibrillation and atrial flutter are occasionally observed, and the ventricular response may be rapid. Ventricular rates as fast as 300 beats/min have been reported.[59] Ventricular tachycardia also has been described.[6,12,61] Ventricular fibrillation may develop in patients with atrial fibrillation and rapid ventricular response.

MAHAIM TYPE OF PREEXCITATION

The Mahaim fibers are muscular bridges with the proximal end located either at the lower portion of the AV node, in the upper part of the bundle of His, or in the bundle branches. Their distal portion ends in the region of the interventricular septum.[53] Depending on the origin of the fibers, these bypass tracts may be called *nodoventricular* (or *nodofascicular*) or *fasciculoventricular* connections.[2] A sinus impulse may therefore travel to the upper part of the AV node with the normal delay, but it is followed by premature excitation of the basal part of the ventricular myocardium, resulting in the inscription of a delta wave. This variant form of preexcitation with a normal PR interval and delta wave (Fig. 20–23) is much less common than the typical WPW pattern and the LGL syndrome. In some cases, the normal PR interval may actually be the result of longer intraatrial conduction time before the impulse reaches the bundle of Kent or slow conduction velocity in the bypass.[89] Figure 20–24 is an example of increased PR interval with advancing age in a patient with the typical WPW pattern. The morphology of the delta wave and QRS complex is unchanged. It may be assumed that the increased PR interval results from prolongation of the conduction time through the accessory bundle.

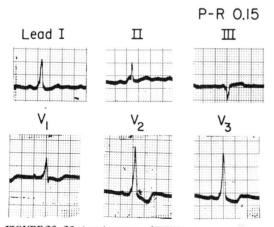

P-R 0.15

Lead I   II   III

V_1 V_2 V_3

FIGURE 20–23. A variant type of WPW pattern with a normal PR interval. The presence of preexcitation is supported by the intermittent appearance of longer PR interval and normal QRS complex (not shown).

11-24-59

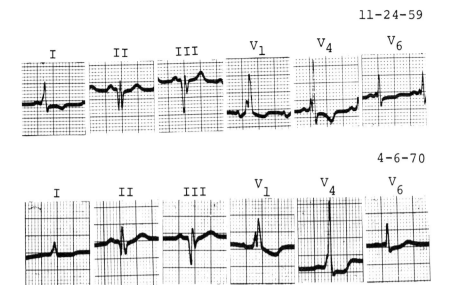

4-6-70

FIGURE 20–24. WPW pattern with prolongation of the PR interval with age. The PR interval in the tracing in 1959 is 0.11 second. It increases to 0.16 second in 1970. The QRS morphology is essentially unchanged.

Reentrant tachycardia with left bundle branch block morphology has been reported in patients with the nodoventricular type of Mahaim fibers. It was postulated that excitation impulse uses a macroreentry circuit, the nodoventricular fibers serving as the antegrade limb and the His-Purkinje system as the retrograde limb.[3,34] Bardy and colleagues suggested that the following findings during tachycardia of left bundle branch block configuration were predictive of the presence of nodofascicular (nodoventricular) fiber: ventricular rate between 134 and 270 beats/min, QRS axis of 0° to −75°, QRS duration of 0.15 second or less, R wave in lead I, rS wave in lead V_1, and a precordial transition from a negative to a positive QRS complex after lead V_4.[3] These findings were present in 12 of the 13 patients they studied. An example of nodofascicular tachycardia is illustrated in Figure 20–25.

CONCEALED WOLFF-PARKINSON-WHITE SYNDROME

An accessory AV pathway may be present but is capable only of retrograde conduction. In the body surface ECG, the features of ventricular preexcitation are absent and the pathway is therefore called *concealed bypass.* The pathway usually can be demonstrated only by intracardiac electrophysiological studies.[37,62,64,79,88] When a reentrant tachycardia occurs in association with such a concealed bypass, the condition is called *concealed WPW syndrome.*

Patients with this syndrome have reciprocating tachycardia when a sinus or an atrial impulse is conducted to the ventricle through the normal AV conduction system. From the ventricle, the impulse is conducted retrograde through the concealed bypass to reactivate the atrium and initiate a reciprocating tachycardia. Such a mechanism may be responsible for many of the reentry tachycardias that were formerly thought to be due to AV nodal reentrant tachycardia. Paroxysms of atrial flutter or fibrillation may develop in such patients if the retrograde activation of the atrium occurs during its vulnerable period.

In most of the recently reported cases of concealed WPW syndrome, the accessory pathway is located on the left side of the cardiac chambers.[37,79] A few cases had right-sided or septal location.

Farshidi and associates considered the following findings during tachycardia to be suggestive of a concealed bypass tract: (1) negative P wave in lead 1 (because of left-sided bypass and early left atrial depolarization), (2) P wave after the QRS complex, and (3) increased cycle length if functional left bundle branch block develops.[27]

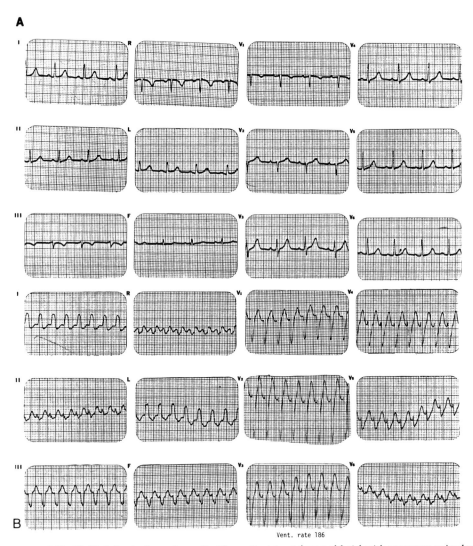

Vent. rate 186

FIGURE 20–25. Nodofascicular tachycardia. The patient is a 14-year-old girl with recurrent episodes of tachycardia but no other evidence of organic heart disease. (A) The resting 12-lead ECG is within normal limits, but the absence of Q waves in leads I, V_5, and V_6 and the small R waves in leads V_1 and V_2 are uncommon at this age. (B) During tachycardia, the QRS complexes have a left bundle branch block appearance. The heart rate is 186 beats/min. The other findings are similar to those described by Bardy and colleagues.[3] Electrophysiological studies supported the diagnosis of nodofascicular tachycardia.

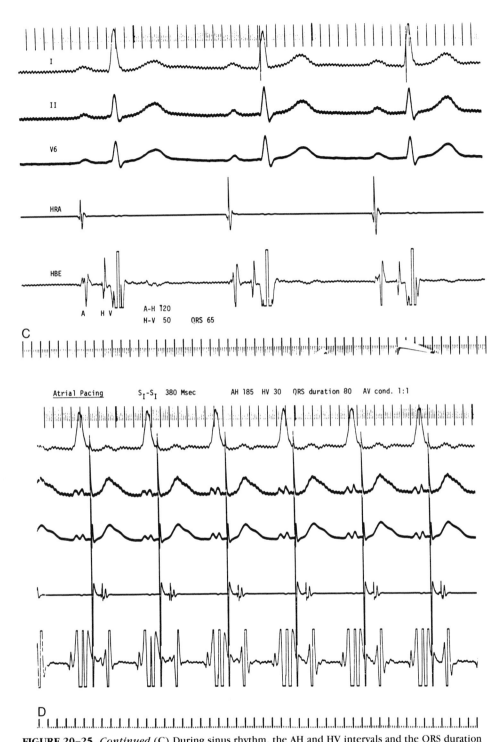

FIGURE 20–25. *Continued* (C) During sinus rhythm, the AH and HV intervals and the QRS duration are normal. With atrial pacing at increasing rates (shorter S_1S_1 interval), there was progressive lengthening of the AH interval, but the HV interval was progressively shortened. The QRS duration gradually increased, but 1:1 AV conduction was maintained. (D) The various measurements when the pacing interval (S_1S_1) was 380 msec. These findings suggest the presence of an accessory pathway (Mahaim fibers) that bypasses the His bundle.

Spontaneous tachycardia following a PVC.

R–R 400 Msec.   Rate 150.

VA 170 Msec.   QRS 130.

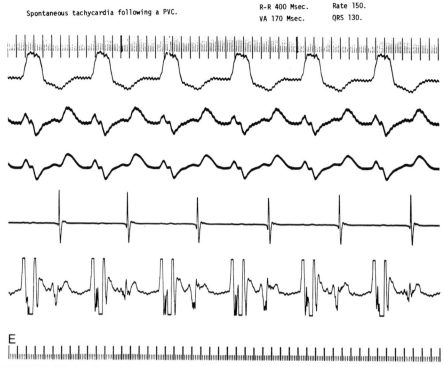

E

FIGURE 20–25. *Continued* (E) During the study, an episode of tachycardia developed spontaneously following a premature ventricular beat. The morphology of the QRS complexes is identical to that in B. The His bundle potential is not seen. There is retrograde atrial activation. HRA = high right atrium; HBE = His bundle electrogram. (Courtesy of Dr. Winston Gaum.)

REFERENCES

1. Akhtar M, Gilbert CJ, Shenasa M: Effect of lidocaine on atrioventricular response via the accessory pathway in patients with Wolff-Parkinson-White syndrome. Circulation 63:435, 1981
2. Anderson RH, Becker AE, Brechenmacher C, et al: Ventricular preexcitation: A proposed nomenclature for its substrates. Eur J Cardiol 3:27, 1975
3. Bardy GH, Fedor JM, German LD, et al: Surface electrocardiographic clues suggesting presence of a nodofascicular Mahaim fiber. J Am Coll Card 3:1161, 1984
4. Bauernfeind RA, Swiryn S, Strasberg B, et al: Analysis of anterograde and retrograde fast pathway properties in patients with dual atrioventricular nodal pathways. Am J Cardiol 49:283, 1982
5. Becker AE, Anderson RH, Durrer D, et al: The anatomic substrates of Wolff-Parkinson-White syndrome. Circulation 57:870, 1978
6. Benditt DG, Pritchett ELC, Smith WM, et al: Characteristics of atrioventricular conduction and the spectrum of arrhythmias in Lown-Ganong-Levine syndrome. Circulation 57:454, 1978
7. Berkman NL, Lamb LE: The Wolff-Parkinson-White electrocardiogram. N Engl J Med 278:492, 1968
8. Brechenmacher C: Atrio-His bundle tracts. Br Heart J 37:853, 1975
9. Burchell HB, Frye RL, Anderson MW, et al: Atrioventricular and ventriculoatrial excitation in Wolff-Parkinson-White syndrome (type B): Temporary ablation at surgery. Circulation 36:663, 1967
10. Campbell RWF, Smith RA, Gallagher JJ, et al: Atrial fibrillation in the preexcitation syndrome. Am J Cardiol 40:514, 1977
11. Caracta AR, Damato AN, Gallagher JJ, et al: Electrophysiologic studies in the syndrome of short P-R interval, normal QRS complex. Am J Cardiol 31:245, 1973
12. Castellanos A, Castillo CA, Agha AS, et al: His bundle electrograms in patients with short P-R intervals, narrow QRS complexes and paroxysmal tachycardias. Circulation 43:667, 1971
13. Castellanos A, Mayer JW, Lemberg L: The electrocardiogram and vectorcardiogram in Wolff-Parkinson-White syndrome associated with bundle branch block. Am J Cardiol 10:657, 1962
14. Childers R: The AV node: Normal and abnormal physiology. Prog Cardiovasc Dis 19:361, 1977
15. Chung EK: Wolff-Parkinson-White syndrome. Current views. Am J Med 62:252, 1977
16. Chung EK: Tachyarrhythmias in Wolff-Parkinson-White syndrome. JAMA 237:376, 1977
17. Chung KY, Walsh TJ, Massie E: Wolff-Parkinson-White syndrome. Am Heart J 69:116, 1965
18. Cobb FR, Blumenschein SD, Sealy WC, et al: Successful surgical interruption of the bundle of Kent in a patient with Wolff-Parkinson-White syndrome. Circulation 38:1018, 1968
19. Colavita PG, Packer DL, Pressley JC, et al: Frequency, diagnosis and clinical characteristics of patients with multiple accessory atrioventricular pathways. Am J Cardiol 59:601, 1987
20. Denes P, Cummings JM, Simpson R, et al: Effect of

propranolol on anomalous pathway refractoriness and circus movement tachycardias in patients with preexcitation. Am J Cardiol 41:1061, 1978

21. Denes P, Wu D, Rosen KM: Demonstration of dual A-V pathways in a patient with Lown-Ganong-Levine syndrome. Chest 65:343, 1974

22. Dreifus LS, Haiat R, Watanabe Y: Ventricular fibrillation: A possible mechanism of sudden death in patients with Wolff-Parkinson-White syndrome. Circulation 43:520, 1971

23. Dreifus LS, Nichols H, Morse D, et al: Control of recurrent tachycardia of Wolff-Parkinson-White syndrome by surgical ligature of the A-V bundle. Circulation 38:1030, 1968

24. Dubuc A, Kus T, Campa MA, et al: Electrophysiologic effects of intravenous propafenone in Wolff-Parkinson-White syndrome. Am Heart J 117:370, 1989

25. Durrer D, Schoo L, Schuilenburg RM, et al: The role of premature beats in the initiation and the termination of supraventricular tachycardia in the Wolff-Parkinson-White syndrome. Circulation 36:644, 1967

26. Durrer D, Schuilenburg RM, Wellens HJJ: Pre-excitation revisited. Am J Cardiol 25:690, 1970

27. Farshidi A, Josephson ME, Horowitz LN: Electrophysiologic characteristics of concealed bypass tracts: Clinical and electrocardiographic correlates. Am J Cardiol 41:1052, 1978

28. Feld GK, Nademanee K, Weiss J, et al: Electrophysiologic basis for the suppression of amiodarone of orthodromic supraventricular tachycardias complicating pre-excitation syndromes. J Am Coll Cardiol 3:1298, 1984

29. Ferrer MI: Pre-excitation, Including the Wolff-Parkinson-White and Other Related Syndromes. Mount Kisco, NY, Futura Publishing, 1976

30. Flowers NV, Horan LG: Electrocardiographic and vectorcardiographic features of myocardial disease. In Fowler NO (ed): Myocardial Diseases. Orlando, Grune & Stratton, 1973

31. Frank S, Braunwald E: Idiopathic hypertrophic subaortic stenosis: Clinical analysis of 126 patients with emphasis on the natural history. Circulation 37:759, 1968

32. Gallagher JJ, Gilbert M, Svenson RH, et al: Wolff-Parkinson-White syndrome: The problem, evaluation, and surgical correction. Circulation 51:767, 1975

33. Gallagher JJ, Pritchett ELC, Sealy WC, et al: The preexcitation syndromes. Prog Cardiovasc Dis 20:285, 1978

34. Gallagher JJ, Smith WM, Kasell JH, et al: Role of Mahaim fibers in cardiac arrhythmias in man. Circulation 64:176, 1981

35. German LD, Gallagher JJ, Broughton A, et al: Effects of exercise and isoproterenol during atrial fibrillation in patients with Wolff-Parkinson-White syndrome. Am J Cardiol 51:1203, 1983

36. Giardina ACV, Ehlers KH, Engle ME: Wolff-Parkinson-White syndrome in infants and children: A long-term follow-up study. Br Heart J 34:839, 1972

37. Gillette PC: Concealed anomalous cardiac conduction pathways: A frequent cause of supraventricular tachycardia. Am J Cardiol 40:848, 1977

38. Grant RB, Tomlison FB, Van Buren JK: Ventricular activation in the pre-excitation syndrome (Wolff-Parkinson-White). Circulation 18:355, 1958

39. Gulamhusein S, Ko P, Carruthers SG, et al: Acceleration of the ventricular response during atrial fibrillation in the Wolff-Parkinson-White syndrome after verapamil. Circulation 65:348, 1982

40. Hejtmancik MT, Herrmann GR: The electrocardio-

graphic syndrome of short P-R interval and broad QRS complexes: A clinical study of 80 cases. Am Heart J 54:708, 1957

41. Holmes DR, Hartzler GO, Merideth J: The clinical and electrophysiologic characteristics of patients with accelerated atrioventricular nodal conduction. Mayo Clin Proc 57:339, 1982

42. Jackman WM, Prystowsky EN, Naccarelli GV, et al: Reevaluation of enhanced atrioventricular nodal conduction: Evidence to suggest a continuum of normal atrioventricular nodal physiology. Circulation 67:441, 1983

43. James TN: Morphology of the human atrioventricular node, with remarks pertinent to its electrophysiology. Am Heart J 62:756, 1961

44. Josephson ME, Kastor JA: Supraventricular tachycardia in the Lown-Ganong-Levine syndrome: Atrionodal versus intranodal reentry. Am J Cardiol 40:521, 1977

45. Josephson ME, Kastor JA, Kitchen JG: Lidocaine in Wolff-Parkinson-White syndrome with atrial fibrillation. Ann Intern Med 84:44, 1976

46. Kerr CR, Prystowsky EN, Smith WM, et al: Electrophysiologic effects of disopyramide phosphate in patients with Wolff-Parkinson-White syndrome. Circulation 65:869, 1982

47. Klein GJ, Bashore TM, Sellers TD, et al: Ventricular fibrillation in the Wolff-Parkinson-White syndrome. N Engl J Med 301:1080, 1979

48. Klein GJ, Gulamhusein SS: Intermittent preexcitation in the Wolff-Parkinson-White syndrome. Am J Cardiol 52:292, 1983

49. Klein GJ, Yee R, Sharma AD: Longitudinal electrophysiologic assessment of asymptomatic patients with the Wolff-Parkinson-White electrocardiographic pattern. N Engl J Med 19:1229, 1989

50. Kou HC, Hung JS, Lee YS, et al: Effects of oral disopyramide phosphate on induction and sustenance of atrioventricular reentrant tachycardia incorporating retrograde accessory pathway conduction. Circulation 66:454, 1982

51. Lemery R, Hammill SC, Wood DL, et al: Value of the resting 12-lead electrocardiogram and vectorcardiogram for locating the accessory pathway in patients with the Wolff-Parkinson-White syndrome. Br Heart J 58:324, 1987

52. Lev M, Fox SM, Bharati S, et al: Mahaim and James fibers as a basis for a unique variety of ventricular preexcitation. Am J Cardiol 36:880, 1975

53. Lev M, Gibson S, Miller RA: Ebstein's disease with Wolff-Parkinson-White syndrome. Am Heart J 49:724, 1955

54. Lindsay BD, Crossen KJ, Cain ME: Concordance of distinguishing electrocardiographic features during sinus rhythm with the location of accessory pathways in the Wolff-Parkinson-White syndrome. Am J Cardiol 59:1093, 1987

55. Lown B, Ganong WF, Levine SA: The syndrome of short P-R interval, normal QRS complex and paroxysmal rapid heart action. Circulation 5:693, 1952

56. Mahaim I: Kent fibers and the A-V paraspecific conduction through the upper connections of the bundle of His-Tawara. Am Heart J 33:651, 1947

57. Mahaim I, Winston MR: Recherches d'anatomie comparee et de pathologie experimentale sur les connexions hautes du faisceau de His-Tawara. Cardiologia 5:189, 1941

58. Mandel WJ, Danzig R, Hayakawa H: Lown-Ganong-Levine syndrome: A study using His bundle electrograms. Circulation 44:696, 1971

59. Moleiro F, Mendoza I, Medina-Ravell V, et al: One to

one atrioventricular conduction during atrial pacing at rates of 300/minute in absence of Wolff-Parkinson-White syndrome. Am J Cardiol 48:789, 1981

60. Moller P: Criteria for the LGL syndrome. Am Heart J 91:539, 1976
61. Myerburg RJ, Sung RJ, Castellanos A: Ventricular tachycardia and ventricular fibrillation in patients with short P-R intervals and narrow QRS complexes. Pace 2:568, 1979
62. Narula OS: Retrograde pre-excitation. Comparison of antegrade and retrograde conduction intervals in man. Circulation 50:1129, 1974
63. Neuss H, Schlepper BM, Berthold R, et al: Effects of flecainide on electrophysiological properties of accessory pathways in the Wolff-Parkinson-White syndrome. Am Heart J 4:347, 1983
64. Neuss H, Schlepper M, Thormann J: Analysis of reentry mechanisms in three patients with concealed Wolff-Parkinson-White syndrome. Circulation 51:75, 1975
65. Newman BJ, Donoso E, Freidberg CK: Arrhythmias in the Wolff-Parkinson-White syndrome. Prog Cardiovasc Dis 9:147, 1966
66. Prystowsky EN, Klein GJ, Rinkenberger RL, et al: Clinical efficacy and electrophysiologic effects of encainide in patients with Wolff-Parkinson-White syndrome. Circulation 69:278, 1984
67. Przybylski J, Chiale PA, Halpern MS, et al: Unmasking of ventricular preexcitation by vagal stimulation or isoproterenol administration. Circulation 61:1030, 1980
68. Rinkenberger RL, Prystowsky EN, Heger JJ, et al: Effects of intravenous and chronic oral verapamil administration in patients with supraventricular tachyarrhythmias. Circulation 62:996, 1980
69. Robertson PGC, Emslie-Smith D, Lowe KG, et al: The association of type B ventricular pre-excitation and right bundle branch block. Br Heart J 25:755, 1963
70. Rosen KM, Barwolf C, Ehsani A, et al: Effects of lidocaine and propranolol on the normal and anomalous pathways in patients with preexcitation. Am J Cardiol 30:801, 1972
71. Rosenbaum FF, Hecht HH, Wilson FN, et al: The potential variations of the thorax and the esophagus in anomalous atrioventricular excitation (Wolff-Parkinson-White syndrome). Am Heart J 29:281, 1945
72. Ruskin JN, Akhtar M, Damato AN, et al: Abnormal Q waves in Wolff-Parkinson-White syndrome. JAMA 235:2727, 1976
73. Sanberg L: Studies on electrocardiographic changes during exercise tests. Acta Med Scand (Suppl) 1961, p 365
74. Schiebler GL, Adams P, Anderson RC: The Wolff-Parkinson-White syndrome in infants and children. Pediatrics 24:585, 1959
75. Schiebler GL, Adams P, Anderson RC, et al: Clinical study of twenty-three cases of Ebstein's anomaly of the tricuspid valve. Circulation 19:165, 1959
76. Sealy WC, Gallagher JJ, Pritchett ELC: The surgical anatomy of Kent bundles based on electrophysiological mapping and surgical exploration. J Thorac Cardiovasc Surg 76:804, 1978
77. Sellers TD, Bashore TM, Gallagher JJ: Digitalis in the preexcitation syndrome: Analysis during atrial fibrillation. Circulation 56:260, 1977
78. Sellers TD, Campbell RWF, Bashore TM, et al: Effects of procainamide and quinidine sulfate in the Wolff-Parkinson-White syndrome. Circulation 55:15, 1977
79. Sung RJ, Gelband H, Castellanos A, et al: Clinical and electrophysiologic observations in patients with con-

cealed accessory atrioventricular bypass tracts. Am J Cardiol 40:839, 1977
80. Swiderski J, Lees MH, Nadas AS: The Wolff-Parkinson-White syndrome in infancy and childhood. Br Heart J 24:561, 1962
81. Tonkin AM, Gallagher JJ, Wallace AG: Tachyarrhythmias in Wolff-Parkinson-White syndrome: Treatment and prevention. JAMA 235:947, 1976
82. Tonkin AM, Wagner GS, Gallagher JJ, et al: Initial forces of ventricular depolarization in the Wolff-Parkinson-White syndrome. Circulation 52:1030, 1975
83. Wellens HJJ: Wolff-Parkinson-White syndrome. I. Diagnosis, arrhythmias, and identification of the high risk patient. Mod Concepts Cardiovasc Dis 52:53, 1983
84. Wellens HJJ, Bar FW, Dassen WRM, et al: Effect of drugs in the Wolff-Parkinson-White syndrome: Importance of initial length of effective refractory period of the accessory pathway. Am J Cardiol 46:665, 1980
85. Wellens HJJ, Brugada P, Roy D, et al: Effect of isoproterenol on the anterograde refractory period of the accessory pathway in patients with the Wolff-Parkinson-White syndrome. Am J Cardiol 50:180, 1982
86. Wellens HJ, Durrer D: Effect of digitalis on atrioventricular conduction and circus-movement tachycardias in patients with Wolff-Parkinson-White syndrome. Circulation 47:1229, 1973
87. Wellens HJ, Durrer D: Effect of procaine amide, quinidine and ajmaline in the Wolff-Parkinson-White syndrome. Circulation 50:114, 1974
88. Wellens HJJ, Durrer D: The role of an accessory atrioventricular pathway in reciprocal tachycardia: Observations in patients with and without the Wolff-Parkinson-White syndrome. Circulation 52:58, 1975
89. Wellens HJ, Lie KI: Ventricular tachycardia: The value of programmed electrical stimulation. In Krikler DM, Goodwin JF (eds): Cardiac Arrhythmias: The Modern Electrophysiological Approach. Philadelphia, WB Saunders, 1975, p 182
90. Wiener I: Syndromes of Lown-Ganong-Levine and enhanced atrioventricular nodal conduction. Am J Cardiol 52:637, 1983
91. Willems JL, DeMedina EO, Bernard R, et al: Criteria for intraventricular conduction disturbances and preexcitation. J Am Coll Cardiol 5:1261, 1985
92. Willus FA, Carryer HM: Electrocardiograms displaying short P-R intervals with prolonged QRS complexes: An analysis of sixty-five cases. Proc Staff Meet Mayo Clin 21:438, 1946
93. Wolferth CC, Wood FC: The mechanism of production of short P-R intervals and prolonged QRS complexes in patients with presumably undamaged hearts: Hypothesis of an accessory pathway of auriculoventricular conduction (bundle of Kent). Am Heart J 8:297, 1933
94. Wolff L: Syndrome of short P-R interval with abnormal QRS complexes and paroxysmal tachycardia (WPW syndrome). Circulation 10:282, 1954
95. Wolff L: Anomalous atrioventricular excitation (Wolff-Parkinson-White syndrome). Circulation 19:14, 1959
96. Wolff L, Parkinson J, White PD: Bundle branch block with short P-R interval in healthy young people prone to paroxysmal tachycardia. Am Heart J 5:685, 1930
97. Wu D, Amat-Y-Leon F, Simpson RJ, et al: Electrophysiological studies with multiple drugs in patients with atrioventricular re-entrant tachycardias utilizing an extranodal pathway. Circulation 56:727, 1979

DRUG EFFECTS, ELECTROLYTE IMBALANCE, AND OTHER MISCELLANEOUS CONDITIONS

Effect of Drugs on the Electrocardiogram

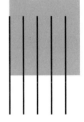

21

DIGITALIS

Digitalis has both direct and indirect electrophysiological effects on the heart. In its direct actions, it inhibits the active transport of sodium and potassium ions across the cell membrane. It acts indirectly by increasing the vagal tone. The combined electrophysiological effects are complex. Digitalis may alter the automaticity, excitability, and conductivity to different degrees and even in opposite directions in the various cardiac tissues.

The administration of therapeutic doses of digitalis decreases the automaticity of the sinoatrial (SA) node. The slowing of the sinus rate is due mostly to the vagal effect of the cardiac glycoside, but its direct action may also be contributory. In toxic doses, digitalis may cause an increase in sinus rate as well as impairment of SA conduction.

In the atrium, the direct effect of digitalis lengthens the effective refractory period and decreases its excitability and conduction velocity, whereas the indirect action of the glycoside tends to have an opposite effect. The automaticity of the subsidiary atrial pacemaker is depressed with low doses of the drug but may be enhanced with higher doses.[41]

At the atrioventricular (AV) junction, the drug causes depression of its conductivity but enhancement of its automaticity. The impairment of impulse conduction is the result of both the vagal and direct effects of the drug. His bundle electrogram shows that the increase in the PR interval is due to prolongation of the AH interval, but the HV interval is unchanged. Digitalis may cause an increase in the automaticity and a decrease in the excitability of the His-Purkinje system by increasing the slope of diastolic depolarization in the Purkinje fibers. This direct action is responsible for the production of digitalis-induced AV junctional and ventricular tachyarrhythmias. In the usual doses, digitalis has no appreciable effect on the excitability of the undifferentiated ventricular myocardial fibers. In high doses, the ventricular refractory period often is shortened, which may not be uniform throughout the ventricle, a fact that may contribute significantly to the appearance of toxic arrhythmias.[56]

The effects of digitalis on ventricular repolarization are responsible for the characteristic ST-segment and T-wave changes associated with the administration of the drug. The recovery process, especially in the subendocardial layer, is accelerated and the QT interval is shortened. With suction electrodes during cardiac catheterization in men, the monophasic action potential recorded from the endocardial surface of the ventricles showed an increase in the slope of phase II and a decrease in its total duration.[94]

Effect of Digitalis on the Electrocardiogram

1. ST-segment depression
2. Decreased amplitude of the T wave, which may become diphasic (negative–positive) or negative
3. Shortening of the QT interval
4. Increase of the U-wave amplitude

After the administration of digitalis, the earliest electrocardiographic (ECG) changes usually consist of a decrease in the amplitude of the T wave and shortening of the QT interval. The more typical finding, however, is the sagging of the ST segment, with the first part of the T wave "dragged down" by the depressed ST segment (Fig. 21–1). Therefore, the T wave becomes diphasic, its initial portion being negative and the terminal portion positive. As the ST-segment depression becomes more pronounced, the entire T wave may become inverted. In some patients, the typical sagging of the ST segment is not seen, but there is a slight upward convexity of the depressed ST segment that resembles that of the so-called strain pattern. These changes are usually more pronounced in leads with tall R

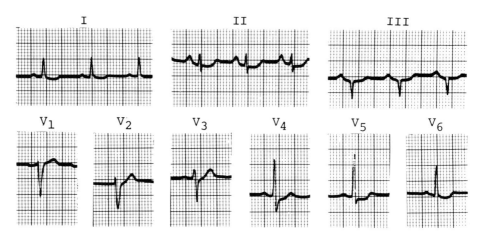

2494   50M

FIGURE 21–1. Digitalis effect. The patient is a 50-year-old man with no evidence of heart disease who took about 5 mg of digoxin for suicidal purpose 1 day before the tracing was recorded. The plasma digoxin level at the time of the recording was 4.1 ng/ml. Note the sagging of the ST segment, especially in leads I, II, and V_4 through V_6. The T waves in leads II and V_5 are biphasic. No arrhythmia was observed.

waves. If the ECG is otherwise normal, these ST-segment and T-wave changes are more prominent in the inferior and left precordial leads. In the right precordial leads, they are less marked, and the ST segment may be elevated with upright T waves in these leads in some instances.

The T-wave changes that result from digitalis may appear in less typical forms. The T waves may be pointedly inverted, simulating those in myocardial ischemia or pericarditis.[107] The QT interval is shortened by digitalis, however, and it is usually normal in pericarditis and prolonged in myocardial ischemia. In about 10 percent of patients receiving digitalis, there is peaking of the terminal portion of the T wave.[60]

The U wave may become more prominent with digitalis therapy. The increased amplitude usually is best seen in the mid-precordial

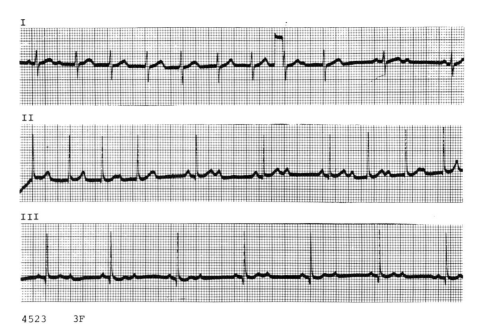

4523   3F

FIGURE 21–2. Digitalis intoxication. The patient is a 3-year-old girl who accidentally ingested 3.5 mg of digoxin. The ECGs obtained after admission showed second-degree AV block with periods of Wenckebach phenomenon, which also is present in this tracing recorded 4 days later. There are no significant ST or T-wave changes.

leads. The degree of increase, however, does not usually approach that resulting from hypokalemia or quinidine.

Although these repolarization abnormalities are the characteristic findings caused by digitalis, they are not always present. Furthermore, the degree of changes has no consistent relation to the amount of digitalis administered or the serum level of the glycoside. Toxic manifestations of the drug, such as gastrointestinal symptoms or arrhythmias, may occur in the absence of any significant ST-segment and T-wave changes (Fig. 21–2). On the other hand, marked repolarization abnormalities may be present when the dosage given is well within the therapeutic range or even below it. These changes also are more likely to be pronounced when there is tachycardia.[107] Digitalis is also one of the causes of false-positive ECG response in exercise testing for ischemic heart disease. Such a false-positive response was reported in 50 percent of normal subjects.[52]

RECOGNITION OF DIGITALIS EFFECT IN THE PRESENCE OF VENTRICULAR HYPERTROPHY OR BUNDLE BRANCH BLOCK

The secondary ST and T-wave changes in patients with ventricular hypertrophy or bundle branch block may simulate or mask the repolarization abnormalities associated with digitalis. Digitalis effect may be recognized, however, if there is definite "sagging" of the ST segment with an upward concavity. The duration of the QT interval is also sometimes helpful. In left ventricular hypertrophy or left bundle branch block, the QT interval is usually prolonged. Digitalis effect may be suspected if the interval is normal or shortened.

Digitalis Intoxication

Digitalis intoxication is common in patients who take the drug. In a prospective study of hospitalized patients receiving the drug reported in 1971, 23 percent developed definite toxic manifestations.[8] The incidence is probably lower in recent years since the dosage of the drug used is generally lower than that used previously. Although gastrointestinal symptoms are common and neurologic manifestations may occur, cardiac complications are the most serious toxic effect of digitalis. Digitalis is known to be capable of producing almost all types of cardiac arrhythmias, resulting from either a disturbance of the impulse formation or an impairment of its conduction. The only exception is bundle branch block, which is rarely caused by digitalis. Table 21–1 gives the relative incidence

TABLE 21–1. Relative Incidence of Digitalis-induced Arrhythmias*

Rhythm		No. of Patients†	% of Total
Frequent PVCs	Total multifocal bigeminy	327	48
		107	16
		165	24
Junctional tachycardia		90	13
Junctional rhythm		30	4
AV dissociation		62	9
Heart block	First degree	84	12
	Second degree	77	11
	Third degree	77	11
PAT	Total	91	13
	With block	70	10
Atrial fibrillation		72	10
Atrial flutter		11	1.6
Premature atrial contractions		34	5
Premature junctional contractions		4	0.6
Sinus arrest		11	1.6
Sinus bradycardia		16	2.3
Sinus tachycardia		30	4
Wandering pacemaker		16	2.3
Ventricular tachycardia		71	10
Ventricular fibrillation		8	1.2

*Irons GV, Orgain ES: Digitalis-induced arrhythmias and their management. Prog Cardiovasc Dis 8:539, 1966, by permission.
†Total number of patients, 688.
PAT = paroxysmal atrial tachycardia; PVCs = premature ventricular contractions.

of digitalis-induced arrhythmias summarized by Irons and Orgain.[47] Different types of arrhythmias are often seen in the same patient within a relatively short time. Digitalis toxicity should be suspected especially when evidence of increased automaticity and impaired conduction are present at the same time. Although some of the arrhythmias are characteristic of digitalis toxicity, none is pathognomonic. As mentioned, the ECG signs of digitalis effect consisting of sagging of the ST segment, shortening of the QT interval, and T-wave inversion do not correlate well with the degree of digitalization and may be absent in obvious cases of intoxication.

Digitalis-Induced Arrhythmias

VENTRICULAR ARRHYTHMIAS: PREMATURE VENTRICULAR BEATS, VENTRICULAR TACHYCARDIA, AND VENTRICULAR FIBRILLATION

Ventricular ectopic beats are the most common arrhythmia and often the earliest manifestation of digitalis intoxication. They account for almost half of the arrhythmias caused by digitalis. They may be unifocal or multifocal. Bigeminal and trigeminal rhythms are particularly characteristic. Premature ventricular beats, however, are the most common arrhythmia in the absence of digitalis. In a patient who has not received an adequate amount of digitalis, additional doses of the drug may reduce or abolish the ectopic beats, probably by improving the cardiac status. When premature ventricular beats due to digitalis are not recognized and administration of the drug is continued, more serious ventricular arrhythmias, such as ventricular tachycardia and ventricular fibrillation, may develop. The latter, however, may occur without the warning premature beats. Digitalis also may cause nonparoxysmal ventricular tachycardia, which usually is not associated with serious hemodynamic consequences.

ATRIOVENTRICULAR BLOCK

Various degrees of AV block are the next most common arrhythmias induced by digitalis. The percentage probably has been lower in recent years. This is not surprising, since conduction delay at the AV junction is one of its known electrophysiological effects. This property is used therapeutically to slow the ventricular rate in patients with atrial fibrillation or atrial flutter. In patients with sinus rhythm, a slight prolongation of the PR interval is generally considered a therapeutic effect, but a definite prolongation of the PR interval should be regarded at least as a warning sign of toxicity. Second- and third-degree AV block, when caused by digitalis, are definite evidence of intoxication. Digitalis-induced second-degree AV block usually presents the Wenckebach phenomenon (see Fig. 21–2). Mobitz type II second-degree AV block is rare.

Monitor lead

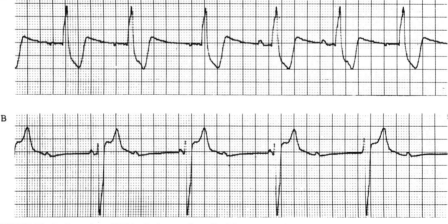

FIGURE 21–3. Complete AV block due to digitalis. The patient had coronary artery disease and complete right bundle branch block. (A) Tracing showing sinus bradycardia. The variation of the P-wave morphology probably is due to wandering of the pacemaker. (B) Tracing showing complete AV block with idioventricular rhythm and a ventricular rate of 43 beats/min. The serum digoxin level was 5 ng/ml. (The electrode placement was the same in A and B.)

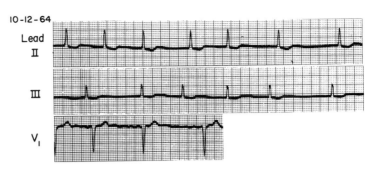

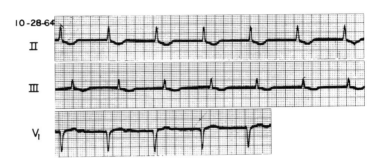

FIGURE 21–4. Atrial fibrillation with complete AV block. The tracing on 10-12-64 shows atrial fibrillation with controlled ventricular response. The ST and T-wave changes are consistent with digitalis effect. The regular RR interval in tracing of 10-28-64 suggests the development of complete AV block with junctional escape rhythm. Digitalis toxicity is strongly suspected. (Reproduced from Chou TC: Digitalis-induced arrhythmias. *In* Fowler NO (ed): Cardiac Arrhythmias: Diagnosis and Treatment. New York, Harper & Row, 1977, by permission.)

Complete AV block that results from digitalis is, as a rule, associated with narrow QRS complexes unless intraventricular conduction defect preexists. The level of the block is proximal to the bifurcation of His bundle. The ventricular escape rate is usually faster than that due to other causes. Exceptions occur, however (Fig. 21–3). In patients with atrial fibrillation, an advanced degree of AV block is manifested by an excessive slowing of the ventricular rate. A regular ventricular rhythm in the presence of atrial fibrillation suggests complete AV block (Fig. 21–4). In patients with atrial flutter, complete AV block is diagnosed by a slow ventricular rate with regular RR interval and varying FR interval.

NONPAROXYSMAL JUNCTIONAL TACHYCARDIA, AV DISSOCIATION, AND JUNCTIONAL ESCAPE RHYTHM

Digitalis may cause an abnormal enhancement of impulse formation at the AV junction, resulting in nonparoxysmal junctional tachycardia. The rate of the junctional discharge is usually between 70 and 130 beats/min, and the rhythm is regular. If the junctional pacemaker fails to capture the atria, AV dissociation occurs. The atrial and ventricular rhythms are independent, and the ventricular rate is generally faster than the atrial rate.

Although nonparoxysmal junctional tachy-

cardia with or without AV dissociation is most commonly the result of digitalis intoxication, it also may be seen in patients with myocarditis or acute myocardial infarction, or following intracardiac surgery. In the 30 cases reported on by Pick and Dominguez, digitalis was responsible for the arrhythmia in 16 patients.[82]

Digitalis is the most frequent cause of bidirectional tachycardia[86] (Fig. 21–5). This arrhythmia is probably AV junctional in origin, with regular alternation of two types of QRS complexes. There is a right bundle branch block pattern in every beat, but the mean QRS axis of the alternate ventricular complexes has opposite directions, probably because of alternate aberrant conduction in the two divisions of the left bundle branch. Well-documented cases of bidirectional ventricular tachycardia have been reported, however.[75]

AV junctional escape rhythm occurs in digitalis intoxication when there is a suppression or failure of impulse formation at the SA node or when there is SA block. When the rate of the sinus discharge or conducted sinus impulse is slower than the inherent rate of the AV junction, the latter assumes the role of pacemaker. The ventricular rate usually varies between 40 and 60 beats/min. As in the case of nonparoxysmal junctional tachycardia, AV dissociation may be present if there is a failure of retrograde atrial capture.

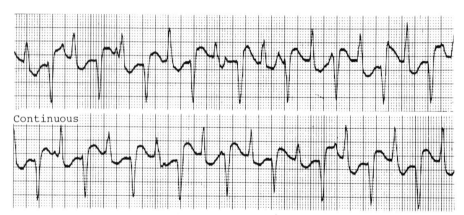

FIGURE 21–5. Bidirectional tachycardia resulting from digitalis. The patient is a 54-year-old man with cardiomyopathy. The rhythm strip shows an atrial rate of 72 beats/min and a ventricular rate of 168 beats/min. There is AV dissociation. The alternate QRS complexes have opposite direction. The 12-lead ECG (not illustrated) showed a right bundle branch block pattern in all complexes.

PAROXYSMAL ATRIAL TACHYCARDIA WITH BLOCK

The importance of digitalis in the production of paroxysmal atrial tachycardia (PAT) with block was emphasized by Lown and associates.[61] It was estimated that, in hospitalized patients with this arrhythmia, about 73 percent of the cases were induced by digitalis. The percentage probably has been lower in recent years. Loss of potassium may be responsible for the precipitation of PAT with block in many digitalized patients.

The atrial rate in PAT with block is usually between 150 and 200 beats/min. The degree of AV block varies (Fig. 21–6), second-degree block and Wenckebach phenomenon being most common. Occasionally there is a 1:1 conduction with normal PR interval, and the AV block is demonstrated only during carotid sinus massage. This particular variant is called PAT with latent block (Fig. 21–7).

ATRIAL FIBRILLATION (see Fig. 21–7)

Although the literature indicates that atrial fibrillation accounts for about 10 percent of the arrhythmias induced by digitalis, it is uncommon in my experience. Their association may be suspected when the arrhythmia develops in a digitalized patient who previously had sinus rhythm. In most instances, however, the arrhythmia is caused by the underlying disease rather than by the drug. Only if sinus rhythm returns after the drug is discontinued can their relation be assumed.

Atrial flutter is rarely caused by digitalis. I have not encountered any proven cases.

SINUS BRADYCARDIA, SINUS ARREST, SINOATRIAL BLOCK, AND SINUS TACHYCARDIA

The ECG diagnosis of these abnormal rhythms usually can be made without difficulty. The reader is referred to Chapter 15 for more detailed description of the changes in sinus arrest and SA block. Figure 21–8 is an example of SA block and AV block resulting from digitalis. The association of digitalis toxicity and sinus tachycardia, however, is often not recognized.

Correlation of Digitalis Intoxication with the Serum Glycoside Level

The serum glycoside level is of considerable value in the confirmation and diagnosis of digitalis-induced arrhythmias. With digoxin, a value above 2 ng/mL is generally considered to be consistent with digitalis intoxication. Considerable overlap of the serum glycoside concentration is found, however, in toxic and nontoxic patients. Toxic manifestations may be seen in some patients with serum levels of 1.6 ng/mL but not in others with concentrations of 3.0 ng/mL.[99]

ANTIARRHYTHMIC AGENTS: CLASSIFICATION

Class I

    A: Quinidine, procainamide, disopyramide

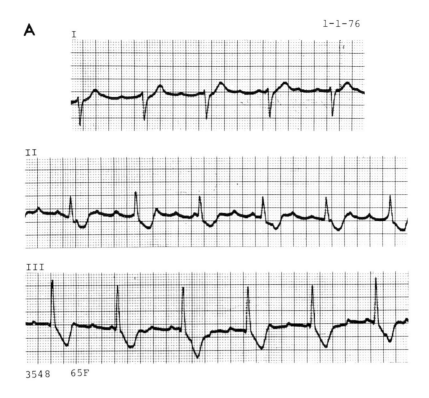

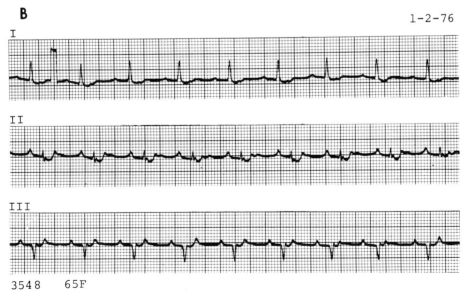

FIGURE 21–6. PAT with block caused by digitalis. (A) The tracing from 1-1-76 shows an atrial rate of 200 beats/min and a ventricular rate of 60 beats/min. There is complete AV block, and the lower pacemaker is idioventricular in origin. (B) On 1-2-76, the rhythm is PAT with 2:1 block. The serum digoxin level was 3.7 ng/ml on 1-2-76.

A

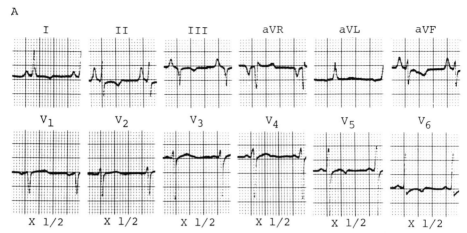

FIGURE 21–7. Atrial arrhythmias caused by digitalis. (A) Tracing showing the 12-lead ECG of a patient who had aortic insufficiency and congestive heart failure. The tracing shows abnormal P waves and left ventricular hypertrophy. A total dosage of 1.5 mg of digoxin was given intravenously to the patient in 36 hours.

B: Lidocaine, tocainide, mexiletine, phenytoin
C: Encainide, flecanide, propafenone
Class II: Propranolol and other beta-adrenergic blocking agents
Class III: Amiodarone, bretylium, sotalol
Class IV: Verapamil, diltiazem

QUINIDINE

Quinidine, the prototype of class I antiarrhythmic agents, blocks the fast sodium channels in cell membrane. It depresses maximum rate of depolarization, lengthens the action potential duration, and increases the refractory periods of the His-Purkinje fibers and myocardium. In addition, it also is anticholinergic.

Therapeutic doses of quinidine have little effect on the SA node. Although its direct effect decreases the automaticity of the pacemaker tissue at the SA node, this is usually counterbalanced by the vagolytic action of the drug, which tends to increase the sinus rate. At the AV junction, the conduction velocity is often decreased because of the direct action of the drug but may be increased because of its vagolytic effect. In the Purkinje system, the automaticity is depressed, the conduction velocity is decreased, and the refractory period is prolonged. The automaticity, excitability, and conductivity of the atrial and ventricular tissues are depressed by quinidine. Their effective refractory period is prolonged. The total duration of the action potential of the ventricular muscle fibers is increased but that

of the atrial fibers is not unless the atrial rate is rapid.

With higher or toxic doses of the drug, the automaticity of the SA node may be depressed, resulting in sinus bradycardia or sinus arrest, or it may be increased, resulting in sinus tachycardia. SA and AV conduction may be impaired and intraventricular conduction time markedly prolonged. The automaticity of the ventricular myocardial fibers may be paradoxically increased with the appearance of ventricular arrhythmias.

Electrocardiographic Findings

THERAPEUTIC EFFECTS

1. Decrease in the amplitude of the T wave or T-wave inversion
2. ST-segment depression
3. Prominent U waves
4. Prolongation of the QTc interval
5. Notching and widening of the P waves

TOXIC EFFECTS

1. Widening of the QRS complex
2. Various degrees of AV block
3. Ventricular arrhythmias, syncope, and sudden death
4. Marked sinus bradycardia, sinus arrest, or SA block

One of the earliest changes in the ECG after the administration of quinidine is often the appearance of prominent U waves. This may occur in the presence of a relatively low

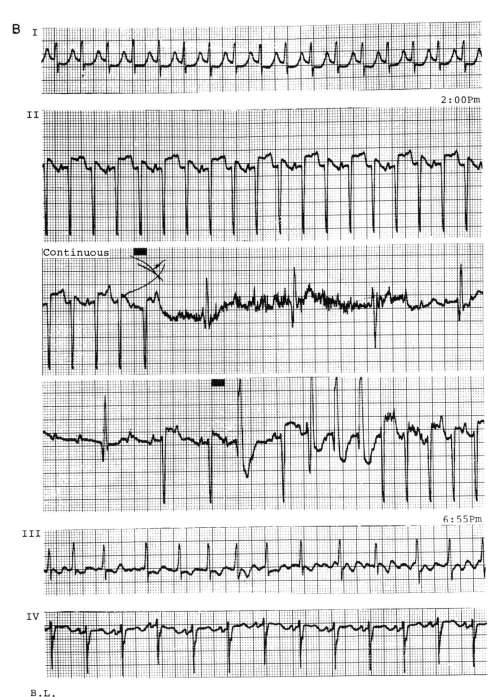

B.L.

FIGURE 21–7 *Continued* (B) He developed various arrhythmias. In I and II of B, the rhythm is PAT with latent block, which is revealed by carotid sinus massage (between the marks). Idioventricular escape rhythm appears during the period of vagal stimulation. The last four abnormal QRS complexes in II are probably due to aberrant ventricular conduction. Note also the presence of T-wave alternans during tachycardia. Strip III of B shows atrial fibrillation, and IV shows normal sinus rhythm. Digoxin blood level at 2 P.M. was 3.5 ng/ml.

plasma quinidine level (Fig. 21–9). Prolongation of the QTc interval is related to the increase in the duration of action potential of the ventricular muscle fibers. The degree of

prolongation may give some indication of the intensity of the quinidine effect, but it cannot be used as a reliable sign to guide the therapy. Because the U wave is often prominent and su-

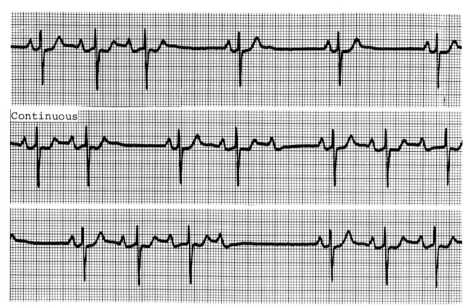

FIGURE 21–8. SA and AV block caused by digitalis. The tracing shows second-degree SA block and Mobitz type I second-degree AV block. The serum digoxin level was 2.8 ng/ml.

perimposed on the T wave, accurate determination of the QT interval is often difficult. In fact, the apparent prolongation of the QT interval in some patients is probably due to the inclusion of the U wave. In 121 patients receiving quinidine for the treatment of atrial fibrillation and atrial flutter, Cheng was able to demonstrate actual prolongation of the QTc interval in only 18 (15 percent).

Figure 21–10 illustrates the prolongation of the QT interval as a result of quinidine, but the exact measurement of the interval is difficult because of the prominent U waves. The ST-segment, T-wave, and U-wave changes caused by quinidine often closely mimic those seen in patients with hypokalemia.

In patients with sinus rhythm, notching and widening of the P waves may occur. Although these changes may be seen with therapeutic doses of the drug, they are observed most often when the plasma level is in the toxic range (Fig. 21–11). In patients with coarse atrial fibrillation or atrial flutter, a widening of the fibrillatory or flutter waves may be seen with a decrease of the atrial rate (see Fig. 16–21). This may occur even when the plasma level of the drug is low (e.g., 1.7 to 2.7 mg/L).[116]

With large doses and higher blood concentration of quinidine the QRS complex may widen progressively. The widening is diffuse, affecting the entire QRS complex. Although

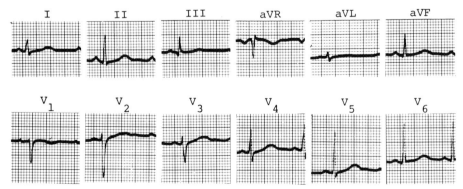

FIGURE 21–9. Prominent U waves due to quinidine. The patient is a 24-year-old woman who had paroxysmal ventricular tachycardia of unknown cause. The arrhythmia was controlled by quinidine, 200 mg given every 6 hours. The plasma level of quinidine was 2 mg/L. The prominent U waves are seen best in leads V_2 and V_3.

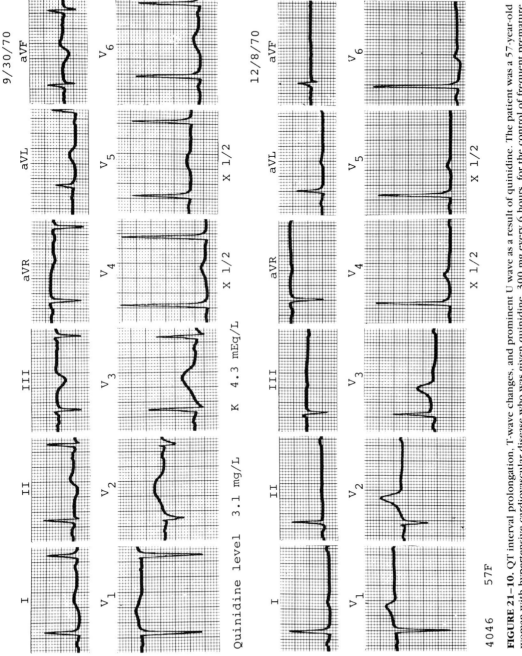

FIGURE 21–10. QT interval prolongation, T-wave changes, and prominent U wave as a result of quinidine. The patient was a 57-year-old woman with hypertensive cardiovascular disease who was given quinidine, 300 mg every 6 hours, for the control of frequent premature ventricular contractions. The tracing from 9-30-70 shows prolongation of the QT interval, even though the exact measurement is difficult because of the prominent U waves. There is T-wave inversion in leads II, III, and aVF. The ECG also suggests left ventricular hypertrophy. The tracing of 12-8-70 was recorded 4 days after quinidine was discontinued. The QT interval has shortened. The U waves are less prominent, and the T waves in the inferior leads have become essentially isoelectric.

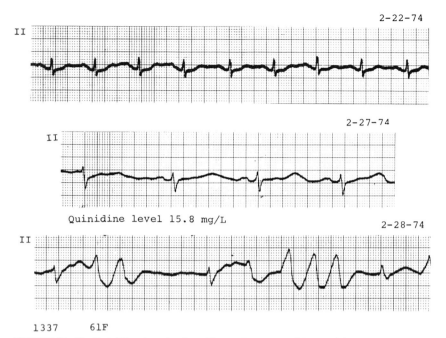

FIGURE 21-11. Quinidine intoxication. The patient was a 61-year-old woman with rheumatic mitral and aortic valve disease. The top strip (2-22-74) represents a baseline tracing. She was receiving digitalis but not quinidine. The P wave is notched with a duration of 0.13 second. The PR interval is 0.20 second, and the QRS duration is 0.06 second. On 2-27-74, she ingested an unknown amount of quinidine and was brought to the hospital in a comatose state. The ECG shows a slow sinus rate of 45 beats/min. The duration of the P wave is increased to 0.20 second, and the PR interval to 0.28 second. There is a diffuse widening of the QRS complex to 0.12 second, with prominent U waves. The quinidine plasma level was 15.8 mg/L. During the subsequent 24 hours, the patient developed ventricular arrhythmias. The strip recorded on 2-28-74 reveals frequent multifocal premature ventricular beats with couplet and triplet. The first and fourth QRS complexes are probably supraventricular in origin. No atrial activities can be identified. With supportive measures, she gradually returned to normal sinus rhythm, and the ECG on the following day was similar to the one recorded on 2-22-74.

this is generally considered a late change, careful measurements by Heissenbuttel and Bigger in 20 patients receiving quinidine revealed increased QRS duration in every patient.[38] The mean increase was 12 msec, and the plasma concentration of the drug was between 2 and 5 mg/L. A prolongation of the duration above 25 percent of the control value, however, usually is considered a toxic sign. Examples are given in Figures 21–11 and 21–12.

Prolongation of the PR interval represents a late and toxic change and occurs only when the serum concentration of quinidine reaches a very high level, usually above 10 mg/L (see Fig. 21–11). Indeed, the study of Josephson and associates using His bundle electrograms showed that therapeutic levels of quinidine (mean value of 4.6 mg/L) tended to shorten the AV nodal conduction time.[51]

Premature ventricular beats, paroxysmal ventricular tachycardia (Fig. 21–13), and ventricular fibrillation occasionally may result from the toxic effect of quinidine. Cases of sudden death have been reported.[108] Selzer and Wray documented 8 cases of quinidine syncope as a result of paroxysmal ventricular fibrillation.[93] Quinidine is one of the common causes of torsades de pointes, a rhythm between ventricular tachycardia and ventricular fibrillation.[52,100] This arrhythmia, paroxysmal ventricular tachycardia, and ventricular fibrillation, often develop while the quinidine blood level is in the therapeutic range and are the cause of syncope (see section on proarrhythmia).

In large doses, quinidine decreases the automaticity of the sinus node. Marked sinus bradycardia or sinus arrest may occur (see Fig. 21–11). SA block also has been reported. Rarely, atrial tachycardia may be the result of quinidine toxicity.

Considerable variation exists in ECG changes in response to the same plasma quin-

4/23/73

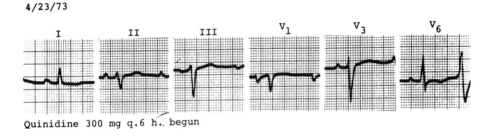

Quinidine 300 mg q.6 h. begun

4/25/73

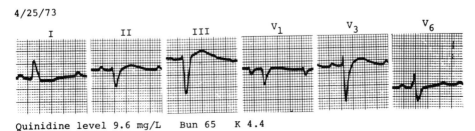

Quinidine level 9.6 mg/L   Bun 65   K 4.4

FIGURE 21–12. Marked widening of the QRS complexes in the presence of high plasma quinidine level. Quinidine, 300 mg every 6 hours, was given to this 65-year-old woman with idiopathic cardiomyopathy, congestive heart failure, and frequent premature ventricular beats on 4-23-73. The ECGs taken on 4-25-73 reveal diffuse widening of the QRS complexes. The QRS duration increases from 0.10 second (on 4-23-73) to 0.13 second. There is also a slight increase of the PR interval from 0.20 second to 0.22 second. The quinidine blood level on 4-25-73 was 9.6 mg/L.

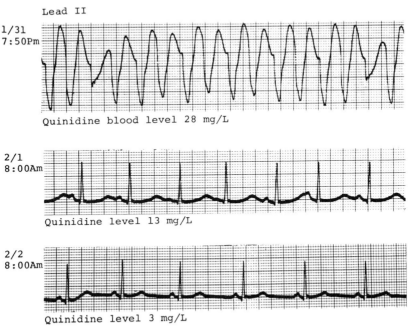

FIGURE 21–13. Quinidine intoxication. The patient was a 20-year-old woman who ingested 4 g of quinidine sulfate in a suicidal attempt. The first rhythm strip (7:50 P.M. 1-31-68) was recorded about 3 hours after the ingestion and shortly after she had a syncopal episode. The rhythm is probably paroxysmal ventricular tachycardia. The third and fifteenth QRS complexes are probably captured beats. The plasma quinidine level at that time was 28 mg/L. At 8 A.M. the following day, the quinidine level decreased to 13 mg/L. The rhythm is normal sinus rhythm with a PR interval of 0.18 second. The QRS duration is normal. There is a prolongation of the QT interval with prominent U waves. A premature atrial beat is present. The tracing recorded at 8 A.M. on 2-2-68 is within normal limits and the quinidine plasma level was 3 mg/L.

idine concentration in different individuals. Patients with advanced heart disease may be particularly sensitive to the drug. Both the quinidine plasma level and the ECG should be used to guide the therapy.

PROCAINAMIDE

The electrophysiological effects of procainamide are similar to those of quinidine except it is not anticholinergic.[42,50,112] The ECG changes that result from therapeutic doses of procainamide are usually less pronounced than are those from quinidine. The sinus rate is not affected in a predictable way. The P wave may be slightly widened and the PR interval slightly prolonged. The QRS duration is increased generally in proportion to the plasma level of the drug but usually does not exceed the normal range. The QTc interval is prolonged (Fig. 21–14) but usually to a lesser degree than the prolongation caused by quinidine. The T waves are lower in amplitude or notched. The U waves become more prominent.[55]

In high or toxic doses, procainamide may cause high-degree AV block, marked widening of the QRS duration (Fig. 21–15), ventricular premature beats, ventricular tachycardia, torsades de pointes, ventricular fibrillation, or asystole.[17,104,106] These manifestations are more frequently seen with intravenous than with oral administration of the drug.

DISOPYRAMIDE PHOSPHATE

Disopyramide phosphate has cardiac effects similar to those of quinidine.[6,22] ECG changes are infrequent when the usual therapeutic doses of the drug are given.[57] In patients with sinus node disease, however, marked depression of the sinus node function may occur.[58] Preexisting AV block or intraventricular conduction defect also may be aggravated by disopyramide.[96] Occasionally, there is QRS complex widening and QTc interval prolongation. Cases of ventricular tachycardia, ventricular fibrillation, and torsades de pointes have been reported in patients receiving the drugs, especially in those with QTc interval prolongation.[67,73,96]

A

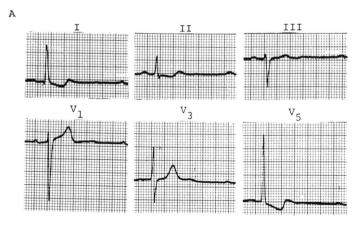

B

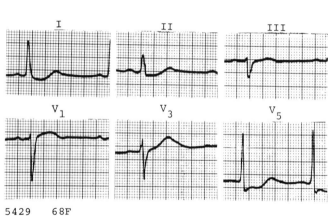

FIGURE 21–14. ECG effects of procainamide. (A) Tracing recorded when the patient was receiving digoxin and propranolol. It shows sinus bradycardia and left ventricular hypertrophy. (B) Tracing recorded when procainamide was given intravenously at a rate of 7 mg/min for the control of ventricular tachycardia. Note the increase in the duration of QRS complex, lowering of the T waves in leads V_1 and V_3, prolongation of the QT interval, and increase in the amplitude of the U wave in tracing B.

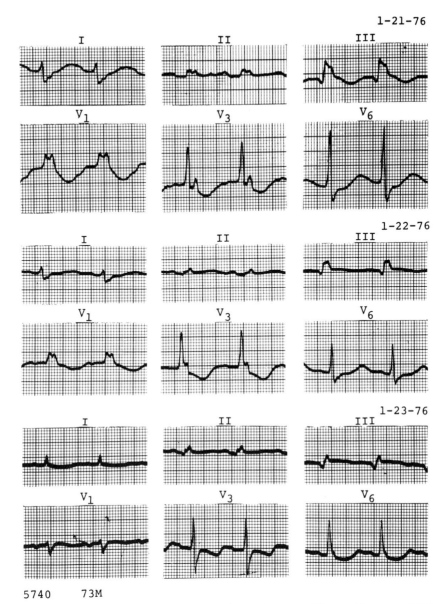

5740   73M

FIGURE 21–15. Procainamide intoxication. The patient was a 73-year-old man receiving procainamide, 6 mg/min intravenously, on 1-21-76. The tracing recorded on that date reveals first-degree AV block and marked prolongation of the QRS complex, with a duration of 0.20 second. The morphology of the QRS complexes resembles that of right bundle branch block. Additional primary ST and T-wave changes are present. On 1-22-76, after procainamide was discontinued, the PR interval and QRS duration have shortened. There are less ST and T-wave changes. The QT interval, which now can be measured more accurately, is prolonged. On the next day (1-23-76), the PR interval is within normal limits. The pattern of right bundle branch block is no longer present, and the QRS duration has decreased to 0.12 second. ST and T-wave abnormalities are still present, especially in the precordial leads.

LIDOCAINE

Lidocaine and other type IB antiarrhythmic agents differ from the type IA agents electrophysiologically in that they shorten the action potential duration of the His-Purkinje fibers and ventricular muscle.[112] The effective refractory period in relation to the action potential duration is, however, lengthened. The conduction velocity of the His-Purkinje and myocardium is not significantly affected. In therapeutic doses, lidocaine has no apprecia-

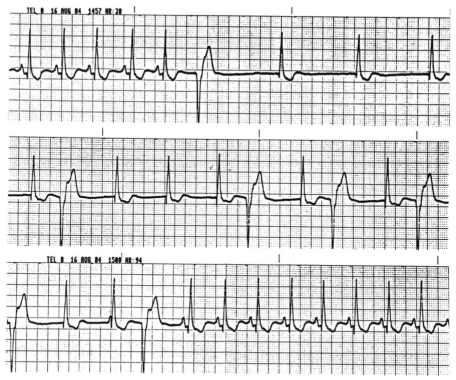

FIGURE 21–16. Sinus arrest due to lidocaine. The patient is a 56-year-old man who underwent aortocoronary artery bypass surgery. Lidocaine, 100 mg, was administered intravenously as a bolus postoperatively for the treatment of ventricular arrhythmias. The tracing was recorded 2 minutes after the injection. There is normal sinus rhythm followed by the appearance of sinus arrest with junctional escape rhythm and premature ventricular beats. Normal sinus rhythm resumed after about 3 minutes.

ble effect on the sinus rate but may slow the rate or cause sinus arrest when administered in very high doses. An unusual case of sinus arrest after the administration of an average therapeutic dose is illustrated in Figure 21–16. The drug slightly decreases the excitability of the atrial muscle. The automaticity of the ectopic atrial pacemakers may be suppressed.[63] The conduction velocities of the atrial muscle, AV node, His-Purkinje fibers, and ventricular muscle are not affected.[21] Lidocaine depresses the automaticity of the Purkinje fibers and the excitability of the ventricular muscle.

In clinical use, the administration of the drug is not associated with noticeable changes of the P wave, PR interval, QRS complex, QT interval, or T wave.[32]

TOCAINIDE AND MEXILETINE

Tocainide is an analogue of lidocaine and can be administered orally. Its electrophysiological properties are similar to those of lidocaine.[3] In therapeutic doses it has no effect on

the PR interval or QRS duration,[3,88,122] but the QT interval may be shortened.[62,122]

Mexiletine also is structurally similar to lidocaine. In therapeutic doses, it has no effect on the PR interval, QRS duration, or QT interval.[1,115]

PHENYTOIN

The usual therapeutic doses of phenytoin do not affect the sinus rates. Its effect on the atrial tissue is minimal. It may shorten the AV conduction time.[39] The automaticity of the Purkinje fibers is decreased.[11] In the ECG, Bigger and associates found that the PR interval tends to be shortened.[11] The QRS duration is not significantly altered, but the QTc interval is decreased in most patients. ST-segment or T-wave changes usually are not observed.[12] Rosen and colleagues found, however, that the PR interval may be increased.[83] Another study revealed no consistent ECG changes in patients treated with phenytoin, 0.3 g daily.[8]

In patients with severe heart disease, intravenous administration of therapeutic doses of phenytoin may produce bradycardia, AV block, asystole, or ventricular fibrillation.[107]

ENCAINIDE, FLECAINIDE, AND PROPAFENONE

Encainide, flecainide, and propafenone are class IC antiarrhythmic agents that differ from other sodium channel blockers in that they have more pronounced effects on intracardiac conduction but cause limited changes in the duration of repolarization.

The electrophysiological effects of chronic oral administration of encainide are significantly different from those of acute therapy. The difference is due to the fact that some of the metabolites of encainide are active and more potent than the parent compound.[5] Intravenous administration (not used clinically at this time) of encainide prolongs the HV interval with no significant changes in the AH interval, refractory periods of the atrium, AV node, or right ventricle. With chronic oral therapy, the AH interval (AV nodal conduction time) and atrial and ventricular refractory periods also are increased.[48] In patients with the

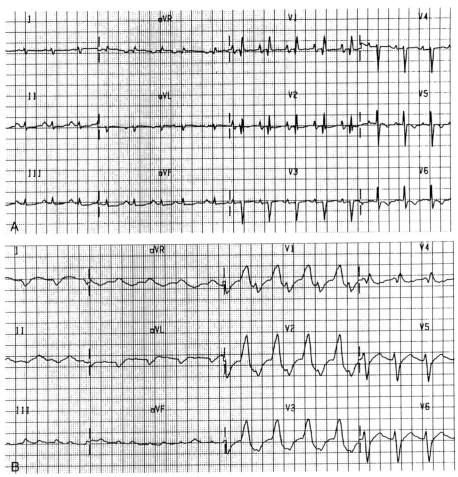

FIGURE 21–17. Encainide toxicity. The patient is a 53-year-old man with dilated cardiomyopathy, nonsustained ventricular tachycardia, and history of syncope. (A) Tracing obtained before encainide was administered. It shows sinus tachycardia, biatrial enlargement, low QRS voltage in the limb leads, right axis deviation, and right ventricular hypertrophy or incomplete right bundle branch block. The Q waves in leads V_1 through V_3 probably represent a pseudoinfarction pattern due to myocardial fibrosis. Nonspecific T-wave abnormalities are present. (B) Tracing recorded 4 days after encainide therapy was begun, at first at the dosage of 25 mg three times daily for 3 days, followed by 50 mg three times daily for 1 day when the ECG was obtained. Compared with the baseline tracing, the PR interval has prolonged from 0.19 to 0.32 second. The QRS complexes have widened from 0.09 to 0.25 second. Both the PR interval and QRS duration returned to the baseline value after the drug was discontinued.

Wolff-Parkinson-White (WPW) syndrome, the refractory period of the accessory pathway also is increased.[79]

In the ECG, the sinus rate is unaffected. The PR interval and QRS duration are prolonged. The QT interval may or may not be appreciably increased.[48,65] The QRS duration may be excessively prolonged even though the dosage of encainide given may be within the recommended therapeutic range. An example is given in Figure 21–17.

The basic and clinical electrophysiological effects of flecainide are similar to those of encainide except it has a greater effect on ventricular repolarization.[28] Unlike encainide, its metabolites are inactive.[65] In the ECG, flecainide has little effect on the sinus rate except in patients with sinus node dysfunction.[114] The PR interval and QRS duration are prolonged. The QT interval is increased slightly, but this increase may be due to prolongation of the QRS duration.[26,40,114] In patients with the WPW syndrome, flecainide also depresses the conduction in the accessory pathway both antegrade and retrograde.

The electrophysiological effects of propafenone are similar to the other class IC agents except it also has beta-adrenergic blocking properties.[101] It may cause sinus node slowing. The PR interval and QRS duration are increased. The QT interval may be prolonged.[19,101] The effective refractory period of the accessory pathway in patients with the WPW syndrome is increased, and, therefore, its conduction capacity may be decreased.[13]

All class IC antiarrhythmic agents, as in the case of class IA agents, may be proarrhythmic. Serious ventricular arrhythmias may occur as a result of their use.

PROPRANOLOL AND OTHER BETA-ADRENERGIC BLOCKING AGENTS

Many beta-adrenergic blocking agents are available for clinical use. Because their electrophysiological actions are similar, only one of them, propranolol, is discussed here. Other than beta-adrenergic blockade, propranolol also has a direct quinidine-like effect on the heart. The drug depresses the automaticity of the SA node and Purkinje fibers. It prolongs the AV conduction time and the effective refractory period of the AV node.[9]

Therapeutic doses of propanolol given orally decrease the sinus rate but otherwise have no significant effect on the P, QRS, T, and U waves or the PR interval.[30] The QTc interval is sometimes shortened. In patients with atrial tachyarrhythmias, especially atrial fibrillation and atrial flutter, it decreases the ventricular rate.[25] Propranolol may cause various degrees of AV block in patients with preexisting disease of the AV conduction system or in those receiving digitalis.

Intravenous administration of propranolol was reported to produce AV block, SA block, shortening of the QTc interval, and occasionally slight peaking and larger amplitude of the T wave.[92,105]

AMIODARONE

The electrophysiological effects of amiodarone consist of depression of the sinus node automaticity and prolongation of the conduction time and refractory period of the atrium, AV node, His-Purkinje system, and ventricle.[90,96] In patients with the WPW syndrome, the administration of amiodarone prolongs the refractory period of the accessory pathway, being more consistently in the antegrade than in the retrograde direction.[118,123]

Sinus bradycardia is commonly seen in the ECGs of patients receiving amiodarone, and occasional cases of SA block and sinus arrest have been described.[37,66,84,111] The PR interval may be prolonged.[90,118] An increase in the QRS duration was noted by some investigators.[90] The QTc interval is often lengthened.[35,84,90] The T waves may become wider and notched and the U waves prominent.[85] These repolarization changes usually begin to appear after the fourth day of treatment, become pronounced in 7 to 10 days, and persist for 15 to 21 days after the drug is discontinued.[85] In a study by Mitchell and co-workers, it was found that the effect of amiodarone on the sinus node automaticity and atrial and AV nodal conduction reached its maximum within 2 weeks.[71] Its effect on ventricular repolarization (and therefore on the QTc interval) and ventricular refractory periods, however, did not become maximal until 10 weeks after oral administration of the drug was begun.

BRETYLIUM

After intravenous administration of bretylium, there is a brief initial sympathomimetic phase of action followed by adrenergic neuronal blockade. It lengthens the duration of the action potential and refractory periods of the atrial, ventricular, and Purkinje fibers. In the ECG, bretylium causes an initial transient increase in the heart rate followed by a later decrease. The QRS duration and QTc interval are unchanged.[24]

SOTALOL

Sotalol is not available for clinical use in the United States. It differs from the other class III antiarrhythmic agents in that it also has beta-adrenergic blocking effects.

In the ECG, sotalol decreases the heart rate but causes no significant changes in the PR interval and QRS duration. The QTc interval is prolonged.[76,87]

CALCIUM-CHANNEL BLOCKING AGENTS

Verapamil, Diltiazem, Nifedipine

The electrophysiological effects of the calcium-channel blocking agents are mainly on the AV node. The effects, however, vary among the different agents. Verapamil and diltiazem slow AV conduction in both antegrade and retrograde directions. Both drugs cause similar degree of lengthening of the AH interval.[70] In contrast, nifedipine either has no effect on, or may even facilitate, AV nodal conduction.[70] The expected depressant effect of the drug is probably counterbalanced by the sympathetic reflexes activated by its more potent hypotensive actions.[58] The refractory period of the AV node is lengthened by both verapamil and diltiazem but to a greater degree by the former. It is shortened by nifedipine. These differences in the electrophysiological effects on the AV node account for the greater effectiveness of verapamil in the termination of paroxysmal supraventricular tachycardia and the slowing of the ventricular response in atrial flutter and atrial fibrillation.

In patients with normal sinus nodes, the calcium-channel blockers do not have significant direct effect on its automaticity.[70] In patients with sinus node disease, however, verapamil and diltiazem may cause severe sinus bradycardia and occasionally sinus arrest.[14,16] The calcium-channel blocking agents have no effect on infranodal conduction (as indicated by the HV interval) or the effective refractory period of the atria, ventricles, or the His-Purkinje system.[97] The effects of these drugs on the accessory pathway in patients with the WPW syndrome are variable.[102] In some patients, verapamil may shorten the antegrade effective refractory period of the accessory pathway and increase the ventricular response.[33]

In the 12-lead ECG, the effect of the administration of calcium-channel blockers on the sinus rate varies depending on the balance between the direct action of the drugs and the antagonistic sympathetic reflex secondary to their hypotensive action. The PR interval is lengthened by verapamil and diltiazem. Rarely, second- and third-degree AV blocks may develop. The PR interval is unchanged with nifedipine. The calcium-channel blocking agents have no effect on the QRS duration or QTc interval.[97]

ADENOSINE AND ADENOSINE TRIPHOSPHATE

Both adenosine and adenosine triphosphate (ATP) depress the automaticity of the sinus node and AV nodal conduction.[23,27] The AV conduction delay is caused by a prolongation of the atrial-to-His bundle (AH) interval without any demonstrable effect on the His-to-ventricle (HV) conduction time. After rapid bolus injection of the drugs, AV block of various degrees usually occurs within 20 seconds and lasts for about 10 to 20 seconds.[23,27] The exact mechanism by which the AV conduction is delayed is not fully understood, but it has been demonstrated in humans that the action is not due to vagal activation.[23,27]

Adenosine and ATP have been used for the termination of paroxysmal AV nodal reentrant tachycardia and orthodromic AV reentrant tachycardia using an accessory pathway.[7,95] The incidence of transient second-degree AV block and various supraventricular and ventricular arrhythmias after the termination of the paroxysmal reentrant tachycardia is high.[7]

SUMMARY OF EFFECTS OF DIGITALIS AND ANTIARRHYTHMIC AGENTS ON THE ELECTROCARDIOGRAM

See Table 21–2.

PROARRHYTHMIC EFFECTS OF ANTIARRHYTHMIC DRUGS

The administration of antiarrhythmic agents may, paradoxically, aggravate the arrhythmias that are being treated or cause new rhythm disorders. Such effect, which is often called *proarrhythmia,* usually occurs when the dosage of the drugs used is in the therapeutic range.[113] Its incidence varies with different agents. It usually appears within a few hours or a few days after the initiation of the treatment.[113] Proarrhythmia is described as *pri-*

TABLE 21–2. Effects of Antiarrhythmic Agents and Digitalis on the Electrocardiogram

Agent	Sinus Rate	PR Interval	QRS Duration	QTc Interval	Conduction by Accessory Pathway in WPW Syndrome
Digitalis	↓	0 or ↑	0	↓	0 or ↑
Quinidine	0 or ↑	↓, 0, or ↑	↑	↑↑	↓
Procainamide	0	0 or ↑	↑	↑	↓
Disopyramide	0	0	↑	↑	↓
Lidocaine	0	0	0	0	0
Tocainide	0	0	0	0	0
Mexiletine	0	0	0	0	0
Phenytoin	0	0	0	↓	0
Encainide	0	↑	↑↑	↑	↓
Flecainide	0	↑	↑↑	↑	↓
Propranolol	↓	0 or ↑	0	0 or ↓	0
Amiodarone	↓	0 or ↑	↑	↑↑	↓
Bretylium	0 or ↓	0	0	0	0
Verapamil	↓	↑	0	0	0 or ↑
Diltiazem	↓	↑	0	0	0
Adenosine	↓	↑	0		

↑ = increase; ↓ = decrease; WPW = Wolff-Parkinson-White.

mary when it is unrelated to any identifiable arrhythmogenic factor other than the underlying arrhythmia or heart disease. It is called *secondary* when its occurrence requires the presence of an adjunctive factor, such as high plasma concentration of the antiarrhythmic drug, concomitant medications, electrolyte disturbances, or myocardial ischemia.[45] Aggravation of the preexisting arrhythmias may be manifested by an increase in the duration or frequency of the arrhythmia. The rate of the tachycardia being treated may be increased.[45,123] New arrhythmias may develop in the form of bradycardia due to sinus node dysfunction or AV block. The drugs also may provoke the development of tachyarrhythmia, either supraventricular or ventricular.

Ventricular proarrhythmia has received the most attention because of its potential serious consequences. Aggravation of preexisting ventricular ectopies is often difficult to recognize because of the marked variation of the number and complexity of premature ventricular beats in patients who are not receiving any antiarrhythmic drugs. Velebit and associates suggested the following changes as evidence of drug-induced aggravation of arrhythmia[113]:

1. A fourfold increase in the hourly frequency of premature ventricular beats compared with the control period
2. A tenfold increase in the hourly frequency of couplets or ventricular tachycardia compared with the control period

3. The first occurrence of sustained ventricular tachycardia not present during control studies

Some investigators question the accuracy of these criteria especially when the premature ventricular ectopic beats are infrequent during the control period and refinement of the criteria has been proposed.[74] In patients who are treated for ventricular tachycardia, a 10 percent shortening of the tachycardia cycle length also is considered evidence of aggravation of the arrhythmia.[123]

New ventricular arrhythmias that may develop after the administration of antiarrhythmic agents include sustained ventricular tachycardia, polymorphic ventricular tachycardia, torsades de pointes, and ventricular fibrillation.[45,123] Figures 18–31 through 18–33 in Chapter 18 are examples of quinidine-induced torsades de pointes, which is probably the most generally recognized form of drug-induced ventricular tachyarrhythmia. As was stated previously, no correlation has been established between the development of these arrhythmias and the dosage or serum concentrations of the drugs. Although the QT interval is often prolonged in these patients, there is no critical value of the QT interval that can be related to the development of the arrhythmias. The reported incidence of proarrhythmia ranges from 3.4 to 16.4 percent depending to a large extent on the antiarrhythmic agents used and the type of proarrhythmia included in the study.[74,103,113] The incidence of ventricular proarrhythmia is highest with the class IC drugs (encainide, flecainide, propafenone) and low with class IB drugs (tocainide, mexiletine).[44,45,103,113,123] Although the percentage of patients who develop proarrhythmic events while receiving class IA drugs (quinidine, procainamide, disopyramide) is lower than that due to the class IC drugs, the total number of cases of proarrhythmia is larger with the former because of the more frequent use of these drugs. This is especially true with quinidine.

PSYCHOTROPIC DRUGS (PHENOTHIAZINES, TRICYCLIC ANTIDEPRESSANTS, LITHIUM)

The electrophysiological effects of the phenothiazines are similar to those of quinidine. The most common ECG changes caused by the phenothiazines include widening, flattening,

notching, or inversion of the T wave; prolongation of the QTc interval; and prominence of the U wave (Fig. 21–18).[46,119] These repolarization abnormalities are seen more frequently in patients receiving thioridazine (Mellaril) than in those receiving chlorpromazine (Thorazine) or, even less, trifluoperazine (Stelazine).[4] The changes are dose-related. With thioridazine, repolarization abnormalities are usually not seen when the dosage is less than 100 mg/day. Such abnormalities are present in about half of the patients when the dosage level is between 100 and 300 mg/day and in about three fourths when the dosage is above 300 mg/day.[46] The effects usually appear within 1 or 2 days after the beginning of therapy and reach their maximum in 4 or 5 days. They are seen more often in women than in men.[46] Although intraventricular conduction defects may be seen, they are not common. Supraventricular and ventricular tachycardia may be observed in pa-

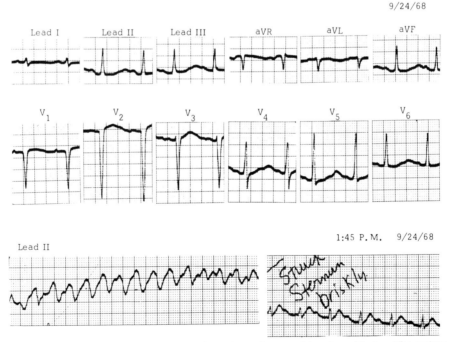

FIGURE 21–18. ECG changes and ventricular tachycardia caused by phenothiazine. The patient was a 36-year-old woman who was treated with Mellaril, 250 mg four times daily; Stelazine, 4 times daily; Thorazine, 300 mg at bedtime; and Cogentin, 1 mg twice daily. The 12-lead ECG was recorded after she had a syncope episode. The PR interval and QRS duration are within normal limits. QS deflections are present in leads V₁ and V₂. There is a prolongation of the QTc interval with prominent U waves in most of the leads, especially in leads II, III, aVF, and V₄ through V₆. Subsequently, she developed many episodes of ventricular tachycardia and ventricular fibrillation. One of the episodes of ventricular tachycardia is illustrated and was converted to sinus rhythm by thumping of the chest. Ventricular tachycardia and fibrillation recurred, however, and she died on the same date. At autopsy, routine gross and microscopic examinations of the heart revealed no abnormality. (Reproduced from Fowler NO, McCall D, Chou TC, et al: Electrocardiographic changes and cardiac arrhythmias in patients receiving psychotropic drugs. Am J Cardiol 37:223, 1976, by permission of Dun-Donnelley Publishing Corp.)

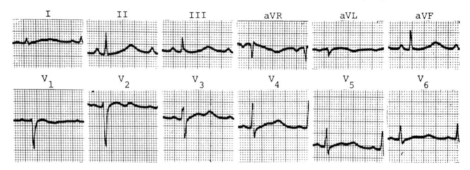

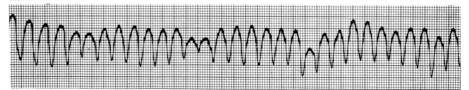

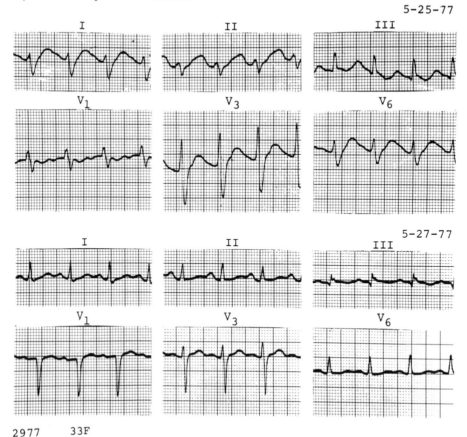

FIGURE 21-19. Phenothiazine overdose. The patient was a 40-year-old woman who took more than 2 g of Mellaril 3 hours before the 12-lead ECG was recorded. The tracing shows prominent U waves. The QT interval is prolonged, but the exact measurement is difficult to obtain because of the superimposed U wave. The patient developed multiple episodes of ventricular tachycardia during the next 2 days. One of the episodes is illustrated.

2977   33F

FIGURE 21-20. Tricyclic antidepressant and phenothiazine overdose. The patient was a 33-year-old woman who took 85 tablets of Triavil (containing amitriptyline and perphenazine) a few hours before the tracing of 5-25-77 was recorded. The tracing shows sinus tachycardia. The P waves are difficult to identify but can be seen best in lead I. There is intraventricular conduction defect, with widening of the QRS complex to 0.16 second. The frontal plane QRS axis is displaced to the right. Two days later (5-27-77), the tracing shows only minimal nonspecific ST and T-wave changes. The QRS duration is now 0.10 second.

tients who take high doses of the drug.[29] Ventricular tachycardia and fibrillation were responsible for sudden death in some of the these patients.[2,43,47]

The ECG changes produced by the tricyclic antidepressants are generally similar to those caused by the phenothiazines. They occur in about 20 percent of patients who take therapeutic doses of the drug.[20] Prolongation of the QTc interval, displacement of the ST segment, T-wave abnormalities, QRS widening, and supraventricular and ventricular tachycardias may all be observed.[29,31,64,70] One study, however, revealed that increased heart rate, lengthening of the PR interval, and flattening of T waves are the only significant changes associated with the administration of the drug.[14] Other than the heart rate, the other findings returned to normal when the therapy was continued.

In overdose of the psychotropic drugs, cardiac arrhythmias are common (Figs. 21–18 through 21–21). These include sinus tachycardia, atrial fibrillation, ventricular tachycardia, ventricular fibrillation, AV block, and bizarre QRS complexes.[20,72,120] In my experience, abnormal widening of the QRS complex is seen more commonly with tricyclic drug intoxication (see Fig. 21–21). Niemann and associates found that sinus tachycardia, pro-

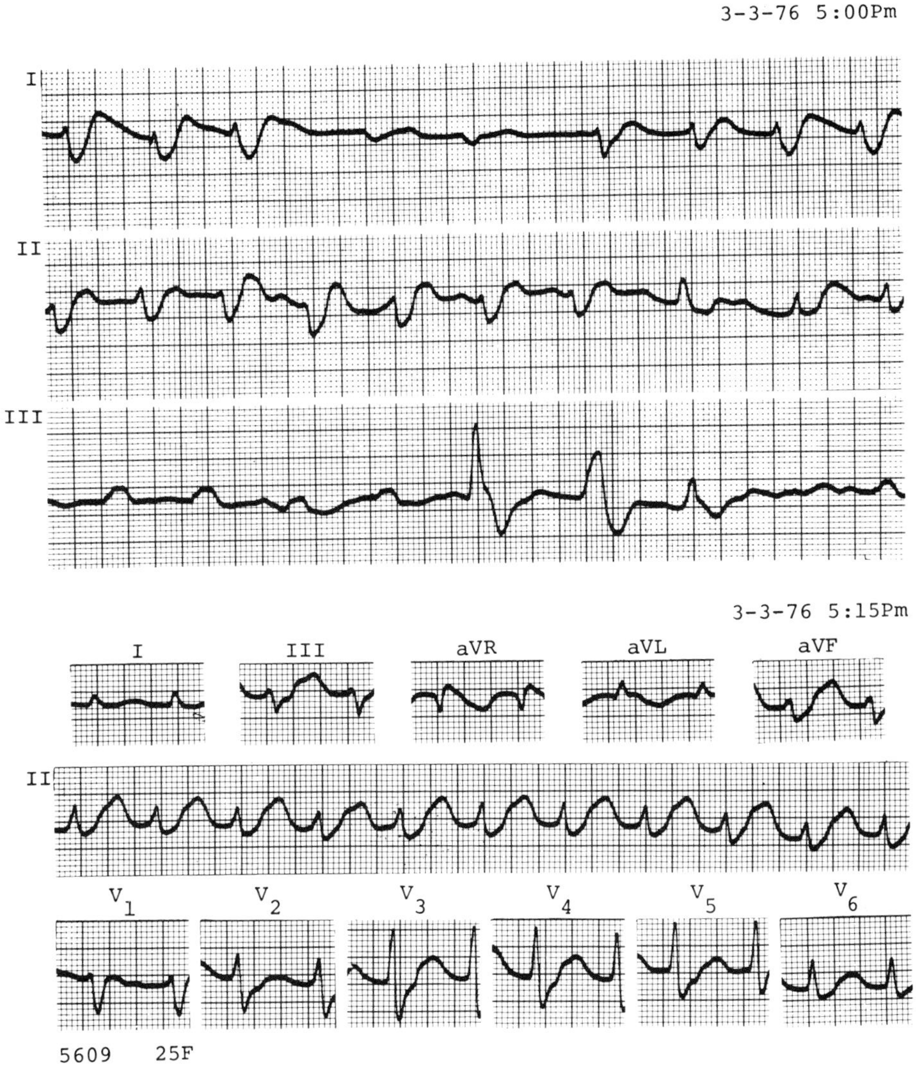
3-3-76 5:00Pm
I
II
III
3-3-76 5:15Pm
I
III
aVR
aVL
aVF
II
V1
V2
V3
V4
V5
V6
5609 25F

FIGURE 21–21. Tricyclic antidepressant overdose. The patient was a 25-year-old woman who took 500 mg of Tofranil (imipramine) 4 hours before the 5 P.M. tracing was recorded. The three standard limb leads show wide QRS complexes of varying morphology. The exact rhythm cannot be determined. She had severe hypotension at this time. Fifteen minutes later, the tracing shows probable supraventricular rhythm with intraventricular conduction defect.

longed QRS duration, prolonged QTc interval, and rightward shift of the terminal 40-msec QRS vector are useful ECG signs of tricyclic antidepressant cardiotoxicity.[76] Their absence practically ruled out the possibility of overdose of the drug.

The most common ECG changes associated with the administration of therapeutic dosage of lithium carbonate are the T-wave abnormalities.[69,109] Flattening or occasional inversion of the T wave may be seen in 20 to 30 percent of the patients who take these drugs.[69] The T-wave changes are reversible within 2 weeks after the drug is discontinued. Partial displacement of intracellular potassium by lithium is believed to be the mechanism by which the repolarization abnormalities develop. The QT interval is not prolonged. Ischemic ST-segment depression is not observed during exercise.[110]

Sinus node dysfunction, including marked sinus bradycardia, sinus pauses, and SA block, may be caused by lithium.[34,69,81,109,117,121] It is uncommon, however. In 97 consecutive patients on lithium therapy examined by Hagman and colleagues, sinus node depression possibly caused by the drug was found in only 2.[34] Both patients had no symptoms. Occasional cases of premature ventricular beats and first-degree AV block also have been attributed to the drug, but many of them are not well documented.

In patients with lithium intoxication, sinus node dysfunction and isolated cases of various supraventricular and ventricular tachyarrhythmias, AV and intraventricular conduction defects, and QT prolongation have been described.[69]

REFERENCES

1. Abinader EG, Cooper M: Use in control of chronic drug-resistant ventricular arrhythmia. JAMA 242:337, 1979
2. Alexander CS, Nini A: Cardiovascular complications in young patients taking psychotropic drugs. Am Heart J 78:757, 1969
3. Anderson JL, Manson JW, Winkle RA, et al: Clinical electrophysiologic effects of tocainide. Circulation 57:685, 1978
4. Banta TA, St Jean A: The effect of phenothiazines on the electrocardiogram. Can Med Assoc J 91:537, 1964
5. Barbey JT, Thompson KA, Echt DS, et al: Antiarrhythmic activity, electrocardiographic effects and pharmacokinetics of the encainide metabolites 0-desmethyl encainide and 3-methoxy-0-desmethyl encainide in man. Circulation 77:380, 1988
6. Blefeler B, Castellanos A, Wells DE, et al: Electrophysiologic effects of the antiarrhythmic agent disopyramide phosphate. Am J Cardiol 35:282, 1975
7. Belhassen B, Glick A, Laniado S: Comparative clinical and electrophysiologic effects of adenosine triphosphate and verapamil on paroxysmal reciprocating junctional tachycardia. Circulation 77:795, 1988
8. Beller GA, Smith TW, Abelmann WH, et al: Digitalis intoxication: A prospective clinical study with serum level correlations. N Engl J Med 284:989, 1971
9. Berkowitz WD, Wit AL, Lau SH, et al: Effects of propranolol on cardiac conduction. Circulation 40:855, 1969
10. Bernstein H, Gold H, Lang TW, et al: Sodium diphenylhydantoin in the treatment of recurrent cardiac arrhythmias. JAMA 191:695, 1965
11. Bigger JT, Bassett AL, Hoffmann BF: Electrophysiological effects of diphenylhydantoin on canine Purkinje fibers. Circ Res 22:221, 1968
12. Bigger JT, Schmidt DH, Kutt H: Relationship between the plasma level of diphenylhydantoin sodium and its cardiac antiarrhythmic effects. Circulation 38:363, 1968
13. Breithardt G, Borggrefe M, Wiebringhaus E, Seipel L: Effect of propafenone in the Wolff-Parkinson-White syndrome: Electrophysiologic findings and long-term follow-up. Am J Cardiol 54:29, 1984
14. Breithardt G, Seipel L, Wiebringhaus E, et al: Effects of verapamil on sinus node function in man. Eur J Cardiol 8:379, 1978
15. Burckhardt D, Raeder E, Muller V, et al: Cardiovascular effects of tricyclic and tetracyclic antidepressants. JAMA 239:213, 1978
16. Carrasco HA, Fuenmayor A, Barboza JS, et al: Effect of verapamil on normal sino-atrial node function and on sick sinus syndrome. Am Heart J 96:760, 1978
17. Castellanos A, Salhanick L: Electrocardiographic patterns of procaine amide toxicity. Am J Med Sci 253:52, 1967
18. Cheng TO, Sutton GC, Swisher WP, et al: Effect of quinidine on the ventricular complex of the electrocardiogram with special reference to the duration of the Q-T interval. Am Heart J 51:417, 1956
19. Chilson DA, Heger JJ, Zipes DP, et al: Electrophysiologic effects and clinical efficacy of oral propafenone therapy in patients with ventricular tachycardia. J Am Coll Cardiol 5:1407, 1985
20. Crane GE: Cardiac toxicity and psychotropic drugs. Dis Nerv Syst 31:534, 1970
21. Damata AN, Lau SH: Clinical value of the electrogram of the conduction system. Prog Cardiovasc Dis 13:119, 1970
22. Danilo P, Rosen MR: Cardiac effects of disopyramide. Am Heart J 92:532, 1976
23. DiMarco JP, Sellers D, Berne RM, et al: Adenosine: Electrophysiologic effects and therapeutic use for terminating paroxysmal supraventricular tachycardia. Circulation 68:1254, 1983
24. Duff HJ, Roden DM, Yacobi A, et al: Bretylium: Relations between plasma concentrations and pharmacologic actions in high-frequency ventricular arrhythmias. Am J Cardiol 55:395, 1985
25. Epstein SE, Braunwald E: Beta-adrenergic receptor blocking drugs: Mechanism of action and clinical applications. N Engl J Med 275:1175, 1966
26. Estes NAM, Garan H, Ruskin JN: Electrophysiologic properties of flecainide acetate. Am J Cardiol 53:26B, 1984
27. Favale S, DiBiase M, Rizzo U, et al: Effect of adenosine and adenosine-5'-triphosphate on atrioventric-

ular conduction in patients. J Am Coll Cardiol 5:1212, 1985

28. Flecainide-Quinidine Research Group: Flecainide versus quinidine treatment of chronic ventricular arrhythmias. Circulation 67:1117, 1983

29. Fowler NO, McCall D, Chou TC, et al: Electrocardiographic changes and cardiac arrhythmias in patients receiving psychotropic drugs. Am J Cardiol 37:223, 1976

30. Gettes LS, Surawicz B: Long-term prevention of paroxysmal arrhythmias with propranolol therapy. Am J Med Sci 254:257, 1967

31. Giardina E, Bigger JT, Glassman AH, et al: The electrocardiographic and antiarrhythmic effects of imipramine hydrochloride at therapeutic plasma concentrations. Circulation 60:1045, 1979

32. Grossman JI, Cooper JA, Frieden J: Cardiovascular effects of infusion of lidocaine on patients with heart disease. Am J Cardiol 24:191, 1969

33. Gulamhusein S, Ko P, Carruthers SG, et al: Acceleration of the ventricular response during atrial fibrillation in the Wolff-Parkinson-White syndrome after verapamil. Circulation 65:348, 1982

34. Hagman A, Arnman K, Ryden L: Syncope caused by lithium treatment: Report of two cases and a prospective investigation of the prevalence of lithium-induced sinus node dysfunction. Acta Med Scand 208:467, 1979

35. Harris L, McKenna WJ, Rowland E, et al: Side effects of long-term amiodarone therapy. Circulation 67:45, 1983

36. Harrison DC: Antiarrhythmic drug classification: New science and practical applications. Am J Cardiol 56:185, 1985

37. Heger JJ, Prystowsky EN, Jackman WM, et al: Amiodarone: Clinical efficacy and electrophysiology during long-term therapy for recurrent ventricular tachycardia or ventricular fibrillation. N Engl J Med 305:539, 1981

38. Heissenbuttel RH, Bigger JT: The effect of oral quinidine on intraventricular conduction in man: Correlation of plasma quinidine with changes in QRS duration. Am Heart J 80:453, 1970

39. Helfant RH, Scherlag BJ, Damato AN: The electrophysiological properties of diphenylhydantoin sodium as compared to procaine amide in the normal and digitalis intoxicated heart. Circulation 36:108, 1967

40. Hellestrand KJ, Bexton RS, Nathan AW, et al: Acute electrophysiological effects of flecainide acetate on cardiac conduction and refractoriness in man. Br Heart J 48:140, 1982

41. Hoffman BF: Effects of digitalis on electrical activity of cardiac fibers. In Fisch C, Surawicz R (eds): Digitalis. New York, Grune & Stratton, 1969

42. Hoffman BF, Rosen MR, Wit AL: Electrophysiology and pharmacology of cardiac arrhythmias. VII. Cardiac effects of quinidine and procaine amide. Am Heart J 89:804, 1975

43. Hollister LE, Kosek JC: Sudden death during treatment with phenothiazine derivatives. JAMA 192:93, 1965

44. Horowitz LN: Drugs and proarrhythmia. In Zipes DP, Rowlands DJ (eds): Progress in Cardiology. Philadelphia, Lea & Febiger, 1988; p 109

45. Horowitz LN, Zipes DP, Bigger JT, et al: Proarrhythmia, arrhythmogenesis or aggravation of arrhythmia: A status report, 1987. Am J Cardiol 59:54E, 1987

46. Huston JR, Bell GE: The effect of thiordiazine hy-

drochloride and chlopromazine on the electrocardiogram. JAMA 198:134, 1966

47. Irons GV, Orgain ES: Digitalis-induced arrhythmias and their management. Prog Cardiovasc Dis 8:539, 1966

48. Jackman WM, Zipes DP, Naccarelli GV, et al: Electrophysiology of oral encainide. Am J Cardiol 49:1270, 1982

49. Jacob EI, Hope RR: Prolongation of the Q-T interval in lithium toxicity. J Electrocardiol 12:117, 1979

50. Josephson MD, Caracta AR, Jau SH, et al: Electrophysiological evaluation of disopyramide in man. Am Heart J 86:721, 1973

51. Josephson M, Seides S, Batsford W, et al: The electrophysiological effects of intramuscular quinidine on the atrioventricular conducting system in man. Am Heart J 87:55, 1974

52. Kawai C, Hultgren HN: The effect of digitalis upon the exercise electrocardiogram. Am Heart J 68:409, 1964

53. Kawai C, Konishi T, Matsuyama E, et al: Comparative effects of three calcium antagonists, diltiazem, verapamil and nifedipine, on the sinoatrial and atrioventricular nodes. Circulation 63:1035, 1981

54. Kay GN, Plumb VJ, Arciniegas JG, et al: Torsade de pointes: The long-short initiating sequence and other clinical features. Observations in 32 patients. J Am Coll Cardiol 2:806, 1983

55. Kayden HT, Brodie BB, Steele JM: Procaine amide: A review. Circulation 15:118, 1957

56. Koch-Weser J: Mechanism of digitalis action on the heart. N Engl J Med 277:188, 1967

57. Koch-Weser J: Drug therapy: Disopyramide. N Engl J Med 300:957, 1979

58. LaBarre A, Strauss HC, Scheinman MM, et al: Electrophysiologic effects of disopyramide phosphate on sinus node function in patients with sinus node dysfunction. Circulation 59:226, 1979

59. Lal R, Chapman PD, Naccarelli GV, et al: Short- and long-term experience with flecainide acetate in the management of refractory life-threatening ventricular arrhythmias. J Am Coll Cardiol 6:772, 1985

60. Levine HD, Angelakos ET: Late peaking of the T wave as a digitalis effect. Am Heart J 68:320, 1964

61. Lown B, Wyatt NF, Levine HD: Paroxysmal atrial tachycardia with block. Circulation 21:129, 1960

62. Maloney JD, Nissen RG, McColgan JM: Open clinical studies at a referral center: Chronic maintenance tocainide therapy in patients with recurrent sustained ventricular tachycardia refractory to conventional antiarrhythmic agents. Am Heart J 100:1023, 1980

63. Mandel WJ, Bigger JT: Effect of lidocaine on sinoatrial node and atrial fibers. Am J Cardiol 25:113, 1970

64. Marshall JB, Forker AD: Cardiovascular effects of tricyclic antidepressant drugs: Therapeutic usage, overdose, and management of complications. Am Heart J 103:401, 1982

65. Mason JW: Basic and clinical cardiac electrophysiology of encainide. Am J Cardiol 58:18C, 1986

66. McGovern B, Garan H, Ruskin JN: Sinus arrest during treatment with amiodarone. Br Med J 284:160, 1982

67. Meltzer RS, Robert EW, McMorrow M, et al: Atypical ventricular tachycardia as a manifestation of disopyramide toxicity. Am J Cardiol 42:1049, 1978

68. Minardo JD, Heger JJ, Miles WM, et al: Clinical characteristics of patients with ventricular fibrillation

during antiarrhythmic drug therapy. N Engl J Med 319:257, 1988

69. Mitchell JE, MacKenzie TB: Cardiac effects of lithium therapy in man: A review. J Clin Psychiatry 43:47, 1982

70. Mitchell LB, Schroeder JS, Mason JW: Comparative clinical electrophysiologic effects of diltiazem, verapamil and nifedipine: A review. Am J Cardiol 49:629, 1982

71. Mitchell LB, Wyse G, Gillis AM, et al: Electropharmacology of amiodarone therapy initiation: Time courses of onset of electrophysiologic and antiarrhythmic effects. Circulation 80:34, 1989

72. Moir DC: Annotations: Tricyclic antidepressants and cardiac disease. Am Heart J 86:841, 1973

73. Morady F, Scheinman MM, Desai J: Disopyramide. Ann Intern Med 96:337, 1982

74. Morganroth J: Risk factors for the development of proarrhythmic events. Am J Cardiol 59:32E, 1987

75. Morris SN, Zipes DP: His bundle electrocardiography during bidirectional tachycardia. Circulation 48:32, 1973

76. Nademanee K, Feld G, Hendrickson J, et al: Electrophysiologic and antiarrhythmic effects of sotalol in patients with life-threatening ventricular tachyarrhythmias. Circulation 72:555, 1985

77. Niemann JT, Bessen HA, Rothstein RJ, et al: Electrocardiographic criteria for tricyclic antidepressant cardiotoxicity. Am J Cardiol 57:1154, 1986

78. Opie LH: Antiarrhythmic agents. Lancet 1:861, 1980

79. Pick A, Dominguez P: Nonparoxysmal A-V nodal tachycardia. Circulation 16:1022, 1957

80. Prystowsky EN, Klein GJ, Rinkenberger, et al: Clinical efficacy and electrophysiologic effects of encainide in patients with Wolff-Parkinson-White syndrome. Circulation 69:278, 1984

81. Reiter MJ, Higgins ST, Payne AG, et al: Effects of quinidine versus procainamide on the QT interval. Am J Cardiol 58:512, 1986

82. Roose SP, Nurnberger JI, Dunner DL, et al: Cardiac sinus node dysfunction during lithium treatment. Am J Psychiatry 136:804, 1979

83. Rosen M, Lisak R, Rubin IL: Diphenylhydantoin in cardiac arrhythmias. Am J Cardiol 20:674, 1967

84. Rosenbaum MB, Chiale PA, Halpern MS, et al: Clinical efficacy of amiodarone as an antiarrhythmic agent. Am J Cardiol 38:934, 1976

85. Rosenbaum MB, Chiale PA, Ryba D, et al: Control of tachyarrhythmias associated with Wolff-Parkinson-White syndrome by amiodarone hydrochloride. Am J Cardiol 34:215, 1974

86. Rosenbaum MB, Elizari MV, Lazzari JO: Mechanism of bidirectional tachycardia. Am Heart J 78:4, 1969

87. Ruder MA, Ellis T, Lebsack C, et al: Clinical experience with sotalol in patient with drug-refractory ventricular arrhythmias. J Am Coll Cardiol 13:145, 1989

88. Ryan W, Engler R, LeWinter M et al: Efficacy of a new oral agent (tocainide) in the acute treatment of refractory ventricular arrhythmias. Am J Cardiol 43:285, 1979

89. Sachs MH, Bonforte RJ, Lasser RP, et al: Cardiovascular complications of imipramine intoxication. JAMA 205:588, 1968

90. Saksena S, Rothbart ST, Shah Y, et al: Clinical efficacy and electropharmacology of continuous intravenous amiodarone infusion and chronic oral amiodarone in refractory ventricular tachycardia. Am J Cardiol 54:347, 1984

91. Sami M, Mason JW, Peters F, et al: Clinical electro-

physiologic effects of encainide, a newly developed antiarrhythmic agent. Am J Cardiol 44:526, 1979

92. Schamroth L: Immediate effects of intravenous propranolol on various cardiac arrhythmias. Am J Cardiol 18:438, 1966

93. Selzer A, Wray HW: Quinidine syncope: Paroxysmal ventricular fibrillation occurring during treatment of chronic atrial arrhythmias. Circulation 30:17, 1964

94. Shabetai R, Surawicz B, Hammill W: Monophasic action potentials in man. Circulation 38:341, 1968

95. Sharma AD, Klein GJ: Comparative quantitative electrophysiologic effects of adenosine triophosphate on the sinus node and atrioventricular node. Am J Cardiol 61:330, 1988

96. Singh BH, Collett JT, Chew CYC: New perspectives in the pharmacologic therapy of cardiac arrhythmias. Prog Cardiovasc Dis 22:243, 1980

97. Singh BH, Hecht HS, Nademanee K, et al: Electrophysiologic and hemodynamic effects of slow-channel blocking drugs. Prog Cardiovasc Dis 25:103, 1982

98. Singh BN, Opie LH, Harrison DC, et al: Antiarrhythmic agents. In Opie LH, et al (eds): Drugs for the Heart, ed 2. Orlando, Grune & Stratton, 1987, p 54

99. Smith TW, Haber E: Digoxin intoxication: The relationship of clinical presentation to serum digoxin concentration. J Clin Invest 49:2377, 1970

100. Soffer K, Dreifus LS, Michelson EL: Polymorphous ventricular tachycardia associated with normal and long Q-T intervals. Am J Cardiol 49:2021, 1982

101. Somberg JC, Tepper D, Landau S: Propafenone: A new antiarrhythmic agent. Am Heart J 115:1274, 1988

102. Spurrell RAJ, Krikler DM, Sowton E: Effects of verapamil on electrophysiological properties of anomalous atrioventricualr connection in Wolff-Parkinson-White syndrome. Br Heart J 36:256, 1974

103. Stanton MS, Prystowsky EN, Fineberg NS, et al: Arrhythmogenic effects of antiarrhythmic drugs: A study of 506 patients treated for ventricular tachycardia or fibrillation. J Am Coll Cardiol 14:209, 1989

104. Stearns NS, Callahan EJ, Ellis LB: Value and hazards of IV procaine amide therapy. JAMA 148:360, 1952

105. Stern S, Eisenberg S: The effect of propranolol (Inderal) on the electrocardiogram of normal subjects. Am Heart J 77:192, 1969

106. Strasberg S, Sclarovsky S, Erdberg A, et al: Procainamide-induced polymorphous ventricualr tachycardia. Am J Cardiol 47:1309, 1981

107. Surawicz B, Lasseter KC: Effect of drugs on the electrocardiogram. Prog Cardiovasc Dis 13:26, 1970

108. Thomason GW: Quinidine as a cause of sudden death. Circulation 14:757, 1956

109. Tilkian AG, Schroeder JS, Kao JJ, et al: The cardiovascular effects of lithium in man. Am J Med 661:665, 1976

110. Tilkian AG, Schroeder JS, Kao J, et al: Effect of lithium on cardiovascular performance: Report on extended ambulatory monitoring and exercise testing before and during lithium therapy. Am J Cardiol 38:701, 1976

111. Touboul P, Atallah G, Gressard A, et al: Effects of amiodarone on sinus node in man. Br Heart J 42:573, 1979

112. Vaughan Williams EM: A classification of antiarrhythmic actions reassessed after a decade of new drugs. J Clin Pharmacol 24:129, 1984

113. Velebit V, Podrid P, Lown B, et al: Aggravation and

provocation of ventricular arrhythmias by antiarrhythmic drugs. Circulation 65:886, 1982

114. Vik-Mo H, Ohm OJ, Lundjohansen P: Electrophysiological effects of flecainide acetate in patients with sinus nodal dysfunction. Am J Cardiol 50:1090, 1982

115. Waspe LE, Waxman HL, Buxton AE, et al: Mexiletine for control of drug-resistant ventricular tachycardia: Clinical and electrophysiologic results in 44 patients. Am J Cardiol 51:1175, 1983

116. Wegria R, Boyle MN: Correlation between effects of quinidine sulfate on heart and its concentration in blood plasma. Am J Med 4:373, 1948

117. Wellens HJJ, Cats VM, Duren DR: Sympatomatic sinus node abnormalities following lithium carbonate therapy. Am J Med 59:285, 1975

118. Wellens HJJ, Lie KI, Bar FW, et al: Effect of amiodarone in the Wolff-Parkinson-White syndrome. Am J Cardiol 38:189, 1976

119. Wendkos MH: Cardiac changes related to phenothiazine therapy, with special reference to thioridazine. J Am Geriatr Soc 15:20, 1967

120. William RB, Sherter C: Cardiac complications of tricyclic antidepressant therapy. Ann Intern Med 74:395, 1971

121. Wilson JR, Kraus ES, Bailas MM, et al: Reversible sinus-node abnormalities due to lithium carbonate therapy. N Engl J Med 294:1223, 1976

122. Young M, Hadidian Z, Horn HR: Treatment of ventricular arrhythmias with oral tocainide. Am Heart J 100:1041, 1980

123. Zipes DP: Proarrhythmic effects of antiarrhythmic drugs. Am J Cardiol 59:26E, 1987

124. Zipes DP, Prystowsky EN, Heger JJ: Amiodarone: Electrophysiologic actions, pharmacokinetics and clinical effects. J Am Coll Cardiol 3:1059, 1984

Electrolyte Imbalance

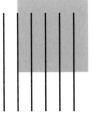

22

The action potential generated by the cardiac cells is the result of transmembrane movement of ions. Abnormalities of electrolytes alter the normal ionic concentration gradient across the cellular membrane, which in turn affects the movement of the ions. The configuration, duration, and amplitude of the action potential may be changed. In the body surface electrocardiogram (ECG), evidence of repolarization, depolarization, or conduction abnormalities often is observed.

The ECG is a useful clinical tool for the recognition of electrolyte imbalance, especially in relation to potassium and calcium. The severity of the imbalance and the serum concentration of the electrolyte sometimes may be estimated. Frequently, however, an accurate prediction cannot be made because of many limiting factors. Multiple electrolytes may be involved, and their effects on the ECG are modified by one another. The baseline tracing may be abnormal because of underlying heart disease. Similar ECG changes may be caused by drugs or extracardiac pathologic states. Once the diagnosis of a specific electrolyte abnormality is made, however, the ECG may provide a convenient and rapid guide to the assessment of the status of the imbalance during the course of therapy.

HYPERKALEMIA

Electrocardiographic Changes

1. Tall, narrow, and peaked T waves
2. Intraventricular conduction defect
3. Decrease of the amplitude of the P waves or absent P wave
4. ST-segment changes simulating current of injury
5. Cardiac arrhythmias: bradyarrhythmias, tachyarrhythmias, atrioventricular (AV) conduction defect

T-WAVE CHANGES

Tall, narrow, and peaked tent-shaped T waves are the earliest ECG sign of hyperkalemia.[13]

They are often seen when the serum potassium level exceeds 5.5 mEq/L.[24,29] The corrected QT (QTc) interval is either normal or decreased.[24] These repolarization changes have been attributed to the decreased duration of the transmembrane action potential and the increased velocity of its phase 3 associated with increased extracellular potassium concentration. The typical morphology of the T waves, however, is encountered only in a minority (22 percent) of patients with hyperkalemia.[3] In most cases, the T waves are tall and peaked but not narrow (Fig. 22–1) or they are peaked but of normal amplitude. The morphology of the T waves also may be modified when intraventricular conduction defect develops as a result of increasing degrees of hyperkalemia.

The tall T waves in hyperkalemia may be simulated by the T waves of many healthy, especially young individuals. Patients with bradycardia, subendocardial ischemia, cerebrovascular accident, or left ventricular volume overload also may have prominent T waves. In patients with myocardial disease or cerebrovascular accident, the QTc interval is usually prolonged, whereas it may be normal or decreased in patients with hyperkalemia. Prominent U waves speak against hyperkalemia but are common in patients with cerebrovascular accident.

INTRAVENTRICULAR CONDUCTION DEFECT

As the serum level of potassium increases further, the QRS complex becomes prolonged (see Fig. 22–1). This is usually seen only when the serum potassium concentration exceeds 6.5 mEq/L[24] and there is some correlation between the degree of QRS prolongation and severity of hyperkalemia. As a rule, the widening of the QRS is diffuse, involving the entire complex. Prominent S waves are often recorded in lead I and in the left precordial leads. As the widening progresses, the QRS

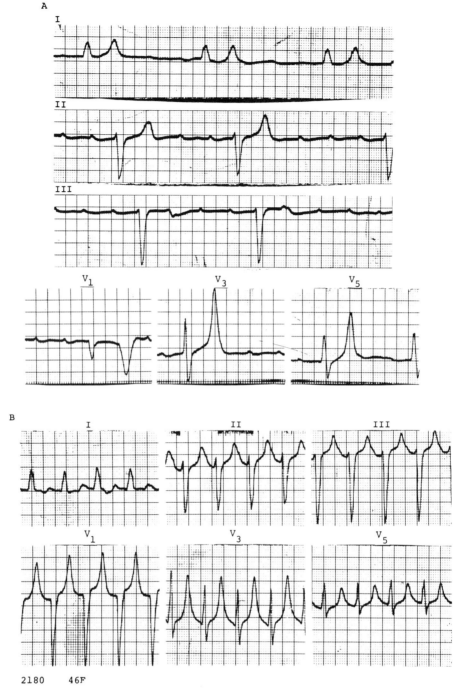

2180   46F

FIGURE 22–1. Hyperkalemia. The patient is a 46-year-old woman with metabolic acidosis. The serum potassium was 8.3 mEq/L; calcium, 5 mEq/L; and blood pH, 7.09. (A) Tracing showing sinus tachycardia with high-degree AV block, intraventricular conduction defect, abnormal left axis deviation, and tall, peaked T waves, especially in the precordial leads. (B) After intravenous administration of sodium bicarbonate and calcium gluconate, the ECG shows first-degree AV block. The QRS duration decreases to 0.14 second. The T waves remain tall and peaked.

complexes may appear as sine waves (Fig. 22–2). Occasionally, left or right axis deviation or a pattern that resembles left or right bundle branch block may develop[10,12,18] (Figs. 22–3 through 22–5).

The intraventricular conduction defect in hyperkalemia is the result of decreased transmembrane concentration gradient of potassium. The resting transmembrane potential is reduced, which in turn decreases the upstroke

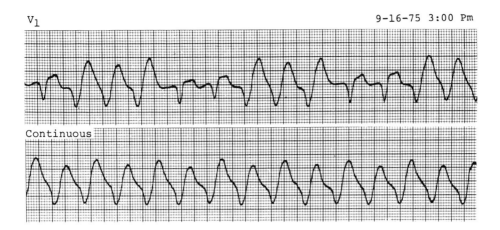

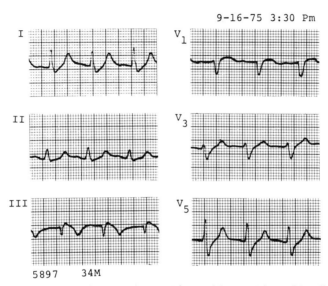

FIGURE 22–2. Hyperkalemia. The patient was a 34-year-old man with renal insufficiency. The 3 P.M. tracing shows wide QRS complexes, which resemble sine waves with intermittent, narrower QRS complexes. A serum potassium level obtained 6 hours before the tracing was recorded was 7.4 mEq/L. He was treated with intravenous calcium chloride, sodium bicarbonate, glucose, and insulin. Thirty minutes later, the ECG shows first-degree AV block and considerable reduction in the QRS duration.

velocity of the action potential and slows intraventricular conduction.

P-WAVE CHANGES

The P-wave amplitude usually decreases, and its duration increases as the serum potassium level rises (see Fig. 22–4). According to Surawicz, these changes usually appear only when the serum potassium concentration exceeds 7.0 mEq/L, and the P wave frequently becomes invisible as the potassium level exceeds 8.8 mEq/L.[24] When the atrial activity can no longer be detected, the site of the cardiac pacemaker becomes difficult to determine. Evidence suggests that there is sino-

ventricular conduction, and impulses are still being generated in the sinoatrial node and are conducted to the ventricles through specialized atrial fibers without depolarizing the atrial muscle.[26] The possibility of AV junctional or ventricular escape rhythm cannot be excluded, however (Fig. 22–6).

ST-SEGMENT CHANGES

In advanced hyperkalemia, ST-segment elevation that simulates myocardial injury or pericarditis may occur. Such ST-segment changes have been called the dialyzable current of injury by Levine and associates.[14] A remarkable example of such a phenomenon is given in

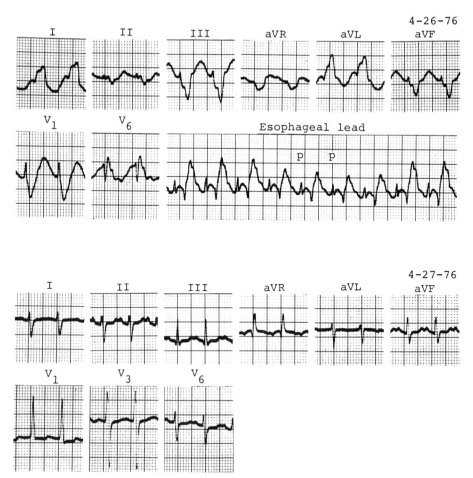

FIGURE 22–3. Left bundle branch block pattern caused by hyperkalemia. The patient was a 2-day-old infant who had profound hypoglycemia with a potassium level of 9.6 mEq/L when the upper tracing (4-26-76) was recorded. The tracing shows abnormally wide QRS complexes with a morphology simulating complete left bundle branch block. After therapy, the tracing on 4-27-76 shows nearly normal QRS complexes and minor T-wave changes. (Courtesy of Drs. Winston Gaum and Samuel Kaplan.)

Figure 22–7. In patients with coexisting QRS abnormalities, an erroneous diagnosis of transmural acute myocardial infarction may be made (see Figs. 9–53 and 9–54).

CARDIAC ARRHYTHMIAS

Mild to moderate degrees of hyperkalemia usually are not associated with ectopic rhythms or AV conduction defect. Marked elevation of the serum potassium level may be accompanied by AV block of various degrees, including complete AV block.[23] As discussed, the P wave may become invisible. Sinoventricular conduction without atrial depolarization or sinus arrest with AV junctional or ventricular escape rhythm may occur. Death may result from ventricular arrest.[12] More commonly, death in patients with hyperkalemia results from ventricular tachycardia and ventricular fibrillation. The impaired intraventricular conduction, with the resultant disparity of recovery in the different areas of the ventricles, favors reentry and precipitation of ventricular tachyarrhythmias.

HYPOKALEMIA

Electrocardiographic Findings

1. ST-segment depression, decreased T wave amplitude, prominent U waves
2. Prolongation of the QRS duration, P-wave changes
3. Cardiac arrhythmias and AV block

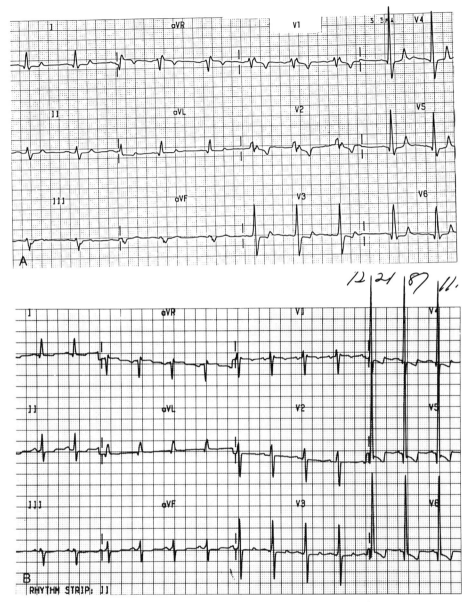

FIGURE 22–4. Right bundle branch block caused by hyperkalemia. The patient was a 46-year-old man with chronic renal failure. (A) Tracing recorded when his serum potassium level was 9.6 mEq/L. It shows first-degree AV block and flat but wide P waves. The QRS duration is increased to 0.16 second. The QRS morphology resembles that of right bundle branch block. ST and T-wave changes secondary to the conduction defect are present in leads V_1 and V_2. The T waves in leads V_4 through V_6 are peaked. Ten hours after the treatment was initiated, the serum potassium level decreased to 6.0 mEq/L, and the ECG (B) shows normal P waves, PR interval, and QRS duration. The right bundle branch block is no longer present. The QRS voltage and ST and T-wave changes are consistent with left ventricular hypertrophy. The tracing is similar to that recorded before the development of hyperkalemia.

REPOLARIZATION ABNORMALITIES

The typical electrocardiographic changes in hypokalemia include depression of the ST segment, lowering of the T-wave amplitude, and prominent U waves (Figs. 22–8 and 22–9).

These changes are related to lengthening and changes in the shape of the ventricular action potential, mainly its phase 3, associated with lowering of serum potassium concentration.[11] The genesis of the U wave is still not well understood, however. Because the ST-segment

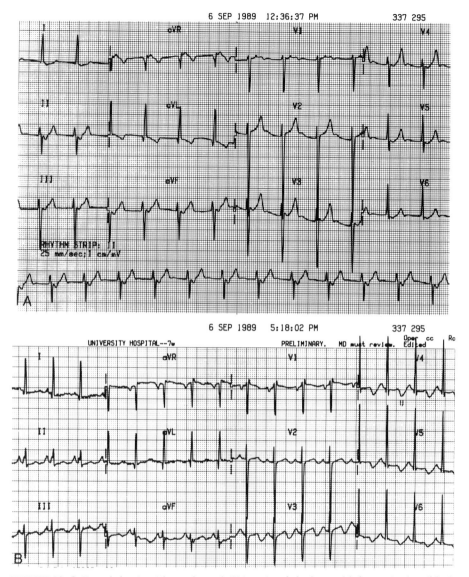

FIGURE 22–5. Hyperkalemia with accelerated AV junctional rhythm and left anterior hemiblock followed by hypokalemia. The patient was a 51-year-old woman with end-stage renal disease. (A) Tracing showing accelerated AV junctional rhythm with a rate of 86 beats/min. Left anterior hemiblock and left ventricular hypertrophy are present. The serum potassium level at the time was 7.7 mEq/L. The patient underwent hemodialysis. The serum potassium level decreased to 2.9 mEq/L. (B) The ECG made at that time shows sinus tachycardia and normal QRS axis, suggesting that the junctional rhythm and left anterior hemiblock in A are probably related to hyperkalemia. The P-wave changes are consistent with left atrial enlargement. Prominent inverted U waves are present in leads V_4 through V_6. The inverted U waves probably are due to left ventricular hypertrophy, but myocardial ischemia cannot be excluded, since the patient had a history of non–Q-wave myocardial infarction. The inverted U waves are prominent because of hypokalemia.

and T-wave changes are common in many pathologic states, the presence of hypokalemia is usually first suspected because of the prominent U waves. They are usually best seen in the mid-precordial leads. The U wave is generally considered prominent when its amplitude is greater than 1 mm or is taller than the T wave in the same lead. Surawicz

and associates found the typical ST-, T-, and U-wave changes of hypokalemia in 78 percent of patients with serum potassium levels below 2.7 mEq/L, in 35 percent of patients with levels between 2.7 and 3.0 mEQ/L, and in 10 percent with levels between 3.0 and 3.5 mEq/L.[24] Similar correlations were found by other investigators.[9,27]

8:30 AM   9/15/72

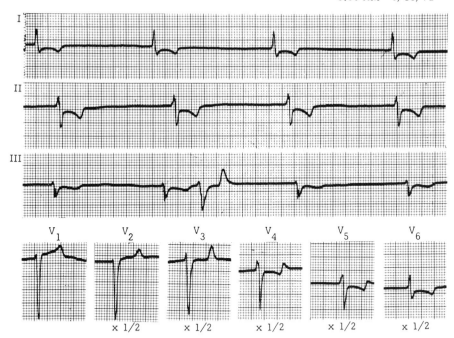

FIGURE 22–6. Hyperkalemia in a patient with chronic renal insufficiency. The serum potassium was 8.5 mEq/L. In the ECG, the P wave cannot be identified. The rhythm may be junctional in origin, or there may be sinoventricular conduction without atrial depolarization. The QRS duration is increased to 0.11 second. There are ST and T-waves changes, some of which are not related to hyperkalemia. One premature ventricular beat is present in lead III.

Contrary to the widespread impression, the QTc interval is not prolonged in hypokalemia. The apparent prolongation of the QTc interval in many cases results from the U wave's being superimposed on the descending limb of the T wave; thus, the measured QT interval is actually the QU interval. The presence of a superimposed U wave should be suspected whenever the T wave appears exceptionally broad. The U wave usually is smallest in lead aVL, and the QT interval can be determined more accurately in this lead.[24] In many instances, however, the fusion of the T and U waves renders an accurate measurement of the QT interval impossible. The recognition of prominent U waves also may be difficult in the presence of tachycardia. The U-wave amplitude generally decreases when the heart rate is rapid. Occasionally, it is superimposed on the succeeding P wave and is overlooked (Fig. 22–10).

The prominent U waves in hypokalemia may be simulated by many other conditions. The U-wave amplitude is increased in bradycardia, but the T waves are usually normal or tall, which is uncommon in hypokalemia. The U-wave amplitude is increased in left ventric-

ular hypertrophy. The recognition of hypokalemia in the presence of left ventricular hypertrophy is often difficult. Low serum potassium levels may be suspected under such circumstance if there is ST-segment depression in the right precordial leads in addition to the prominent U waves. In uncomplicated left ventricular hypertrophy, the ST segment is either normal or elevated in these leads. Quinidine, procainamide, and phenothiazines may cause large U waves. Patients who receive both digitalis and quinidine may have ST-, T-, and U-wave changes indistinguishable from those that result from hypokalemia. Prominent U waves also are seen in patients with cerebrovascular accidents. In these patients, however, the T-wave amplitude is usually normal or increased rather than decreased.

QRS CHANGES

In advanced hypokalemia, the QRS duration may be prolonged, but this is uncommon. In adults, the increase in duration is seldom more than 0.02 second. In children, the widening of the QRS complex may be more pronounced.[7]

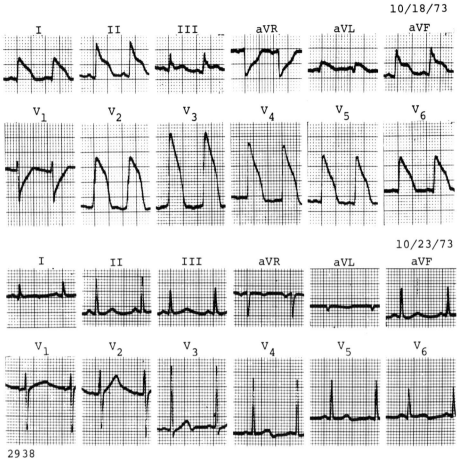

FIGURE 22–7. Current of injury caused by hyperkalemia. The patient had diabetes mellitus with ketoacidosis. The serum potassium level on 10-18-73 was 6.9 mEq/L. In the ECG, there is marked diffuse ST-segment elevation involving all leads except aVR and V_1, in which it is depressed. The morphology of the complexes resembles monophasic action potential. The tracing on 10-23-73 was recorded after the electrolyte imbalance was corrected.

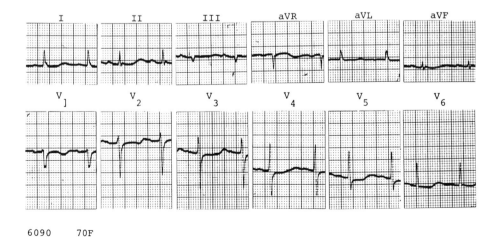

FIGURE 22–8. Hypokalemia produced by diuretics. The serum potassium level was 2.7 mEq/L; sodium, 124 mEq/L; and calcium, 9.2 mg/dl. The ECG shows diffuse ST-segment depression, T-wave flattening, and prominent U waves. The prominent U waves may be mistaken for T waves.

2-23-74

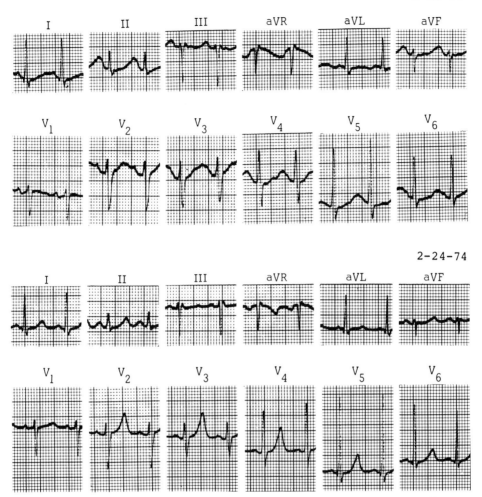

FIGURE 22–9. Hypokalemia associated with periodic paralysis. The patient was a 33-year-old woman with periodic paralysis. The upper tracing (2-23-74) was recorded when the serum potassium level was 2.4 mEq/L. ST-segment depression and low amplitude of the T wave are seen in leads I, II, aVF, and V_4 through V_6. Prominent U waves are best seen in leads II, III, aVF, and V_3 through V_6. The bottom tracing was recorded the next day, after the serum potassium level was restored to normal.

An increase in the amplitude and duration of the P wave also has been reported in hypokalemia.[24]

CARDIAC ARRHYTHMIAS AND AV BLOCK

Many types of arrhythmias may be caused by hypokalemia. They include paroxysmal atrial tachycardia with block, AV dissociation, first- and second-degree AV block with Wenckebach periods, ventricular arrhythmias including premature ventricular beats, and ventricular tachycardia and fibrillation. It is generally known that patients receiving digitalis are especially susceptible to the development of such arrhythmias in the presence of hypokalemia. Indeed, the incidence of these arrhythmias caused by hypokalemia alone is relatively low.

HYPERCALCEMIA

The major ECG change in hypercalcemia is a decrease in the QTc interval (Fig. 22–11). The decrease is at the expense of the ST segment, which becomes shortened or absent. According to Bronsky and colleagues, the QTc interval is inversely proportional to the serum calcium level up to 16 mg/100mL.[6] At levels greater than this, prolongation of the T wave occurs, and the QT interval becomes more normal. The interval between the onset of the QRS and that of the T wave (QoTc interval)

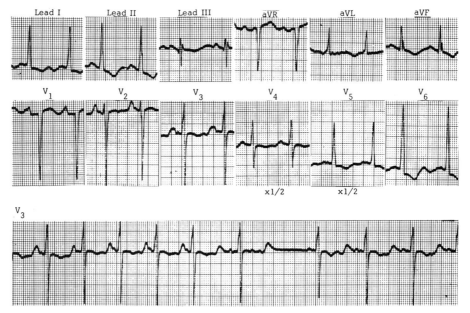

FIGURE 22–10. Hypokalemia. The patient has hypertensive cardiovascular disease. The serum potassium level was 1.6 mEq/L. The tracing shows left ventricular hypertrophy with abnormal ST and T waves. Prominent U waves are present. They are inverted in leads I, V_5, and V_6 and upright in leads V_1 through V_4. U-wave inversion in the anterolateral leads probably is related to left ventricular hypertrophy. The marked increase in amplitude is probably caused by hypokalemia. In the right and mid-precordial leads, the U waves may be mistaken for P waves. The prominent U wave is well demonstrated in the bottom strip (V_3) during carotid sinus massage. The U wave is separated from the succeeding P wave when the heart rate is slower.

remains short, however. Nierenberg and Ransil found that the interval from the beginning of the QRS complex to the apex of the T wave (QaTc) correlated more closely than the QTc or QoTc interval with the serum calcium levels.[17] A QaTc interval of 0.27 second or less was associated with hypercalcemia in more than 90 percent of the cases they studied.

The reported effect of hypercalcemia on the QRS complex varies. Some investigators noted a slight prolongation of the QRS duration.[24] Others described no change.[6] In either event,

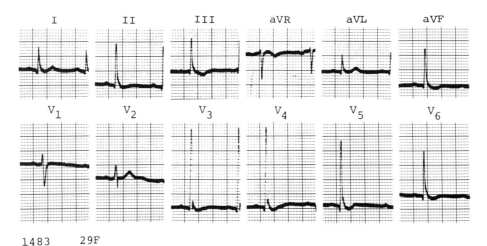

1483   29F

FIGURE 22–11. Hypercalcemia. The patient was a 29-year-old woman with malignant lymphoma involving multiple organs, including the bones. The serum calcium level was 17.4 mg/dl. She was not receiving digitalis. The heart was found to be normal at autopsy. Note the short QT interval in the ECG. The ST segment is almost absent. The flat T waves may or may not be related to hypercalcemia.

the changes are minor. A high serum calcium level usually does not alter the morphology of the P and T waves, but the amplitude of the U wave may increase.[24] Flattening or inversion of the T or P wave, however, has been noted in patients receiving calcium gluconate solution intravenously.[2]

Cardiac arrhythmias are uncommon in patients with hypercalcemia. Slight prolongation of the PR interval is occasionally observed, and cases of second- or third-degree AV block have been reported.[8,25] Other types of arrhythmias, including sinus arrest, SA block, premature beats, paroxysmal ventricular tachycardia, and sudden death, have been reported, most often in patients receiving rapid intravenous injections of calcium solution.[1] The administration of intravenous calcium in a fully digitalized patient may be particularly dangerous. Various and sometimes fatal arrhythmias may develop.

In my experience, the ECG recognition of hypercalcemia is often disappointing. Moderate or even marked elevation of the serum calcium level is often not accompanied by any significant changes in the QTc interval.

HYPOCALCEMIA

Prolongation of the QTc interval is the major ECG effect of hypocalcemia (Fig. 22–12). The prolongation is the result of an increase in the duration of the ST segment, whereas that of the T wave is unchanged. The degree of ST-segment lengthening is about proportional to the lowering of the serum calcium concentration, and it is the ionic form of the calcium in the blood that is electrophysiologically active. According to Surawicz, the QTc interval in hypocalcemia seldom exceeds 140 percent of normal[24]; otherwise, additional electrolyte abnormality is probably present and the QT interval is probably a QU interval. He also maintained that, with the possible exception of hypothermia, there are no other agents or metabolic abnormalities that would prolong the duration of the ST segment without changing the duration of the T wave. According to Bronsky and associates, changes in the morphology of the T waves are common in patients with hypocalcemia.[5] In some patients, there is peaking of the T waves; others show flattening or sharp inversion of the T waves. These changes are most pronounced in the right precordial leads.

Although hypocalcemia may decrease the QRS duration, the changes are minor and usually not recognized clinically. P waves, PR interval, and U waves are usually not affected by hypocalcemia. Cardiac arrhythmias are uncommon.

HYPERMAGNESEMIA AND HYPOMAGNESEMIA

Whether abnormal concentration of magnesium in the blood is associated with significant ECG changes is uncertain. Surawicz stated that the effect is unlikely to be detected in the ECG.[24] Others reported an increase in the PR interval and QRS duration and occasionally SA and AV block when magnesium sulfate was administered intravenously.[16,22]

In hypomagnesemia, slight narrowing of the QRS complex and tall, peaked T waves with normal QT interval may be observed.[20] In chronic magnesium deficiency, the ECG often resembles that of hypokalemia, showing ST-

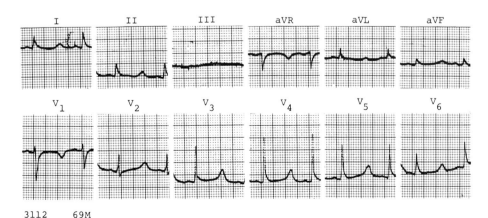

3112   69M

FIGURE 22–12. Hypocalcemia. The patient is a 69-year-old man with uremia. The serum calcium level was 5.6 mg/dl, and the potassium level was 5.6 mEq/L. In the ECG, there is a prolongation of the QT interval, mainly because of the lengthening of the ST segment.

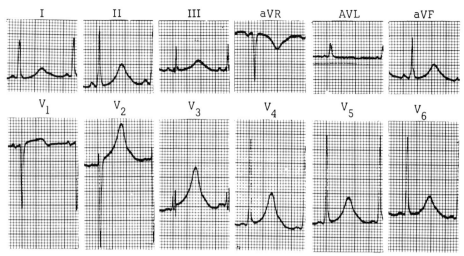

FIGURE 22–13. Hypomagnesemia. The serum magnesium level was 1.1 mg/dl. The serum potassium and calcium levels were normal. The tracing shows tall T waves in most of the leads. The QT interval is prolonged, but the exact interval is difficult to measure because of the U waves on the descending limb of the T waves.

segment depression, flattening of the T wave, and sometimes slight prolongation of the PR interval and QRS duration. Prominent U waves also may be seen. Nonspecific ST-segment and T-wave changes were reported by others.[19] Loeb and associates described prolongation of the QT interval and ventricular fibrillation in 2 patients with hypomagnesemia.[15] On reviewing their illustrated tracings, however, the apparent prolongation of the QT interval is probably the result of prominent U waves, and the QU instead of the QT interval was measured. Hypomagnesemia also is known to potentiate digitalis toxicity.[21] The effect of ab-

normal plasma magnesium concentration on the ECG has been attributed to its action on adenosine triphosphatase (ATPase), which is an essential energy source for the sodium–potassium pump. The exact mechanism for the ECG changes is unclear, however.

Figures 22–13 and 22–14 are examples of hypomagnesemia and hypermagnesemia, respectively, that I encountered. Figure 22–13 was recorded from a 36-year-old woman with chronic alcoholism, acute pancreatitis, and carpopedal spasm. She had an episode of ventricular fibrillation followed by atrial fibrillation. The 12-lead ECG taken after the resump-

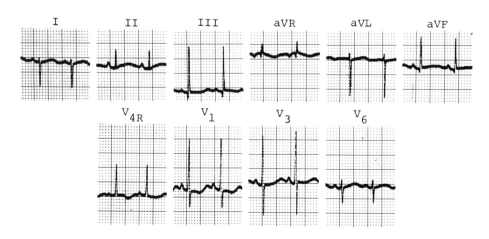

5240   New Born

FIGURE 22–14. Hypermagnesemia. The patient was a 12-hour-old-infant. The serum magnesium level was 4.1 mg/dl. The serum calcium concentration was 9.4 mg/dl. The tracing shows prolongation of the QT or QU interval.

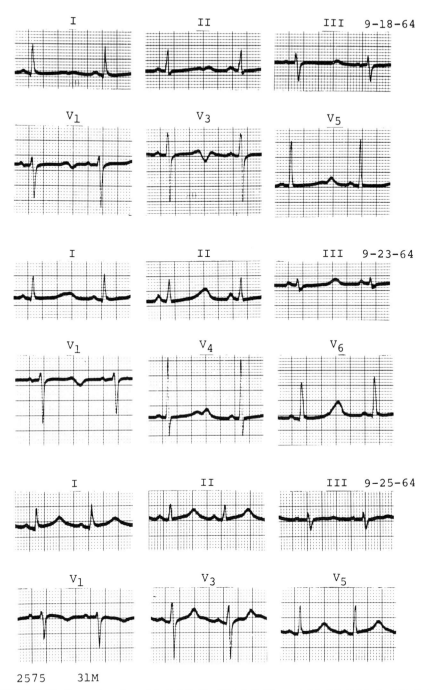

FIGURE 22-15. Hypocalcemia and hypokalemia. The patient was a 31-year-old man with chronic renal failure. The tracing on 9-18-64 shows prolongation of the QT interval, especially the ST segment. The U waves are prominent. The serum calcium level was 5.8 mg/dl, and potassium was 3.3 mEQ/L. On 9-23-64, the serum potassium level was 2.8 mEq/L. The U waves become more prominent and, in most of the leads, they are superimposed on the T waves. The ST segment remains prolonged. On 9-25-64, the serum calcium level was increased to 6.5 mg/dl, and the potassium level was increased to 3.5 mEq/L. The tracing shows definite shortening of the ST segment, and the U waves are less prominent.

tion of sinus rhythm (not illustrated) revealed tall T waves in leads V_2 through V_4 and prominent U waves in leads V_1 through V_6. Serum sodium, potassium, and calcium levels were within normal limits. On the following day, the ECG (illustrated) showed an increase in the T-wave amplitude. The U waves remained prominent. The serum magnesium level was 1.1 mg/100 mL (normal range, 1.7–2.8 mg/ 100 mL). The serum potassium level was 3.8 mEq/L. Figure 22–14 was recorded from a 12-hour-old infant whose mother received intravenous drip of magnesium sulfate during labor because of preeclampsia. The significant finding is the prolongation of the QT or QU interval. The serum magnesium level was 4.1 mg/100 mL, and the calcium level was 9.4 mg/100 mL.

ABNORMALITIES OF SODIUM CONCENTRATION

Neither hypernatremia nor hyponatremia appreciably affects the ECG.[24] In patients with intraventricular conduction defect due to hyperkalemia or quinidine, however, intravenous injections of sodium solution are known to shorten the duration of the QRS complex.[24]

ABNORMALITIES OF BLOOD pH

Acidosis and alkalosis are usually associated with abnormalities of serum potassium or calcium levels. The ECG findings usually reflect the changes of the electrolyte concentrations. The change in the pH value per se is difficult to identify by the ECG.

ELECTROCARDIOGRAPHIC CHANGES IN MULTIPLE ELECTROLYTE ABNORMALITIES

The ECG effects of one ion may be affected by alterations of other electrolytes. The action of potassium is antagonized by that of calcium and sodium ions. Therefore, ECG manifestations of hyperkalemia are less pronounced in the presence of a high serum calcium or sodium level, but they are exaggerated when serum calcium or sodium concentrations are low. The combination of hyperkalemia and hypocalcemia is frequently seen in patients with uremia, and the ECG usually displays a prolongation of the ST segment as a result of hypocalcemia and peaked T waves as a result of hyperkalemia. In patients with hypocalcemia and hypokalemia, the prolonged ST seg-

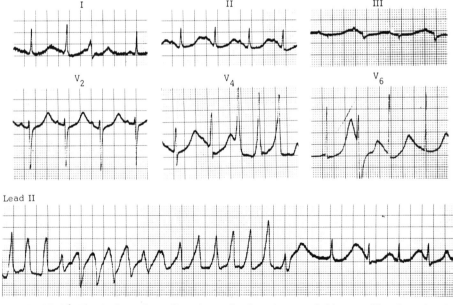

FIGURE 22–16. Ventricular tachycardia and torsades de pointes, probably caused by electrolyte imbalance. The patient was a 63-year-old woman who had hypertension, diabetes mellitus, and chronic alcoholism. The tracing shows prolongation of the QT or QU interval, with probable prominent U waves and an episode of ventricular tachycardia in lead V_4. Long lead II shows an episode of torsades de pointes. The serum potassium level was 2.9 mEq/L, and the calcium level was 7.9 mg/dl. Serum magnesium level determined 2 days later was 0.7 mg/dl. It is likely that the hypokalemia and hypomagnesemia are responsible for the ventricular arrhythmias.

ment is accompanied by prominent U waves that are often superimposed on the T waves. An example is given in Figure 22–15. Figure 22–16 is an example of ventricular tachycardia and torsades de pointes associated with low serum concentrations of potassium, calcium, and magnesium.

REFERENCES

1. Bellet S: Clinical Disorders of the Heart Beat, ed 3. Philadelphia, Lea & Febiger, 1971
2. Berliner K: Effect of calcium infections on human heart. Am J Med Sci 191:117, 1936
3. Braun HA, Surawicz B, Bellet S: T waves in hyperpotassemia. Am J Med Sci 230:147, 1955
4. Bronsky D, Dubin A, Kushner DS, et al: Calcium and the electrocardiogram. III. The relationship of the intervals of the electrocardiogram to the level of serum calcium. Am J Cardiol 7:840, 1961
5. Bronsky D, Dubin A, Waldstein SS, et al: Calcium and the electrocardiogram. I. The electrocardiographic manifestations of hypoparathyroidism. Am J Cardiol 7:823, 1961
6. Bronsky D, Dubin A, Waldstein SS, et al: Calcium and the electrocardiogram. II. The electrocardiographic manifestations of hyperparathyroidism and of marked hypercalcemia from various other etiologies. Am J Cardiol 7:833, 1961
7. Cherry JC, Surawicz B: Unusual effects of potassium deficiency on the heart of a child with cystinosis. Pediatrics 30:414, 1962
8. Crum WD, Till HJ: Hyperparathyroidism with Wenckebach's phenomenon. Am J Cardiol 6:838, 1960
9. Dreifus LS, Pick A: A clinical correlative study of the electrocardiogram in electrolyte imbalance. Circulation 14:815, 1956
10. Ewy GA, Karliner J, Bedynek JL: Electrocardiographic QRS axis shift as a manifestation of hyperkalemia. JAMA 215:429, 1971
11. Gettes LS, Surawicz B, Shiu JC: Effect of high K, low K, and quinidine on QRS duration and ventricular action potential. Am J Physiol 203:1135, 1962
12. Levine HD, Merrill JP, Somerville W: Advanced disturbances in cardiac mechanisms in potassium poisoning. Circulation 3:899, 1951
13. Levine HD, Vazifdar JP, Lown B, et al: "Tent-shaped" T waves of normal amplitude in potassium intoxication. Am Heart J 43:437, 1952
14. Levine HD, Wanzer SH, Merrill JP: Dialyzable currents of injury in potassium intoxication resembling acute myocardial infarction of pericarditis. Circulation 13:29, 1956
15. Loeb HS, Pietras RJ, Gunnar RM, et al: Paroxysmal ventricular fibrillation in two patients with hypomagnesemia: Treatment by transvenous pacing. Circulation 37:210, 1968
16. Miller JR, Van Dellen TR: Electrocardiographic changes following the intravenous administration of magnesium sulfate. J Lab Clin Med 26:1116, 1941
17. Nierenberg DW, Ransil BJ: Q-aTc interval as a clinical indicator of hypercalcemia. Am J Cardiol 44:243, 1979
18. Pryor R, Blount SG: The clinical significance of true left axis deviation, left intraventricular blocks. Am Heart J 72:391, 1966
19. Randall RE, Rossmeisl EC, Bleifer H: Magnesium depletion in man. Ann Intern Med 50:257, 1959
20. Seelig MS: Electrocardiographic patterns of magnesium depletion appearing in alcoholic heart disease. Ann NY Acad Sci 162:902, 1969
21. Seller RH, Cangiano J, Kim KE, et al: Digitalis toxicity and hypomagnesemia. Am Heart J 79:57, 1970
22. Smith PK: Pharmacologic actions of parenterally administered magnesium salts. Anesthesiology 3:323, 1942
23. Surawicz B: Role of electrolytes in etiology and management of cardiac arrhythmias. Prog Cardiovasc Dis 8:364, 1966
24. Surawicz B: Relationship between electrocardiogram and electrolytes. Am Heart J 73:814, 1967
25. Vass DM, Drake EH: Cardiac manifestations of hyperparathyroidism with presentation of a previously unreported arrhythmia. Am Heart J 73:235, 1967
26. Vassalle M, Hoffman BF: The spread of sinus activation during potassium administration. Circ Res 17:285, 1965
27. Weaver WF, Burchell HB: Serum potassium and electrocardiogram in hypokalemia. Circulation 21:505, 1960
28. Weidner RJ, Gaum W, Chou TC, et al: Hyperkalemia: Electrocardiographic abnormalities. J Pediatr 93:462, 1978
29. Winkler AW, Hoff HE, Smith PK: Electrocardiographic changes and concentrations of potassium in serum following intravenous injection of potassium chloride. Am J Physiol 124:478, 1938

Diseases of the Central Nervous System; Hypothermia

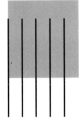

23

DISEASES OF THE CENTRAL NERVOUS SYSTEM

An association between electrocardiographic (ECG) abnormalities and cerebrovascular accidents has long been noted.[3,4,7,9] This is particularly true of subarachnoid and intracranial hemorrhage. In one series, ECG changes were seen in 71.5 percent of patients with subarachnoid hemorrhage and in 57.1 percent with cerebral hemorrhage.[18] Abnormal ECGs also are observed in other types of central nervous system disease. These include head injuries, tumor, and infections.[13,14] ECG changes are also seen after neurosurgical procedures.[10] The pattern of the ECG abnormalities is such that if the association is not recognized, an erroneous diagnosis of organic heart disease (especially ischemic heart disease), electrolyte imbalance, or drug effect is often made.

The most characteristic ECG findings in patients with central nervous system disease are large, upright, or deeply inverted T waves; prolongation of the QTc interval; and prominent U waves (see Figs. 9–50, 23–1, and 23–2). These changes may persist for as long as 11 days.[3] In some instances, the T-wave changes are less typical, consisting of lowering of the amplitude or notching.[2] ST-segment elevation or depression may occur, and the former simulates the injury pattern of ischemic heart disease.[7] Occasionally, the ST elevation is diffuse, mimicking acute pericarditis (Fig. 23–3). In some cases, abnormal Q waves develop, and the erroneous diagnosis of acute myocardial infarction may be made[5,7] (see Figs. 9–50 and 23–4). One case report described the appearance of camel-hump sign (J wave) following head injury that simulated that seen in hypothermia.[1] Tall P waves were frequently encountered in one series.[14]

Rhythm disturbances may occur in patients with central nervous system disease. These include sinus bradycardia, sinus tachycardia, wandering pacemaker, AV junctional rhythm, premature ventricular beats (see Fig. 23–4),

and ventricular tachycardia.[12] I have seen atrial fibrillation develop after head injury in two young persons (Fig. 23–5).

The pathogenesis of the characteristic ECG changes in central nervous system disease has been a subject of considerable interest. The most generally accepted explanation is altered autonomic tone, which affects ventricular repolarization.[2] In animal studies, stimulation of the left stellate ganglion or ablation of the right stellate ganglion results in large T waves and prolongation of the QT interval, similar to those seen in central nervous system disease. Direct stimulation of areas with known sympathetic connections—midbrain, posterior diencephalon, and hypothalamus—can produce ECG abnormalities.[2] In human subjects, the characteristic ECG findings were reported in a patient following right radical neck surgery, presumably due to destruction of the sympathetic nerve fibers.[16] An anatomic basis for the ECG changes also has been suggested, however. Subendocardial hemorrhage was found in patients with subarachnoid hemorrhage and ECG changes but without evidence of significant coronary artery disease.[17] In a series of 231 patients who died of intracranial lesions, microscopic focal myocytolysis was found in 8 percent.[6] Left ventricular wall motion abnormalities have been demonstrated by echocardiograms in some patients with subarachnoid hemorrhage.[20] It is possible that a combination of factors is responsible for the ECG manifestations.

HYPOTHERMIA

Hypothermia is associated with characteristic ECG changes from which the condition can often be diagnosed. As the body temperature falls, there is a progressive slowing of the sinus rate and prolongation of the PR and QTc intervals.[8,15] Although the duration of the QRS complex also is increased, the prolongation is often caused by the appearance of a J wave

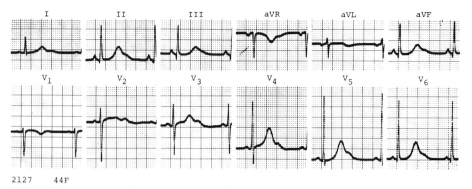

FIGURE 23–1. Subarachnoid hemorrhage. The ECG was recorded from a 44-year-old woman who had hypertension and subarachnoid hemorrhage. The tracing shows the characteristic tall and wide T waves, prolongation of the QT interval, and prominent U waves.

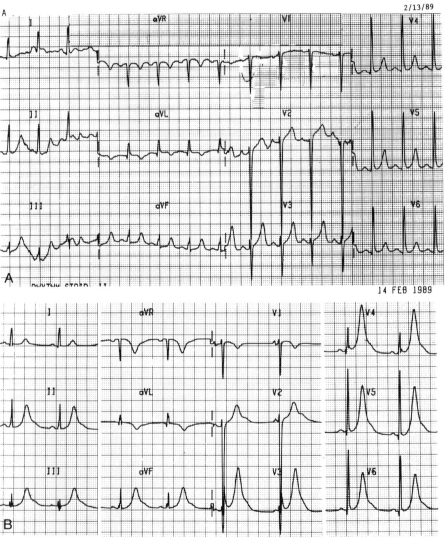

FIGURE 23–2. Postoperative changes following intracranial surgery. The patient was a 39-year-old woman with a history of hypertension who was admitted on 2-13-89 with the diagnosis of ruptured internal carotid artery aneurysm. (A) The ECG shows high QRS voltage consistent with left ventricular hypertrophy. There are no significant changes in the ST segment or T waves. Clipping of a ruptured right anterior choroidal artery aneurysm was performed on that day. (B) A repeat tracing on the next day shows tall and peaked T waves in most of the leads. The U waves are prominent, but the QTc interval is not prolonged. The electrolytes, including potassium, were normal and so were the cardiac enzymes. The T waves returned to normal a few days later.

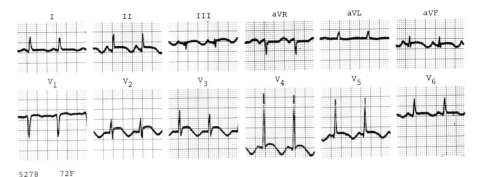

5278   72F

FIGURE 23–3. Cerebral thrombosis. The patient was a 72-year-old woman who was comatose on admission when this ECG was obtained. There is diffuse ST-segment elevation involving all leads except leads aVR and aVL. There also is T-wave inversion in most of the leads, with prolongation of the QT interval. The ECG may suggest the possibility of acute pericarditis, but the prolongation of the QT interval is against the diagnosis. At autopsy, there was extensive cerebral atherosclerosis, with scattered large infarcts in the cerebral and cerebellar hemispheres and pons. Although there also was generalized atherosclerosis of the coronary arteries, there was no evidence of either pericarditis or myocardial infarction.

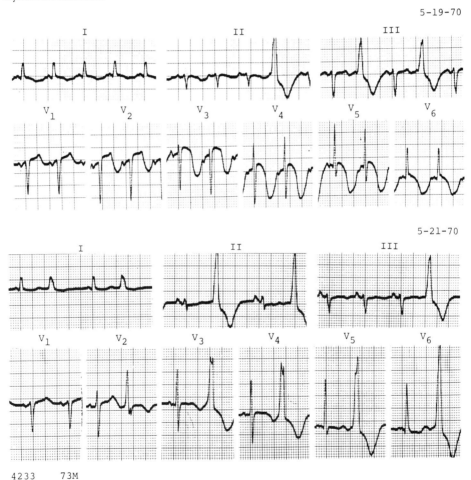

4233   73M

FIGURE 23–4. Head injury. The patient was a 73-year-old man with fracture of the skull. The tracings were recorded after the patient underwent craniotomy with evacuation of epidural, subdural, and left temporal lobe hematoma. There are frequent premature ventricular beats, with periods of bigeminal rhythm. The tracing on 5-19-70 shows sinus tachycardia and left anterior hemiblock. There are QS complexes in leads V_1 and V_2. ST-segment elevation and wide and inverted T waves are present in all the precordial leads except lead V_1, which shows an upright T wave. Inverted U waves can be seen in leads I and V_6. It was uncertain whether these abnormalities were due to the original head injury or the intracranial surgical procedure. The tracing on 5-21-70 shows the appearance of R waves in leads V_1 and V_2, and the ST and T-wave changes have much improved. At autopsy, the heart showed left ventricular hypertrophy, with 60 percent narrowing of the left circumflex artery. No evidence of myocardial infarction was found.

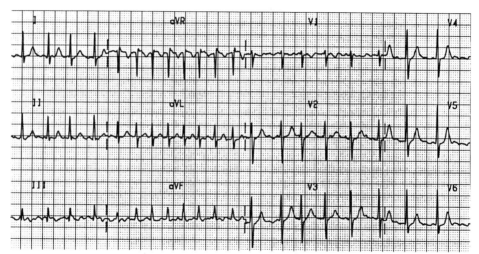

FIGURE 23–5. Atrial fibrillation due to head injury. The tracing was recorded from a 29-year-old man shortly after he received a severe blow on the head with a blunt object. It shows atrial fibrillation with rapid ventricular response. The morphology of the ventricular complexes is normal. An ECG recorded 6 days before the head injury for an unrelated reason was normal. The patient had no history or evidence of organic heart disease.

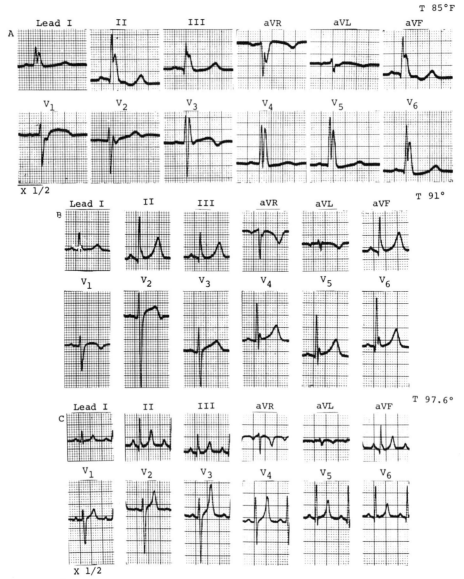

FIGURE 23–6. Legend on facing page.

Age: 45   T. 80°

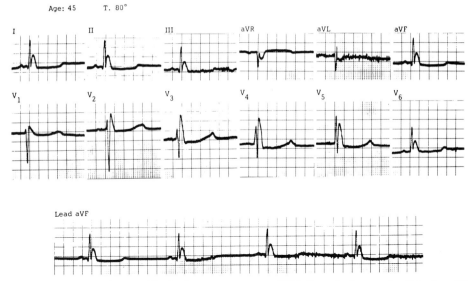

Lead aVF

FIGURE 23-7. Hypothermia. The body temperature was 80°F. Note the J waves in all leads, with prolonged QT interval and low T waves. Intermittent baseline oscillation is present as a result of somatic muscle tremors. The heart rate is 32 beats/min.

(see later discussion) rather than widening of the QRS per se.[8]

The most typical ECG finding in patients with hypothermia is the J wave (also called Osborn wave[19] or camel-hump sign). The J wave is a slowly inscribed extra deflection between the QRS complex and the early part of the ST segment (Figs. 23-6 and 23-7). It was first described by Grosse-Brockhoff and Schoedel[11] and is consistently found when the body temperature is below 25°C.[20] It is upright and more prominent in leads that face the left ventricle and increases in amplitude as temperature falls. When the J wave becomes very tall, the T wave in the same lead usually becomes inverted. The origin of the J wave is unclear. It was thought by various investigators to represent injury current, delayed ventricular depolarization, or early repolarization occurring in a portion of the ventricle before delayed depolarization is completed in another portion.[21] Indeed, a small J wave may be simulated by the deflection following the terminal portion of the QRS in subjects with the early repolarization pattern. The camel-hump sign also has been described in patients with

cerebral injuries.[1] I have seen a case of Prinzmetal's angina with ST-segment elevation simulating the J wave during the anginal episode.

About 50 to 60 percent of patients with hypothermia develop atrial fibrillation.[15] In one series, it appeared at a mean body temperature of 29°C.[8] Other ectopic rhythms, such as atrial flutter, AV junctional rhythm, ventricular ectopic beats, and ventricular fibrillation, also may occur. A constant or intermittent oscillation of the baseline as a result of muscle tremors may be present in the ECG, even though shivering may not be clinically evident (see Fig. 23-5). Both the rhythm and morphologic changes are reversible with rewarming.

REFERENCES

1. Abbott JA, Cheitlin MD: The nonspecific camel-hump sign. JAMA 235:413, 1976
2. Abildskov JA, Millar K, Burgess MJ, et al: The electrocardiogram and the central nervous system. Prog Cardiovasc Dis 13:210, 1970
3. Burch GE, Meyers R, Abildskov JA: A new electrocardiographic pattern observed in cerebrovascular accidents. Circulation 9:719, 1954

FIGURE 23-6. Hypothermia. The patient is a 24-year-old man. (A) Tracing recorded when his body temperature was 85°F. The heart rate at the time was 53 beats/min. J waves are prominent in all the leads. There is a prolongation of the QT interval, with T-wave changes in many of the leads. (B) Tracing recorded as the body temperature was raised to 91°F. The amplitude of the J waves has markedly decreased. The T waves are now within normal range. (C) Tracing recorded when the body temperature was 97.6°F. The tracing is now within normal limits except for sinus tachycardia. The slurring of the terminal part of the QRS complex in leads II, III, aVF, and V₆ is probably caused by early repolarization. It persisted in the later tracings.

4. Byer E, Ashman R, Toth LA: Electrocardiogram with large upright T waves and long QT intervals, Am Heart J 33:796, 1947

5. Chou TC, Susilavorn B: Electrocardiographic changes in intracranial hemorrhage. J Electrocardiol 2:193, 1969

6. Connor RCR: Heart damage associated with intracranial lesions. Br Med J 3:29, 1968

7. Cropp GJ, Manning GW: Electrocardiographic changes simulating myocardial ischemia and infarction associated with spontaneous intracranial hemorrhage. Circulation 22:25, 1960

8. Emslie-Smith D, Sladden GE, Stirling GR: The significance of changes in the electrocardiogram in hypothermia. Br Heart J 21:343, 1959

9. Fentz V, Gormsen J: Electrocardiographic patterns in patients with cerebrovascular accidents. Circulation 25:22, 1962

10. Finkelstein D, Nigaglioni A: Electrocardiographic alterations after neurosurgical procedures. Am Heart J 66:772, 1961

11. Grosse-Brockhoff F, Schoedel W: Das Bild der akuten Unterkuhlung im Tierexperiment. Arch Exp Pathol Pharmakol 201:417, 1943

12. Grossman MA: Cardiac arrhythmias in acute central nervous system disease. Arch Intern Med 136:203, 1976

13. Hersch C: Electrocardiographic changes in head injuries. Circulation 23:853, 1961

14. Hersch C: Electrocardiographic changes in subarachnoid hemorrhage, meningitis and intracranial space occupying lesions. Br Heart J 26:785, 1964

15. Hicks CE, McCord MC, Blount SG: Electrocardiographic changes during hypothermia and circulatory occlusion. Circulation 13:21, 1956

16. Hugenholtz PG: Electrocardiographic changes typical for central nervous system disease after right radical neck dissection. Am Heart J 74:438, 1967

17. Koskelo P, Punsar S, Sipila W: Subendocardial hemorrhage and ECG changes in intracranial bleeding. Br Med J 1:1479, 1964

18. Kreus KE, Kemila SJ, Takala JK: Electrocardiographic changes in cerebrovascular accidents. Acta Med Scand 185:327, 1969

19. Osborn JJ: Experimental hypothermia: Respiratory and blood pH changes in relation to cardiac function. Am J Physiol 175:389, 1953

20. Pollick C, Cujec B, Parker S, et al: Left ventricular wall motion abnormalities in subarachnoid hemorrhage: An echocardiographic study. J Am Coll Cardiol 12:600, 1988

21. Trevino A, Razi B, Beller B: The characteristic electrocardiogram of accidental hypothermia. Arch Intern Med 127:470, 1971

Mitral Valve Prolapse Syndrome; Skeletal Deformities

24

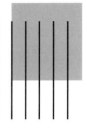

MITRAL VALVE PROLAPSE SYNDROME

The typical clinical manifestations of the mitral valve prolapse syndrome include the auscultatory findings of nonejection mid-systolic clicks and a late systolic murmur heard over the mitral area. Electrocardiographic (ECG) changes are present in many of these patients, and the term *auscultatory-electrocardiographic* syndrome was once suggested.[17] The syndrome is one of the most common cardiac abnormalities.[6,25] Its cause is unknown in most cases. It may be associated with cardiac diseases such as Marfan's syndrome, atrial septal defect, rheumatic endocarditis, obstructive and congestive cardiomyopathy, ischemic heart disease, and traumatic heart disease.[21,24] In some cases, there is a familial incidence.

The prolapse usually involves either the posterior leaflet or both leaflets. Involvement of the anterior leaflet alone also occurs but is less common.[18] The most characteristic histologic findings in autopsied cases is myxomatous infiltration of the leaflets.[22] The most common ECG abnormalities consist of ST-segment and T-wave changes and arrhythmias.

Electrocardiographic Findings

1. Morphology of the ventricular complex
   a. ST-segment and T-wave abnormalities
   b. Prominent U waves, QT prolongation
   c. Abnormal Q waves
   d. Preexcitation
2. Arrhythmias
   a. Premature ventricular beats, ventricular tachycardia, torsades de pointes
   b. Premature atrial beats, supraventricular tachycardia
   c. Atrial fibrillation
   d. Sinus node dysfunction
   e. Atrioventricular (AV) block

MORPHOLOGY OF THE VENTRICULAR COMPLEX

The most typical morphologic changes in the ECG of patients with the mitral valve prolapse syndrome are flattening or inverted T waves in leads II, III, and aVF, with or without ST-segment depression. They are often mistaken as signs of myocardial ischemia (Fig. 24–1). They occur in 15 to 42 percent of the larger reported series.[2,18,25] In some patients, similar changes also are present in the left precordial leads. Occasionally, the T-wave abnormalities are confined to the precordial leads. T-wave changes in the right precordial leads were said to be usually associated with prolapse of both leaflets.[18] Diffuse T-wave inversion also has been described but is uncommon.[2,27] Spontaneous variation of the T-wave changes may occur, and, in some cases, the T waves may become normal.[1,18] Inhalation of amyl nitrite may cause the development or worsening of inverted T waves, whereas exercise usually normalizes the T waves.[2,18] Horizontal ST-segment depression may occur with exercise in patients with normal coronary arteriogram to simulate the positive exercise test in ischemic heart disease.[2,13] In patients with this syndrome and chest pain, a false-positive response was found in 53 percent.[23]

Prominent U waves, especially in the right precordial leads, are common in some reported series[3,16] but are less so in others[18] (Fig. 24–2). The incidence of QT prolongation is a subject of debate.[2] In 54 patients with idiopathic mitral valve prolapse reported by Bekheit and Ali, all but 1 had prolonged QT intervals.[4]

The pathogenesis of the T-wave abnormalities is still unclear. Barlow and Pocock suggested that the increased traction from the chordae attached to the billowing leaflet might interfere with the rather tenuous vascular supply of the papillary muscle, which in turn could cause ischemia or infarction of that papillary muscle and adjacent myocardium.[2] It is a common observation, however, that there is a lack of correlation between symptoms, intensity of the auscultatory signs, or severity of the mitral valve prolapse and the extent of ECG abnormalities.

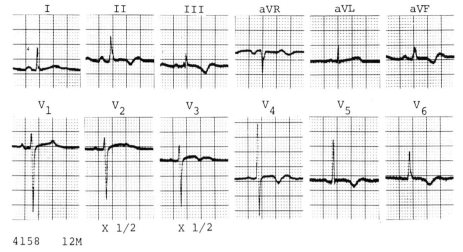

FIGURE 24–1. Mitral valve prolapse syndrome in a 12-year-old asymptomatic boy. A mid-systolic click and a late systolic murmur were heard in the mitral area. Rhythm strips showed frequent premature supraventricular beats. The 12-lead ECG shows T-wave inversion in the inferior leads and leads V_3 through V_6 and prominent U waves.

A few instances of abnormal Q waves suggestive of transmural myocardial infarction have been described in patients with normal coronary arteriograms.[29] The location of the infarction pattern may be either anterior or inferior. Chesler and associates reported 4 young adults with mitral valve prolapse, acute transmural or nontransmural infarction, and normal coronary arteriogram.[5] They suggested that coronary artery spasm in reflex response to billowing of the posterior mitral leaflet was a possible cause.

ARRHYTHMIAS

Cardiac arrhythmias are common in patients with mitral valve prolapse and are observed in the routine resting ECG in about 50 percent of the cases.[15,31] The incidence is lower in my own experience. The arrhythmias include ventricular and supraventricular ectopic rhythms and occasional conduction disturbances. They are observed more frequently when ambulatory monitoring or exercise testing is used.

Premature ventricular beats are the most common arrhythmia in this syndrome. They are seen by some authors in about one third of the routine ECGs.[10] They may be unifocal or multifocal; in bigeminy, trigeminy, or couplets (Fig. 24–3); or displaying the R-on-T phenomenon. During exercise, they may increase or decrease in frequency, but, in the latter case, they reappear in larger number immediately after exercise.[15,28] Ambulatory mon-

itoring with the Holter monitor reveals even a higher incidence of the arrhythmia. In 24 unselected patients with this syndrome monitored for 24 hours, Winkle and associates found frequent premature ventricular beats (defined by them as more than 425 per 24 hours) in 50 percent, infrequent premature ventricular beats in 25 percent, and no premature ventricular beats in 25 percent.[31] DeMaria and associates compared the results of ambulatory monitoring in 31 patients with mitral valve prolapse and 40 normal subjects.[8] Premature ventricular beats occurred in 58 percent of the patients with mitral valve prolapse and in 25 percent of the normal subjects. The incidence of premature ventricular beats in patients with mitral valve prolapse decreases during sleep.[31]

Paroxysmal ventricular tachycardia, torsades de pointes, and ventricular fibrillation occur occasionally and may be responsible for syncope or sudden death in some patients[26] (see Fig 24–2B).

Premature atrial or junctional beats are seen less frequently than are premature ventricular beats. They occur in about 10 percent of the routine ECGs and in up to 62 percent by ambulatory monitoring.[31] DeMaria and co-workers found supraventricular premature beats in 35 percent of patients with mitral prolapse and in 10 percent of normal subjects by Holter monitoring.[8]

Paroxysmal supraventricular tachycardia is the most common paroxysmal tachycardia in this syndrome (see Figs. 24–2C and 24–4). It was detected by ambulatory monitoring in 7 of the 24 patients examined by Winkle and associates[31] but less often by others,[8] including me. Other supraventricular tachycardias encountered include atrial fibrillation and atrial flutter[2,18] (see Fig. 24–4).

Evidence of sinus node dysfunction has been noted in various frequency by different

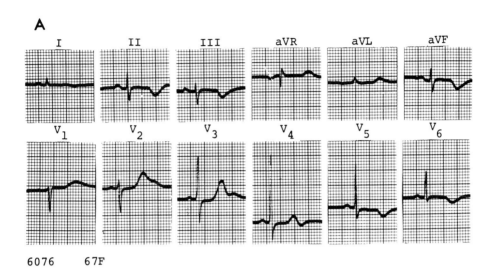

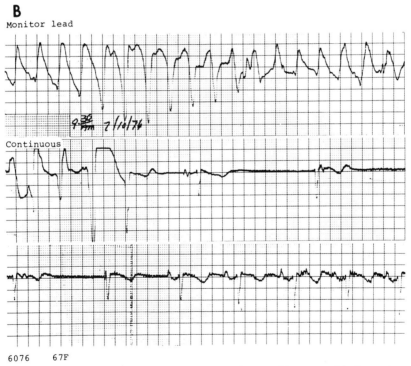

FIGURE 24–2. Mitral valve prolapse. The patient was a 67-year-old woman with chest pain, paroxysmal atrial tachycardia, premature beats, and syncope. Her coronary arteriogram was normal, but left ventriculogram revealed prolapse of the mitral valve. (A) The ECG shows T-wave inversion in the inferior and left precordial leads. There also is prolongation of the QT interval and prominent U waves in the right precordial leads (the heart rate at the time of the recording was 56 beats/min). On physical examination, mid-systolic clicks and late systolic murmur were heard in the mitral area. (B) The rhythm strip was recorded from the same patient shortly after a syncopal episode. It shows an episode of torsades de pointes followed by marked sinus bradycardia or periods of sinus arrest with junctional escape rhythm.

C

Monitor lead

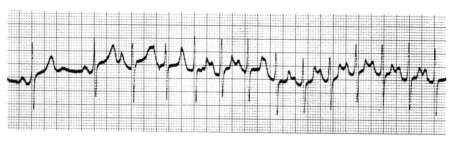

6076   67F

FIGURE 24–2 *Continued* (C) An episode of paroxysmal atrial tachycardia observed in the same patient.

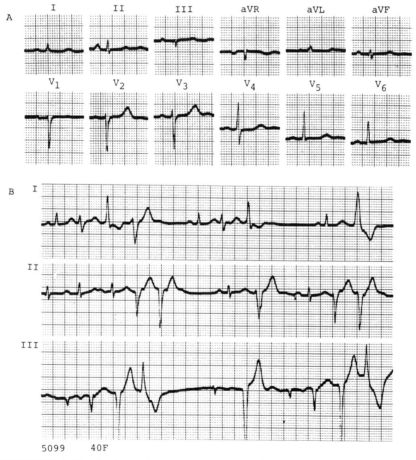

5099   40F

FIGURE 24–3. Mitral valve prolapse. The patient was a 40-year-old woman with auscultatory, echocardiographic, and angiographic findings of mitral valve prolapse. She had recurrent episodes of ventricular tachycardia and fibrillation resistant to drugs. She died suddenly. Autopsy revealed myxomatous degeneration of the mitral leaflets and chordae tendineae. (A) The 12-lead ECG reveals low voltage of the QRS complexes in the limb leads. The QT interval is prolonged (heart rate, 52 beats/min), and there are slightly prominent U waves in many of the leads. (B) Tracing showing premature atrial beats and multifocal premature ventricular beats with couplets and triplets.

authors. This includes sinus bradycardia, sinus arrest, and sinoatrial (SA) block.[2,8] Although AV block of various degrees and bundle branch block have been reported, it is uncertain whether they are merely coincidental or represent a real association.[10] The incidence of Wolff-Parkinson-White (WPW) syndrome in patients with mitral prolapse, however, appears to be higher than in normal subjects. All 7 patients with mitral valve prolapse in the series of WPW syndrome reported by Gallagher and associates had type A WPW pattern with left ventricular bypass.[14]

The genesis of arrhythmia in mitral valve prolapse syndrome is unclear. The ectopic rhythms may be the result of mechanical stress on the ventricle and atrium. It also has been suggested that the abnormal tension on the papillary muscle with secondary ischemia may cause ventricular arrhythmias, but atrial arrhythmias cannot be explained on this basis.[2] There is also no apparent relationship between the arrhythmias and the ST-segment and T-wave abnormalities.[10] Extensive postmortem examination of the conduction system in 1 patient with mitral valve prolapse who died suddenly showed no abnormalities.[26] Electrophysiological studies in patients with paroxysmal supraventricular tachycardia have demonstrated a high incidence of bypass tracts that would facilitate reentrant tachycardia.[19] As in the patient with the WPW syndrome and mitral valve prolapse, the accessory pathways in these patients also were left-sided.

ELECTROCARDIOGRAPHIC CHANGES RESULTING FROM SKELETAL DEFORMITIES

Pectus Excavatum (Funnel Chest)

In pectus excavatum, there is posterior displacement and depression of the sternum and costal cartilages. The heart is often compressed and displaced leftward. Although the condition by itself is rarely responsible for cardiac dysfunction, the ECG often simulates that of organic heart disease.

P WAVE

An entirely negative P wave is a frequent finding in lead V_1 (Fig. 24–5). It was found in 11 of 13 cases reported by deOliveira and colleagues.[9] As the heart is displaced leftward because of the chest deformity, the relation between the atria and the location of lead V_1 electrode is altered. Lead V_1 now records mostly negative potential as atrial activation proceeds in a direction away from the site of the electrode. The electrical potential at lead V_1 becomes similar to that at the right shoulder (lead aVR).

QRS-T COMPLEX

An rSr' pattern in lead V_1 is one of the characteristic ECG changes in pectus excavatum. It has been observed in most patients in some series.[9,30] In some patients, a Qr rather than an rSr' pattern is recorded (see Fig. 24–5). These

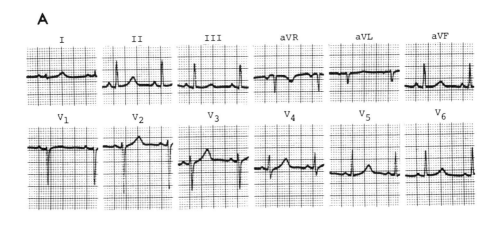

A

| I | II | III | aVR | aVL | aVF |

| V_1 | V_2 | V_3 | V_4 | V_5 | V_6 |

5737   38F

FIGURE 24–4. Mitral valve prolapse in a 38-year-old woman. The diagnosis was based on the presence of apical mid-systolic clicks and echocardiographic findings of mitral valve prolapse. She had a history of chest pain, recurrent palpitations, dizziness, and near syncope. (A) The 12-lead ECG is within normal limits.

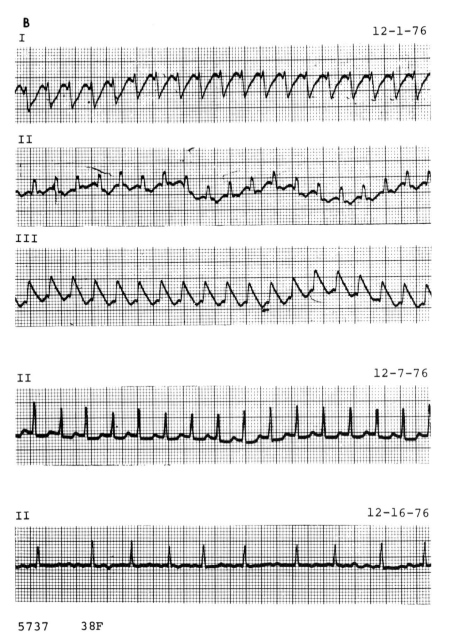

5737   38F

FIGURE 24–4 *Continued* (B) Various types of tachyarrhythmias were observed. The rhythm on 12-1-76 is probably supraventricular tachycardia with aberrant ventricular conduction. Paroxysmal supraventricular tachycardia with normal QRS complex is present on the tracing of 12-7-76. Atrial fibrillation is present on the tracing of 12-16-76. Atrial flutter also was observed but is not shown here.

changes also may be explained by the altered relation between the position of the electrode and that of the heart. In addition, there also may be a clockwise rotation of the heart. The late QRS forces from the basal portions of the ventricles are displaced more rightward and appear in lead V_1 as the r′ of the rSr′ pattern, or the r wave of the Qr complex. The duration of the QRS complex is usually normal, but oc-

casional cases of complete right bundle branch block have been reported.[12]

Abnormal Q waves that simulate either anterior or inferior myocardial infarction may be observed.[12] The former is more common, and the Q waves are seen most often in the right and mid-precordial leads. T-wave inversion in these leads also may occur.[11] Although mechanical injury as a result of compression of

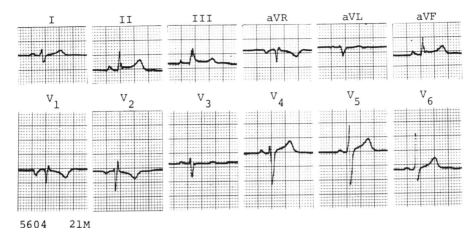

5604   21M

FIGURE 24–5. Pectus excavatum in a 21-year-old man. Note the prominent negative P wave and Qr pattern in V_1 and rSr′ in V_2.

the right ventricle has been suggested as the cause of the T-wave inversion, the changes also may be related to cardiac displacement. False-positive exercise test results also have been described in patients with pectus excavatum.[20]

RHYTHM

Paroxysmal tachycardias were reported in patients with pectus excavatum.[12] It is uncertain whether they are coincidental findings or truly related to the deformity.

Because pectus excavatum may be seen in patients with Marfan's syndrome, other ECG changes may be observed because of the cardiac anomalies associated with the latter disease. Pectus excavatum and other types of chest deformity, such as the straight back syndrome, also are seen more frequently in pa-

tients with the mitral valve prolapse syndrome.[10]

Straight Back Syndrome

In the straight back syndrome, there is a loss of normal upper thoracic kyphosis. The anteroposterior diameter of the chest is reduced, causing compression of the heart between the dorsal spine and sternum. The heart may appear enlarged ("pancake" heart) in the posteroanterior review of the chest roentgenogram. It is often displaced leftward. An erroneous diagnosis of organic heart disease may be made, because pulmonary ejection systolic murmur and expiratory splitting of the second heart sound are frequently heard in these patients. The ECG findings further confuse the problem.

As in pectus excavatum, most of the ECG

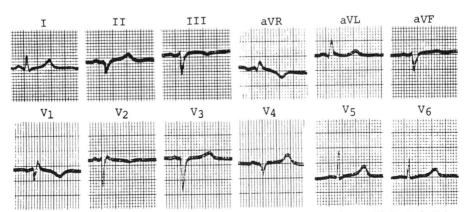

FIGURE 24–6. Straight back syndrome in a 25-year-old woman. There is abnormal left axis deviation, rSr′ pattern in V_1, and pseudoinfarction pattern in the mid-precordial leads.

changes are probably related to the cardiac displacement. An rSr′ pattern was observed in 6 of 23 cases reported by DeLeon and co-workers.[7] A small terminal r wave was present in lead aVR in 12 cases. Nonspecific T-wave changes were seen in 2 patients.

Pseudoinfarction pattern also is encountered occasionally (Fig. 24–6). I have seen several cases with abnormal left axis deviation (see Fig. 24–6), the explanation for which is lacking.

Kyphoscoliosis

Kyphoscoliosis may cause compression of the lungs and atelectasis. In advanced cases, alveolar hypoventilation results in arterial hypoxemia, which in turn causes pulmonary hypertension. Chronic cor pulmonale commonly develops in such patients. Their ECGs may show right atrial enlargement and right ventricular hypertrophy.

REFERENCES

1. Barlow JB, Bosman CK, Pocock WA, et al: Late systolic murmurs and non-ejection (mid-late) systolic clicks: An analysis of 90 patients. Br Heart J 30:203, 1968
2. Barlow JB, Pocock WA: The problem of non-ejection systolic clicks and associated mitral systolic murmurs: Emphasis on the billowing mitral leaflet syndrome. Am Heart J 90:636, 1975
3. Behar VS, Whalen RE, McIntosh HD: The ballooning mitral valve in patients with the "precordial honk" or "whoop." Am J Cardiol 20:789, 1967
4. Bekheit S, Ali A: QT interval in idiopathic prolapsed mitral valve. Am J Cardiol 41:374, 1978
5. Chesler E, Matison RE, Lakier JB, et al: Acute myocardial infarction with normal coronary arteries: A possible manifestation of the billowing mitral leaflet syndrome. Circulation 54:203, 1976
6. Darsee JR, Mikolich JR, Nicoloff NB, et al: Prevalence of mitral valve prolapse in presumably healthy young men. Circulation 59:619, 1979
7. DeLeon AC, Perloff JK, Twigg H, et al: The straight back syndrome: Clinical cardiovascular manifestations. Circulation 32:193, 1965
8. DeMaria AN, Amsterdam EA, Vismara LA, et al: Arrhythmias in the mitral valve prolapse syndrome. Ann Intern Med 84:656, 1976
9. deOliveira JM, Sambhi MP, Zimmerman HA: The electrocardiogram in pectus excavatum. Br Heart J 20:495, 1958
10. Devereux RB, Perloff JK, Reichek N, et al: Mitral valve prolapse. Circulation 54:3, 1976
11. Dressler W, Roesler H: Electrocardiographic changes in funnel chest. Am Heart J 40:877, 1950
12. Elisberg EI: Electrocardiographic changes associated with pectus excavatum. Ann Intern Med 49:130, 1958
13. Engel PJ, Alpert BL, Triebwasser JH, et al: Exercise testing in mitral valve prolapse. Am J Cardiol 41:430, 1978
14. Gallagher JJ, Gilbert M, Svenson RH, et al: Wolff-Parkinson-White syndrome. Circulation 51:767, 1975
15. Gooch AS, Vicencio F, Maranhao V, et al: Arrhythmias and left ventricular asynergy in the prolapsing mitral leaflet syndrome. Am J Cardiol 29:611, 1972
16. Hancock EW, Cohn K: The syndrome associated with midsystolic click and late systolic murmur. Am J Med 41:183, 1966
17. Humphries JO, McKusick VA: The differentiation of organic and "innocent" systolic murmurs. Prog Cardiovasc Dis 5:152, 1962
18. Jeresaty RM: Mitral valve prolapse–click syndrome. Prog Cardiovasc Dis 15:623, 1973
19. Josephson ME, Horowitz LN, Kastor JA: Paroxysmal supraventricular tachycardia in patients with mitral valve prolapse. Circulation 57:111, 1978
20. Kattus AA: Exercise electrocardiography: Recognition of the ischemia response, false positive and negative patterns. Am J Cardiol 33:721, 1974
21. Leachman RD, Cokkinos DV, Cooley DA: Association of ostium secundum atrial septal defects with mitral valve prolapse. Am J Cardiol 38:167, 1976
22. Marshall CE, Shappell SD: Sudden death and the ballooning posterior leaflet syndrome. Arch Pathol 98:134, 1974
23. Massie B, Botvinick EH, Shames D, et al: Myocardial perfusion scintigraphy in patients with mitral valve prolapse. Circulation 57:19, 1978
24. Pocock WA, Barlow JB: Etiology and electrocardiographic features of the billowing posterior mitral leaflet syndrome. Am J Med 51:731, 1971
25. Procacci PM, Savran SV, Schreiter SL, et al: Prevalence of clinical mitral valve prolapse in 1169 young women. N Engl J Med 294:1086, 1976
26. Shappell SD, Marshall CE, Brown RE, et al: Sudden death and the familial occurrence of the midsystolic click, late systolic murmur syndrome. Circulation 48:1128, 1973
27. Shell WE, Walton JA, Clifford ME, et al: The familial occurrence of the syndrome of mid-late systolic click and late systolic murmur. Circulation 39:327, 1969
28. Sloman G, Wong M, Walker J: Arrhythmias on exercise in patients with abnormalities of the posterior leaflet of the mitral valve. Am Heart J 83:312, 1972
29. Tuqan AK, Mau RD, Schwartz MJ: Anterior myocardial infarction patterns in the mitral valve prolapse–systolic click syndrome. Am J Med 58:719, 1975
30. Wachtel FW, Ravitch MM, Grishman A: The relation of pectus excavatum to heart disease. Am Heart J 52:121, 1956
31. Winkle RA, Lopes MG, Fitzgerald JW, et al: Arrhythmias in patients with mitral valve prolapse. Circulation 52:73, 1975

Nonspecific ST-Segment and T-Wave Changes; Abnormal QT Interval; Abnormal U Wave

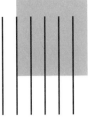

25

NONSPECIFIC ST-SEGMENT AND T-WAVE CHANGES

Nonspecific ST-segment and T-wave changes are among the most common electrocardiographic (ECG) interpretations. The phrase is used to indicate that the ST segment and T wave are abnormal, but the cause of the repolarization changes is not apparent to the electrocardiographer. The multiple factors that may affect repolarization process is well illustrated by Levine's list of 67 causes of ST-segment and T-wave abnormalities, which he said was "very incomplete."[22] The physician attending the patient is in a much better position to determine the clinical significance of such a finding. An excellent review of this subject was given by Surawicz.[35]

Nonspecific ST-segment and T-wave changes may be seen in patients with ischemic heart disease in whom the typical symmetrical T-wave inversion is not demonstrated. Patients with left or right ventricular hypertrophy may present repolarization abnormalities without the characteristic QRS changes. They may have the so-called strain pattern without the QRS voltage suggestive of ventricular hypertrophy. Acute right-sided heart strain caused by pulmonary embolism may cause ST-segment and T-wave changes that require clinical correlation and serial tracings before their significance becomes apparent. Acute and chronic pericarditis may not be associated with the typically diffuse ST-segment and T-wave changes to make one suspect their presence. ST-segment and T-wave changes may be the only abnormal findings in patients with various types of myocardial diseases. The repolarization abnormalities produced by various drugs or electrolyte imbalance may not be recognized when the clinical information is not available. The ST-segment and T-wave changes of mitral valve prolapse are nonspecific, and their association will not be realized unless the auscultatory findings of click and murmur are known. T-wave inversion may develop after ventricular pacing.

The repolarization abnormalities seen in patients with central nervous system disease were described in Chapter 22. In many cases, the changes are less typical and are interpreted as nonspecific. Other extracardiac causes of ST-segment and T-wave changes apparently caused by dysfunction of the autonomic nervous system include endocrine disorders such as pheochromocytoma, adrenal insufficiency, hypothyroidism, and hypopituitarism.[35] Fear, tension, and stress are known to cause ST and T-wave changes.[33] Visceral reflexes are thought to be responsible for the ST and T-wave changes associated with acute abdominal processes such as gallbladder disease[11,16] and acute pancreatitis,[2,6] as well as truncal vagotomy.[7]

The significance of ST-segment and T-wave changes is particularly difficult to determine when they occur in a patient without symptoms who has no clinical evidence of organic heart disease. The following are some of the conditions that may be associated with "benign" repolarization abnormalities. Failure to recognize their relationship may result in the creation of iatrogenic heart disease.

Hyperventilation

Wasserburger and associates reported T-wave inversion occurring in about 10 percent of 350 healthy adults after 10 to 15 seconds of hyperventilation.[40] Other studies revealed T-wave inversion in about 70 percent of healthy young individuals after 30 to 60 seconds of hyperventilation.[1,17] The longer period of hyperventilation and monitoring of multiple leads during the procedure was believed to be responsible for the higher incidence.[1] Various factors have been suggested as the contributing causes for the T-wave changes associated with hyperventilation. These include respiratory alkalosis, change in extracellular potassium concentration, change in heart position, tachycardia, and vagally mediated reflex. Biberman and associates proposed that asynchronous shortening of ventricular repolarization during sympathetic stimulation produced by hyperventilation may be the responsible factor.[1]

Orthostatic Changes

Lepeschkin and Surawicz found orthostatic T-wave changes in 3 percent of 179 normal subjects.[21] A higher incidence (23 percent) was observed by Kemp and Ellestad.[17] In my own experience, the changes occur most frequently in the inferior leads. Whether the changes occur more often in patients with ischemic heart disease is a subject of debate.[17] Increased sympathetic activity in response to the standing position is believed to be the responsible mechanism.

Postprandial T-Wave Changes

T-wave changes after food intake are one of the most common causes for such abnormalities in the resting ECGs of healthy individuals.[14,32] As many as 50 percent of healthy persons with nonspecific T-wave changes may have normal ECGs when the tracings are repeated in the fasting state.[14,34]

Normal Variant

T-wave inversion may occur in healthy individuals as a normal variant. The T waves in the right precordial leads and sometimes also in the mid-precordial leads may be inverted in the adult because of a persistent juvenile pattern. This is more common in the black population, especially women. Benign T-wave inversion also is seen occasionally in healthy young adults in the mid- and left precordial leads. These changes with or without ST-segment elevation may simulate those of myocardial injury or ischemia. This pattern is more common in young black men, especially trained athletes[10,12,13,23,27,37] (see Fig. 9–69).

To differentiate benign from pathologic T wave, Sleeper and Orgain suggested the use of certain physiological manipulations.[34] They found that fasting, deep inspiration, hyperventilation, or exercise normalized the T waves in most healthy persons. In patients with organic heart disease, the T-wave changes were less labile in response to the various maneuvers. A follow-up study in these patients after an average period of 8 years supported their previous conclusion.[29] In 10 highly trained athletes with abnormal ECGs examined by Oakley and Oakley, the T waves were normalized with exercise in 5, all of whom had normal coronary arteriograms.[27]

Oral administration of potassium salts also has been used to differentiate "functional" T-wave abnormalities from those due to organic heart disease, the former being likely to be normalized and the latter to be unchanged.[40] This procedure is not in common use because of the question of safety. Serious arrhythmias have been reported after its administration.[30,40]

ABNORMAL QT INTERVAL

Prolongation of the QT Interval

The QT interval represents the time required for the completion of ventricular depolarization and repolarization. It is abnormally long when the QTc interval is greater than 0.44 second. Prolongation of the QT interval is seen when there is lengthening of the ventricular activation time as a result of intraventricular conduction defects or left ventricular hypertrophy. Secondary repolarization abnormalities in such instances contribute further to the prolongation of the interval. Other conditions may prolong the QT interval by affecting primarily the ventricular recovery phase, while the QRS complex may or may not be abnormal. These conditions include the following[26,35,36]:

A. Idiopathic long QT interval syndrome
  1. The Jervell-Lange-Nielson syndrome
  2. The Romano-Ward syndrome
  3. Sporadic long QT syndrome
B. Secondary (acquired) types of QT prolongation
  1. Coronary artery disease—myocardial ischemia, myocardial infarction
  2. Mitral valve prolapse, cardiomyopathy
  3. Central nervous system disease, especially intracranial hemorrhage
  4. Autonomic nervous system dysfunction secondary to radical neck dissection, carotid endarterectomy, transabdominal truncal vagotomy
  5. Metabolic disturbances—electrolyte imbalance (such as hypocalcemia), liquid protein diet, intracoronary injection of contrast agents
  6. Cardiac drugs—quinidine, procainamide, disopyramide, encainide, flecainide, propafenone, amiodarone

7. Psychotropic drugs—phenothiazines, tricyclic antidepressants
8. Miscellaneous conditions—severe bradycardia, high degree AV block, post–Stokes-Adams seizures, hypothyroidism, hypothermia, pheochromocytoma, organophosphorus poisoning

The prolongation of the QT interval has attracted increasing attention because of its relation to serious ventricular arrhythmias (especially torsade de pointes), syncope, and sudden cardiac death in some patients. The association is particularly evident in patients with the idiopathic (congenital) long QT syndrome and in patients receiving antiarrhythmic agents such as quinidine, procainamide, encainide, and flecainide. Marked asynchrony of ventricular repolarization has been proposed as the principal underlying cause of the life-threatening ventricular arrhythmias.[36]

LONG QT SYNDROME

The Jervell-Lange-Nielson syndrome is the clinical entity of prolonged QT interval, congenital deafness, syncope, and sudden death.[15] The syndrome is apparently transmitted as an autosomal recessive trait. Heterozygous persons may be clinically normal or have a slightly prolonged QT interval.[5] Schwartz and associates found that its incidence among deaf-mute children is about 0.25 percent.[31] The Romano-Ward syndrome is clinically similar to the Jarvell-Lange-Nielsen syndrome except that hearing is normal.[28,39] It is apparently an autosomal dominant disorder. Homozygous and heterozygous persons may have similar clinical symptoms. An example of the idiopathic long QT syndrome without deafness is given in Figure 25–1.

Moss and associates reported a prospective international study of 196 patients with the idiopathic long QT syndrome.[25] One hundred eighty seven patients had QTc intervals greater than 0.44 second. Nine had intervals ranging from 0.40 to 0.44 second but had unexplained syncope or at least one blood relative who had a QTc interval of greater than 0.44 second. The average age of the patients was 24 ± 16 years. There were almost twice as many females as males. Congenital deafness was present in 6 percent of the patients. Eighty-eight percent of the subjects had family members with QT prolongation. Twenty-one percent had a history of torsades de pointes or ventricular fibrillation documented by ECG. A history of syncope was obtained from 57 per-

cent of the patients, and there was a strong association between the syncopal episodes and intense emotions (anger or fright), vigorous activity, or loud noises. In an average follow-up period of 26 months, 27 patients had one or more episodes of syncope and 4 patients died suddenly. The authors also found that congenital deafness, history of syncope, female gender, and prior occurrence of torsades de pointes or ventricular fibrillation were each associated with a significantly increased likelihood of syncope or sudden death.

Although the pathogenesis of the long QT syndrome is still unclear, the most favored theory is that there is an imbalance between various components of the cardiac sympathetic innervation. In patients with the long QT syndrome, left stellate ganglion block, right stellate ganglion stimulation, and administration of propranolol shorten the QT interval. Right stellate ganglion block and left stellate ganglion stimulation have the opposite effect.[3] This neurogenic theory is further supported by the fact that the most effective therapy is the administration of beta-adrenergic blocking agents or left stellate ganglion ablation. Electronic cardiac pacing also has been effective in some patients with the long QT syndrome and syncope, perhaps by decreasing the dispersion of refractoriness.[4]

Shortening of the QT Interval

The QT interval is shortened in patients receiving digitalis and in those with hypercalcemia.

ABNORMAL U WAVE

The normal U wave has the same polarity as the T wave. Its amplitude is generally proportional to that of the T wave in the same lead, ranging between 5 and 25 percent of the T-wave amplitude.[20] It is tallest in leads V_2 and V_3, where it may reach 2.0 mm but usually does not exceed 1 mm.

Prominent U Wave

A U wave is generally considered abnormally large when its amplitude is greater than 1.5 mm in any lead. The common causes of prominent U wave are as follows:

1. Bradycardia
2. Electrolyte imbalance, such as hypokalemia, hypomagnesemia, and hypercalcemia

A

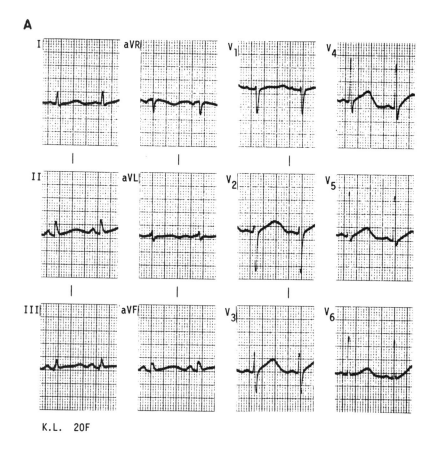

K.L.   20F

B

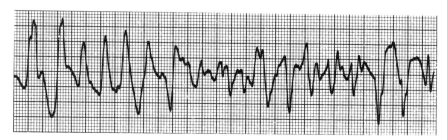

K.L.   20F

FIGURE 25–1. Idiopathic long QT syndrome. The patient was a 20-year-old woman with a history of recurrent syncope. She had no hearing defect. (A) The 12-lead ECG reveals prolonged QT interval with prominent U waves. The QT interval cannot be measured precisely because of the superimposed U waves. The QRS complexes are normal. (B) She developed torsade de pointes and ventricular fibrillation and died on the same day the 12-lead ECG was obtained.

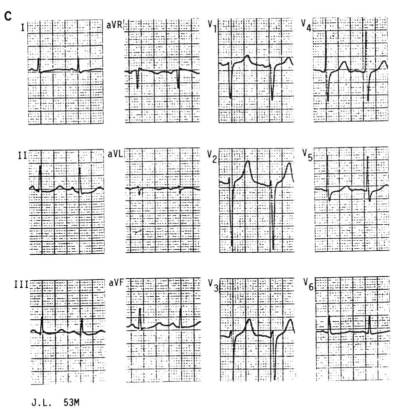

J.L. 53M

FIGURE 25–1 *Continued* (C) The ECG of her 53-year-old father reveals a QTc interval of 0.6 second. (Courtesy of Dr. John Held.)

3. Drugs, such as quinidine, procainamide, disopyramide, amiodarone, digitalis, phenothiazines, and epinephrine
4. Central nervous system disease
5. Left ventricular hypertrophy
6. Hyperthyroidism
7. Mitral valve prolapse syndrome
8. The long QT syndrome

U-Wave Inversion

A negative U wave is highly specific for the presence of organic heart disease.[18] The U wave polarity may become abnormal in ventricular hypertrophy. In left ventricular hypertrophy, the U wave may be inverted in leads I, V_5, and V_6. According to Lepeschkin, it occurs more commonly in cases with volume overload of the left ventricle, such as aortic insufficiency, than in those with pressure overload, such as aortic stenosis.[19,20] The U wave may be inverted with or without concurrent inversion of the T wave in the same lead. Indeed, in some instances, inverted U waves in the left precordial leads provide the only evidence of abnormality in patients with left ventricular hypertrophy.

In right ventricular hypertrophy, the U wave is sometimes inverted in the right precordial leads and in leads II and III. As in the cases of left ventricular hypertrophy, an inverted U wave is seen more commonly in patients with volume overload of the right ventricle (such as atrial septal defect) than in those with pressure overload (such as mitral stenosis and chronic cor pulmonale).

U-wave inversion also is seen in patients with ischemic heart disease. It is observed in myocardial infarction as well as in myocardial ischemia without infarction. It may be the only ECG abnormality in patients with coronary artery disease. In some patients, the U wave becomes inverted only during an anginal episode.[19] Exercise-induced U-wave inversion is considered a reliable sign of ischemic heart disease.[24] Gerson and associates found that U-wave inversion at rest or induced by exercise is a marker of severe stenosis of the left anterior descending coronary artery.[8,9]

Lepeschkin reviewed 181 patients with isolated U-wave inversion but with otherwise normal ECG.[19] He found that 56 percent of the patients had left ventricular hypertrophy or conditions that usually cause left ventricular hypertrophy. Twenty percent had angina pectoris, 14 percent had both, and the cause was uncertain in 10 percent.

REFERENCES

1. Biberman L, Sarma RN, Surawicz B: T-wave abnormalities during hyperventilation and isoproterenol infusion. Am Heart J 81:166, 1971
2. Cohen MH, Rotsztain A, Bowen PJ, et al: Electrocardiographic changes in acute pancreatitis resembling acute myocardial infarction. Am Heart J 82:672, 1971.
3. Crampton R: Preeminence of the left stellate ganglion in the long Q-T syndrome. Circulation 59:769, 1979
4. Eldar M, Griffin JC, Abbott JA, et al: Permanent cardiac pacing in patients with the long QT syndrome. J Am Coll Cardiol 10:600, 1987
5. Fraser G, Eroggatt P, Murphy T: Genetical aspects of the cardio-auditory syndrome of Jervell and Lange-Nielson (congenital deafness and electrocardiographic abnormalities). Ann Hum Genet 28:133, 1964
6. Fulton MC, Marriott HJL: Acute pancreatitis simulating myocardial infarction in the electrocardiogram. Ann Intern Med 59:730, 1963
7. Gallivan GJ, Levine H, Canzonetti AJ: Ischemic electrocardiographic changes after truncal vagotomy. JAMA 211:798, 1970
8. Gerson MC, McHenry PL: Resting U wave inversion as a marker of stenosis of the left anterior descending coronary artery. Am J Med 69:545, 1980
9. Gerson MC, Phillips JF, Morris SN, et al: Exercise-induced U wave inversion as a marker of stenosis of the left anterior descending coronary artery. Circulation 60:1014, 1979
10. Goldman MJ: Normal variants in the electrocardiogram leading to cardiac invalidism. Am Heart J 59:71, 1960
11. Hampton AG, Beckwith JR, Wood JE: The relationship between heart disease and gallbladder disease. Ann Intern Med 50:1135, 1959
12. Hanne-Paparo N, Drory Y, Schoenfeld Y, et al: Common ECG changes in athletes. Cardiology 61:267, 1976
13. Hanne-Paparo N, Wendkos MH, Brunner D: T wave abnormalities in the electrocardiograms of top-ranking athletes without demonstrable organic heart disease. Am Heart J 81:743, 1971
14. Hiss RG, Averill KH, Lamb LE: Electrocardiographic findings in 67,375 asymptomatic individuals. Part VIII. Nonspecific T wave changes. Am J Cardiol 6:178, 1960
15. Jervell A, Lange-Nielsen F: Congenital deaf-mutism, functional heart disease with prolongation of the Q-T interval and sudden death. Am Heart J 54:59, 1957
16. Kaufman JM, Lubera R: Preoperative use of atropine and electrocardiographic changes. JAMA 200:197, 1967
17. Kemp GL, Ellestad MH: The significance of hyperventilation and orthostatic T-wave changes on the electrocardiogram. Arch Intern Med 121:518, 1968
18. Kishida H, Cole JS, Surawicz B: Negative U wave: A highly specific but poorly understood sign of heart disease. Am J Cardiol 49:2030, 1982
19. Lepeschkin E: The U wave of the electrocardiogram. Mod Concepts Cardiovasc Dis 38:39, 1969
20. Lepeschkin E: Physiologic basis of the U wave. In Schlant RC, Hurst JW (eds): Advances in Electrocardiography. New York, Grune & Stratton, 1976, p 353
21. Lepeschkin E, Surawicz B: Characteristics of true-positive and false-positive results of electrocardiographic Master two-step exercise test. N Engl J Med 258:511, 1958
22. Levine HD: Non-specificity of the electrocardiogram associated with coronary artery disease. Am J Med 15:344, 1953
23. Lichtman J, O'Rourke RA, Kelin A, et al: Electrocardiogram of the athlete: Alterations simulating those of organic heart disease. Arch Intern Med 132:763, 1973
24. McHenry PL, Fisch C: Clinical applications of the treadmill exercise test. Mod Concepts Cardiovasc Dis 46:21, 1977
25. Moss AJ, Schwartz PJ, Crampton RS, et al: The long QT syndrome: A prospective international study. Circulation 1:17, 1985
26. Moss AJ, Schwartz PJ: Delayed repolarization (QT or QTU prolongation) and malignant ventricular arrhythmias. Mod Conc Cardiovasc Dis 51:85, 1982
27. Oakley DG, Oakley CM: Significance of abnormal electrocardiograms in highly trained athletes. Am J Cardiol 50:985, 1982
28. Romano C, Gemme G, Pongiglione R: Aritmie Cardiache rare dell'eta pediatrica. II. Accessi sinopali per fibrillazione ventricolare parassistics (presentazione del primo case della letteratura pediatrica italiana). Clin Paediate 45:656, 1963
29. Rotman M, Colvard MC, Ruskin J, et al: Nonspecific T-wave changes. Arch Intern Med 130:895, 1972
30. Schneider RG, Lyon AF: Use of oral potassium salts in the assessment of T-wave abnormalities in the electrocardiogram: A clinical test. Am Heart J 77:721, 1969
31. Schwartz PJ, Periti M, Malliani A: The long Q-T syndrome. Am Heart J 89:378, 1975
32. Sears GA, Manning GW: Routine electrocardiography: Postprandial T wave changes. Am Heart J 56:591, 1956
33. Simonson E, Baker C, Burns N, et al: Cardiovascular stress (electrocardiographic changes) produced by driving an automobile. Am Heart J 75:125, 1968
34. Sleeper JC, Orgain ES: Differentiation of benign from pathologic T waves in the electrocardiogram. Am J Cardiol 11:338, 1963
35. Surawicz B: The pathogenesis and clinical significance of primary T-wave abnormalities. In Schlant RC, Hurst JW (eds): Advances in Electrocardiography. New York, Grune & Stratton, 1972, p 377
36. Surawicz B, Knoebel SB: Long QT: Good, bad or indifferent? J Am Coll Cardiol 4:398, 1984
37. Thomas J, Harris E, Lassiter G: Observations on the T wave and S-T segment changes in the precordial electrocardiograms of 320 negro adults. Am J Cardiol 5:468, 1960
38. Vincent AM, Abildskov JA, Burgess MJ: Q-T interval syndromes. Prog Cardiovasc Dis 16:523, 1974
39. Ward OC: New familial cardiac syndrome in children. J Ir Med Assoc 54:103, 1964
40. Wasserburger RH, Siebecker KL, Lewis WC: The effect of hyperventilation on the normal adult electrocardiogram. Circulation 13:850, 1956

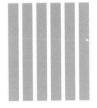

TRAUMATIC HEART DISEASE, CARDIAC TRANSPLANTATION, ARTIFICIAL ELECTRONIC PACEMAKERS, AND AMBULATORY ELECTROCARDIOGRAM

IV

Traumatic Heart Disease and Cardiac Transplantation

26

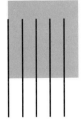

TRAUMATIC HEART DISEASE

Cardiac trauma may be the result of penetrating wound or nonpenetrating injury. The clinical presentation associated with penetrating cardiac injury depends mostly on the location of the penetration and the cardiac structures involved. Although the electrocardiogram (ECG) is helpful in the evaluation of this type of cardiac damage, it is usually not as important as the physical and roentgenographic findings. The ECG is, however, more valuable in the detection of cardiac injuries due to nonpenetrating trauma. The latter entity is the subject of discussion in this text. Electrical injuries to the heart also are included.

Nonpenetrating Cardiac Injury

Most of the nonpenetrating cardiac injuries are the results of motor vehicular impact. The heart usually is compressed by the steering wheel or the latter squeezes the heart between the sternum and the spine. Sudden acceleration or deceleration also may contribute to the cardiac damage. The trauma also may be caused by a direct blow to the chest with a blunt object, a clenched fist, or a kick by an animal. It often occurs during cardiac resuscitation procedures. Serious cardiac damage may be present in the absence of fractures of the bony structures of the chest wall.

The following cardiac lesions may be caused by nonpenetrating chest trauma, myocardial contusion being the most common pathology[31,37]:

1. Pericardium
   a. Disruption
   b. Hemopericardium and tamponade
   c. Pericarditis
2. Myocardium
   a. Contusion
   b. Rupture
   c. Septal perforation
   d. Late aneurysm
3. Valves, chordae tendineae, and papillary muscles: rupture
4. Coronary arteries
   a. Contusion and thrombosis
   b. Laceration

ELECTROCARDIOGRAPHIC CHANGES

1. ST-segment and T-wave changes
2. Reduction of QRS voltage
3. Pseudoinfarction pattern
4. Intraventricular conduction defect
5. Supraventricular and ventricular arrhythmias

The most common ECG changes seen in patients with nonpenetrating cardiac trauma are ST-segment and T-wave abnormalities (Fig. 26–1). The reported incidence of such changes ranges from 17 to 58 percent.[14,31,37,38,47] The different figures are probably related to the severity of the trauma sustained by the patients included in the studies and the timing and frequency of the ECG recordings. The presence of such repolarization abnormalities before the injury cannot be excluded in many of the patients. The ST-segment and T-wave changes usually develop within 24 to 48 hours after injury and often mimic changes due to myocardial ischemia or injury.[31] In most cases, the changes are transient but they may persist. Myocardial contusion or traumatic pericarditis usually is the underlying abnormality. When abnormalities persist, extensive myocardial scarring may be present. Potkin and colleagues cautioned that the ST-segment and T-wave changes are nonspecific for the diagnosis of cardiac injury.[38] They may be noncardiac in origin (Fig. 26–2). Concomitant contusion of the lung, severe hypoxia, head injury, and electrolyte imbalance are some of the possible causes for these repolarization abnormalities. In the series of 100 consecutive patients with nonpenetrating

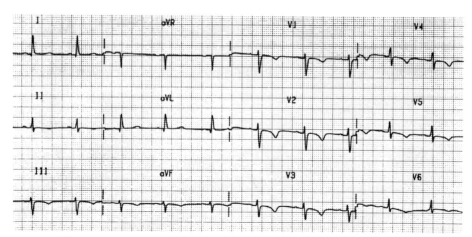

FIGURE 26–1. T-wave abnormalities in nonpenetrating trauma. The patient is a 30-year-old woman involved in an automobile accident in which her chest hit the dashboard of the car. The ECG recorded immediately after the accident showed diffuse T-wave changes that became more marked by the next day, when this tracing was obtained. The T-wave inversion is most pronounced in the precordial leads.

chest trauma reported by Potkin and co-workers, 10 patients had transient ECG abnormalities but no evidence of myocardial contusion at autopsy. Blair and colleagues reported normal ECGs in some patients with autopsy-proven myocardial contusion.[6] Other noninvasive tests of cardiac damage such as cardiac enzymes (CPK-MB) and technetium-99m pyrophosphate scintigraphy have been found to be even less sensitive than the ECG in the diagnosis of myocardial contusion.[38] In the series of Potkin and associates, most patients with documented myocardial contusion at autopsy had normal enzyme values and normal scintigraphic findings.[38]

In patients with pericardial injury, hemopericardium, pericardial effusion, and cardiac tamponade may develop. Their presence may

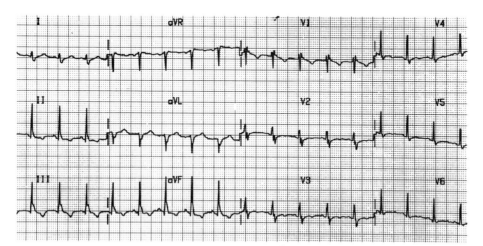

FIGURE 26–2. Abnormal ECG after nonpenetrating trauma without pathologic evidence of cardiac damage. The patient was a 15-year-old boy involved in an automobile accident with multiple trauma, including trauma to the chest. This ECG was obtained shortly after the accident. It shows sinus tachycardia with ST-segment and T-wave abnormalities in the inferior leads and the precordial leads. There is an RSR' pattern in lead V_1 that may be a normal variant, but incomplete right bundle branch block cannot be excluded. Six days after the accident, the patient had cardiac arrest. Although a clinical diagnosis of myocardial contusion was made, the cardiac enzymes, an echocardiogram, and a radionuclide ventriculogram were all normal. The patient died 12 days after the accident. At autopsy, no evidence of cardiac damage could be found. The patient had intracranial hemorrhage, which was probably the cause of death and which might account for the ST and T-wave changes in the ECG.

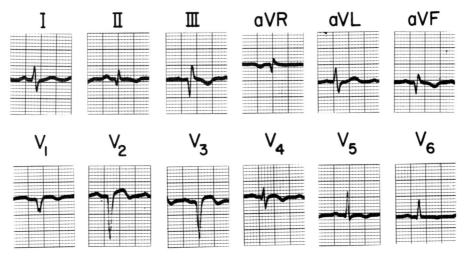

FIGURE 26–3. Myocardial infarction pattern due to myocardial contusion. The tracing was recorded from a 34-year-old man who sustained a nonpenetrating trauma to the chest while riding a motorcycle. The ECG is suggestive of anteroseptal and inferior myocardial infarction. The coronary arteriogram was normal. (This tracing is the same as in Figure 9–52.)

be suggested by a diffuse reduction of the QRS voltage. Recurrent pericardial effusion and chronic constrictive pericarditis also have been reported.[11,15,21]

ECG changes that mimic those of acute myocardial infarction may rarely be seen in patients with severe myocardial contusion. I have seen such changes in a patient involved in a motorcycle accident (Fig. 26–3). His coronary arteriogram was normal. Myocardial infarction as a result of laceration or thrombosis

of the coronary arteries may occur but is uncommon.[36]

Intraventricular conduction defect may occasionally occur in patients with nonpenetrating trauma. The high incidence of 23 percent reported in one series[38] is not observed by most other investigators, including me.[14,17,47] Among patients with such defects, transient right bundle branch block is seen most frequently (Fig. 26–4), but left bundle branch block, bifascicular block, and nonspecific in-

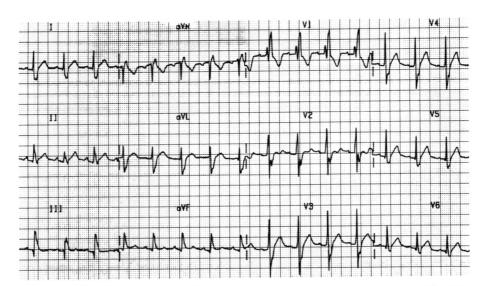

FIGURE 26–4. Right bundle branch block due to nonpenetrating trauma. The patient is a 21-year-old man who was involved in an automobile accident in which his chest hit the steering column. He sustained multiple trauma including laceration of the liver and spleen. The ECG shows complete right bundle branch block, which resolved 4 days later.

traventricular conduction defect also have been reported.[15,22,30,31] Injury, including rupture of the interventricular septum, may be the cause, but the intraventricular conduction defect may appear in the absence of other evidence of myocardial contusion.[15,30,37]

Various cardiac arrhythmias, both supraventricular and ventricular, may develop after nonpenetrating trauma. Sinus tachycardia, sinoatrial (SA) block, sinus arrest, paroxysmal supraventricular tachycardia, atrial flutter and fibrillation, premature ventricular beats, ven-

tricular tachycardia, and ventricular fibrillation have been described[16,31,38] (Fig. 26–5). Ventricular fibrillation may be responsible for sudden death in these patients. Atrioventricular (AV) block of various degrees has been observed.[7,31] Most of these rhythm disorders are transient. In an autopsy case of third-degree AV block due to nonpenetrating trauma, examination of the conduction system revealed hemorrhage in the region of the AV node and AV bundle.[42] The AV bundle was transsected at one point.

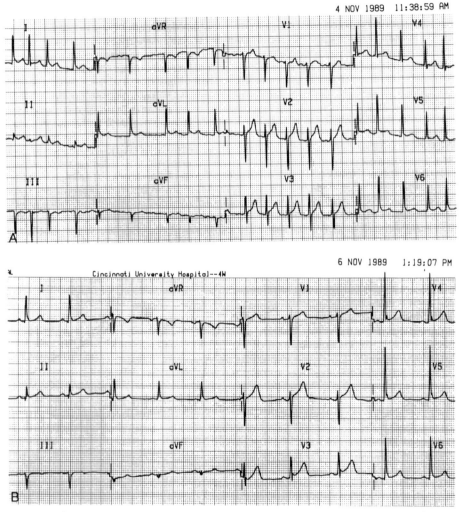

FIGURE 26–5. Atrial fibrillation due to nonpenetrating trauma. The patient was a 32-year-old man who was involved in a head-on automobile collision. He had external evidence of chest injury. He had no previous history of cardiac disease. (A) The ECG taken shortly after the accident shows atrial fibrillation with rapid ventricular response. There is a slight flattening of the T waves in the left precordial leads. Later tracings proved the slight diffuse ST-segment elevation to be due to early repolarization instead of pericarditis. No pericardial rub was heard. Cardiac enzymes and an echocardiogram were normal. The rhythm converted to normal sinus rhythm on the next day. (B) The tracing taken on the third day is normal with rather diffuse ST-segment elevation due to early repolarization.

Electrical Injury

Cardiac damage is an important complication of electrical injury. Sudden death from electrocution is usually due to ventricular fibrillation or cardiac standstill. Alternating current with 40 to 60 cycles/sec is most dangerous to the heart. Cardiac muscle is progressively more tolerant to current of higher frequency.[28] Current flow produces tissue damage by heat, which causes tissue coagulation. The tissue damaged is directly related to the voltage of the electricity, the resistance of the tissue involved, and the duration of the current flow. Most electrical injuries are the results of high-tension (500 volts or greater) alternating current.[13] Lightning also accounts for some cases.[8,27,35] Injury from lightning may result from direct stroke or side flashes in which current discharges from a vertical object through the air to a nearby vertical object. In addition to severe local changes at the points of entry and exit of the current, electrical injury is typically deep and involves skeletal muscle, nervous system, and internal organs, including the heart.

ECG abnormalities have been reported in 10 to 46 percent of patients who have sustained electrical injuries.[9,13,26,43,48] Various arrhythmias, including atrial fibrillation, ventricular tachycardia, and ventricular fibrillation, may develop.[29,34,43] The arrhythmias may appear many hours after the injury and may be recurrent for several months.[29] ST-segment and T-wave changes, some of which resemble those of myocardial ischemia or injury, may occur.[8,9] The QT interval may be prolonged.[8] ECG changes consistent with acute myocardial infarction have been observed in some cases.[9,27,35,43] Right bundle branch block was seen in 3 of 65 cases of electrical injuries reported by DiVincenti and associates.[13]

Figure 26–6 illustrates the myocardial injury pattern and paroxysmal supraventricular tachycardia seen in a patient who sustained electrical injury from a high-tension wire.

CARDIAC TRANSPLANTATION

In orthotopic cardiac transplantation, the recipient heart is removed but the posterior walls of the atria with their venous connections are left in situ. Although removal of the coronary blood supply to the residual atrial tissue may lead to ischemic necrosis in occasional cases, viability of the atrial remnants is maintained in most patients by bronchial collateral vessels that penetrate the atria posteriorly.[45] The donor heart is implanted by suturing its atria to the corresponding structures of the recipient residual atria and anastomosis of the great vessels. The transplanted heart is denervated and lacks autonomic neural control.

The ECG changes seen in cardiac transplant patients are mainly due to persistent electrical activity of the recipient atrial remnants, injury to the donor heart during the transplant procedures, and increased pulmonary vascular resistance in the recipient. Atrial arrhythmias may occur, and ventricular conduction defects are common. The role of the ECG in the diagnosis of acute rejection is controversial. Myocardial infarction may occur as a result of accelerated coronary artery atherosclerosis.

Electrocardiographic Findings After Cardiac Transplantation

1. Two sets of P waves
2. Right bundle branch block, complete or incomplete
3. Left anterior hemiblock
4. Bradyarrhythmias due to sinus node dysfunction; atrial, junctional, and ventricular arrhythmias
5. ST-segment and T-wave changes

TWO SETS OF P WAVES

The activation of the atrial remnants from the preserved sinus node of the recipient heart generates P waves of small amplitude. The excitation of the donor atria from its sinus node gives rise to P waves that usually have normal amplitude and configuration (Figs. 26–7 through 26–9). The suture line between the donor and recipient atria blocks any interchange of the electrical impulses from the two sources. Atrial dissociation is present. The donor atrial impulse is conducted and activates the ventricles, whereas the impulses from the recipient atrial remnants are not conducted. Unless sinus node dysfunction is present, the resting atrial rate of the denervated donor heart is usually faster than the recipient atrial rate.[2]

In the first 63 cardiac transplantation patients who had satisfactory serial 12-lead ECGs at the University of Cincinnati Hospital, two sets of P waves could be identified in 54 (86 percent). The P waves from the recipient atrial remnants may not be seen because of their small amplitude or the presence of sinus node dysfunction or atrial fibrillation prior to the transplantation (Fig. 26–8). Relative isch-

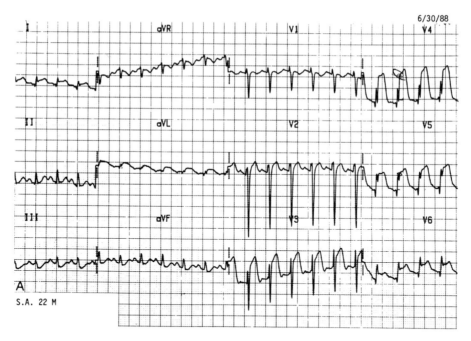

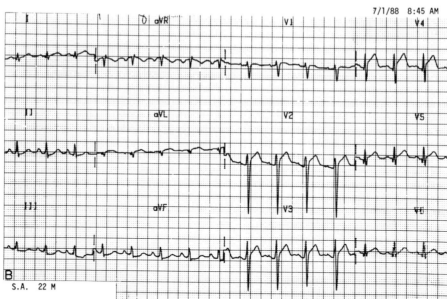

FIGURE 26–6. Electrical injury. The patient was a 22-year-old painter who hit a 4400-volt power line while moving an aluminum ladder. He lost consciousness, and cardiopulmonary resuscitation was applied within a few minutes. After he was transported to a nearby hospital, he was found to have ventricular tachycardia and ventricular fibrillation. Normal sinus rhythm resumed after direct current countershock. (A) The 12-lead ECG shows sinus tachycardia with marked ST-segment elevation in the anterolateral leads to suggest myocardial injury. Anterolateral myocardial infarction may be present. (B) On the next day, the heart rate is slower. The ST-segment elevation in the anterolateral leads is less pronounced. (*Figure continues on next page.*)

emia of the recipient sinus node due to loss of sinus node artery during surgery also may contribute to its dysfunction. Bexton and coworkers described two patients in whom no electrical activity of the recipient atria could be detected despite extensive and careful mapping of the posterior atrial wall.[4]

The absence of any relation between the atrial activities of the two sets of atria may create some perplexing atrial rhythms. Sinus

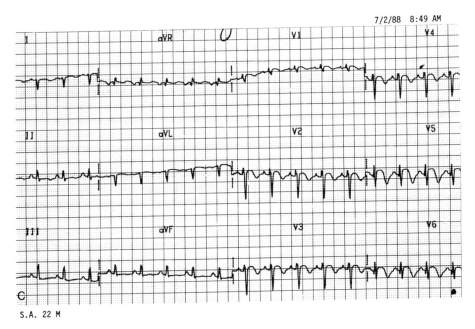

S.A. 22 M

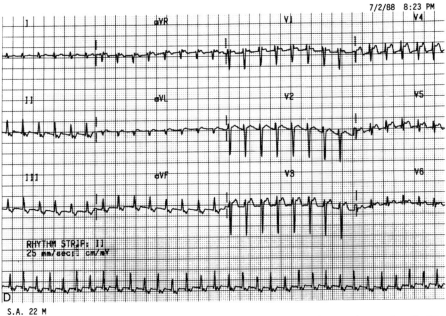

S.A. 22 M

FIGURE 26–6 *Continued* (C) The T waves in the anterolateral leads become inverted on the tracing recorded the next day. The QRS axis is shifted rightward. (D) In the evening of that day, he had paroxysmal supraventricular tachycardia with a rate of 220 beats/min. The mechanism of the tachycardia is most likely AV nodal reentry. Electrical alternans of the QRS complex is present and can be seen best in the rhythm strip. The tachycardia was converted to normal sinus rhythm after intravenous administration of verapamil. The patient's ECG gradually returned to normal in the next few days. His serum creatine phosphokinase level was 5000 IU/L with a MB fraction of 5 percent (normal, 0 to 3 percent) at 6 hours after the accident. It increased to 11,000 IU/L at 24 hours with a MB fraction of 2 percent. An echocardiogram and radionuclide ventriculogram were performed a week after the accident. The findings of both tests were normal.

rhythm may be present in the recipient atrial remnants while atrial flutter or fibrillation is present in the donor atria, or vice versa.[45] Figure 26–9 gives an example of sinus rhythm from the donor heart and atrial flutter from the recipient atrial remnants. Rarely, synchronization of the recipient and donor atria is observed.[4]

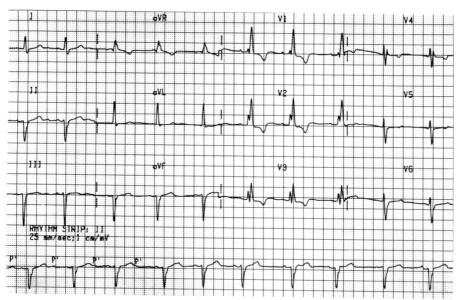

FIGURE 26–7. Two sets of P waves, complete right bundle branch block, and left anterior hemiblock after cardiac transplantation. The patient is a 42-year-old man, and the tracing was obtained 18 months after orthotopic cardiac transplantation. The P waves from the recipient atrial remnants (P's) are small. They are dissociated from the P waves of the donor heart and are not followed by ventricular depolarization.

RIGHT BUNDLE BRANCH BLOCK, COMPLETE OR INCOMPLETE

Right bundle branch block, complete or incomplete, is common after cardiac transplantation (see Figs. 26–7, 26–8, and 26–10). In the 63 cases I reviewed, it occurred in 52 (83 percent). Thirty-four patients had complete right bundle branch block, and 18 patients had incomplete right bundle branch block. In two patients, it was uncertain whether this conduction defect was present because electronic ventricular pacing was required postoperatively. In 5 patients, right bundle branch block (3 complete, 2 incomplete) did not appear in the first postoperative ECG but did appear within a few days. Twelve of the 34 cases of complete right bundle branch block were transient, 11 of them converting to incomplete block and 1 to normal conduction within 60 days. In others, the conduction defect persisted for the duration of the follow-up period (up to 3 years). One of the 18 cases of incomplete right bundle branch block was transient. In a larger series of posttransplantation patients, the incidence of complete right bundle branch block was much lower.[40] It was present at the time of discharge from the hospital in 10 percent of the 191 patients in this series, whereas incomplete right bundle branch block was present in 35 percent. The pathogenesis of the right bundle branch block

is uncertain. Ischemic time and preoperative pulmonary vascular resistance do not appear to be important contributing factors[40] (Fig. 26–10). Sandhu and associates suggested that the conduction defect may be related to posterior rotation of the heart and right ventricular dysfunction.[40]

LEFT ANTERIOR HEMIBLOCK

Left anterior hemiblock occurred in 15 of the 63 transplant patients I reviewed. A lower incidence of 7 percent was reported by Sandhu and colleagues.[40] In 12 of our cases, the hemiblock was present in association with right bundle branch block; in 3, it was isolated (see Figs. 26–7 through 26–11). Because right bundle branch block is common in patients after transplantation, the coexistence of these conduction abnormalities does not necessarily suggest that they had the same cause. Two of the 15 cases of left anterior hemiblock were transient, lasting for less than 3 days. In the other 13 cases, this conduction defect persisted. Complete left bundle branch block was not observed in any of our patients.

POSTTRANSPLANTATION ARRHYTHMIAS

Romhilt and colleagues reported sinus bradycardia in 5 and sinus pauses in 1 of 13 trans-

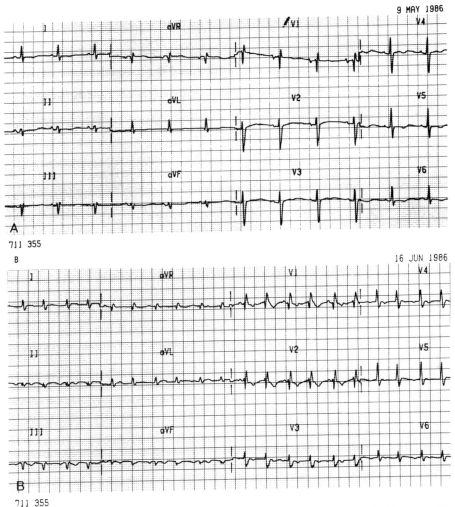

FIGURE 26–8. Atrial flutter and marked decrease in the QRS voltage associated with severe allograft rejection. The patient was a 47-year-old man with dilated cardiomyopathy. Orthotopic cardiac transplantation was performed on April 23, 1986. (A) Tracing obtained 16 days after the surgery. It shows sinus rhythm. P waves from the recipient atrial remnants cannot be identified. There is borderline abnormal left axis deviation and incomplete right bundle branch block. Nonspecific ST and T-wave changes are present. (B) Tracing recorded the day before the patient died. The rhythm is atrial flutter with alternating 1:1 and 2:1 AV conduction. Compared with the tracing on 5-9-86, there is a marked reduction of the QRS voltage in all of the leads. At autopsy the heart weighed 835 g. All four heart chambers were markedly dilated, and the left and right ventricular wall thickness was markedly increased. There was severe myocardial edema. Microscopic examination revealed signs of severe rejection.

plant patients they carefully followed.[39] Mackintosh and associates observed evidence of sinus node dysfunction by electrophysiological studies in 5 of 10 patients in the first 3 weeks after cardiac transplantation.[33] The dysfunction could not be explained solely by the degree of rejection as assessed by endomyocardial biopsy or by the ischemic time of the heart during procurement.[33] Because the subsidiary pacemakers in the denervated heart may be unreliable in providing an escape rhythm, sudden death may occur.[33] In some patients, the sinus node dysfunction persists and permanent electronic pacemakers are needed.[39] Even in the asymptomatic long-term survivors of cardiac transplantation, Bexton and co-workers found prolonged donor sinus node recovery and SA conduction time in 4 of 14 patients.[4]

Premature atrial beats, paroxysmal supraventricular tachycardia, and atrial flutter and fibrillation are seen both during the postoperative period and in long-term survivors.[39,41] Although earlier data suggest that atrial ar-

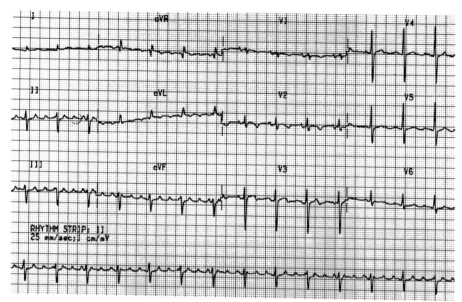

FIGURE 26–9. Atrial flutter originated from the recipient atrial remnants. Sinus P waves from the donor atria can best be seen preceding the QRS complexes in leads V_1 and V_2. In the other leads, they are distorted or masked by the flutter waves generated from the recipient atrial remnants. The tracing also demonstrates left anterior hemiblock and nonspecific T-wave changes.

rhythmias often are associated with rejection episodes,[41] we have not observed such a relationship to any degree of consistency. Occasional cases of atrial flutter that developed in the long-term survivors of transplantation did have biopsy evidence of moderate or severe rejection, however. An example is given in Figure 26–8B.

AV junctional rhythm was observed in 67 percent of Romhilt's series during the early posttransplantation period (within 70 days), usually within the first week after transplant.[39] The junctional rates ranged from 27 to 120 beats/min (Fig. 26–10B).

The electrophysiological characteristics of the AV conduction system of the denervated transplanted heart are similar to those of the innervated heart.[5] First-degree AV block is occasionally seen in patients after transplantation. I have encountered only 2 patients with second-degree AV block on the 12-lead ECG in the 63 cases reviewed. One of them was found to have severe coronary artery disease at autopsy 2 months after the appearance of the conduction defect. A case of complete AV block attributed to acute rejection has been described.[32]

Premature ventricular beats are common after transplantation but usually are few in number.[1,39] The development of complex ven-

tricular ectopies in the late posttransplantation period (greater than 70 days) and in long-term survivors (more than 6 months) usually is associated with the presence of severe coronary artery disease and high mortality.[39] An example is given in Figure 26–11.

ST-SEGMENT AND T-WAVE CHANGES

ST-segment and T-wave abnormalities are common in patients who have received cardiac transplants. Some patients may develop diffuse ST-segment elevation followed by evolutionary changes of the ST segment and T waves consistent with acute pericarditis in the early postoperative period. The pericarditis is probably traumatic in origin, related to the transplantation procedures. As a rule, such ST-segment and T-wave changes are transient.

Not uncommonly, marked ST-segment and T-wave changes suggestive of myocardial ischemia are seen postoperatively or in long-term survivors (Fig. 26–12). The cause of these repolarization abnormalities is often not apparent. In most cases, they are not associated with biopsy evidence of acute rejection and their coronary arteriograms are normal (see Fig. 26–12). In some cases, however, the ST-segment and T-wave changes may be the only ECG signs of myocardial infarction.[20]

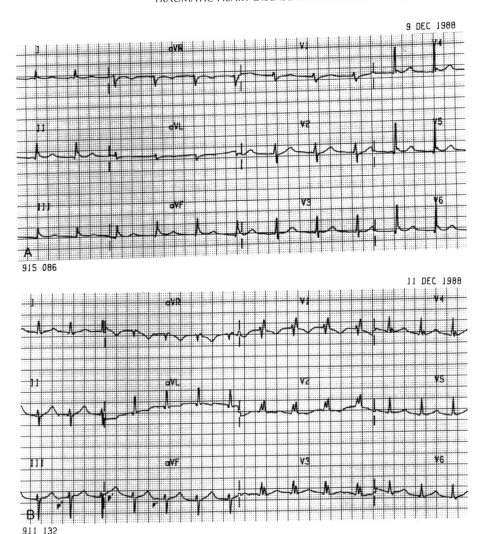

FIGURE 26–10. The donor's ECG and the ECG of the recipient after cardiac transplantation. (A) Tracing obtained from the donor (aged 37 years) the day before he died of severe head injuries. It shows abnormal P waves and slight prolongation of the QT interval. (B) Tracing recorded 1 day after the donor heart was transplanted to the 51-year-old recipient. It shows an accelerated AV junctional rhythm. A separate and dissociated set of P waves from the recipient atrial remnants (P's) can be seen. There is also left anterior hemiblock and complete right bundle branch block. The donor and the recipient were located in the same hospital at the time of transplantation. The ischemic time was relatively short.

Electrocardiographic Signs of Acute Rejection

A significant reduction in the QRS voltage was held as a reliable predictor of cardiac rejection in the early days of cardiac transplantation.[44] Its diagnostic value has been questioned in recent years.[10,12,24] Locke and associates followed 10 patients with daily ECGs, and 600 tracings were recorded during this study.[32] The tracings were analyzed and correlated with the findings of 147 endomyocardial biopsies. A 20 percent reduction in the summated QRS voltages from leads I, II, III, V_1, and V_6 was used as the criterion for a significant decrease in the voltage. During the study period, there were 18 episodes of acute rejection based on the biopsy findings. Only 3 episodes of rejection were accompanied by a significant decrease in the QRS voltage. Conversely, 20 other ECGs showed such a decrease in the voltage but were not associated with biopsy evidence of rejection. Pericardial or pleural effusion, generalized edema, and pulmonary and systemic infection were suggested as the possible causes for the false-pos-

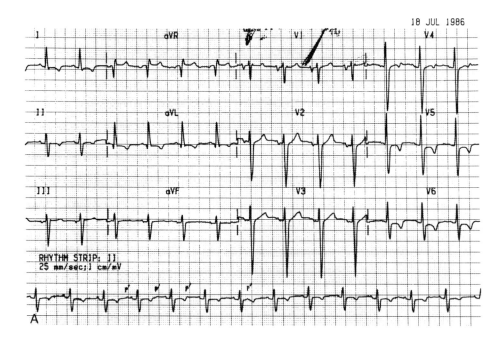

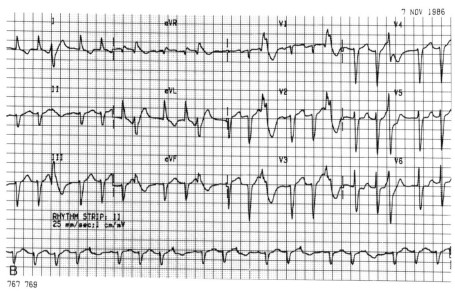

767 769

FIGURE 26–11. Frequent premature ventricular beats associated with severe acute allograft rejection and diffuse coronary artery disease. The patient was a 50-year-old man with a history of idiopathic dilated cardiomyopathy. Orthotopic cardiac transplantation was performed 3 days before tracing A was recorded. The tracing shows two sets of P waves. The P waves from the recipient atrial remnants (P's) are small. The donor P waves show a large negative component in lead V_1 suggestive of left atrial abnormality. There is left anterior hemiblock. ST-segment depression and T-wave inversion are present in the anterolateral leads. Endomyocardial biopsy on that day revealed no evidence of rejection. (B) Tracing recorded while the patient was having severe rejection. It shows sinus tachycardia with frequent premature ventricular beats and episodes of trigeminal rhythm. There is left anterior hemiblock with additional intraventricular conduction defect. The QRS duration is longer than that on the previous tracing. There is poor R-wave progression in the precordial leads, with clockwise rotation, which probably is related to the conduction defects. The patient deteriorated clinically and underwent retransplantation 10 days later. The explanted heart showed severe acute allograft rejection. The major coronary arteries had diffuse atherosclerosis with 80 percent luminal narrowing of the distal right coronary artery and 50 percent narrowing of the proximal anterior descending artery. The lumens of the distal branches of the left anterior descending and circumflex arteries also were reduced considerably.

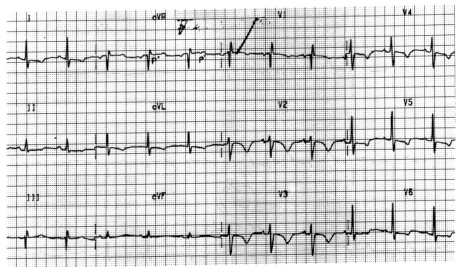

FIGURE 26–12. Ischemic ST-segment and T-wave changes in the absence of coronary artery disease or signs of allograft rejection. The tracing was obtained 1 week after orthotopic cardiac transplantation. Two sets of P waves are present, but the P waves from the recipient atrial remnants are small. There is incomplete right bundle branch block. The QT interval is prolonged. The T waves in leads V_2 through V_4 are deeply inverted. Slight ST-segment depression and T-wave inversion also are present in the anterolateral leads. These ST and T-wave abnormalities are more pronounced than those in the previous tracings obtained postoperatively. Endomyocardial biopsy performed on the same day when this tracing was recorded showed no evidence of rejection. Two yearly coronary arteriograms made since that time were normal.

itive diagnosis. They concluded that the ECG is unreliable in the diagnosis of cardiac rejection. Its value in this regard has diminished in recent years probably because different immunosuppressive agents are being used.

In the 63 cases I reviewed, a *marked* reduction of the QRS voltage in all leads was seen in 4 patients. They all had severe rejection resulting in death (see Fig. 26–8). Quantitative analysis of the voltage changes was not performed in this series.

A rightward shift of the QRS axis, ST-segment depression, T-wave inversion, and atrial arrhythmias also were suggested as signs of acute rejection in the early years of cardiac transplantation.[23,41] No evidence supports their value in the prediction of rejection in patients who have undergone cardiac transplantation in recent years.

Accelerated Coronary Artery Atherosclerosis

The development of accelerated coronary artery disease is a major complication in long-term survivors of cardiac transplantation. Postoperative coronary arteriograms have demonstrated diseased vessels in about 40 percent of the patients at 3 years.[18,46] The ac-

celerated coronary artery disease is equally frequent in patients who initially had idiopathic cardiomyopathy and in those who had ischemic heart disease. Immunologic injury of the coronary endothelium was suggested as one of the major causes of this pathologic process.

Angiographically, the accelerated coronary artery disease in the transplanted heart is a mixture of "ordinary" proximal lesions and unusual diffuse obliterative disease.[19] The latter is characterized by concentric and longitudinal narrowing with distal pruning, vessel obliteration, and absence of collateral vessels.

In patients with cardiac transplants, ischemic heart disease is usually clinically silent because the allograft is denervated and lacks afferent pain fibers. Among the 22 cases of acute myocardial infarction diagnosed by autopsy or from the explanted hearts at Stanford University, only 3 patients had chest or arm pain.[20] The ECGs showed abnormal Q waves in 11 of the cases. Pathologically, 14 hearts had transmural myocardial infarction. Among the hearts with nontransmural infarct, 4 had multiple infarcts.

Figure 26–13 illustrates a case of acute myocardial infarction after transplantation in a patient from our institution.

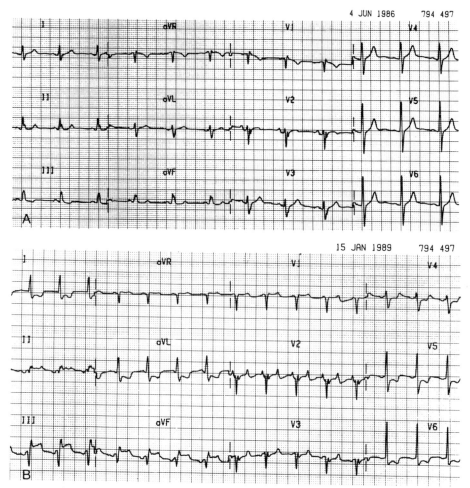

FIGURE 26–13. Accelerated coronary atherosclerosis with acute inferior myocardial infarction after cardiac transplantation. The patient was a 28-year-old man with a history of idiopathic dilated cardiomyopathy. Cardiac transplantation was performed 2 years before the recording of tracing A. The tracing shows two sets of P waves and incomplete right bundle branch block. Coronary arteriogram performed at that time was normal. In June 1988, a repeat coronary arteriogram revealed 20 percent narrowing in the proximal portion of the dominant right coronary artery. The left coronary artery was normal. The patient complained of shortness of breath 2 days before the recording of tracing B. The ECG revealed atrial flutter with changes of acute inferior myocardial infarction. The tracing also shows poor R-wave progression in the right precordial leads. The ST-segment depression and T-wave inversion in the anterolateral leads probably represent reciprocal changes of the acute inferior infarction. Coronary arteriogram performed 4 days later revealed complete occlusion of the right coronary artery in its midportion. The patient died 25 days later. At autopsy, the heart weighed 685 g, with dilatation of both atria and ventricles and left ventricular hypertrophy. The coronary arteries showed atherosclerosis. The right coronary artery was occluded at its proximal portion. A transmural inferior myocardial infarction was found extending from the apex to the base. Microscopic examination revealed acute cellular and chronic vascular rejection of the allograft.

REFERENCES

1. Alexopoulos D, Yusuf S, Bostock J, et al: Ventricular arrhythmias in long-term survivors of orthotopic and heterotopic cardiac transplantation. Br Heart J 59:648, 1988
2. Alexopoulos D, Yusuf S, Johnston JA, et al: The 24-hour heart rate behavior in long-term survivors of cardiac transplantation. Am J Cardiol 61:880, 1988
3. Bexton R, Nathan AW, Hellestrand KJ, et al: Electrophysiological abnormalities in the transplanted human heart. Br Heart J 50:555, 1983
4. Bexton RS, Nathan AW, Hellestrand KJ, et al: Sino-atrial function after cardiac transplantation. J Am Coll Cardiol 3:712, 1984
5. Bexton RS, Nathan AW, Hellestrand KJ, et al: The electrophysiologic characteristics of the transplanted human heart. Am Heart J 107:1, 1984

6. Blair E, Topuzlu C, Davis JH: Delayed or missed diagnosis of cardiac damage in blunt chest trauma. J Trauma 11:129, 1971

7. Brennan JA, Field JM, Liedtke J: Reversible heart block following nonpenetrating chest trauma. J Trauma 19:784, 1979

8. Burda CD: Electrocardiographic changes in lightning stroke. Am Heart J 72:521, 1966

9. Butler ED, Gant TD: Electrical injuries, with special reference to the upper extremities. Am J Surg 134:95, 1977

10. Cooper DKC, Charles RG, Rose AG, et al: Does the electrocardiogram detect early acute heart rejection. Heart Transplant IV:546, 1985

11. Deterling RA, Humphreys GH: Factors in the etiology of constrictive pericarditis. Circulation 12:30, 1955

12. Deviveni R, McKenzie N, Kostuk WJ, et al: Cyclosporine in cardiac transplantation: Observations on immunologic monitoring, cardiac history, and cardiac function. Heart Transplant 2:219, 1983

13. DiVincenti FC, Moncrief JA, Pruitt BA: Electrical injuries: A review of 65 cases. J Trauma 9:497, 1969

14. Dolara A, Morando P, Pampaloni M: Electrocardiographic findings in 98 consecutive non-penetrating chest injuries. Dis Chest 52:50, 1967

15. Dolara A, Pazzi L: Atrioventricular and intraventricular conduction defects after nonpenetrating trauma. Am Heart J 72:138, 1966

16. Fox KM, Rowland E, Krikler DM, et al: Electrophysiological manifestations of non-penetrating cardiac trauma. Br Heart J 43:458, 1980

17. Frazee RC, Mucha P, Farnell MB, Miller FA: Objective evaluation of blunt cardiac trauma. J Trauma 26:510, 1986

18. Gao S, Alderman EL, Schroeder JS, et al: Accelerated coronary vascular disease in the heart transplant patient: Coronary arteriographic findings. J Am Coll Cardiol 12:334, 1988

19. Gao S, Schroeder JS, Alderman EL, et al: Clinical and laboratory correlates of accelerated coronary artery disease in the cardiac transplant patient. Circulation 76(Suppl V):V-56, 1987

20. Gao S, Schroeder JS, Hunt SA, et al: Acute myocardial infarction in cardiac transplant recipients. Am J Cardiol 64:1093, 1989

21. Goodkind MJ, Bloomer WE, Goodyer A: Recurrent pericardial effusion after nonpenetrating chest trauma: Report of two cases treated with adrenocortical steroids. N Engl J Med 263:874, 1960

22. Gozo EG, Cohen HC, Pick A: Traumatic bifascicular intraventricular block. Chest 61:294, 1972

23. Griepp RB, Stinson EB, Dong E, et al: Acute rejection of the allografted human heart. Ann Thorac Surg 12:113, 1971

24. Griffith BP, Hardesty RL, Thompson ME, et al: Cardiac transplantation with cyclosporine: The Pittsburgh experience. Heart Transplant 2:251, 1983

25. Guest JL, Hall DP, Yeh TJ, Ellison RG: Late manifestations of trauma to the pericardium. Surg Gynecol Obstet 120:787, 1965

26. Hammond J, Ward G: Myocardial damage and electrical injuries: Significance of early elevation of CPK-MB isoenzymes. South Med J 79:414, 1986

27. Jackson SHD, Parry DJ: Lightning and the heart. Br Heart J 43:454, 1980

28. Jaffe RH: Electropathology: A review of the pathologic changes produced by electric currents. Arch Pathol 5:837, 1928

29. Jensen PJ, Thomsen P, Bagger J, et al: Electrical injury causing ventricular arrhythmias. Br Heart J 57:279, 1987

30. Kumpuris AG, Casale TB, Mokotoff DM, et al: Right bundle-branch block: Occurrence following nonpenetrating chest trauma without evidence of cardiac contusion. JAMA 242:172, 1979

31. Liedtke AJ, DeMuth WE: Nonpenetrating cardiac injuries: A collective review. Am Heart J 86:687, 1973

32. Locke TJ, Karnik R, McGregor CGA, Bexton RS: The value of the electrocardiogram in the diagnosis of acute rejection after orthotopic heart transplantation. Transplant Int 2:143, 1989

33. Mackintosh AF, Carmichael DJ, Wren C, et al: Sinus node function in first three weeks after cardiac transplantation. Br Heart J 48:584, 1982

34. Morgan ZV, Headley RN, Alexander EA, Sawyer CG: Atrial fibrillation and epidural hematoma associated with lightning stroke. N Engl J Med 259:956, 1956

35. Myers GJ, Colgan MT, VanDyke DH: Lightning-strike disaster among children. JAMA 238:1045, 1977

36. Oliva PB, Hilgenberg A, McElroy D: Obstruction of the proximal right coronary artery with acute inferior infarction due to blunt chest trauma. Ann Intern Med 91:205, 1979

37. Parmley LF, Manion MW, Mattingly TW: Nonpenetrating traumatic injury of the heart. Circulation 18:371, 1958

38. Potkin RT, Werner JA, Trobaugh GB, et al: Evaluation of noninvasive tests of cardiac damage in suspected cardiac contusion. Circulation 66:627, 1982

39. Romhilt DW, Doyle M, Sagar KB, et al: Prevalence and significance of arrhythmias in long-term survivors of cardiac transplantation. Circulation 66(Suppl I):I-219, 1982

40. Sandhu JS, Curtiss EI, Follansbee WP, et al: The scalar electrocardiogram of the orthotopic heart transplant recipient. Am Heart J 119:917, 1990

41. Schroeder JS, Berke DK, Graham AF, et al: Arrhythmias after cardiac transplantation. Am J Cardiol 33:604, 1974

42. Sims BA, Geddes JS: Traumatic heart block. Br Heart J 31:140, 1969

43. Solem L, Fischer RP, Strate RG: The natural history of electrical injury. J Trauma 17:487, 1977

44. Stinson EB, Dong E, Bieber CP, et al: Cardiac transplantation in man. I. Early rejection. JAMA 207:2233, 1969

45. Stinson EB, Schroeder JS, Griepp RB, et al: Observations on the behavior of recipient atria after cardiac transplantation in man. Am J Cardiol 30:615, 1972

46. Uretsky BF, Murali S, Reddy S, et al: Development of coronary artery disease in cardiac transplant patients receiving immunosuppressive therapy with cyclosporine and prednisone. Circulation 76:827, 1987

47. Watson JH, Bartholomae WM: Cardiac injury due to nonpenetrating chest trauma. Ann Int Med 52:871, 1960

48. Wilkinson C, Wood M: High voltage electric injury. Am J Surg 136:693, 1978

Artificial Electronic Pacemakers

27

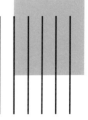

An electronic pacemaker system has two major components, the pulse generator and the lead. The many types of artificial pacemakers differ mainly in the characteristics of the pulse generator, whereas the lead is either bipolar or unipolar. For temporary pacing, an external pulse generator is used. The lead, in most instances, is introduced intravenously to the endocardium of the right heart, usually the right ventice. In postoperative patients, the lead may be connected transthoracically to the myocardium. For permanent pacing, the pacemaker is implanted and the site of stimulation may be either endocardium by the transvenous route or epicardium-myocardium through thoracotomy. This chapter focuses mainly on the electrocardiographic (ECG) findings in patients with implanted pacemakers.

As a result of rapid advance of pacemaker technology, many types of implantable pacemakers are available. Pacing of the heart may involve one or two chambers. Spontaneous depolarization of the ventricle or atrium or both may be sensed and, in turn, may inhibit or trigger pacing. All modern pacemakers can be programmed at the time of implantation or later by noninvasive means to obtain the desired features such as the pacing rate, the duration and amplitude of the stimulating pulse, the minimal voltage to be sensed, the pacing mode, and other functions of the pacemaker. Many pacemakers also have telemetry functions to provide information such as programmed and present parameter values, pulse generator battery status, lead resistance, intracardiac electrograms, and implantation data entered by the physician.

PACEMAKER CODE

Because of the increasing complexity of the designs of some of the newer pacemakers, the interpretation of the ECGs of patients with these pacemakers may be difficult. This is es-
pecially true if the characteristics of the pacemaker are not known to the electrocardiographer. Pacemakers used for the treatment of tachyarrhythmias and automatic implantable cardioverter–defibrillators (AICDs) also have been developed. Discussion of these devices is beyond the scope of this text. The advantages and disadvantages of the various types of pacemakers also are not dealt with.

To identify the types of implantable cardiac pacemakers, a three-position code was proposed by the Intersociety Commission for Heart Disease Resources (ICHD) in 1974.[33] The code has been widely used by both physicians and pacemaker manufacturers. The first letter of the code indicates the chamber paced, the second the chamber sensed, and the third the mode of response. For example, the code for the commonly used ventricular demand (ventricular inhibited) pacemaker is VVI. The pacemaker paces the ventricle (V), senses the ventricle (V), and is inhibited (I) by a sensed signal. Table 27–1 lists the three positions and the letter used under each category.

In 1981, to accommodate the newer developments involving noninvasive programming and pacing to control tachyarrhythmias, a five-position pacemaker code was proposed by ICHD (Table 27–2).[34] The symbols placed in the first three positions are the same as they were previously in the three-position code, except an *S* (single-chamber) may be used by the manufacturer in the first and second positions to label programmable pacemaker that is adaptable for either atrial or ventricular use. The letter *R* (reverse) is added in the third position to indicate a function in which the pacemaker is silent when the intrinsic rate is slow but discharges when the rate is faster than a preset value to terminate tachycardia. The fourth position gives the programmable functions. The letter *C* (communicating) indicates a telemetric function to provide information for record keeping, regarding the state

TABLE 27–1. Three-Position Pacemaker Code (ICHD)

Position	I	II	III
Category	Chamber Paced	Chamber Sensed	Mode of Response
Letters used	V—ventricle A—atrium D—double chamber	V—ventricle A—atrium D—double chamber O—none	I—inhibited T—triggered D—double O—none

of the pacemaker hardware and physiological data such as intracardiac electrogram. The fifth position indicates special antitachyarrhythmia functions. For example, the code VVI,M (or VVIM, a comma separating the third and fourth positions is optional) indicates ventricular pacing, ventricular sensing, inhibited mode, and multiprogrammable. The code AOO,OE is used for a pacemaker that is atrial pacing, nonsensing, nonprogrammable, and externally activated.

As most of the pacemakers are implanted for the treatment of bradycardia and are programmable, the three-position code remains in common use because of its simplicity. It also meets our needs in this chapter.

PACEMAKER SPIKE (PACEMAKER STIMULUS, ARTIFACT, IMPULSE, PULSE)

The pacemaker impulse is recognized in the ECG as a sharp narrow spike (Fig. 27–1). Its duration is generally less than 2 msec,[21] and it appears as a vertical line on the routine ECG. When the pacing spike is large, however, it is often followed by an exponential voltage decay curve that may distort or even mask the depolarization waveform induced by the pacemaker[27] (Fig. 27–2).

As a rule, pacemakers with a unipolar lead give much larger pacing spikes than those produced by bipolar pacemakers (Fig. 27–3). Bipolar epicardial–myocardial leads given even smaller spikes than do bipolar endocardial leads[21] (see Fig. 27–4). In bipolar leads, the negative electrode usually is located at the tip of the catheter and the positive electrode is 1 cm proximal to the tip. The electric current flows from the negative toward the positive electrode to complete the electrical circuit. In unipolar pacemakers, the active electrode, the cathode, is located at the tip of the catheter, and the indifferent electrode, the anode, is the exposed metal portion of the pulse generator. The electrical current flows from the tip of the electrode catheter to the indifferent electrode through the body tissue and fluid. Because of the greater distance between the two electrodes and, therefore, the bigger electric dipole, the magnitude of the spike from unipolar pacemakers is larger. The longer distance between the electrodes also renders the pacemaker more vulnerable to extrinsic signal interference, such as electromagnetic and myopotential interference from skeletal muscles.

TABLE 27–2. Five-Position Pacemaker Code (ICHD)*

Position	I	II	III	IV	V
Category	Chamber paced	Chamber sensed	Modes of Response	Programmable Functions	Special Antitachyarrhythmia Functions
Letters used	V—ventricle	V—ventricle	T—triggered	P—programmable (rate and/or output)	B—bursts
	A—atrium	A—atrium	I—inhibited	M—multiprogrammable	N—normal rate competition
	D—double	D—double	D—double†	C—communicating	S—scanning
		O—none	O—none		
			R—reverse	O—none	E—external
Manufacturer's designation only	S—single chamber	S—single chamber	↓ Comma optional here		

*Reproduced from Parsonnet V, Furman S, Smyth NPD, et al: Optimal resources for implantable cardiac pacemakers. Circulation 68:227A, 1983, by permission.
†Triggered and inhibited response.

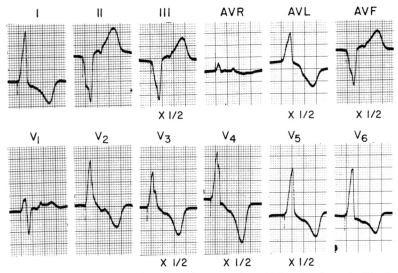

FIGURE 27-1. Transvenous right ventricular pacemaker with bipolar electrode. The tip of the electrode is located at the apex of the right ventricle. The pacemaker spikes are narrow and relatively small in amplitude. The QRS-T morphology resembles that of complete left bundle branch block. Retrograde capture of the atria is present.

FIGURE 27-2. Pacemaker spike decay curve. The tracing was recorded from a patient with malfunctioning ventricular demand pacemaker (VVI). It was selected to demonstrate pure pacer artifacts without being altered by depolarization potential. There is constant failure to capture and intermittent failure of sensing. The gradual downward inscriptions following the spikes represent the spike decay curves, one of which is indicated by an arrow. They are more prominent than those produced by most pacemakers.

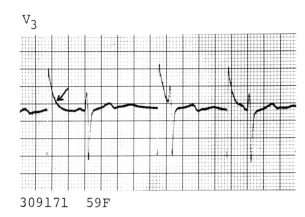

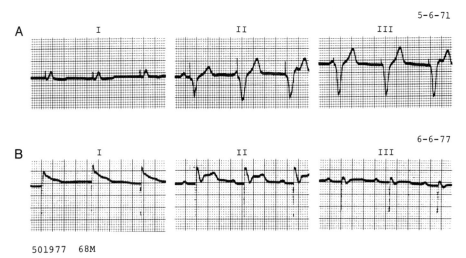

FIGURE 27-3. Pacemaker spikes from bipolar and unipolar leads. Both tracings were recorded from the same patient. (A) Tracing obtained when the patient had a transvenous bipolar lead. The amplitude of the pacemaker spikes is relatively small. The first complex in lead II is a fusion beat. (B) Tracing recorded after a transvenous unipolar lead was used. The amplitude of the spikes is much larger. Spike decay curves are present, causing distortion of the QRS complexes.

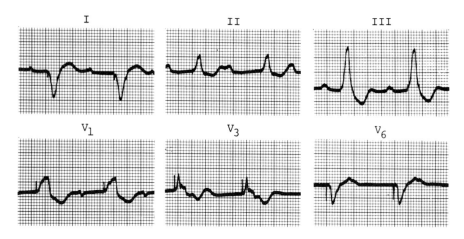

417352   65F

FIGURE 27–4. Left ventricular epicardial pacemaker with a bipolar lead. Note the small amplitude of the pacemaker spikes. The QRS complexes show right axis deviation and a right bundle branch block pattern.

Tracings recorded with digital electrocardiography may display unusually large pacemaker spikes because they are artificially simulated. Therefore, they do not have the same implications.

Whether the pacemaker is endocardial or epicardial–myocardial, unipolar or bipolar, the voltage and polarity of the pacing impulse differ in the various leads of the ECG. The amplitude and polarity of the spike in a certain lead depend on the relation between the axis of the lead and the spatial orientation of the spike vector. For example, with a transvenous bipolar electrode located at the apex of the right ventricle the vector of the pacing impulse is directed toward the negative side of lead II (because the negative electrode is at the tip of the catheter and the positive electrode is proximal to it). Therefore, lead II usually records a large negative spike and lead aVR, a large positive spike. Leads that are perpendicular to the spike vector record a small deflection. With a unipolar electrode the vector of the pacer impulse has an orientation

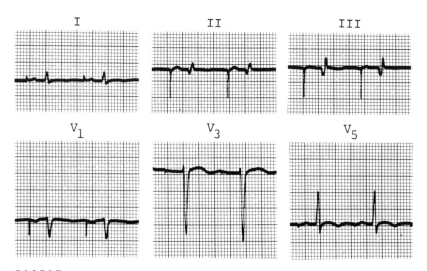

502537

FIGURE 27–5. Fixed-rate atrial pacemaker (AOO). The lead (bipolar) was implanted, through thoracotomy, in the region of the sinoatrial node of the right atrium. The morphology of the P waves resembles that of normal sinus beats.

parallel to a line joining the tip of the catheter to the pulse generator, the latter having the positive polarity. The actual direction of the vector therefore depends on the location of the pulse generator as well as on the pacing site.

Morphology of the Electrocardiographic Complexes Induced by Artificial Pacing

ATRIAL PACING

The morphology of the waveform induced by pacing depends on the site of stimulation. With atrial pacing, the pacer artifacts are followed by ectopic P waves. If the right atrium is stimulated, the P-wave morphology resembles that of sinus beats if the site of stimulation is near the sinus node (Fig. 27–5). If a transvenous catheter is implanted in the coronary sinus, the P-wave axis is directed superiorly, and inverted P waves are recorded in the inferior leads.

VENTRICULAR PACING

With ventricular pacing, the pacer impulse is followed by an abnormal QRS complex, the characteristics of which usually give a fairly good indication of the location of the stimulating electrode. Right ventricular pacing is accompanied by QRS complexes similar to those of complete left bundle branch block (see Figs. 27–1 and 27–20). In most cases of transvenous ventricular pacing, the tip of the electrode is located at the apex of the right ventricle. The induced sequence of ventricular activation is from right to left and from apex to base. The apex-to-base sequence of depolarization results in a superior orientation of the QRS vector and abnormal left axis deviation in the front plane. In many patients, although typical complete left bundle branch block pattern is seen in the limb leads and lead V_1, lead V_6 has an essentially downward deflection (Fig. 27–6). This finding is due to the direction of lead axis of V_6, which is not only leftward but also slightly downward. When there is marked superior displacement of the QRS forces, they may project on the negative side of the lead axis of V_6.

If the site of stimulation is at the inflow or outflow tract of the right ventricle, the frontal plane QRS axis is usually normal. If it is immediately below the pulmonary valve, the QRS axis becomes vertical or even rightward.[7]

With left ventricular epicardial–myocardial pacing the 12-lead ECG displays a complete right bundle branch block pattern. When the electrode is implanted in the mid- to high lateral portions of the left ventricle, there is right axis deviation, leads I and V_6 having an essentially negative deflection and lead V_1 having an R wave (see Figs. 27–4 and 27–20). When the stimulation site is near the apex, an $S_1S_2S_3$ pattern is seen as the activation front advances rightward and superiorly. Occasionally, left ventricular pacing near the apex may produce an essentially negative QRS deflection in lead V_1. In that case, it may be impossible to determine from the ECG whether the left or right ventricle is being paced.[7]

PACING-INDUCED T-WAVE CHANGES

In patients with artificial ventricular pacemakers, striking T-wave inversion may develop in the spontaneous beats that simulate those

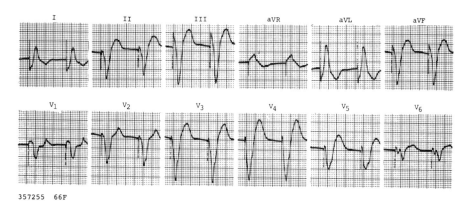

357255 66F

FIGURE 27–6. Transvenous right ventricular pacemaker. The QRS complex in lead V_6 has a predominantly negative deflection rather than an upright deflection that would be expected in left bundle branch block.

caused by myocardial ischemia. The inverted T waves are usually broad and associated with QT prolongation. They are seen most commonly in the inferior leads and left precordial leads[9,10,20] (see Fig. 9–71).

TYPES, MODES, AND CODES OF IMPLANTABLE PACEMAKERS

Atrial pacing
  Atrial asynchronous AOO
  Atrial demand
    Atrial inhibited AAI
    Atrial triggered AAT
Ventricular pacing
  Ventricular asynchronous VOO
  Ventricular demand
    Ventricular inhibited VVI
    Ventricular triggered VVT
  Atrial synchronous VAT
  Atrial synchronous ventricular inhibited VDD
Dual chamber pacing
  AV sequential DVI
  AV universal DDD

Most available pacemakers can be programmed noninvasively through a radiofrequency or an electromagnetic signal to the mode of cardiac pacing best suited to the needs of the individual patient. Although a single-chamber pacemaker has limited programmable options, a dual-chamber pacemaker such as DDD can be programmed to all the modes of pacing listed above.

ATRIAL ASYNCHRONOUS PACEMAKERS (AOO) (see Fig. 27–5)

The atrial asyncrhonous pacemaker is also called *fixed-rate atrial pacemaker.* It has no sensing function. Its lead is connected to the right atrium, which it paces at a preset rate regardless of the patient's own heart rate or rhythm. Normal ventricular activation depends on an intact AV conduction system. This type of pacemaker is rarely used today.

ATRIAL DEMAND PACEMAKERS (AAI, AAT)

Atrial demand pacemakers, either atrial inhibited or atrial triggered, pace the atrium and sense the atrial impulse. In the case of atrial inhibited pacemakers (AAI), the presence of spontaneous atrial activity with a rate greater than (or the PP interval less than) a predetermined level no stimulus would be delivered.

With the atrial triggered pacemakers (AAT), the pacer senses the atrial impulse and stimulates the atrium when the atrial rate falls below a certain level, but it also delivers stimuli when it senses native P waves. As in the case of atrial asynchronous pacemakers, both types of atrial demand pacemakers are seldom used today.

VENTRICULAR ASYNCHRONOUS PACEMAKERS (VOO)

Asynchronous ventricular pacemakers also are called *fixed-rate ventricular pacemakers.* The pacer delivers stimuli at a constant rate regardless of the patient's own heart rate or rhythm. The artificial impulses compete with the patient's spontaneous ventricular beats if the latter are present. The pacemaker spikes are seen regularly at a preselected interval, and each stimulus is followed by a QRS complex unless the stimulus occurs during the ventricular refractory period (Fig. 27–7). The resulting rhythm is similar to ventricular parasystole. Fusion beats may be seen, part of the ventricles being depolarized by the artificial pacemaker and part by the patient's own impulse.

The fixed-rate ventricular pacemakers are rarely used. In many patients, the bradyarrhythmia for which the pacemaker is used is intermittent. There is a risk that the artificial stimulus may fall within the vulnerable period, resulting in ventricular fibrillation. Although this risk is low in most patients, it increases if there is myocardial ischemia, electrolyte imbalance, or drug toxicity.[15]

During the follow-up of patients with ventricular demand pacemaker, an ECG is often obtained while a magnet is applied to the pulse generator. The magnet converts the pacemaker from the demand mode to a fixed-rate mode. It is mostly under this condition that ventricular asynchronous pacing is observed clinically (see Fig. 27–7).

VENTRICULAR DEMAND PACEMAKERS (VVI, VVT)

Ventricular Inhibited Pacemakers (VVI)

Ventricular demand pacemakers are the most popular pacemakers in use. This is especially true for the ventricular inhibited type (VVI). It is a common practice among clinicians to imply ventricular *inhibited* pacemaker when they use the more general term ventricular *demand* pacemaker. The VVI pacemaker gener-

lead II

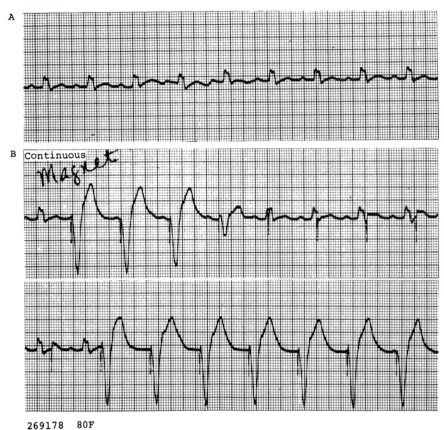

269178   80F

FIGURE 27-7. Ventricular demand pacemaker (VVI) converted to a fixed-rate pacemaker by magnet. (A) Tracing showing sinus rhythm with a rate of 80 beats/min. There is a borderline first-degree AV block and intraventricular conduction defect. The pacemaker is suppressed as the spontaneous heart rate is greater than 72 beats/min, which is the automatic rate of the demand pacemaker. (B) Tracing recorded while a magnet was applied. The pacemaker was converted from the demand to fixed-rate mode. The pacemaker fires at a rate of 74 beats/min regardless of patient's spontaneous rhythm. Many of the pacemaker stimuli are ineffective, falling on various portions of the QRS-T complex of the spontaneous beats. The fifth QRS complex is a fusion beat.

ates impulses whenever the patient's own ventricular rate falls below a predetermined level (Fig. 27-8). The artificial stimulus is suppressed if the patient's own ventricular rate is above this level. The spontaneous ventricular beats may originate from the sinus node or from an ectopic focus in the atrium or ventricle. The artificial pacing is noncompetitive and occurs only when it is needed. Therefore, the ability to sense the ventricular activity is an important function of the ventricular demand pacemakers.

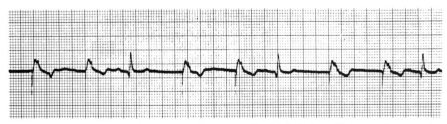

FIGURE 27-8. Ventricular inhibited pacemaker (VVI). The third, sixth, and last complexes are sinus beats that suppress the pacemaker. The spike-to-spike interval is 840 msec.

The ECGs of patients with properly functioning ventricular inhibited pacemaker may present the following findings:

1. All the ventricular complexes are the results of pacemaker stimulation. The spike-to-spike interval (pace interval, automatic interval) remains constant. In adults, the pacing rate is commonly set at about 72 beats/min. When a demand pacemaker is pacing uninterruptedly, it is indistinguishable from a fixed-rate pacemaker on the ECG.

2. All ECG complexes are the patient's spontaneous complexes, and the existence of an artificial pacemaker cannot be detected. This occurs when the spontaneous ventricular rate is faster than the pacemaker's pacing rate and all the spontaneous RR intervals are shorter than the pace interval. The presence of pacing function can be demonstrated by applying an external magnet to the pulse generator to inactivate its sensing device and convert it to the fixed rate mode (see Fig. 27-7). Depending on the manufacturer of the pacemaker, the pacing rate during its fixed-rate mode may or may not be the same as the pacing rate during its demand mode.

3. Both spontaneous and paced beats are present. The spontaneous beats may be conducted supraventricular complexes or ventricular extrasystoles. If a spontaneous beat is followed by a paced beat, the interval from the onset of the spontaneous QRS complex to the pacemaker spike is called the *escape interval*. The escape interval need not be the same as the pace interval (spike-to-spike interval) and is usually longer (Fig. 27-9). Depending on the origin of the spontaneous impulse, its potential may not be sensed by the electrode until the later part of the depolarization process. The pacemaker is therefore not reset until part of the QRS complex in the surface ECG is already inscribed. In certain pacemakers, the escape interval is deliberately set longer than the pacing interval, a feature called *hysteresis* (see later part of this chapter).

4. Fusion beats and pseudofusion beats may be seen. As in the case of a fixed-rate pacemaker, fusion beats may be present. The ventricles are simultaneously depolarized by two activation fronts, one from the pacing impulse and one from the spontaneous focus. The morphology of the fusion beats varies, depending on the portion of the ventricles each of the activation fronts depolarizes (Fig. 27-10).

Occasionally, patients with ventricular inhibited pacemakers may have an ineffective

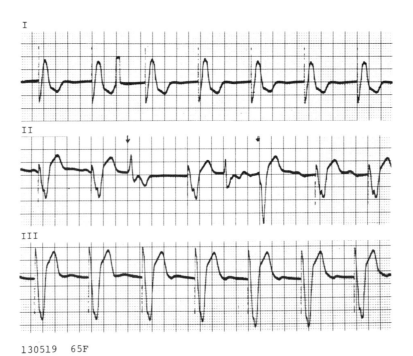

130519 65F

FIGURE 27-9. Right ventricular demand pacemaker (VVI) illustrating escape intervals. The pace interval is 880 msec. In lead II, there are three spontaneous beats. The two escape intervals are 1000 and 960 msec.

I

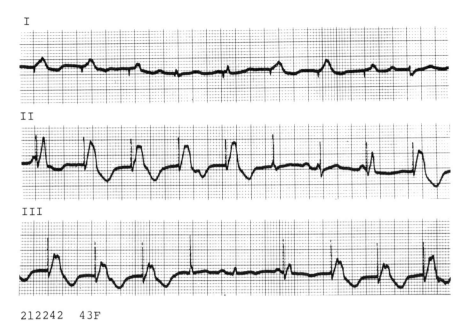

212242   43F

FIGURE 27–10. Right ventricular demand pacemaker (VVI) showing fusion beats. Depending on the proportion of spontaneous and pacer-induced ventricular activation, the morphology of the QRS-T complex varies. The pacemaker rate is 92 beats/min.

pacing impulse superimposed on a spontaneous complex. Such a complex is called *pseudofusion beat* (Fig. 27–11). The pacemaker impulse does not induce ventricular depolarization, and the QRS complex, other than the superimposed spike, has the same morphologic characteristics of a pure spontaneous beat. Pseudofusion beats occur when the pacemaker discharges during the absolute refractory period of the heart after the onset of spontaneous ventricular depolarization but before sufficient intracardiac voltage has been

generated to activate its sensing circuit. The pacemaker spike falls within the QRS complex because the surface ECG does not correspond precisely to the electrical changes recorded from the pacing catheter.[4]

Pseudofusion beats are more likely to be seen in patients with intraventricular conduction defect or ectopic ventricular beats.[41] In patients with complete right bundle branch block and a right ventricular artificial pacemaker, there is a delay in the arrival of the activation front of the spontaneous beats at the

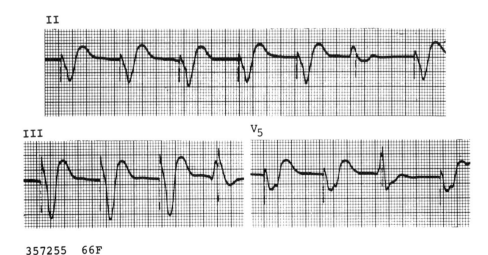

357255   66F

FIGURE 27–11. Pseudofusion beats. There is an ineffective pacemaker stimulus falling on the premature beat in each of the three leads.

site of the electrode. The pacemaker may discharge its stimulus at its preset interval in the initial part of the QRS complex because it has not yet sensed the event in progress in the left ventricle. The same phenomenon may be seen in patients with complete left bundle branch block and left ventricular artificial pacemaker. Pseudofusion beats may be seen in patients with left ventricular premature ventricular beats and a right ventricular pacemaker (see Fig. 27–11) or right ventricular premature beats and a left ventricular pacemaker by similar mechanism. Pseudofusion beats do not indicate malfunction of the sensing device of the pacemaker but are normal manifestations of a demand pacemaker.

Occasionally, certain ventricular ectopic beats may not be sensed at all by an otherwise properly functioning demand pacemaker. The abnormal depolarization impulse does not generate adequate signal at the site of the intracardiac electrode to be sensed by the pacemaker. The local electrical voltage may be low or its rate of discharge (dv/dt) may be too slow to inhibit the pacemaker.

VENTRICULAR INHIBITED PACEMAKER (VVI) IN THE MAGNET MODE

The application of a magnet against the skin over the pacemaker implant site while the ECG is being recorded is useful in the evaluation of the function of the VVI pacemakers. The magnet converts the pacemaker from the demand to asynchronous (fixed-rate) mode. If the patient's spontaneous ventricular rate is faster than the programmed pacing rate during the time of examination, the pacemaker is inhibited and no pacing spikes are seen until the magnet is applied. In the magnet mode, the pacing rate can be determined regardless of the patient's native rate. A significant decrease in the pacing rate usually indicates a decrease

in the pacemaker's battery voltage. In most pacemakers, the pacing rate in the magnet mode is the same as that during automatic pacing. In some pacemakers, however, the rates are different. In either case, the response of the ventricle to the pacing stimuli can be evaluated. Ventricular capture should occur if the ventricle is stimulated after its refractory period. Some manufacturers of pacemakers incorporate "threshold margin test" during the initial part of the magnet mode. The application of a magnet to such pacemakers initiates three asynchronous pacing pulses at the rate of 100 times/min. The pulse width of the third stimulus is reduced by 25 percent (Fig. 27–12). The purpose of this reduction is to ensure that the pacemaker's output is providing at least 25 percent more energy than is required to capture the ventricle.

RATE-RESPONSIVE VENTRICULAR INHIBITED PACEMAKERS (VVI + ACTIVITY)

The rate-responsive pacemakers are designed to increase the pacing rate and therefore the cardiac output in response to increased physical activity. One of the available devices has a piezoelectric crystal activity sensor fixed to the inside of the pacemaker case. The crystal detects vibration generated by body motion. Circuitry inside the pacemaker then converts these detected vibrations into an increased pacing rate in response to the level of activity being performed.[5,12,26] Figure 27–13 gives an example of this type of pacemaker.

Other rate-responsive pacemakers use the right ventricular blood temperature, minute ventilation, the QT interval, mixed venous oxygen saturation, and other physiological parameters as variables to modulate the pacing rate.[16] They are either available only in Europe or still under clinical evaluation.

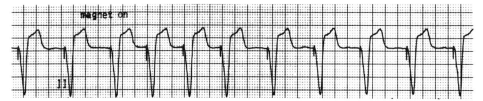

FIGURE 27–12. Ventricular inhibited pacemaker (VVI) in the magnet mode demonstrating the "threshold margin test." With the application of a magnet, this pacemaker (manufactured by Medtronic) generates the first three stimuli at the rate of 100 times per minute. The pulse width of the third stimulus is reduced by 25 percent, but this measurement cannot be made on the routine ECG because of the slow paper speed. The pacing rate after the first three stimuli is identical to that during automatic pacing.

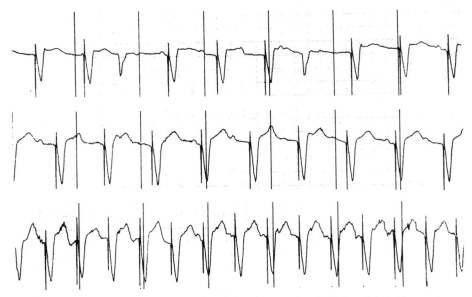

FIGURE 27–13. Rate-responsive ventricular inhibited pacemaker (VVI + activity). The tracing was obtained with Holter monitoring. The upper and middle strips show a ventricular pacing rate of 80 times per minute. The pacemaker senses and captures properly. The bottom strip was recorded during exercise and the pacing rate was increased to 124 times per minute.

VENTRICULAR TRIGGERED PACEMAKERS (VVT)

The ventricular triggered type of demand pacemakers (VVT) functions similarly to the inhibited type (VVI) in that it delivers a stimulus at a preset interval if no spontaneous ventricular depolarization is detected. It differs from the ventricular inhibited pacemakers, however, by also delivering a stimulus immediately after a spontaneous QRS is sensed. In the ECG, each QRS complex is accompanied by a pacing spike. When there is a spontaneous ventricular complex, the pacing spike appears shortly after the onset of the QRS, therefore, during the absolute refractory period of the ventricle. If there is no spontaneous ventricular activation, the pacemaker spike appears at the end of the escape or pacing interval. In the paced beats, the stimulus spike initiates rather than falls on the QRS complex (Fig. 27–14).

The ventricular triggered pacemakers were originally designed to avoid the potential problem of pacemaker inhibition by extracardiac electrical signals such as those that originated from the skeletal muscles or radio transmitters, especially when unipolar leads were used. Modern pacemaker circuitry has reduced the likelihood of such interferences. Because of the additional power drain and the distortion of the native QRS complexes by the pacing spikes, the triggered mode of pacing is used infrequently.

ELECTROCARDIOGRAPHIC SIGNS OF MALFUNCTION OF VENTRICULAR DEMAND PACEMAKERS

Although other procedures may be employed to evaluate the functions of ventricular demand pacemakers, only those findings that are detectable by routine ECG are discussed here. With demand pacemakers, the malfunction may involve sensing or pacing or both. Loss of sensing ability usually occurs before loss of pacing ability.[27,35] The source of malfunction may be in the pulse generator, in the lead, or at the junction of the cardiac tissue and electrode. The more commonly implanted ventricular inhibited pacemakers (VVI) are discussed here.

SENSING MALFUNCTION[2]

UNDERSENSING. A malfunctioning ventricular demand pacemaker may be undersensing or oversensing. When it has completely lost its ability to sense, it performs like a fixed-rate asynchronous pacemaker (Fig. 27–15). Such dysfunction cannot be detected if the patient has consistent bradycardia and spontaneous ventricular complexes are not present. In some patients, exercise or drugs may accelerate the heart rate and expose spontaneous QRS complexes. The sensing ability of the pacemaker may then be determined. In some instances, the undersensing is intermittent and may or may not be associated with pacing

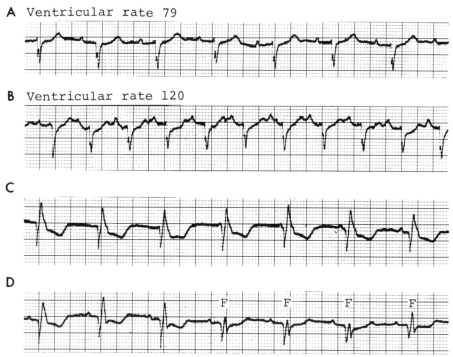

FIGURE 27–14. Ventricular triggered pacemaker (VVT). (A) Tracing recorded during normal sinus rhythm. The pacemaker senses the R waves of the spontaneous beats and generates stimuli that are superimposed on the initial part of the QRS complexes. The same phenomenon occurs when the heart rate increases during walking (B). In C, the spontaneous ventricular rate falls below 76 beats/min. The pacemaker operates in its demand mode with a rate of 76 beats/min. All ventricular complexes are paced beats. In D, fusion beats (F) are present. These fusion beats are the result of ventricular depolarization by impulses coming from both the pacemaker and conducted spontaneous impulse. The spontaneous ventricular rate and the pacemaker rate in its demand mode are nearly the same.

failure (Fig. 27–16). Failure of sensing does not always indicate malfunction of the pulse generator. In newly implanted pacemakers, the electrical potential to be sensed may be too low because of underlying myocardial scar, inadequate myocardial or endocardial contact, poor orientation of a bipolar electrode, or inappropriate programming of amplifier sensitivity.[15] Later loss of signal potential may be the result of acute myocardial infarction, growth of an insulating tissue around the electrode, or myocardial perforation with the electrode migrated to a poor signal area.[15] Broken leads or wire insulation

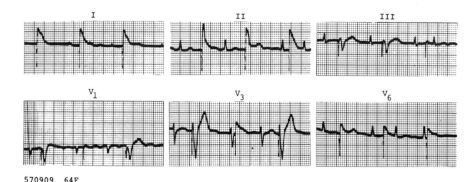

570909   64F

FIGURE 27–15. Ventricular demand pacemaker (VVI) with sensing malfunction. The pacemaker operates like a fixed-rate pacemaker. The spontaneous ventricular beats are not sensed. The spontaneous rhythm is atrial fibrillation.

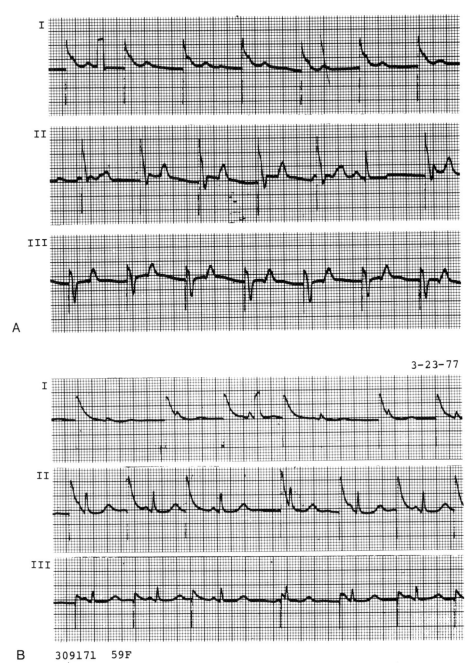

3-23-77

B   309171   59F

FIGURE 27-16. Pacemaker malfunction. (A) Tracing showing a properly functioning transvenous right ventricular demand pacemaker (VVI). Retrograde capture of the atria is present and is most clearly seen in lead III. In B, there is failure of sensing of most of the spontaneous QRS complexes. There also is a complete failure of capture. Note the prominent pacemaker spike decay curves, which are larger than the spontaneous waveforms in leads I and II.

tears with current leakage have been uncommon in recent years as the quality of the lead wire has been improved.

In a previous section, findings that may be mistaken for a sensing malfunction have been discussed. These include pseudofusion beats and certain unsensed ventricular ectopic beats.

OVERSENSING. Oversensing of physiological intracardiac voltage is uncommon with implanted pacemakers. Occasionally, very tall P or T waves may be mistaken for R waves and thereby cause the pacing to be reset[2,4] (Fig. 27–17). Myopotential inhibition of implanted unipolar demand pacemakers during pectoralis muscle contraction, however, is common and may cause symptoms.[6,18,30,38] An example is given in Figure 27–18. Electromagnetic interference may come from nonphysiological sources such as radar, television, and radio transmitters. Electrocautery may inhibit the pacemaker output if it is used within a few inches of the pulse generator. Microwave ovens and weapon detector equipment no longer cause potential problems for proper function of the modern pacemakers. Although their effects are not restricted to the sensing function, it is pertinent to mention that direct current countershock and therapeutic radiation may damage the pulse generator.[28]

PACING MALFUNCTION

Pacing failure cannot be recognized if the patient is in a spontaneous rhythm with a ventricular rate faster than the pacemaker's preset pacing rate. A magnet may be applied to convert the pacemaker to the fixed-rate mode, and the pacing rate can be examined. Depending on the manufacturer of the pacemaker, the pacing rate in its magnet mode may not be the same as its automatic rate. In some patients, slowing of the heart rate may be accomplished by carotid sinus stimulation to allow the pacemaker to escape. Such a procedure, however, is associated with the potential risk of ventricular asystole if pacing malfunction does exist.

The pacing rate is by far the most valuable indicator of battery power of the pulse generator. When specially constructed electronic counters are used, a change in the spike-to-spike interval of more than 10 msec (or less than 1 per minute in pacing rate) may indicate early battery depletion. Such a small change in rate is difficult to determine from the routine ECG, however. An increase or decrease of 1 or 2 beats/min in pacing rate is often due to variation in the ECG paper speed. Pacemaker battery failure is usually manifested by a slowing of the pacing rate (Fig. 27–19). With some pacemakers, the slowing of the pacing rate appears first in the magnet (fixed-rate) mode instead of during automatic pacing. In most pacemakers, a reduction of 4 or more beats per minute in the automatic or magnet rate is an indication of battery depletion. The exact number varies with different

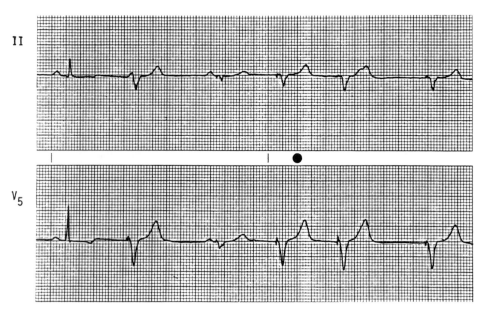

FIGURE 27–17. Oversensing of T wave. The two leads were recorded simultaneously. The VVI pacemaker is programmed to have a pacing rate of 70 beats/min. The first QRS complex is spontaneously conducted. The second, fourth, fifth, and sixth QRS complexes are paced. The third QRS complex is a fusion beat. The spike-to-spike interval of the fourth and fifth complexes is 860 msec, which is the equivalent of the programmed pacing rate. The spike-to-spike interval of the fifth and sixth complexes is much longer. The interval between the last pacing spike and the apex of the preceding T wave is, however, 860 msec. The delay of the last pacing spike is, therefore, most likely the result of sensing of the preceding T wave. The long spike-to-spike interval that involves the second and third complexes can be explained on the same basis.

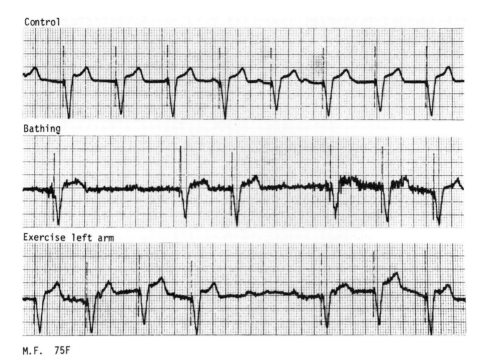

Control

Bathing

Exercise left arm

M.F.   75F

FIGURE 27–18. Myopotential inhibition of a ventricular demand pacemaker (VVI). The ECG was obtained during telemetry monitoring. In the control tracing, while the patient was inactive, the pacemaker is pacing regularly at the rate of 73 beats/min. Intermittent inhibition of the pacemaker occurred while the patient was taking a shower and during left arm exercise. Baseline artifacts due to skeletal muscle potential are present. The pulse generator was implanted overlying the pectoralis muscle, and the lead was unipolar.

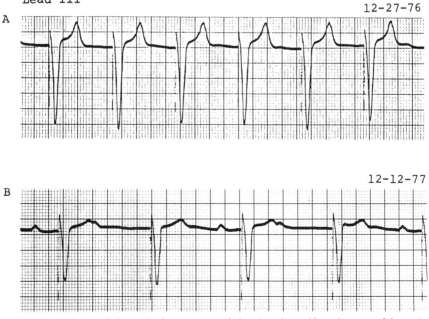

Lead III   12-27-76

A

                                           12-12-77

B

FIGURE 27–19. Battery failure. The battery power failure is indicated by a decrease of the pacing rate from 70 to 47 beats/min.

manufacturers as well as different models from the same manufacturer. In patients with intermittent spontaneous rhythm, improper pacing function may be indicated by the failure of the pacemaker to discharge an impulse when its escape interval has been exceeded. With modern pacemakers, marked increase in the pacing rate (runaway pacemaker) is seldom seen as a sign of battery depletion. Oscilloscopic analysis of the amplitude, duration, and configuration of the pacemaker impulse may be used in the early detection of battery exhaustion,[35] as well as impending lead fracture or insulation disruption.

Pacing malfunction also may be manifested by failure of the pacemaker impulse to depolarize the ventricles. The failure may be consistent or intermittent. It may be the result of inadequate voltage output from the pulse generator, or it may be caused by wire fracture (Fig. 27–20), electrode displacement (inadequate local potential of stimulation), or an increase in the stimulation threshold at the site of electrode. As was mentioned, some pacemakers have incorporated additional features in the magnet mode to test the adequacy of voltage output. The pulse width or pulse amplitude of one of the stimuli is reduced by a certain percentage. The altered impulse would fail to initiate ventricular depolarization if the originally programmed stimulus strength is marginal.

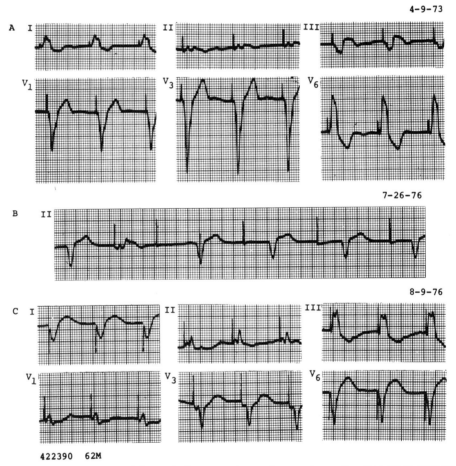

FIGURE 27–20. Right and left ventricular pacemakers and pacemaker malfunction. These tracings were obtained from the same patient. (A) Tracing recorded when the patient had a transvenous right ventricular demand pacemaker that was functioning properly. Because there are no spontaneous beats the demand function of the pacemaker cannot be demonstrated. (B) Tracing showing intermittent pacing failure. The first QRS complex is a spontaneous beat. The second complex is pacemaker induced. The next pacemaker spike appears prematurely and is not followed by ventricular depolarization. A pseudofusion beat follows. None of the last three pacemaker stimuli captures the ventricle. The sensing function of the pacemaker appears intact. The pacing malfunction was found to be the result of broken lead. (C) Tracing recorded after the patient received an epicardial left ventricular pacemaker.

Lead II

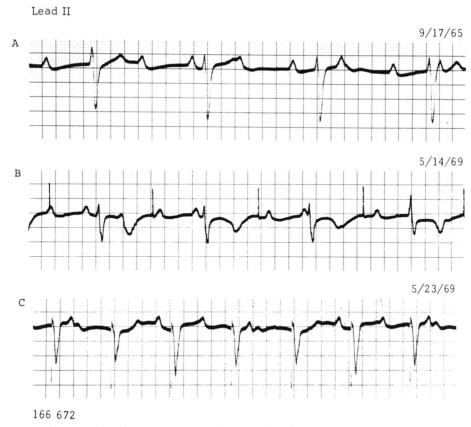

166 672

FIGURE 27–21. Failure of pacing as a result of myocardial perforation. (A) Tracing showing complete AV block with idioventricular rhythm recorded before pacemaker implantation. (B) Tracing obtained after a new transvenous electrode was inserted. It shows that the pacemaker is sensing properly, but the stimuli do not depolarize the ventricles. The malfunction is the result of myocardial perforation, and the electrode was lying on the epicardium of the left ventricle. (C) Tracing recorded after the lead was replaced.

Myocardial perforation may occasionally be responsible for pacing failure and occurs most frequently during the first few weeks of implantation (Fig. 27–21). A right ventricular endocardial lead may perforate the interventricular septum or more commonly the free wall of the right ventricle. The electrode may migrate and rest on the epicardial surface of the left ventricle. In the ECG, the paced beats may change from a left bundle branch block to a right bundle branch block pattern. Indeed, if such morphologic changes occur spontaneously in a patient with right ventricular transvenous electrode, the diagnosis of myocardial perforation can be made (Fig. 27–22).

ATRIAL SYNCHRONOUS PACEMAKERS (VAT)

An atrial synchronous pacemaker is a ventricular stimulating pacemaker with its pacing rate dependent on the atrial rate. It is rarely used today. It has two leads, one of which senses the atrial potential and, one that, following a preset PR interval, stimulates the ventricle. If the atrial potential is inadequate or absent within a preset interval, the pacemaker becomes an asynchronous ventricular pacemaker with a pacing rate usually between 60 and 70 beats/min for adults. If the atrial rate becomes abnormally rapid, the pacemaker is programmed to produce 2:1, 3:1, or 4:1 block to protect the ventricles from excessive rate.[14]

ATRIAL SYNCHRONOUS VENTRICULAR INHIBITED PACEMAKERS (VDD)[29]

The atrial synchronous ventricular inhibited pacemaker is similar to the atrial synchronous pacemakers in that it senses the atrium and paces the ventricle. The pacemaker is refined

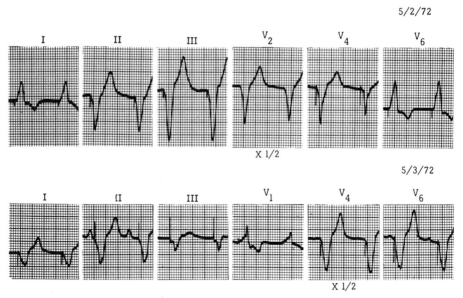

FIGURE 27-22. Perforation of the heart by a pacemaker electrode. The patient had a transvenous right ventricular pacemaker implanted for the treatment of complete AV block. On 5-2-72, the tracing shows functioning right ventricular pacing with QRS-T morphology similar to that of complete left bundle branch block. The following day, the ECG reveals a sudden change in the QRS-T complexes from a left bundle branch block to a right bundle branch block pattern. The changes were the result of right ventricular perforation, with the tip of the electrode resting on the epicardial surface of the left ventricle.

by the addition of ventricular sensing and to provide ventricular demand pacing during sinus bradycardia. It also prevents competitive pacing when ventricular ectopic beats are present.

ATRIOVENTRICULAR SEQUENTIAL PACEMAKERS (DVI)

The atrioventricular (AV) sequential pacemaker is a dual-chamber pacemaker that paces both the atrium and ventricle but senses only the ventricle.[8,15] If conducted supraventricular beats occur at a rate above a preset level, all activities of the pacemaker are suppressed. If no ventricular potential is sensed by the ventricular electrode at a predetermined interval, atrial pacing occurs. The subsequent ventricular pacing activity depends on the type of the AV sequential pacemaker, committed or uncommitted. In the uncommitted type, ventricular pacing is inhibited by the native QRS interval if the spontaneous AV conduction time is shorter than the programmed pacemaker AV interval. If there is AV block or prolongation of the PR interval beyond the preset pacemaker AV interval, however, the ventricular electrode senses the delay of ventricular response and paces the ventricle to provide AV sequential stimulation (Fig. 27–

23). In the committed type, ventricular pacing occurs at the programmed AV interval regardless whether there is spontaneous AV conduction (Fig. 27–24). In both types, the pacemaker restores normal AV sequence only when the native atrial rate is slower than the pacemaker's automatic rate. Because the pacemaker does not sense the atrium and the pacing interval is reset by ventricular depolarization, the atrial stimulus is competitive with the native atrial impulse. Atrial fibrillation may develop if the atrial stimulus is delivered during the vulnerable period (Fig 27–25).

ATRIOVENTRICULAR UNIVERSAL PACEMAKERS (DDD)[23] Figs. 27–26 through 27–28)

The AV universal pacemaker is the most common dual-chamber pacing device implanted today. It senses and paces both the atrium and the ventricle. From the sensed events, it may be inhibited or triggered to pace the atrium or ventricle or both according to the programmed rate limits and AV interval. Most of the DDD pacemakers can be programmed and function in other pacing modes.

Because of the many possible modes of presentation, the ECGs of patients with an AV universal pacemaker are often difficult to inter-

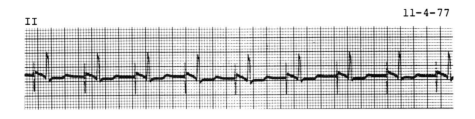

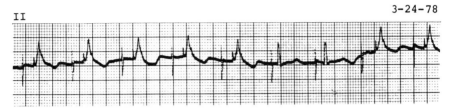

234426   33M

FIGURE 27-23. AV sequential pacemaker (DVI), uncommitted. The patient was a 33-year-old man with rheumatic mitral and aortic valve disease. He also had the sick sinus syndrome with sinus bradycardia, for which the pacemaker was implanted. In the tracing of 11-4-77, only atrial pacing is present. The atrial impulse is conducted to the ventricles with a PR interval of 0.16 second. Artificial ventricular pacing is inhibited because spontaneous AV conduction occurs within the preset pacemaker AV interval of 0.16 second. The pacing rate is 80 beats/min. On 3-24-78, the patient developed atrial fibrillation. Atrial stimulation continued at the same rate. Because of the underlying atrial fibrillation, however, the stimuli were not effective in inducing atrial depolarization. In the first five complexes, AV sequential pacing occurs with an atrial to ventricular spike interval slightly greater than 0.16 second. In the sixth and seventh complexes, the interval between the atrial spike and the onset of QRS complex is shorter because of spontaneous AV conduction.

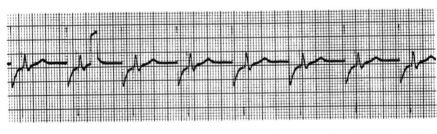

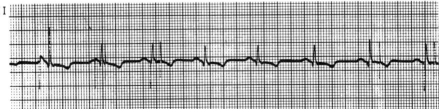

FIGURE 27-24. AV sequential pacemaker (DVI), committed. The pacemaker's pacing rate is 73 beats/min and the AV interval is 160 msec. Lead I shows atrial and ventricular pacing at the programmed rate and AV interval. In the first three beats of lead II, atrial and ventricular stimuli fall on or after the spontaneous P and QRS complexes. The spontaneous heart rate is slightly faster than the pacing rate. Because there is no atrial sensing, atrial stimuli are delivered according to the programmed VA interval (660 msec), even though the next native P wave already has appeared. Because this DVI pacemaker is of the committed type, the ventricular stimuli follow the atrial stimuli at the end of 160 msec despite the presence of conducted native QRS. The fourth native QRS appears before the end of the pacer's VA interval and therefore inhibits the AV pacing. The delayed appearance of the fourth pair of stimuli is due to hysteresis.

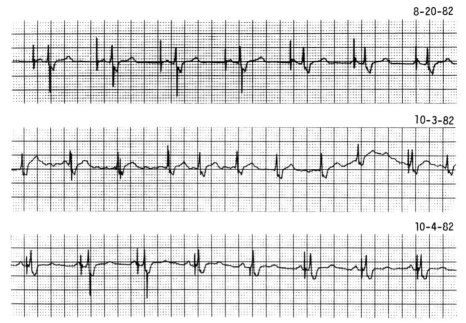

FIGURE 27–25. DVI pacemaker induced atrial fibrillation. The patient was a 34-year-old man who had an implanted AV sequential pacemaker of the uncommitted type. The pacing rate in the tracing made on 8-20-82 is 62 beats/min and the AV interval 250 msec. The first four P waves are pacemaker induced and the last three are not. Ventricular stimuli are not present in the last three complexes since this DVI pacemaker is uncommitted. The spontaneous QRS complexes are sensed within 250 msec of the atrial stimuli and inhibit ventricular pacing. In the first four complexes, ventricular pacing still occurs because of the presence of right bundle branch block. The right ventricular electrode has not yet sensed the activation potential, but the surface ECG already has begun to inscribe the QRS as a result of left ventricular depolarization. On 10-3-82, atrial fibrillation developed. The arrhythmia probably was induced by atrial stimulation because the DVI pacemaker was unable to sense atrial activity. The atrial mechanism returned to normal sinus on 10-4-82. Before 10-3-82, the pacemaker was reprogrammed, and the pacing rate on 10-3-82 and 10-4-82 is 70 beats/min and AV interval is 140 msec.

pret. There also are some built-in safety features for the prevention of pacemaker-induced arrhythmias. The specifics of the features, such as the atrial and ventricular refractory periods of the pulse generator during which the demand or sensing mechanism becomes unresponsive to cardiac or external signals, vary with different manufacturers and are often programmable. It is essential that such information is known to the interpreter. Without such information, an incorrect diagnosis of pacemaker malfunction may be made.

In the following section, some of the common modes of presentation of the DDD pacemaker are described. They are illustrated by schematic diagrams in Figure 27–26. To simplify the discussion, the programmed lower rate limit is assumed to be 60 pulses/min, the upper rate limit to be 150 pulses/min, and the AV interval to be 200 msec.

In the absence of spontaneous atrial or ventricular activity, both atrial and ventricular pacing occur at the programmed lower rate of 60 pulses/min with an AV interval of 200 msec. The ventricular activation resets the timing of the next atrial pacing stimulus (spike), and the VA interval is 800 msec (1000 − 200 msec). If the spontaneous atrial rate is faster than 60 beats/min and AV conduction occurs in less than 200 msec (the programmed interval), no pacing stimulus is seen. The tracing shows no signs to indicate the presence of a pacemaker.

If a spontaneous P wave appears in less than 800 msec from the preceding QRS, atrial pacing is inhibited. Ventricular stimulus is delivered at the end of 200 msec if spontaneous AV conduction is delayed or absent. No ventricular stimulus is delivered in less than 400 msec from the preceding QRS interval, however, regardless how early the native P wave appears as the programmed upper rate limit is 150 pulses/min (equivalent to a VV interval of 400 msec).

If a premature ventricular beat is sensed in less than 800 msec after the preceding QRS,

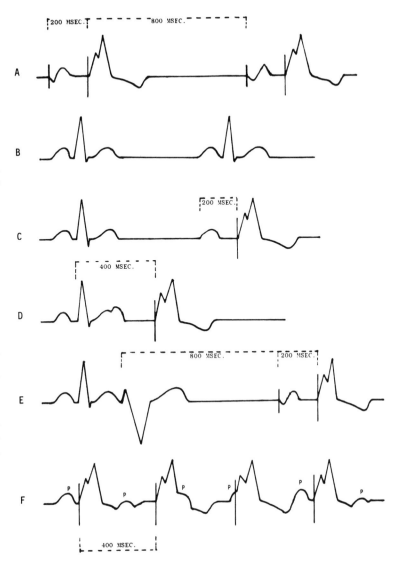

FIGURE 27–26. AV universal pacemaker (DDD). Schematic diagrams depicting some of the modes of presentation of DDD pacemakers. The pacemaker is assumed to be programmed with a lower rate limit of 60 beats/min, an upper rate limit of 150 beats/min, and an AV interval of 200 msec. (A) AV pacing at the lower rate limit. (B) Spontaneous sinus rhythm inhibiting both atrial and ventricular pacing. (C) Spontaneous P wave followed by ventricular pacing at the end of the programmed AV interval. (D) Premature atrial activation that is not followed by ventricular pacing at the programmed AV interval because of the upper rate limit. Ventricular stimulus occurs with an interval of 400 msec (equivalent to the rate of 150 beats/min) from the preceding QRS. (E) A premature ventricular beat inhibits both atrial and ventricular pacing until the lower rate limit is reached. (F) Ventricular pacing at the upper rate limit (150 beats/min) in the presence of faster spontaneous atrial rate.

both atrial and ventricular pacing is inhibited. The atrial and ventricular pacing response is reset by this ventricular ectopic beat.

If the spontaneous atrial rate is faster than 150 beats/min, atrial pacing is inhibited. Unless spontaneous AV conduction and ventricular depolarization occur within 200 msec, ventricular pacing is triggered. The ventricular rate is limited, however, to the programmed upper limit of 150 beats/min, which is slower than the spontaneous atrial rate.

DDD PACEMAKER IN THE MAGNET MODE

As discussed in the section on ventricular inhibited (VVI) pacemakers, the application of a magnet against the skin over the implanted

pacemaker site serves to reveal the programmed pacing mode, verify capture, and evaluate the status of the pacemaker's power source. The magnet mode also may be helpful to identify the specific pulse generator, since pacemakers from different manufacturers respond differently to magnet application. Conversely, the specific response to magnet application must be known for each pacemaker to determine whether the response is normal. Otherwise, interpretation of the findings will often be erroneous.

The application of a magnet to an AV universal (DDD) pacemaker results in asynchronous pacing in both the atrial and ventricular chambers (DOO mode). In some models, magnet application results in asynchronous atrial pacing but ventricular sensing is retained.[24] In most devices, however, the atrial

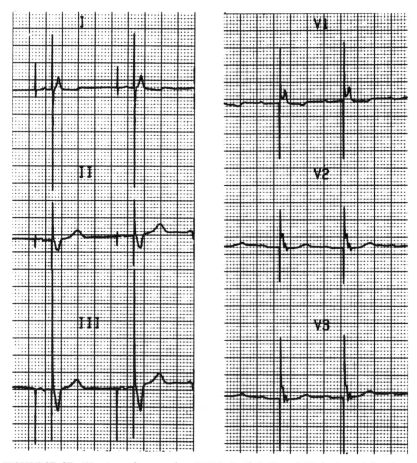

FIGURE 27–27. AV universal pacemaker (DDD). Leads I, II, and III depict atrial and ventricular pacing at the rate of 60 beats/min (lower limit) with an AV interval of 200 msec. Leads V_1 through V_3 depict sinus rhythm with a rate of 78 beats/min. Atrial pacing is inhibited. Ventricular pacing still occurs because of the delayed spontaneous AV conduction beyond 200 msec.

and ventricular pacing spikes appear at a specific interval regardless of whether spontaneous beats are present. The pacing rate varies depending on the model and the manufacturer of the pacemaker. A significant decrease in the rate from that of the expected usually indicates battery depletion. Atrial and ventricular captures should occur consistently if there are no spontaneous beats. They occur intermittently if spontaneous beats are present

and the chambers are stimulated outside of their refractory periods. Certain DDD pacemakers respond to magnet application with two different pacing rates. During the initial part of the magnet mode several beats are paced at a faster rate, the last of which being stimulated with reduced pulse width. The AV interval during this period is shortened to avoid competitive depolarization from spontaneous AV conduction (Fig. 27–29).

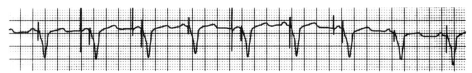

FIGURE 27–28. AV universal (DDD) pacemaker. The tracing shows consistent ventricular pacing. Atrial stimulation is seen intermittently depending on whether the native P wave appeared before the programmed VA interval, which is 700 msec.

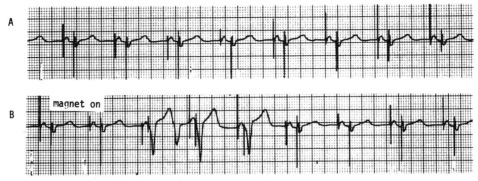

FIGURE 27–29. AV universal (DDD) pacemaker with and without magnet application. (A) Tracing recorded without the magnet. The pacing rate is 71 times/min and the AV interval is 180 msec. There is consistent atrial capture. The ventricular pacing spikes, however, occur at the same time as when spontaneous ventricular depolarization begins, resulting in pseudofusion beats. (B) Tracing obtained while a magnet was applied. There are three pairs of AV stimuli occurring at a rate of 78 times/min with an AV interval of 100 msec (threshold margin test). There is both atrial and ventricular capture. After these three beats, the pacing rate and AV interval return to the same values seen before the magnet was applied.

DDD PACEMAKER–RELATED ARRHYTHMIAS

Because of the characteristics of the DDD pacemaker, certain tachycardias and irregular rhythms may be seen even though the pacemaker is functioning normally.

Wenckebach Pacemaker Response[3,39]

Wenckebach pacemaker response is observed when the spontaneous atrial rate is faster than the programmed DDD pacemaker upper rate limit. The atrial impulses are sensed (unless they occur during the pacemaker's atrial refractory period) and atrial pacing is inhibited. Ventricular pacing does not occur at the preset AV interval but is delayed until the upper rate limit (the shortest VV interval) is reached (Fig. 27–30). Therefore, there is a prolongation of the P-to-V interval, the degree of which is inversely proportional to the preceding VP interval. This shortening of the VP interval and lengthening of the PV interval is progressive until the P wave falls within the postventricular portion of the atrial refractory period, during which the P wave is not sensed. The unsensed P wave is not followed by a ventricular stimulus. The succeeding P wave, however, is sensed and is followed by ventricular pacing at the programmed AV interval. A long VV interval is observed. The progressive lengthening of the PV interval until a P wave is no longer followed by a paced QRS complex superficially resembles the Wenckebach type of second-degree AV block.

Pacemaker Circus Movement Tachycardia[17,19,37]

The reentry tachycardia occasionally seen in patients with normal functioning DDD pacemakers is sometimes also called *endless loop* tachycardia. The underlying cause of this pacemaker-induced tachycardia is the presence of retrograde P waves (Fig. 27–31). Retrograde atrial depolarization from a paced ventricular beat may occur in patients with sick sinus syndrome as well as in those with advanced antegrade AV block. Such retrograde P wave is sensed by the atrial component of the pacemaker, which in turn triggers the delivery of a ventricular stimulus, resulting in a paced QRS complex with retrograde atrial capture. The same event repeats itself, resulting in a reentry or endless loop tachycardia. The rate of the tachycardia is limited by the upper rate limit programmed for the pacemaker. Lengthening of the atrial refractory period of the pacemaker may decrease the incidence of, but does not eliminate, this complication.

HYSTERESIS, FALLBACK RESPONSE, RATE SMOOTHING[3]

AV interval hysteresis is a feature included in some of the DDD pacemakers. The pulse generator has two AV intervals. The AV interval of a sensed atrial event is shorter than that which follows an atrial stimulus. The purpose of this feature is to provide equivalent AV hemodynamic intervals, whether the atrial contrac-

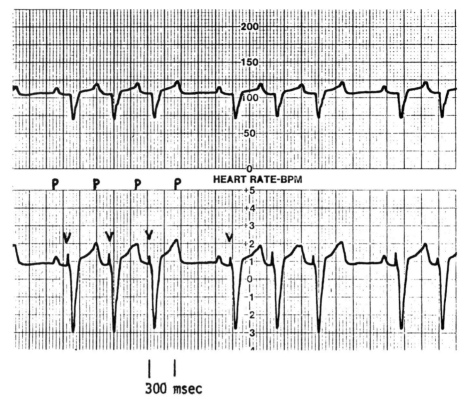

FIGURE 27–30. Wenckebach response of a DDD pacemaker. The programmed lower rate of the pacemaker is 60 and the upper rate is 120 pulses/min. The AV interval is 150 msec, and the post-ventricular atrial refractory period is 325 msec. The two-channel Holter recording shows that the patient's spontaneous atrial rate is 128 beats/min (PP interval, 470 msec). Ventricular pacing occurs at the upper rate limit of 120 pulses/min (VV interval, 480 msec) for three beats followed by a pause. There is a progressive lengthening of the PV interval and shortening of the VP interval until the pause occurs. The last VP interval before the pause measures 300 msec. The P wave preceding the pause, therefore, falls within the postventricular atrial refractory period and is not sensed. Ventricular pacing is not triggered until the next P wave appears and the same sequence is repeated.

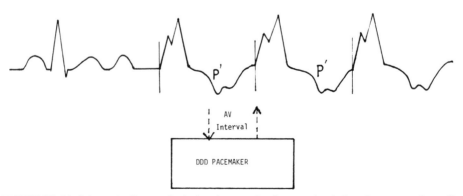

FIGURE 27–31. Schematic diagram depicting the genesis of pacemaker-induced reentry tachycardia. The retrograde P wave (P′) of a paced beat is sensed by the DDD pacemaker and induces the delivery of a ventricular stimulus at the end of the programmed AV interval. The pacemaker serves as a bypass to initiate and perpetuate a reentry tachycardia.

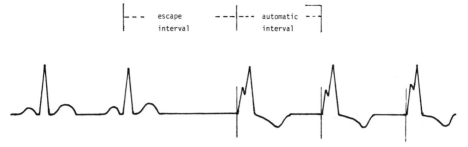

FIGURE 27–32. Hysteresis. Schematic diagram illustrating the longer escape interval after the spontaneous beats. Once pacing begins, the rate returns to the programmed automatic rate.

tion is spontaneous or paced. It is assumed that, in the case of spontaneous atrial beat, the atrial electrode senses the impulse after atrial contraction has already begun. Therefore, a shorter AV interval provides the same mechanical time sequence generated by paced atrial beat with a longer electrical AV interval.

Rate hysteresis is present when the pacemaker's escape interval is longer than the pacing interval (Fig. 27–32). This feature is provided to allow the patient's own sinus rhythm, which is more physiological, to be maintained at a lower rate than the pacing rate. It is more often included in the ventricular demand than other types of pacemakers.

In certain pacemakers, a fallback response is included to limit the time the ventricular rate remains at the programmed upper rate.[3] This option is designed to be used in patients who cannot tolerate a sustained upper rate. The response is activated by the detection of an atrial rate faster than the programmed upper rate. The fallback mechanism then gradually returns the ventricular rate to more tolerable levels. AV synchrony may or may not be maintained during the fallback response.

Rate smoothing is a programmable option available in one particular model of DDD pacemakers (CPI) that is designed to eliminate pronounced variations in the pacing cycle length. The maximum change in the pacing rate from cycle to cycle is limited to some percentage of the previous RR interval. It is intended to be used in patients who cannot tolerate marked fluctuations of paced rate.

DUAL-CHAMBER, RATE-MODULATED (DDDR) PACEMAKERS[24]

The DDDR pacemakers only recently became available. During exercise, the pacemaker is capable not only of tracking the patient's intrinsic P wave but also of responding to the activity sensor fixed in the inside of the pacemaker case. The ECG findings in patients with this type of pacemaker may be complicated. They are not discussed here.

ELECTROCARDIOGRAPHIC SIGNS OF MALFUNCTION OF THE AV UNIVERSAL (DDD) PACEMAKERS

As in the case of ventricular demand (VVI) pacemakers, malfunction of the DDD pacemakers may be indicated by undersensing or oversensing, absence of pacing stimuli when expected, slowing of the pacing rate, and failure to capture. Those problems that involve only the ventricular channel are common to both modes of pacing. They are not repeated here. The ECG diagnosis of malfunction of the DDD pacemakers is usually more difficult because the characteristics of the pulse generators vary with manufacturers and different models from the same manufacturer. Misinterpretation of pacemaker malfunction is often made when the specifics of these characteristics are not known to the electrocardiographer. It also happens if the parameters (e.g., pacing rate, pacing mode) have been reprogrammed since the previous tracing and the interpreter is not informed.

Atrial undersensing is one of the most common problems in DDD pacing.[3,40] It may be due to poor electrode location, lead dislodgement, inadequate P-wave amplitude, or problems that involve the lead itself and pulse generator.

Myopotential interference may occur in as many as 30 to 50 percent of unipolar DDD pacemakers.[3,22,36,42] The myopotentials may be sensed by the atrial electrode and trigger ventricular pacing, resulting in regular or irregular tachycardia. These potentials also may be sensed by the ventricular electrode and may inhibit ventricular pacing.

Unique to the DDD (and DVI) pacemakers is the phenomenon of cross talk, or self-inhibition.[3] Cross talk is the inappropriate detection of the atrial stimulus by the ventricular electrode. Consequently ventricular pacing is inhibited. Cross talk usually is due to high atrial channel output or high sensitivity of the ventricular channel. Most contemporary DDD pacemakers minimize the possibility of cross talk by including a ventricular blanking period. During the ventricular blanking period (usually 10 to 60 msec after the atrial stimulus), the ventricular amplifier is disabled.

PACEMAKER SYNDROME

Patients with single-chamber ventricular pacemaker (e.g., VVI) occasionally complain of dizziness, fatigue, syncope, or near syncope, even though there is no evidence to indicate pacemaker dysfunction. These symptoms are often referred to as the *pacemaker syndrome*.[1] The syndrome is the result of unfavorable hemodynamic consequences of ventricular pacing due to the loss of normal AV synchrony and atrial contribution to ventricular systole.[11] The incidence of the syndrome was found to be higher in patients with ventriculoatrial conduction.[31] Ausubel and Furman have written an excellent review paper on this syndrome.[1]

REFERENCES

1. Ausubel K, Furman S: The pacemaker syndrome. Ann Intern Med 103:420, 1985
2. Barold SS, Falkoff MD, Ong LS, et al: Electrocardiographic diagnosis of pacemaker malfunction. *In* Wellens HJJ, Kulbertus, HE (eds): What's New in Electrocardiography. Boston, Martinus Nijhoff Publishers, 1981, p 236.
3. Barold SS, Falkoff MD, Ong LS, Heinle RA: Basic concepts, upper rate response, retrograde ventriculoatrial conduction, and differential diagnosis of pacemaker tachycardias. *In* Saksena S, Goldschlager N: Electrical Therapy for Cardiac Pacing. Philadelphia, WB Saunders, 1990, p 225–264
4. Barold SS, Gaidula JJ: Evaluation of normal and abnormal sensing functions of demand pacemakers. Am J Cardiol 28:201, 1971
5. Benditt DG, Mianulli M, Fetter J, et al: Single-chamber cardiac pacing with activity-initiated chronotropic response: Evaluation by cardiopulmonary exercise testing. Circulation 75:184, 1987
6. Breivik K, Ohm OJ: Myopotential inhibition of unipolar QRS-inhibited (VVI) pacemakers, assessed by ambulatory Holter monitoring of the electrocardiogram. PACE 3:470, 1980
7. Castellanos A, Ortiz JM, Pastis N, et al: The electrocardiogram in patients with pacemakers. Prog Cardiovasc Dis 13:190, 1970
8. Castillo CA, Berkovitz BV, Castellanos A, et al: Bifocal demand pacing. Chest 59:360, 1971
9. Chatterjee K, Harris AM, Davies JG, et al: T-wave changes after artificial pacing. Lancet 1:759, 1969
10. Chatterjee K, Harris A, Davies G, et al: Electrocardiographic changes subsequent to artificial ventricular depolarization. Br Heart J 31:770, 1969
11. Cohen SI, Frank HA: Preservation of active atrial transport. Chest 81:51, 1982
12. Dulk KD, Bouwels L, Lindemans F, et al: The activitrax rate responsive pacemaker system. Am J Cardiol 61:107, 1988
13. Dulk KD, Lindemans, Bar FW, Wellens HJJ: Pacemaker-related tachycardias. PACE 5:476, 1982
14. Dodinot BP, Petitier A, Gilgenkratz JM, et al: Clinical experience with atrial synchronous pacing. Ann NY Acad Sci 167:1038, 1969
15. Escher DJW: Types of pacemakers and their complications. Circulation 47:1119, 1973
16. Fearnot NE, Smith HJ, Geddes LA: A review of pacemakers that physiologically increase rate: The DDD and rate-responsive pacemakers. Prog Cardiovasc Dis 29:145, 1986
17. Furman S: Newer modes of cardiac pacing. Mod Concepts Cardiovasc Dis 52:1, 1983
18. Furman S: Electromagnetic interference. PACE 5:1, 1982
19. Furman S, Fisher JD: Endless loop tachycardia in an AV universal (DDD) pacemaker. PACE 5:486, 1982
20. Gould L, Venkataraman K, Goswami MK, et al: Pacemaker-induced electrocardiographic changes simulating myocardial infarction. Chest 63:829, 1973
21. Green GD: Assessment of cardiac pacemakers: Pacemaker frontal plane vectors. Am Heart J 81:1, 1971
22. Halperin JL, Camunas JL, Stern EH, et al: Myopotential interference with DDD pacemakers: Endocardial electrographic telemetry in the diagnosis of pacemaker-related arrhythmias. Am J Cardiol 54:97, 1984
23. Hauser RG: The electrocardiography of AV universal DDD pacemakers. PACE 6:399, 1983
24. Hayes DL, Higano ST, Eisinger G: Electrocardiographic manifestations of a dual-chamber, rate-modulated (DDDR) pacemaker. PACE 12:555, 1989
25. Hoffman BF, Cranefield PF: Electrophysiology of the Heart. New York, McGraw-Hill, 1960
26. Dumen DP, Kostuk WJ, Klein GJ: Activity-sensing, rate-responsive pacing: Improvement in myocardial performance with exercise. PACE 8:52, 1985
27. Kastor JA, Leinbach RC: Pacemakers and their arrhythmias. Prog Cardiovasc Dis 13:240, 1970
28. Katzenberg CA, Marcus FI, Heusinkveld RS, et al: Pacemaker failure due to radiation therapy. PACE 5:156, 1982
29. Kruse I, Ryden L, Duffin EL: Clinical evaluation of atrial synchronous ventricular inhibited pacemakers. PACE 3:641, 1980
30. Mymin D, Cuddy TE, Sinha SN, et al: Inhibition of demand pacemakers by skeletal muscle potentials. JAMA 223:527, 1973
31. Nishimura RA, Gersh BJ, Vlietstra RE, et al: Hemodynamic and symptomatic consequences of ventricular pacing. PACE 5:903, 1982
32. Parsonnet V, Furman S, Smyth NPD: Implantable cardiac pacemakers: Status report and resource guidelines. Pacemaker study group (ICHD). Circulation 50:A21, 1974
33. Parsonnet V, Furman S, Smyth NPD: A revised code for pacemaker identification. PACE 4:400, 1981
34. Parsonnet V, Furman S, Smyth NPD, et al: Optimal resources for implantable cardiac pacemakers. Circulation 68:227A, 1983
35. Parsonnet V, Myers GH, Gilbert L, et al: Prediction of impending pacemaker failure in a pacemaker clinic. Am J Cardiol 25:311, 1970

36. Rozanski J, Blankstein RL, Lister JW: Pacer arrhythmias: Myopotential triggering of pacemaker-mediated tachycardia. PACE 6:795, 1983
37. Rubin JW, Frank MJ, Boineau JP, et al: Current physiologic pacemakers: A serious problem with a new device. Am J Cardiol 52:88, 1983
38. Secemsky SI, Hauser RG, Denes P, et al: Unipolar sensing abnormalities: Incidence and clinical significance of skeletal muscle interference and undersensing in 228 patients. PACE 5:10, 1982
39. Sutton R, Perrins EJ, Duffin E: Interpretation of dual chamber pacemaker electrocardiograms. PACE 8:6, 1985
40. Van Mechelen R, Hart C, DeBoer H: Failure to sense P waves during DDD pacing. PACE 9:498, 1986
41. Vera Z, Mason DT, Awan NA, et al: Lack of sensing by demand pacemakers due to intraventricular conduction defects. Circulation 51:815, 1975
42. Zimmern SH, Clark MF, Austin WK: Characteristics and clinical effects of myopotential signals in a unipolar DDD pacemaker population. PACE 9:1019, 1986

Ambulatory Electrocardiography

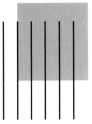

28

Ambulatory electrocardiograms (ECGs), also called *Holter* or *dynamic* ECGs, are commonly used for the detection of cardiac arrhythmias and myocardial ischemia. The ECG is obtained with a portable tape recorder over a prolonged period while the patient continues his or her usual physical activities. The recording is later scanned and the pertinent parts of the data are extracted. The technique was developed in the early 1960s and has become a widely used diagnostic tool.[32] The length of the recording and the feasibility of correlating the ECG with the patient's symptoms and activities are some of the obvious advantages of the ambulatory ECG over the conventional ECG or bedside monitoring

Most Holter monitors are capable of recording two or three leads of the ECG simultaneously and continuously for at least 24 hours. The three-channel monitor decreases the chances of failure to obtain technically satisfactory signals due to artifacts or loose electrode attachment. It facilitates the analysis of abnormal beats. The leads generally used are modified leads V_1 and V_5, and, in the case of three-channel recording, modified lead aVF is used. These are bipolar leads. In two-channel recordings, two negative electrodes are placed in the area of the upper sternum and the two positive electrodes at the conventional lead V_1 and V_5 positions respectively. A ground electrode is placed over the right side of the chest. In three-channel recordings, another negative electrode is placed at the left infraclavicular fossa, and the electrode at the conventional lead V_5 position is used as the positive electrode for the modified lead aVF. In patients who are monitored because of chest pain, a set of control tracings should be taken with the patient in the supine, sitting, and standing positions, and during hyperventilation. These baseline tracings are important and helpful in determining whether any ST-segment changes are significant.

The patient's diary during the monitoring period is an essential part of the information. All of the modern recorders have an event marker to be used by the patient to indicate the areas on the tape when symptoms occur. They also are equipped with a clock so that the time of the patient's symptoms and activities can be noted and correlated with the ECG findings.

Most of the commercially available playback equipment is capable to scan the tape at several different speeds varying from real time to 240 times real time. The various models differ in their features of computerized recognition, classification, and quantification of ectopic beats, which can be edited by the operator. A discussion of the advantages and disadvantages of the various systems is beyond the scope of this text. All units have time identification whenever the ECG is printed out either by automated program or at the discretion of the operator. A 24-hour trend sheet or digital printout is provided to display the heart rate and ST-segment changes in relation to the time of the day, as well as the number and characteristics of ventricular and supraventricular ectopic beats on an hourly basis (Fig. 28–1). Certain playback systems print out the ECG from the entire Holter tape in a condensed form (Fig. 28–2). Some portions of the tracing may be selected for enlargement and detailed examination. This type of equipment serves mainly to detect major abnormalities and cannot be used to quantitate abnormal beats.

The technician who scans the Holter tape plays an important role in obtaining accurate results. Even with the most automated scanning system, the computer interpretation may not be always reliable and artifacts are frequently the cause of errors. Quantitation of ventricular premature beats may have an average error of 24 percent.[68] The computer readout often needs editing. Because of the large amount of data recorded on the tape, the technician should be able to select the perti-

```
PATIENT:                     DCG COMPUTERSCAN REPORT NO. 657753-0344
```

HOUR ENDG	TOTAL BEATS	MIN	MAX	AVG	VE BEATS	VE/ 1000	VBG BEATS	PD VE BEATS	R-on-T BEATS	VT BEATS	VT RUNS	MAX VT RN-BTS
10AM	5610	84	115	96	20	4	2		2			
11	4905	72	89	82	74	15	2					
12PM	4746	77	97	82	23	5						
1PM	4395	71	83	75	8	2						
2	5139	77	99	88	5	1						
3	5027	76	105	85	48	10						
4	5008	80	108	85	59	12						
5	5035	78	94	85	98	19	2					
6	4932	75	105	84	39	8						
7	4791	77	89	81	8	2						
8	4708	75	88	80	1							
9	4683	74	90	79	2							
10	4440	72	77	74	5	1						
11	4467	70	80	75	8	2						
12AM2	4470	72	89	76	9	2						
1AM2	4500	70	94	76	12	3	2					
2	4409	71	77	74	15	3						
3	4465	70	88	76	8	2						
4	4334	66	79	73	10	2						
5	4380	67	77	73	10	2						
6	4196	64	76	70	12	3						
7	4107	62	69	70	10	2						
8	4405	69	87	75	7	2						
9	4800	72	95	83	5	1						
10	5070	78	104	87	20	4						
11	5594	83	116	95	6	1						
1106AM	502	82	93	83								

FIGURE 28–1. A portion of a 24-hour digital print-out from a Holter tape depicting the hourly total number of beats, minimum, maximum, and average heart rate, number of ventricular ectopic (VE) beats, VE per 1000 beats, bigeminal VE beats, paired VE beats, R-on-T VE beats, number of ventricular tachycardia (VT) beats, VT runs, and maximum number of beats in VT runs.

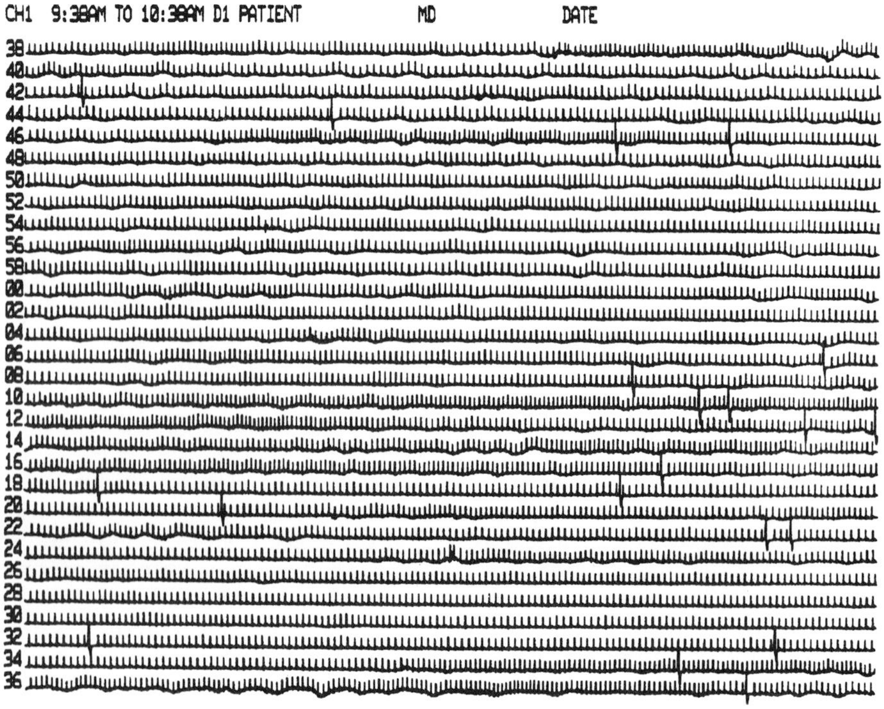

FIGURE 28–2. Condensed print-out of 1 hour of ambulatory ECG from a patient with premature ventricular beats.

nent parts of the tape to print out for the physician to analyze and interpret. The technician should, therefore, be experienced in ECG interpretation and know the clinical significance of the common cardiac arrhythmias.

AMBULATORY ELECTROCARDIOGRAMS IN NORMAL SUBJECTS

Knowledge of the normal variation in the ECG of ambulatory subjects is essential for its proper interpretation. The type and degree of physical activity, the mental status of the individual, and environmental factors may have significant effects on the cardiac rhythm. The ECG recorded during sleep may differ significantly from that of the waking hours. As in the 12-lead resting ECG, the findings in the ambulatory ECG may be affected by age and sex.

Heart Rate

In young and middle aged adults with normal hearts, the heart rate varies widely during a 24-hour period, day and night. In subjects who do not participate in any regular exercise program, the heart rate in a 24-hour period may range from 35 to 190 beats/min, with an overall average rate of about 80 beats/min.[12,43,73] There is a distinct diurnal variation. The maximal heart rate usually occurs in the late morning and the minimal heart rate between 3 and 5 A.M. With increasing age, the maximal heart rate decreases significantly during both day and night. The average heart rate for the 24 hours, however, is essentially unaffected.[43] The decrease in fluctuation of the heart rate is particularly evident in the elderly. In a group of 98 active elderly subjects 75 years of age or older, only 15 had heart rates that exceeded 100 beats/min intermittently in a 24-hour period.[13] In more than one third of the subjects, the heart rate did not vary by more than 10 beats/min during the 24-hour period.

Women generally have faster heart rates than men.[12,17,73] In 50 healthy young men and 50 healthy young women between the age of 22 and 28 years studied by the same institution, the average waking and sleeping heart rates were faster in women by about 10 beats/min.[12,73] The sex-related difference in heart rate persists to a certain degree with advancing age.[17]

The heart rate in normal subjects increases not only with physical exercise but also with mental stress. In a group of house officers presenting cases at medical grand rounds, the average heart rate increased from 73 to 154 beats/min.[56] The fastest heart rate was recorded either in the minutes before or in the first minutes of actual presentation and occasionally reached 187 beats/min.

It is well known that the heart rate of trained athletes is slower than that of the general population. In one study that compared long-distance runners with untrained young adults, the average heart rates during normal activities in a 24-hour period were 61 and 73 beats/min, respectively.[79] The heart rate during sleeping hours in endurance athletes may be as slow as 24 beats/min.[80]

Ectopic Beats

Isolated asymptomatic supraventricular ectopic beats may be observed in up to 64 percent of healthy young subjects.[12,73] In most cases, the premature beats are few. In two groups of young adults studied, less than 2 percent of them had more than 100 such ectopic beats in a 24-hour period. The frequency of the premature beats is higher in the older population.[64] In a group of healthy men and women older than 80 years, they were present in all.[37]

The prevalence of ventricular ectopic beats found in otherwise healthy adults monitored with 24-hour ambulatory ECGs ranged from 17 to 100 percent but most commonly from 40 to 55 percent.[12,17,25,43,73] As in the case of supraventricular ectopic beats their occurrence appears to increase with age, and the highest incidence was encountered in a group of individuals 60 years of age or older.[25,37] They are rare in newborns and young children.[74,75] Increase in the duration of monitoring reveals higher incidence of ventricular ectopic beats.[17] As a rule, the total number of ventricular ectopic beats is small. They are fewer than 100 in a 24-hour period in 96 percent of the cases.[12,43,73] Complex ventricular ectopic beats as are commonly defined (greater than 30 beats/hr, multiforms, bigeminy, couplets, or R-on-T phenomenon) may be present in 7 to 22 percent of the subjects and may be seen in as high as 77 percent of an older population. Ventricular ectopic beats may appear or increase in healthy individuals with physical or nonphysical stress,[46,78] but a relationship between premature ventricular beats and smoking, coffee, tea, or alcohol intake has not been established.[43]

One of the frequently quoted studies of ambulatory ECGs in apparently healthy middle-age men is that reported by Hinkle and associates.[30] Ventricular premature beats were found in 62 percent and complex ventricular arrhythmias including ventricular tachycardia in 19 percent of 283 actively employed men. Because follow-up examination revealed coronary artery disease in many of the subjects however, these data do not represent findings in healthy subjects but rather in middle-aged men who exhibited no symptoms of the rhythm disorders.

Tachyarrhythmias

Short episodes of atrial tachycardia, usually lasting not more than a few seconds, are occasionally seen in the ambulatory ECGs of otherwise healthy persons. A prevalence of 2 to 5 percent was reported in young adults, but the tachycardia was more frequent in the older population.[12,17,64,73] In our experience, it is the most common ectopic tachycardia seen on the ambulatory ECG.[16] It is seen in patients of all ages with or without heart disease. The heart rate is generally between 100 and 150 beats/min. The rhythm is often slightly irregular, suggesting that the tachycardia is probably of the automatic variety. The tachycardia has been referred to as *benign slow paroxysmal atrial tachycardia* or ectopic atrial tachycardia[12,76] (Fig. 28–3). We prefer to call it *accelerated atrial rhythm.* With rare exception it is asymptomatic

Nonsustained ventricular tachycardia also is encountered in apparently healthy young adults but is uncommon.[12,73] It is usually asymptomatic. Its long-term clinical significance is unclear.

Bradyarrhythmias and Conduction Abnormalities

Marked sinus bradycardia is common in the ambulatory ECGs of healthy adults. This is particularly true during sleeping hours. The bradycardia is often associated with transient atrioventricular (AV) junctional escape rhythm, which is observed in 4 to 22 percent of healthy subjects[12,17,73] (Fig. 28–4). Brief periods of sinus pauses or sinoatrial (SA) block may be seen in 28 to 34 percent. First- and second-degree AV blocks with Wenckebach phenomenon have been reported in 1 to 12 and 3 to 6 percent of normal subjects, respectively (Fig. 28–5). They are seen mostly in younger individuals and during sleep. These various types of bradyarrhythmias are more common in trained athletes.[80]

In summary, supraventricular and ventricular ectopic beats are common in the ambulatory ECGs of persons with normal hearts. They are usually few in number and asymptomatic. The frequency of the ectopic beats increases with age. In contrast, bradyarrhythmias and

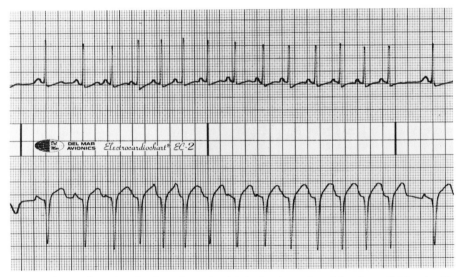

FIGURE 28–3. A short episode of accelerated atrial rhythm (ectopic atrial tachycardia) in a healthy young man. (Reproduced from Chou TC, Ceaser JH: Ambulatory electrocardiogram: Clinical applications. Cardiovas Clin 13(3):321, 1983, by permission of FA Davis, Philadelphia.)

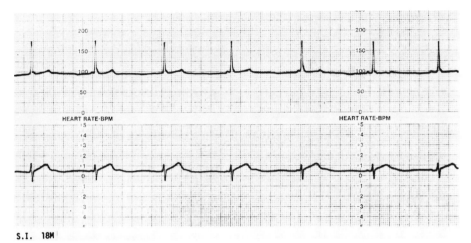

FIGURE 28–4. Sinus bradycardia with AV junctional escape rhythm in a healthy 18-year-old man.

AV block are more common in younger individuals and are seen mostly during sleep. As a rule, these arrhythmias in asymptomatic healthy subjects are benign and require no therapy.

INDICATIONS FOR AMBULATORY ELECTROCARDIOGRAM[41]

Although a large amount of data may be obtained with one or more 24-hour recordings, an ambulatory ECG is not to be considered a routine test for cardiac patients or those who may have heart disease. It is still a time-consuming and relatively expensive procedure. Useful information is more likely to be obtained when the test is performed in the following groups of patients: (1) patients with symptoms of suspected cardiac origin such as palpitation, dizziness, syncope, or chest pain; (2) patients with specific heart disease in whom the presence of arrhythmias, whether symptomatic or not, is thought to be of prognostic and therapeutic importance; and (3) patients receiving antiarrhythmic agent to be evaluated for its therapeutic effect.

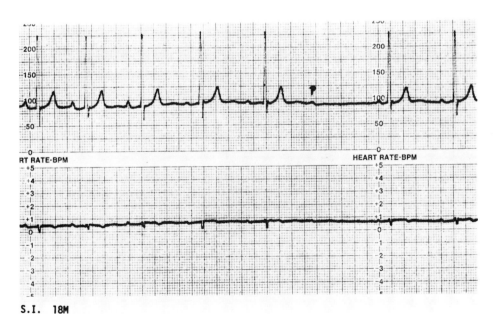

FIGURE 28–5. Second-degree AV block with Wenckebach phenomenon in a healthy young man.

Patients with Symptoms of Suspected Cardiac Origin

The value of ambulatory ECG is most apparent in patients who have episodes of palpitation, dizziness, syncope, or chest pain. The length of the monitoring period and the availability of a permanent record during the entire period often make the ambulatory ECG the only means to correlate symptoms of transient nature with the cardiac rhythm or ST-segment changes. Continuous oscilloscopic monitoring in a hospital requires the expense of hospitalization and has been shown to fail frequently in the identification of ectopic beats.[65] Brief periods of bradyarrhythmia also may be missed. The ambulatory ECG also provides the only means to record cardiac rhythm during normal daily activities, when the subject is exposed to the same stress as when he or she experiences symptoms. Useful information can be easily obtained if the symptoms occur frequently, but prolonged periods of recording may be needed if they do not. The decision of whether to extend the monitoring period depends on the severity of the complaint and the potential seriousness of the underlying cause.

PALPITATION, DIZZINESS, SYNCOPE

In the evaluation of symptoms such as palpitation, fluttering in the chest, and irregular heart beats, most cardiologists are impressed by the poor correlation between the symptoms and the presence or absence of cardiac arrhythmias. Most people do not perceive premature beats, including complex ventricular premature contractions. The occasional patients who experienced the sensation of thumping, jumping, skipped beats, or palpitation may sense only a few of the many premature beats they have. Short episodes of paroxysmal tachycardia are also seldom felt by patients.

Although sustained paroxysmal tachycardias are more likely to be noticed by the patient, frequently they are not. The same patient may have palpitation during some episodes but not during others (Fig. 28–6). Conversely, it is common that patients who complain of such symptom have normal sinus rhythm or sinus tachycardia. Such negative findings, nevertheless, are useful in the management of the patients.

Symptoms suggestive of transient cerebral ischemia such as dizziness and syncope are among the most common indications for ambulatory ECG. However, there are many noncardiac causes for these symptoms. The reported ability of 24-hour ambulatory ECG to correlate a symptomatic episode with cardiac arrhythmia ranges from 10 to 64 percent.[38] Valuable information also is obtained if rhythm disturbances are absent during the symptomatic periods. Indeed, in our experience, in patients with the symptoms of dizziness, the ambulatory ECG has been helpful more often in excluding cardiac arrhythmias as the cause of the symptom than in detecting them. Arrhythmias capable of producing cerebral ischemia include bradycardia less than 40 beats/min, tachycardia greater than 150 beats/min, and asystole longer than 3 to 5 seconds, depending on the patient's body position and activity at the time of the arrhythmias.[66,82] In patients with organic heart disease, the decrease in cardiac output is likely to be greater and symptoms are more likely to occur than in those without heart disease during tachyarrhythmia or bradyarrhythmia. Because of the abnormal sequence of ventricular activation and contraction, ventricular tachycardia can often cause cerebral symptoms at a rate as low as 120 beats/min.[36] Conversely, patients with supraventricular tachycardia seldom develop syncope unless the ventricular rate is rapid. Other causes should be looked for if syncope does occur. One of such causes is the sick sinus syndrome with tachy-bradyarrhythmia: the syncope is due to bradycardia rather than tachycardia even though the latter is the presenting abnormal rhythm (Fig. 28–7). Focal neurologic abnormalities are rarely due to decreased cerebral flow from cardiac arrhythmias alone. The ambulatory ECG is unlikely to be helpful in patients with these signs.[23]

CHEST PAIN

When the ambulatory ECG is used in the evaluation of chest pain, it is important to recognize the limitations of using ST-segment changes for the diagnosis of myocardial ischemia. As in the graded exercise test, horizontal or downsloping ST-segment depression may occur in the ambulatory ECG in the absence of coronary artery disease[42] Body position, hyperventilation, cardiac medications, and other factors may contribute to the appearance of ST-segment depression resembling that of ischemia.[39] Stern and associates studied 50 patients with precordial pain by means of ambulatory ECG and coronary arteriogram.[77] They found that the ambulatory

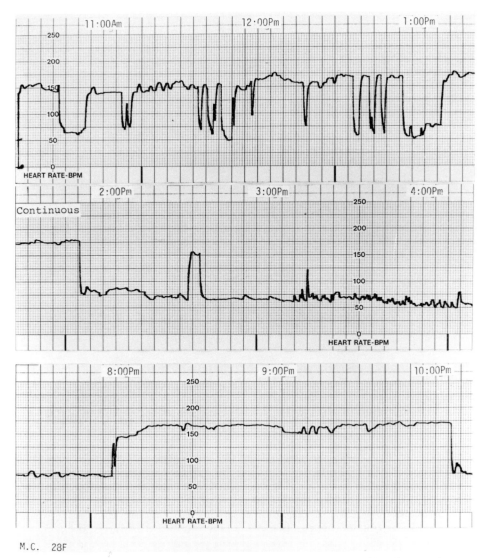

M.C. 28F

FIGURE 28–6. The heart rate trend chart of a 28-year-old woman with the Wolff-Parkinson-White syndrome and frequent episodes of paroxysmal supraventricular tachycardia. Of the many episodes of tachycardia, the patient experienced palpitation only briefly during the 10:45 A.M. episode. (Reproduced from Chou TC, Ceaser JH: Ambulatory electrocardiogram: Clinical applications. Cardiovasc Clin 13(3):321, 1983, by permission of FA Davis, Philadelphia.)

ECG has a sensitivity of 91 percent and a specificity of 78 percent in the diagnosis of significant coronary artery disease. Patients with abnormal resting ECGs, however, were included in this study, and T-wave inversion also was considered a positive sign for myocardial ischemia. Crawford and associates examined 70 patients with histories of chest pain and normal resting ECG with ambulatory monitoring, treadmill exercise test, and coronary arteriogram.[19] They found that the ambulatory ECG showed ischemic type ST-segment depression in 24 of 39 patients with significant coronary artery disease demonstrated by arteriography

(a sensitivity of 62 percent). There were no ischemic ST-segment changes in the Holter recording in 19 of the 31 patients without coronary artery disease (a specificity of 61 percent). Armstrong and associates studied 50 middle-age normal men with 24-hour Holter monitoring.[1] Transient horizontal or downsloping ST-segment depression of 1 mm or more was recorded in 15 (30 percent) of the subjects. The abnormal ST-segment depression lasted from 30 seconds to 2 hours and the magnitude of the depression varied from 1 to 4 mm. These men had no symptoms during an average 36-month follow-up period. This

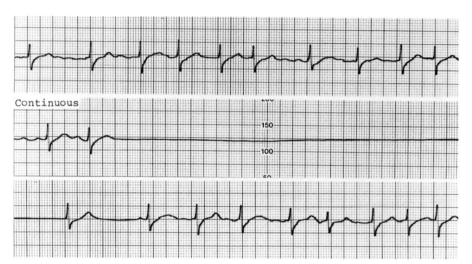

FIGURE 28–7. Tachybradycardia in a patient with the sick sinus syndrome and recurrent syncope. The tracing shows atrial fibrillation, with one probable sinus beat preceding the period of sinus arrest. A junctional escape beat appears before the resumption of atrial fibrillation. (Reproduced from Chou TC, Ceaser JH: Ambulatory electrocardiogram: Clinical applications. Cardiovasc Clin 13(3):321, 1983, by permission of FA Davis, Philadelphia.)

study also demonstrated that isolated T-wave inversion in the ambulatory ECG is a nonspecific finding, since 36 percent of the normal subjects had such a finding intermittently. In contrast, it is generally agreed that transient ST-segment elevation of 1 mm or more on ambulatory ECG is a highly specific sign for myocardial ischemia. It seldom occurs in normal persons without symptoms.[2]

To minimize the incidence of false-positive diagnosis of myocardial ischemia, a set of control tracings should be obtained at the beginning of the Holter recording with the patient in the supine, sitting, and standing positions, and during hyperventilation. It is my practice to interpret transient horizontal or downsloping ST-segment *depression* of 1 mm or more on the ambulatory ECG as probable but not definite evidence of myocardial ischemia unless the changes are associated with symptoms suggestive of angina. If the patient is known to have coronary artery disease, transient asymptomatic ST depression may be considered probably ischemic (silent) if it is not seen in the control tracing. Some of the ambulatory ECGs have only two bipolar leads. Although lead V_5, or modified lead V_5, is the most sensitive lead for the detection of ST-segment changes due to myocardial ischemia, the changes may be limited to other leads and a false-negative diagnosis may therefore be made.[7,8,45] To evaluate patients with chest pain related to exertion, we generally prefer to perform the graded exercise test or the exercise

radionuclide test. The ambulatory ECG is used to monitor patients when their chest pain occurs at rest or at night, or is associated with stresses other than simple exercise. It is particularly useful in patients who have chest pain suggestive of Prinzmetal's or vasospastic angina. The recording technique is best suited for such patients to detect ST-segment elevation during pain at rest. Occasionally, the continuous recording may reveal other mechanisms responsible for the onset of angina. Figure 28–8 illustrates an example in which the patient's angina was precipitated by an episode of supraventricular tachycardia. The tachycardia itself may or may not be perceived by the patient.

PATIENTS WITH SPECIFIC HEART DISEASE

Coronary Artery Disease

EVALUATION OF ISCHEMIC EPISODES

Holter monitoring has been used to examine patients with unstable or vasospastic angina, to detect silent myocardial ischemia, and to evaluate antianginal therapy. Figueras and associates studied 23 patients with coronary artery disease and resting or nocturnal angina with continuous hemodynamic and ECG recording.[22] In 11 patients, recurrent episodes of pain were always preceded by an average of

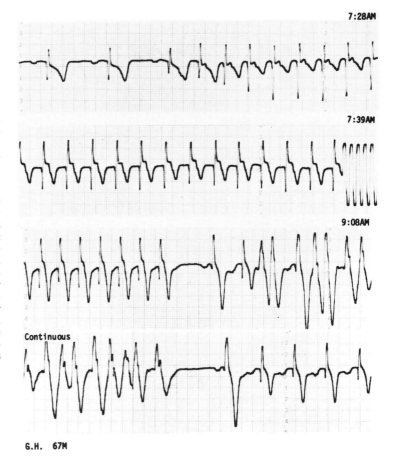

7:28AM

7:39AM

9:08AM

Continuous

G.H. 67M

FIGURE 28–8. Angina pectoris precipitated by paroxysmal supraventricular tachycardia. The patient is a 67-year-old man who was monitored because of chest pain. The ambulatory ECG shows sinus rhythm with first-degree AV block. At 7:28 A.M., while the patient was asleep, the tracing shows the onset of paroxysmal supraventricular tachycardia. At 7:32 A.M. (not shown) ST-segment elevation appears. The patient was awakened by palpitation and chest pain at 7:39 A.M. The symptoms continued while he was up and around until 9:08 A.M., when both the palpitation and chest pain suddenly stopped. The tracing reveals the termination of the supraventricular tachycardia followed by a short run of ventricular tachycardia before sinus rhythm resumes. ST-segment elevation disappears as soon as sinus rhythm is resumed.

8 minutes of ischemic ECG changes and hemodynamic signs of left ventricular dysfunction. Two patients had transient ischemic ECG and hemodynamic changes without pain. In 116 patients with unstable angina, Johnson and co-workers found that the appearance of transient ischemic ST-segment displacement or ventricular tachycardia on the Holter recording is an indicator of severe left main or triple-vessel coronary artery disease, variant angina, or impaired prognosis in the subsequent 3 months.[35]

Vasospastic angina may occur in patients with or without fixed occlusive coronary disease. Prinzmetal's variant angina is the best known form of vasospastic angina. Coronary spasm also is believed to be a possible cause of unstable angina and acute myocardial infarction.[28,49,50,58] In variant angina, the pain usually occurs at rest and the characteristic ECG finding is ST-segment elevation during pain. Continuous ECG monitoring in patients with variant angina reveals serious cardiac arrhythmias in about 50 percent of the cases. These arrhythmias include ventricular tachy-

cardia, ventricular fibrillation, complex ventricular ectopic beats, second- and third-degree AV block, and asystole.[40,51,63] The occurrence of serious arrhythmias has no apparent relationship to the patient's ventricular function or the severity of the coronary artery disease.[40,51] They are, however, seen mostly in patients with marked ST-segment elevation of 4 mm or more.[40,51,63] Serious ventricular arrhythmias are usually associated with ST-segment elevation in the anterior leads, whereas bradyarrhythmias are usually associated with ST elevation in the inferior leads.[40,61] The ventricular arrhythmias may develop during the period of maximal ST-segment elevation or during resolution of the ST-segment changes.[63] Previtali and associates suggested that the arrhythmias seen during ST-segment elevation represented occlusion arrhythmias and that those during resolution represented reperfusion arrhythmias.[63] The later occurred more often when the duration of myocardial ischemia was longer. Patients with variant angina and serious arrhythmias also have been shown to be at a much higher risk for sudden death. In 114 patients with variant angina followed for a mean period of 26 months by Miller and associates, sudden death occurred in 42 percent of patients with serious arrhythmias during their anginal episodes compared with 6 percent of those without such arrhythmias.[51]

Asymptomatic episodes of ischemic type of ST-segment changes are often observed in the ambulatory ECGs of patients with coronary artery disease[3,14,18,53,69] (Fig. 28–9). They are seen in patients with exertional or rest angina. The ST segment may be elevated or depressed. In these patients, up to 90 percent of the ep-

isodes of ST-segment changes may be asymptomatic. In my experience, however, the incidence is much lower. The duration and degree of the ST changes tend to be less with the asymptomatic than the symptomatic episodes.[14] Convincing evidence suggests that these episodes represent silent myocardial ischemia in most instances. Coronary arteriograms performed by Biagini and associates during these asymptomatic ST-segment changes revealed coronary spasm in 6 of 8 patients.[4] Impairment of ventricular function, reduction of coronary oxygen saturation, and reduction of thallium-201 uptake also have

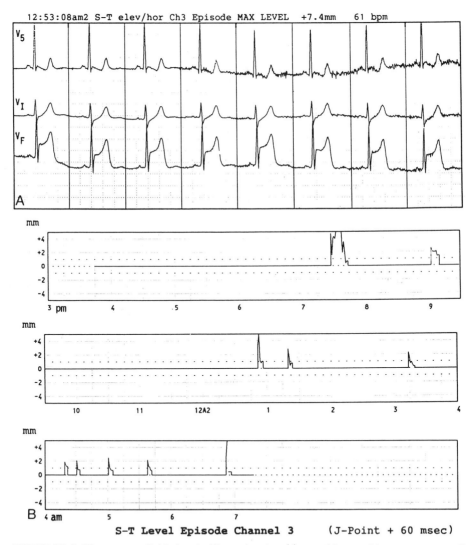

FIGURE 28–9. Silent myocardial ischemia. The patient is a 44-year-old man with coronary artery disease and a history of cardiac arrest. Holter monitoring showed recurrent episodes of ST-segment elevation without angina. (A) Tracing showing the marked ST-segment elevation in modified lead aVF during one of the episodes. (B) Tracing illustrating the time and number of episodes during the recording period as well as the duration and degree of ST-segment elevation of each episode. The Holter monitor also recorded complex ventricular ectopic beats and short episodes of ventricular tachycardia.

been observed during these asymptomatic episodes.[14,15,60] The frequency of the episodes may be reduced by the hourly administration of nitroglycerin.[69] In 93 patients with silent ischemic episodes on ambulatory ECGs, Mody and co-workers found that the patients who had longer cumulative duration (more than 60 minutes per 24 hours) of ischemia were more likely to have three-vessel and proximal coronary artery disease.[53] The absence of prolonged ischemia, however, is of little predictive value.

POSTINFARCTION VENTRICULAR ARRHYTHMIAS

In postmyocardial infarction patients, ambulatory ECGs are often used for the detection of ventricular arrhythmias. Although the occurrence of complex ventricular ectopic beats in the acute phase of myocardial infarction does not appear to have any prognostic implications,[20] their presence 2 or 3 weeks after the acute phase is associated with increased risk of sudden death.[5,33,44,55,67,81] Some studies suggest that the increased risk of sudden cardiac death is related to the decreased left ventricular ejection fraction in these patients.[10,71] Reports based on the study of a relatively large number of patients, however, indicate that complex ventricular arrhythmias in postinfarction patients represent an independent risk factor for sudden death. Ruberman and associates obtained 1 hour of recording in 1739 male survivors of myocardial infarction within 1 year of the acute event.[67] In a 5-year follow-up study, they found that men with the R-on-T phenomenon or runs of ventricular ectopic beats had a sudden cardiac death rate of 25 percent compared with 6 percent of men free of ventricular ectopic beats.[67] Moss and colleagues evaluated 940 postinfarction patients with 6-hour Holter ECG recorded before their hospital discharge.[55] In an average of 36 months of follow-up, the risk of sudden death in patients with complex ventricular arrhythmias increased by threefold when compared with those without. Bigger and associates obtained 24-hour ambulatory ECGs from 430 patients 2 weeks after an acute myocardial infarction and followed them for 1 year.[5,6] The mortality of patients with frequent or repetitive ventricular ectopic beats was 25 percent. In patients with ventricular tachycardia (three or more complexes), the 1-year mortality rate was 38 percent compared with 11.6 percent in patients without ventricular tachycardia.

Sick Sinus Syndrome

SA node dysfunction characterized by marked sinus bradycardia, SA block, or sinus arrest is often accompanied by a failure of lower pacemakers to initiate an escape rhythm. It is one of the common causes of dizziness and syncope. If the diagnosis is not apparent in the routine ECG, ambulatory monitoring is indicated. It is superior to invasive electrophysiological studies for establishing a definitive diagnosis. The presence of sick sinus syndrome is documented if a prolonged sinus pause without an escape rhythm is recorded during the symptomatic episode. Repeated 24-hour monitoring is often needed to establish a temporal relationship between the patient's symptoms and the ECG findings. In some instances, sinus pauses are seen but the patient exhibits no symptoms during the period of monitoring. SA node dysfunction may be suspected, but it is possible that the cause of the patient's symptom is noncardiac. Brief sinus pauses (up to 2 seconds) may occur in normal subjects especially during sleep.

Patients with the sick sinus syndrome and brady-tachyarrhythmias may have the tachyarrhythmia as the presenting abnormality. Sinus arrest often appears at the termination of an episode of supraventricular tachycardia to cause dizziness or syncope (see Fig. 28–7). Ambulatory ECG may disclose the true pathogenesis of the tachyarrhythmia, and pacemaker implantation is needed in these patients before drug therapy is used to control the tachycardia.

Conduction Abnormalities

Conduction abnormalities, including various combinations of fascicular blocks and various degrees of AV block, may be intermittent. A patient with a normal PR interval on the routine ECG may be found by Holter monitoring to have transient high-degree AV block and marked bradycardia. Patients with bifascicular blocks may have transient episodes of second-degree or complete AV block long before the development of permanent complete heart block.[9] The ambulatory ECG may be used to detect such conduction abnormalities if symptoms suggestive of transient cerebral ischemia appear.

Pacemaker Evaluation

Patients with implanted cardiac pacemakers are periodically evaluated with ECGs recorded in the routine manner or by transtelephonic transmission. The ambulatory ECG may be helpful in the evaluation of patients with pacemakers that appear to function properly on routine evaluation but who have symptoms suggestive of pacemaker malfunction. In one study, 18 percent of patients shown to have normal pacemaker function by routine methods were found to have malfunction by ambulatory ECG.[9] Up to 69 percent of patients with unipolar ventricular demand pacemaker (VVI) have been reported to reveal ventricular asystole from myopotential inhibition during their daily activities[11,21] (see Fig. 27–18). The incidence of such myopotential inhibition is, however, much lower in our own experience. In the early post implantation period, Holter monitoring was found to be more effective in detecting pacemaker dysfunction than telemetric monitoring.[34] The ambulatory ECG also has been used to determine whether implanted pacemaker electrodes remain in place during exercise.[9] In some patients, symptoms such as dizziness and syncope are found to be caused by tachyarrhythmias instead of pacemaker malfunction.

Mitral Valve Prolapse

Cardiac arrhythmias, both ventricular and supraventricular, are common in patients with mitral valve prolapse, and sudden death occurs occasionally.[27,86] Many patients with the mitral valve prolapse syndrome are troubled by symptoms of palpitations, lightheadedness, and atypical chest pain. In one study, only 27 percent of the patients with symptoms were found to have arrhythmias associated with their symptoms.[86] In most cases, the negative correlation between symptoms and arrhythmias serves to reassure the patients of the benign nature of their symptoms.

Preexcitation Syndrome

In patients with documented Wolff-Parkinson-White (WPW) pattern, the ambulatory ECG showed that the preexcitation may be intermittent in 65 percent of the cases.[29] When the routine ECG is suggestive but not diagnostic of the WPW pattern, the demonstration of more typical signs of preexcitation intermittently confirms the presence of such an anomaly. Although patients with ventricular preexcitation often complain of palpitations, only a minority of them were found to have cardiac arrhythmias related to the symptoms. If tachyarrhythmias are present, their mechanisms

may be documented and the therapeutic efficacy of the antiarrhythmic agents used evaluated.

Cardiomyopathies

Hypertrophic obstructive cardiomyopathy (or idiopathic hypertrophic subaortic stenosis) is frequently associated with atrial and ventricular arrhythmias and occasionally sudden death.[27,47,48] In a multicenter study of 190 patients with hypertrophic obstructive cardiomyopathy reported by Shah and associates, sudden death was the most common mode of demise.[72] In a prospective study conducted by Maron and associates, 99 patients with hypertrophic cardiomyopathy had 24-hour ambulatory ECGs and were followed for 3 years.[48] There was a significantly increased risk of sudden death in patients with asymptomatic ventricular tachycardia; the annual mortality rate in these patients was 8.6 percent.

Patients with dilated cardiomyopathy are known to have frequent complex ventricular arrhythmias. Patients with complex ventricular arrhythmias or nonsustained ventricular tachycardia and dilated cardiomyopathy were found to have a high risk of sudden death.[24,31] Although the value of antiarrhythmic drugs in the prevention of sudden death in these patients has not been established, Holter monitoring is one of the most sensitive means to document the presence of these arrhythmias.

EVALUATION OF EFFICACY OF DRUG THERAPY

The ambulatory ECG has gained wide use in the evaluation of drug therapy for arrhythmias, especially ventricular arrhythmias. It is obtained before and after the institution of antiarrhythmic therapy. The suppression of episodes of ventricular tachycardia or a significant reduction in ventricular ectopic beats is considered to be an indication of the efficacy of the drug. Ventricular ectopic activity varies widely in frequency from hour to hour and from day to day. The spontaneous variation is even greater when the ambulatory ECG is repeated at weekly or longer intervals.[1] Such fluctuations in frequency have led to difficulties in deciding whether an observed reduction in ectopic activity is due to drug effect or spontaneous variations. It has been proposed that if one 24-hour Holter monitoring is obtained before and one 1 or 2 weeks after the therapy begins, a reduction by more than 85 percent in the total number of premature ventricular contractions is necessary before the changes can be attributed to drug effect.[1,54] It is almost impossible to distinguish drug effect from spontaneous variation of the arrhythmias if the interval is longer than 3 months.[70] Longer monitoring periods require a lower percentage of reduction. In some patients, the drug may be considered effective if their symptoms are relieved even though the percentage of reduction of the arrhythmias shown on the ambulatory ECG does not meet the usual criteria.

SLEEP APNEA SYNDROME

Cardiac arrhythmias and conduction disturbances were reported in patients with the sleep apnea syndrome during sleep.[26,52] In 23 patients with this syndrome monitored with 24-hour ECG, Miller found marked sinus arrhythmia, extreme sinus bradycardia with a heart rate less than 30 beats/min, sinus pauses, and first- and second-degree AV block in a few cases.[52] In the large series of 400 patients reported by Guilleminault and associates, 48 percent of the patients had cardiac arrhythmias during the night of the Holter recording.[26] Nonsustained ventricular tachy-

cardia was seen in 8 patients, sinus arrest lasting for 2.5 to 13 seconds in 43, and second-degree AV block in 31. Seventy-five patients had frequent (more than 2 beats/min) premature ventricular beats during sleep. In 50 patients with significant arrhythmias who had a tracheostomy performed, no arrhythmia other than premature ventricular contractions was seen in the Holter monitoring after surgery.

AMBULATORY ELECTROCARDIOGRAM IN VICTIMS OF CARDIAC ARREST

In recent years, a number of patients who had cardiac arrest or sudden death during Holter monitoring have been reported.[57,59,62,84,85] The terminal event at the time of cardiac arrest is ventricular tachyarrhythmia in most cases (about 80 percent),[59] but bradyarrhythmias and asystole were more common in one reported series of patients without apparent heart disease.[84] The ventricular tachyarrhythmias include ventricular tachycardia or flutter, torsades de pointes, and ventricular fibrillation. Ventricular fibrillation is always preceded by ventricular tachycardia or ven-

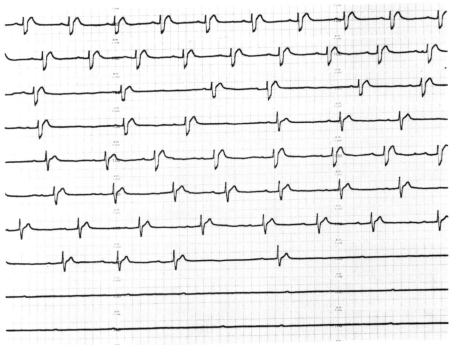

FIGURE 28–10. Ventricular asystole during Holter monitoring. The patient was a 74-year-old man with a history of recurrent dizziness. He had cardiac arrest while the ambulatory ECG was being recorded. The tracing shows sinus bradycardia, sinus pauses or SA block, first-degree and complete AV block, and ventricular asystole.

tricular flutter. In patients who have cardiac arrest due to bradyarrhythmia, the mechanism is mostly sinus arrest (Fig. 28–10), complete AV block being responsible in some cases. In patients with sustained ventricular fibrillation, there is usually an increased frequency of premature ventricular beats in the hour before the event.[62] The premature ventricular beats initiating ventricular tachycardia that leads to ventricular fibrillation do not present the R-on-T phenomenon in most instances. QT prolongation may or may not (often not) be present in the sinus beats.

In patients resuscitated from cardiac arrest, the presence of complex ventricular ectopic beats in their ambulatory ECGs significantly increase the risk of subsequent cardiac arrest. In 144 patients with coronary artery disease resuscitated from ventricular fibrillation, Weaver and associates found that cardiac arrest recurred in 56 percent of those with complex ventricular ectopic beats compared with 28 percent of those without.[84] Although complex ventricular ectopic beats were associated with a history of congestive heart failure or remote myocardial infarction in most patients, they were believed to be an independent predictor of mortality rate.

REFERENCES

1. Anastasiou-Nana MI, Menlove RL, Nanas JN, Anderson JL: Changes in spontaneous variability of ventricular activity as a function of time in patients with chronic arrhythmias. Circulation 78:286, 1988
2. Armstrong WF, Jordan JW, Morris SN, et al: Prevalence and magnitude of S-T segment and T wave abnormalities in normal men during continuous ambulatory electrocardiography. Am J Cardiol 4:1638, 1982
3. Balasubramanian V, Lahiri A, Green HL, et al: Ambulatory ST segment monitoring: Problems, pitfalls, solutions and clinical application. Br Heart J 44:419, 1980
4. Biagini A, Mazzei MG, Carpeggiani C, et al: Vasospastic ischemic mechanism of frequent asymptomatic transient ST-T changes during continuous electrocardiographic monitoring in selected unstable angina patients. Am Heart J 103:13, 1982
5. Bigger JT, Weld FM, Rolnitzky LM: Prevalence, characteristics and significance of ventricular tachycardia (three or more complexes) detected with ambulatory electrocardiographic recording in the late hospital phase of acute myocardial infarction. Am J Cardiol 48:815, 1981
6. Bigger JT, Weld FM, Rolnitzky LM: Which postinfarction ventricular arrhythmias should be treated? Am Heart J 103:660, 1982
7. Blackburn H, Katigbak R: What electrocardiographic leads to take after exercise? Am Heart J 67:184, 1964
8. Blackburn H, Taylor HL, Okamoto N, et al: The exercise electrocardiogram: A systematic comparison of chest lead configurations employed for monitoring during exercise. In Karvonen M, Barry A (eds): Physical Activity and the Heart. Springfield, Ill, Charles C Thomas, 1966
9. Bleifer SB, Bleifer DJ, Hansmann DR, et al: Diagnosis of occult arrhythmias by Holter electrocardiography. Prog Cardiovas Dis 16:569, 1974
10. Borer JS, Rosing DR, Miller RH, et al: Natural history of left ventricular function during 1 year after acute myocardial infarction: Comparison with clinical, electrocardiographic and biochemical determinations. Am J Cardiol 46:1, 1980
11. Breivik K, Ohm OJ: Myopotential inhibition of unipolar QRS-inhibited (VVI) pacemakers, assessed by ambulatory Holter monitoring of the electrocardiogram. Pace 3:470, 1980
12. Brodsky M, Wu D, Denes P, et al: Arrhythmias documented by 24 hour continuous electrocardiographic monitoring in 50 male medical students without apparent heart disease. Am J Cardiol 39:390, 1977
13. Camm AJ, Evans KE, Ward DE, et al: The rhythm of the heart in active elderly subjects. Am Heart J 99:598, 1980
14. Cecchi AC, Dovellini EV, Marchi F, et al: Silent myocardial ischemia during ambulatory electrocardiographic monitoring in patients with effort angina. J Am Coll Cardiol 1:934, 1983
15. Chierchia S, Brunelli C, Simonetti I, et al: Sequence of events in angina at rest: Primary reduction in coronary flow. Circulation 61:759, 1980
16. Chou TC, Ceaser JH: Ambulatory electrocardiogram: Clinical applications. In Fowler NO (ed): Noninvasive Diagnostic Methods in Cardiology, Philadelphia, FA Davis, 1983, p 321
17. Clarke JM, Shelton JR, Hamer J, et al: The rhythm of the normal human heart. Lancet 2:508, 1976
18. Cohn PF: Silent myocardial ischemia in patients with a defective anginal warning system. Am J Cardiol 45:697, 1980
19. Crawford MH, Mendoza CA, O'Rourke RA, et al: Limitations of continuous ambulatory electrocardiogram monitoring for detecting coronary artery disease. Ann Intern Med 89:1, 1978
20. DeSoyza N, Bennett FA, Murphy ML, et al: The relationship of paroxysmal ventricular tachycardia complicating the acute phase and ventricular arrhythmia during the late hospital phase of myocardial infarction in long-term survival. Am J Med 64:377, 1978
21. Famularo MA, Kennedy HL: Ambulatory electrocardiography in the assessment of pacemaker function. Am Heart J 104:1086, 1982
22. Figueras J, Singh BN, Ganz W, et al: Mechanism of rest and nocturnal angina: Observations during continuous hemodynamic and electrocardiographic monitoring. Circulation 59:955, 1979
23. Fisher M: Holter monitoring in patients with transient focal cerebral ischemia. Stroke 9:514, 1978
24. Follansbee WP, Michelson EL, Morganroth J: Nonsustained ventricular tachycardia in ambulatory patients: Characteristics and association with sudden cardiac death. Ann Intern Med 92:741, 1980
25. Glasser SP, Clark PI, Applebaum HJ: Occurrence of frequent complex arrhythmias detected by ambulatory monitoring: Findings in an apparently healthy asymptomatic elderly population. Chest 75:565, 1979
26. Guilleminault C, Connolly SJ, Winkle RA: Cardiac arrhythmia and conduction disturbances during sleep in 400 patients with sleep apnea syndrome. Am J Cardiol 52:490, 1983
27. Harrison DC, Fitzgerald JW, Winkle RA: Ambulatory

electrocardiography for diagnosis and treatment of cardiac arrhythmias. N Engl J Med 294:373, 1976

28. Hellstrom HR: Coronary artery vasospasm: the likely immediate cause of acute myocardial infarction. Br Heart J 41:426, 1979

29. Hindman MC, Last JH, Rosen KM: Wolff-Parkinson-White observed by portable monitoring. Ann Intern Med 79:654, 1973

30. Hinkle LE, Carver ST, Stevens M: The frequency of asymptomatic disturbances of cardiac rhythm and conduction in middle-aged men. Am J Cardiol 24:629, 1969

31. Holmes J, Kubo SH, Cody RJ, Kligfield P: Arrhythmias in ischemic and nonischemic dilated cardiomyopathy: Prediction of mortality by ambulatory electrocardiography. Am J Cardiol 55:146, 1985

32. Holter NJ: New method for heart studies: Continuous electrocardiography of active subjects over long periods is now practical. Science 134:1214, 1961

33. Ivanova LA, Mazur NA, Smirnova TM, et al: Electrocardiographic exercise testing and ambulatory monitoring to identify patients with ischemic heart disease at high risk of sudden death. Am J Cardiol 45:1132, 1980

34. Janosik DL, Redd RM, Buckingham TA, et al: Utility of ambulatory electrocardiography in detecting pacemaker dysfunction in the early postimplantation period. Am J Cardiol 60:1030, 1987

35. Johnson SM, Mauritson DR, Winniford MD: Continuous electrocardiographic monitoring in patients with unstable angina pectoris: Identification of high-risk subgroup with severe coronary disease, variant angina, and/or impaired early prognosis. Am Heart J 103:4, 1982

36. Jonas S, Klein I, Dimant J: Importance of Holter monitoring in patients with periodic cerebral symptoms. Ann Neurol 1:470, 1977

37. Kantelip JP, Sage, E, Duchene-Marullaz P: Findings on ambulatory electrocardiographic monitoring in subjects older than 80 years. Am J Cardiol 57:398, 1986

38. Kennedy HL, Caralis DG: Ambulatory electrocardiography: A clinical perspective. Ann Intern Med 87:729, 1977

39. Kennedy HL, Wiens RD: Ambulatory (Holter) electrocardiography and myocardial ischemia. Am Heart J 117:164, 1989

40. Kerin NZ, Rubenfire M, Naini M, et al: Arrhythmias in variant angina pectoris: Relationship of arrhythmias to ST-segment elevation and R-wave changes. Circulation 60:1343, 1979

41. Knoebel SB, Crawford MH, Dunn MI, et al: Guidelines for ambulatory electrocardiography: A report of the American College of Cardiology/American Heart Association Task Force on Assessment of Diagnostic and Therapeutic Cardiovascular Procedures (Subcommittee on Ambulatory Electrocardiography). J Am Coll Cardiol 13:249, 1989

42. Kohli RS, Cashman PM, Lahiri A, Raftery EB: The ST segment of the ambulatory electrocardiogram in a normal population. Br Heart J 60:4, 1988

43. Kostis JB, Moreyra AE, Amendo MT, et al: The effect of age on heart rate in subjects free of heart disease: Studies by ambulatory electrocardiography and maximal exercise stress test. Circulation 65:141, 1982

44. Kotler MN, Tabatznik B, Mower MM, et al: Prognostic significance of ventricular ectopic beats with respect to sudden death in the late postinfarction period. Circulation 47:959, 1973

45. MacAlpin RN: Correlation of the location of coronary arterial spasm with the lead distribution of ST segment elevation during variant angina. Am Heart J 99:555, 1980

46. McHenry PL, Morris SN, Kavalier M, et al: Comparative study of exercise-induced ventricular arrhythmias in normal subjects and patients with documented coronary artery disease. Am J Cardiol 37:609, 1976

47. McKenna WJ, Chetty S, Oakley CM, et al: Arrhythmia in hypertrophic cardiomyopathy: Exercise and 48 hour ambulatory electrocardiographic assessment with and without beta adrenergic blocking therapy. Am J Cardiol 45:1, 1980

48. Maron BJ, Savage DD, Wolfson JK, et al: Prognostic significance of 24 hour ambulatory electrocardiographic monitoring in patients with hypertrophic cardiomyopathy: A prospective study. Am J Cardiol 48:252, 1981

49. Maseri A, L'Abbate A, Baroldi G, et al: Coronary vasospasm as a possible cause of myocardial infarction. N Engl J Med 299:1281, 1978

50. Maseri A, L'Abbate A, Chierchia S, et al: Significance of spasm in the pathogenesis of ischemic heart disease. Am J Cardiol 44:788, 1979

51. Miller DD, Waters DD, Szlachcic J, et al: Clinical characteristics associated with sudden death in patients with variant angina. Circulation 66:588, 1982

52. Miller WP: Cardiac arrhythmias and conduction disturbances in the sleep apnea syndrome. Am J Med 73:317, 1982

53. Mody FV, Nademanee K, Intarachot V, et al: Severity of silent myocardial ischemia on ambulatory electrocardiographic monitoring in patients with stable angina pectoris: Relation to prognostic determinants during exercise stress testing and coronary angiography. J Am Coll Cardiol 12:1169, 1988

54. Morganroth J, Michelson EL, Horowitz LN, et al: Limitations of routine long-term electrocardiographic monitoring to assess ventricular ectopic frequency. Circulation 58:408, 1978

55. Moss AJ, Davis HT, DeCamilla J, et al: Ventricular ectopic beats and their relation to sudden and nonsudden cardiac death after myocardial infarction. Circulation 60:998, 1979

56. Moss AJ, Wynar B: Tachycardia in house officers presenting cases at grand rounds. Ann Intern Med 72:255, 1970

57. Nikolic G, Bishop RL, Singh JB: Sudden death recorded during Holter monitoring. Circulation 66:218, 1982

58. Olivia PB, Breckinridge JC: Arteriographic evidence of coronary artery spasm in acute myocardial infarction. Circulation 56:366, 1977

59. Panidis IP, Morganroth J: Sudden death in hospitalized patients: Cardiac rhythm disturbances detected by ambulatory electrocardiographic monitoring. J Am Coll Cardiol 2:798, 1983

60. Parodi O, Severi S, Uthurralt N, et al: Angina pectoris at rest: Regional myocardial perfusion during ST segment elevation or depression (abstract). Circulation 55,56(Suppl III):III-229, 1977

61. Plotnick GD, Fisher ML, Becker LC: Ventricular arrhythmias in patients with rest angina: correlation with ST segment changes and extent of coronary atherosclerosis. Am Heart J 105:32, 1983

62. Pratt CM, Francis MJ, Luck JC, et al: Analysis of ambulatory electrocardiograms in 15 patients during spontaneous ventricular fibrillation with special reference to preceding arrhythmic events. J Am Coll Cardiol 2:789, 1983

63. Previtali M, Klersy C, Salerno JA, et al: Ventricular tachyarrhythmias in Prinzmetal's variant angina: Clinical significance and relation to the degree and time course of S-T segment elevation. Am J Cardiol 52:19, 1983

64. Raftery EB, Cashman PMM: Long-term recording of the electrocardiogram in normal population. Postgrad Med J 52(Suppl 7):32, 1976

65. Romhilt DW, Bloomfield SS, Chou TC, et al: Unreliability of conventional electrocardiographic monitoring for arrhythmia detection in coronary care units. Am J Cardiol 31:457, 1973

66. Rossen R, Kabat H, Anderson JP: Acute arrest of cerebral circulation in man. Arch Neurol Psychiat 50:510, 1943

67. Ruberman W, Weinblatt E, Goldberg JD, et al: Ventricular premature complexes and sudden death after myocardial infarction. Circulation 64:297, 1981

68. Salerno DM, Granrud G, Hodges M: Accuracy of commercial 24-hour electrocardiogram analyzers for quantitation of total and repetitive ventricular arrhythmias. Am J Cardiol 60:1299, 1987

69. Schang SJ, Pepine CJ: Transient asymptomatic S-T segment depression during daily activity. Am J Cardiol 39:396, 1977

70. Schmidt G, Ulm K, Goedel-Meinen L, et al: Spontaneous variability of simple and complex ventricular premature contractions during long time intervals in patients with severe organic heart disease. Circulation 78:296, 1988

71. Schulze RA, Strauss HW, Pitt B: Sudden death in the year following myocardial infarction: Relation to ventricular premature contractions in the late hospital phase and left ventricular ejection fraction. Am J Med 62:192, 1977

72. Shah PM, Adelman AG, Wigle ED, et al: The natural (and unnatural) history of hypertrophic obstructive cardiomyopathy. Circ Res 34,35(Suppl II):II-179, 1974

73. Sobotka PA, Mayer JH, Bauernfeind RA, et al: Arrhythmias documented by 24-hour continuous ambulatory electrocardiographic monitoring in young women without apparent heart disease. Am Heart J 101:753, 1981

74. Southall DP, Johnston F, Shinebourne EA, et al: 24-hour electrocardiographic study of heart rate and rhythm patterns in population of healthy children. Br Heart J 45:281, 1981

75. Southall DP, Richards JM, Mitchell P, et al: Study of cardiac rhythm in healthy newborn infants. Br Heart J 43:14, 1980

76. Stemple DR, Fitzgerald JW, Winkle RA: Benign slow proxysmal atrial tachycardia. Ann Intern Med 87:44, 1977

77. Stern S, Tzivoni D, Stern Z: Diagnostic accuracy of ambulatory ECG monitoring in ischemic heart disease. Circulation 52:1045, 1975

78. Taggart P, Carruthers M, Somerville W: Electrocardiogram, plasma catecholamines and lipids, and their modification by oxprenolol when speaking before an audience. Lancet 2:341, 1973

79. Talan DA, Bauernfeind RA, Washley WW, et al: Twenty-four continuous ECG recordings in long-distance runners. Chest 82:19, 1982

80. Viitasalo MT, Kala R, Eisalo A: Ambulatory electrocardiographic recording in endurance athletes. Br Heart J 47:213, 1982

81. Vismara LA, Pratt C, Price JE, et al: Correlation of the standard electrocardiogram and continuous ambulatory monitoring in the detection of ventricular arrhythmias in coronary patients. J Electrocardiol 10:299, 1977

82. Walter PF, Reid SD, Wenger NK: Transient cerebral ischemia due to arrhythmia. Ann Intern Med 72:471, 1970

83. Wang F, Lien W, Fong T, et al: Terminal cardiac electrical activity in adults who die without apparent cardiac disease. Am J Cardiol 58:491, 1986

84. Weaver WD, Cobb LA, Hallstrom AP: Ambulatory arrhythmias in resuscitated victims of cardiac arrest. Circulation 66:212, 1982

85. Winkle RA: Current status of ambulatory electrocardiography. Am Heart J 102:757, 1981

86. Winkle RA, Lopes MG, Fitzgerald JW, et al: Arrhythmias in patients with mitral valve prolapse. Circulation 52:73, 1975

Subject Index

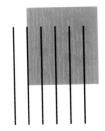

Note: Page numbers in *italics* refer to illustrations;
page numbers followed by "t" refer to tables.